ANIMAL OSTEOPATHY

A comprehensive guide to the osteopathic treatment of animals and birds

ANIMAL OSTEOPATHY

A comprehensive guide to the osteopathic treatment of animals and birds

Editors

Tony NEVIN ▪ Chris COLLES ▪ Paolo TOZZI

Foreword

Joshua M Plotnik

HANDSPRING PUBLISHING

HANDSPRING PUBLISHING LIMITED
The Old Manse, Fountainhall,
Pencaitland, East Lothian
EH34 5EY, United Kingdom
Tel: +44 1875 341 859
Website: www.handspringpublishing.com

First published 2020 in the United Kingdom by Handspring Publishing

3

ISBN 978-1-909141-30-8
ISBN (Kindle eBook) 978-1-912085-27-9

British Library Cataloguing in Publication Data
A catalogue record for this book is available from the British Library

Library of Congress Cataloging in Publication Data
A catalog record for this book is available from the Library of Congress

Commissioning Editor Mary Law
Project Manager Morven Dean
Designer Bruce Hogarth
Indexer Aptara, India
Typesetter DiTech, India
Printer Ashford Colour Ltd

The authorised representative in the EEA is Hachette Ireland, 8 Castlecourt Centre, Dublin 15, D15 XTP3, Ireland (email:info@hbgi.ie)

CONTENTS

DEDICATION

This book is dedicated to the continuing professional development of animal and avian osteopathy and to the future generations of osteopaths around the world using an integrated medicine approach and working with veterinary surgeons.

FOREWORD

I was setting up a group of new elephant cognition experiments in the Golden Triangle of northern Thailand in 2011 when I first heard that an animal osteopath was coming to treat some of the elephants. The Golden Triangle Asian Elephant Foundation, a Thai non-profit charity that is home to more than 20 elephants, was my research base for studying elephant behavior as a way of trying to construct a figurative window into their minds. I design experiments, or 'games for elephants', that aim to *ask* questions of them, despite not having the benefit of a mutually spoken language. For example, are they self-aware? (we set up mirrors to see if they recognize themselves), can they cooperate flexibly? (we placed some food out of their reach to see whether they could coordinate their actions), and can they judge quantity using only their trunks to smell differences? (we provided two buckets with varying quantities of sunflower seeds to see whether they chose the larger amount).

One of our research goals is to try to understand how complex cognitive abilities develop across evolutionarily distant species like primates and elephants. We also aim to use our insight into the elephant mind to discover ways not only of looking after them better when they're in the care of humans but of protecting them when they're under threat in the wild. Over time, I've learned that although our work can contribute to the improvement of elephant welfare and conservation efforts, these are issues that require multidisciplinary approaches.

Pepsi, a 10-year-old bull elephant living at the Foundation in 2011, had done what many young elephant males had foolishly done before him: challenged an older bull and lost. Unfortunately, he had sustained a wound in his front left leg from 40-year-old Phuki's tusks and was clearly in pain. The Foundation's elephant veterinarian treated Pepsi's wound and was meticulously vigilant about a possible growing infection (a common worry in the wet tropics of southeast Asia). When I heard Tony Nevin was coming to take a look, I was initially skeptical. As a scientist, I always question novel approaches to physical ailments, especially when they involve a 90 kg human osteopath massaging and manipulating the muscles of a 3000 kg bull elephant. I had, however, grown quite fond of Pepsi during the first year I had known him. He was an exceptionally intelligent animal and one of my research team's star subjects. The injury was clearly causing him discomfort as he walked. I was therefore as concerned as the Foundation's management and veterinary teams about Pepsi's health and became cautiously optimistic about what Tony could do to help.

I did not introduce myself to Tony when he first arrived at the elephant camp. I wanted to observe his work as an osteopath without any preconceptions of who he was as a person. I was interested to see that Tony spoke to Pepsi as he first approached him, and gently touched his face and the top of his leg before asking the handler to have him lie down. Tony then used the full force of his body weight for the manipulation, massaging the muscles and extending and flexing the leg. He worked on Pepsi's body for some time and then asked him to stand up. As the elephant got to his feet and slowly walked off in the direction of the forest, the change was obvious. Pepsi's limp was considerably reduced, and he no longer shuddered with each step. With each successive treatment over several days, Pepsi's condition continued to improve. Tony had provided a complementary treatment that seemed to help. The work was non-invasive, gentle and deliberate. After observing that first treatment, I told Tony that his work could make a real difference for elephants and that I was interested in reading more scientific research about its efficacy. He explained that animal osteopathy was a field that needed more attention from the international community.

I hope this book, which offers an exciting contribution from a unique perspective, will help attract that attention from a larger veterinary and science research audience. It presents a comprehensive and detailed overview of non-human animal osteopathy that allows medical practitioners, animal behavior experts and members of the public alike to judge the science underlying it for themselves. There is still so much that we do not understand about animals. It is crucially important that future approaches to both welfare and conservation integrate a complement of scientific work related to understanding both an animal's mind and its body. This book is an important contribution for anyone who agrees.

Joshua M. Plotnik, Ph.D.
Department of Psychology, Hunter College,
City University of New York
Think Elephants International, Inc
New York, NY, USA
October, 2019

PREFACE

There are numerous osteopathic texts available on diagnosing and treating the myriad conditions that afflict the human body, but before this book there were only two texts published on animal osteopathy, both of them restricted to the treatment of horses. Although animal osteopathy is a fast-growing part of the profession, until now those involved in treatment and teaching have done little to commit their considerable knowledge and experience to print.

This book has taken considerable time to prepare, with more than 16 contributors from six countries presenting their specialist knowledge. The efforts of everyone involved are testament to the interprofessional support that exists in the field of osteopathic medicine. We have tried to include the most relevant information, while keeping repetition to a minimum. To all of us involved it has reinforced the vocational nature of our professions.

This book includes the culmination of several decades of clinical experience from some of the world's top osteopathic and veterinary specialists who are involved in making osteopathy part of an integrated treatment in animal care. Without the generous contribution of their knowledge this book could not have been written. The book is intended to support the postgraduate osteopath who has a desire to enter this fascinating field of practice, as well as providing support for physiotherapists, chiropractors, veterinary surgeons, and dedicated animal care workers. It is not just a book of techniques, but a comprehensive text providing essential background knowledge on different animals, to help each individual practitioner develop their own skills safely, and to act as a reference source as they build up their animal-based clinics. The editors have done their best to present as much information as possible to try and fulfill this role, but inevitably in a single volume we could not include all the detailed knowledge that was offered to us.

The format and text of each chapter has been standardized as much as possible while maintaining the style of the various contributors. Similarities and also differences between species and genus of patient are given. At the end of each chapter is a list of relevant references so that the reader can refer to other texts to support their learning.

Clearly, we cannot cover everything on all species in a single volume, nor are the views and experiences of the authors the final word in animal osteopathy. We hope, however, that we have managed to provide a starting point for those interested in becoming involved in this fascinating area.

Tony Nevin
Chris Colles
Paolo Tozzi
October 2019

ACKNOWLEDGMENTS

Creating this book would not have been possible without the support and help of countless people, all of whom gave freely of their time and expertise. We have been deeply touched by their generosity and would like to thank them all here.

From the veterinary profession we would like to thank Drs Alessandro Paini, Andrew Prentis, Klaus Friedrich, Stavros Kalpakis, and Tim Partridge, as well as all of the staff at Arvonia Vets, Garston Vets, Masefield Veterinary Centre, Vale Wildlife Hospital, and Weirfield Wildlife Hospital.

From the equine field we would like to thank Kay Humphries for her advice on saddlery and Ron Ware for his life's work in farriery. Jenna Zan, Victoria Dooley, Frances Colles, Trish Thornton, and Alexandra Filmer all assisted with photographs for this book.

From the zoo, safari, and wildlife sectors our thanks go to: Longleat Safari Park and in particular to Darren Beasley, Ryan Hockley, Kevin Knibbs and the elephant team, Mark Tye and the gorilla team, Leah Drury and hoof stock; Rome Zoo veterinary clinic; Bob Lawrence and the staff at West Midlands Safari Park; John Minion and everyone at Yorkshire Wildlife Park; Craig Pritchard, Terri Hill, John Roberts, and the Golden Triangle Asian Elephant Foundation; and Roxy Dankwerts at the Zimbabwe Elephant Nursery.

For stepping in and helping at the eleventh hour we thank Annabel Jenks, Richard Bridges, Jazmine Keane, and Martyn Dixon. Our gratitude and thanks are extended to all of the contributing authors: Brendan Atkin, Julia Brooks, Leonidas Christodoularis, Kate Colles, Jon Cracknell, Vibeke Elbrønd, Caroline Gould, David Gutteridge, Andy Hayton, Richard Hillam, Nadine Hobson, Nic Masters, Sophia Prousali, Andrew Routh, John Hope-Ryan, and Rikke Schultz; to the illustrators Bruce Hogarth and Carol Vincer whose diagrams have greatly enhanced this book; and to the copy editor Sally Davies and to Mary Law and Morven Dean of Handspring Publishing, all of whom have been instrumental in this project.

Our thanks also go to everyone else who has supported our efforts to write this book and who have continually shown faith in us.

Finally, we would like to thank our families and friends, who have had to put up with us being unavailable for events and gatherings while we have been writing and editing this book, for supporting our efforts along the way.

EDITORS

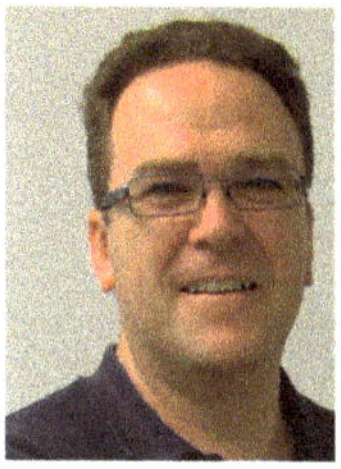

Tony Nevin BSc (Hons) Ost, DO graduated from the European School of Osteopathy, Maidstone, UK in 1988. He has pioneered osteopathic treatment with over 300 different species and breeds of domestic and wild creatures. Based in the UK, he works internationally, both treating and teaching. Tony is passionate about animal osteopathy and is Course Director for an MSc program for postgraduate osteopaths. He runs several equine, small animal, zoo, and wildlife clinics in the UK. His particular interest is chronic problems affecting horses and dogs. Working with veterinary practitioners has allowed him to integrate osteopathy with standard veterinary practice, often achieving remarkable results. He is author of several published papers on his equine, elephant, wildlife and avian work.

He produces and presents his own radio show on osteopathy called 'The Missing Link', for Corinium Radio, and is also a member of the editorial team for Animal Therapy Media.

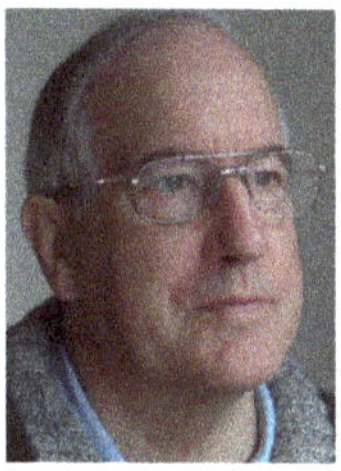

Chris Colles BVetMed PhD HonFWCF MRCVS qualified as a veterinary surgeon from London in 1971. He joined the Animal Health Trust in 1975, where he carried out research into equine lameness. He was head of the equine clinical department when he returned to specialized equine practice in 1988. He was awarded a PhD in 1981, became an RCVS recognized specialist in equine surgery in 1996, and was awarded an Honorary Fellowship of the Worshipful Company of Farriers in 2000.

Chris has written over 40 scientific papers and contributed to, or written, nine text books as well as lecturing to international meetings in many different countries, primarily on equine lameness.

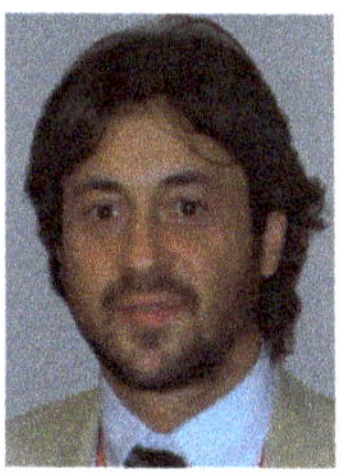

Paolo Tozzi MSc Ost, DO, PT is a leading teacher and practitioner of osteopathy and is well-known and highly regarded throughout Europe, South America, and Japan. He is former Treasurer of the Osteopathic European Academic Network (OsEAN) and former Principal of the School of Osteopathy CROMON in Rome. Paolo is a Member of the Fascia Science and Clinical Applications Advisory Board of the *Journal of Bodywork and Movement Therapies*. He is a regular speaker at national and international congresses of osteopathic medicine and manual therapy, including the International Fascia Research Congresses. Paolo is author of various articles on fascia and fascia research and is an expert on osteopathy applied to domestic and exotic animals.

CONTRIBUTORS

Brendan Atkin BSc (Clin Sci), MHSc (Osteo), MSc Animal Osteopathy, DPO, GCTE
Director, Animal Osteopathy Australia
Faculty of Sutherland Cranial Teaching Foundation ANZ
Lecturer, Osteopathy,
College of Health and Biomedicine, Victoria University,
Melbourne, Australia

Julia Brooks DO (Hons), MSc
Head of Clinic, Haywards Heath, Sussex, UK

Leonidas Christodoularis BSc.Ost (Hons), DO, PGCert.An.Ost
Osteopath, Thessaloniki, Greece

Kate Colles BVet Med, MSc
Retired veterinary surgeon, UK

Jonathan Cracknell BVMS, Cert Zoo Med, CertVA
CEO, Cracknell Wildlife and Veterinary Services,
Potters Bar, UK

Vibeke S. Elbrønd DVM, PhD
Assistant Professor, Section of Pathobiology,
Department of Veterinary and Animal Sciences,
Faculty of Medical and Health Sciences,
University of Copenhagen, Denmark

Caroline Gould
Founder, Vale Wildlife Hospital, Beckford, Tewkesbury,
Gloucestershire, UK

David Gutteridge DO, LicAc
Wheelton, Chorley, Lancashire, UK

Andy Hayton
Longleat Enterprises, retired, UK

CONTRIBUTORS

Richard Hillam BVSc, PhD, CertVR, MRCVS
Partner, Arvonia Vets, Cheltenham, Gloucestershire, UK

Nadine M Hobson DO, Osteopath
British School of Osteopathy (1978)
Consultant Osteopath at Hyde Park
Veterinary Centre for
Integrated Animal Healthcare,
London (1998-2018)

John Hope-Ryan MA, VetMB, MRCVS
Clinical Director, Masefield Veterinary Practice,
Barnards Green, Malvern, UK

Nicholas J. Masters MA, VetMB
MSc, DipECZM, MRCVS
Assistant Director of Wildlife Health Services,
Zoological Society of London,
Regents Park, London, UK

Sophia P. Prousali DVM, MSc
Veterinarian in Charge, Action for Wildlife Rehabilitation Center,
Thessaloniki, Greece

Andrew Routh BVSc, CertZooMed, FRCVS Jersey

Rikke M. Schultz, DVM, IVAS, EVSO, BAHVS
RMS Equine Practice,
Kokkedal, Denmark

GLOSSARY

AA
atlas–axis

ACTH
adrenocorticotropic hormone

ALKP
alkaline phosphatase is tested for in the blood; high levels can denote liver damage, Cushing's disease, or active bone growth in young animals

ALT
alanine transaminase enzyme is normally found in low levels in the blood; high levels suggest liver damage or inflammation

ANS
autonomic nervous system

anterior
toward the front or view from the front

AST
aspartate transaminase, also known as AspAT, ASAT, or AAT, is an enzyme present in the liver

Artiodactyla
even-toed ungulates that weight-bear on the 3rd and 4th toes

autotomy
spontaneous self-amputation of the tail in some reptiles

AZA
Association of Zoos and Aquariums

backed
refers to a horse that has been trained to accept a rider

BECAM 2.0
Animal Osteopathy and Wellness international congress, held on September 29–30, 2018, in Rome, Italy

BIAZA
British & Irish Association of Zoos & Aquariums

binding
where there is a contracture of fascia or shortening of muscle fibers that creates a certain level of friction on movement

biotensegrity
a conceptual model used in biology to look at the way the individual parts of the body function and interact as a whole structure

BLT
balanced ligamentous tension – an osteopathic technique

bow-leg, bow-legged
describes the points of both hocks when viewed from behind when they appear to be too far apart

bowing
a term used to describe the shape of a tendon with tendinitis where the outline is bow-shaped

brachycephalic
from the Greek meaning "short" and "head," describes a skull shorter than typical for a species, as found in certain dog breeds

BVA
British Veterinary Association – the UK authority governing veterinary surgeons

BVOA
British Veterinary Orthopaedic Association

CAE
caprine arthritis and encephalitis – a retroviral disease affecting goats

caudal
toward the tail

caudoventral
toward the tail and ventral surface

CaCL
caudal cruciate ligament; also called the posterior cruciate ligament in humans

carpus
wrist

cauda equina
term used to describe the caudal fibers within the spinal canal that originate from the end of the spinal cord

CCTV
closed-circuit television

CDRM
chronic degenerative radiculomyelopathy

Chelonia
turtles and tortoises

chondrodystrophoid
angular deformity of the limbs, accepted as normal in some breeds of dog

CITES
Convention on International Trade in Endangered Species of Wild Fauna and Flora

CKCS
Cavalier King Charles spaniel – a breed of dog originating in the UK

clays
term used to describe the 3rd and 4th digits of even-toed ungulates

cloaca
a posterior orifice serving as the common opening for the digestive, urinary, and reproductive tracts in amphibians, reptiles, birds, and some mammals

CM
Chiari-like malformation

CMO
craniomandibular osteopathy – an orthopedic disease mostly affecting dogs

CN
cranial nerve

CNS
central nervous system

coccygeal segments
tail vertebrae

cow-hocked
describes the points of both hocks when viewed from behind when they appear to be too close to each other

CPK
creatine phosphokinase enzyme found in the heart, brain, and skeletal muscles

cranial
toward the head and the front proximal half of a limb; also occasionally used as an abbreviation for cranial osteopathy

cranial base
also known as the cranial floor, it separates the brain case from the rest of the skull

cranioventral
toward the head and the ventral surface

CrCL
cranial cruciate ligament; also called the anterior cruciate ligament in humans

CRH
corticotrophin-releasing hormone

Crocodylia
crocodiles and alligators

chromophores
atoms and electrons within a cell that determine which color or colors from the spectrum are reflected or absorbed

Cryptodira
a suborder of turtles that retract their necks by laterally flexing them in an "S" shape caudally into the carapace

CSF
cerebrospinal fluid

CSM
cervical spondylomyelopathy

GLOSSARY

CT
computed tomography; cervicothoracic

CT junction
cervicothoracic junction within the spine

CV4
compression of ventricle 4 in the brain – an osteopathic technique

DDF
deep digital flexor

distal
refers to the lower half of a limb

DJD
degenerative joint disease

DL junction
dorsolumbar junction; *see also* **TL junction**

DLS score
dorsolateral subluxation score

DMSO
dimethyl sulfoxide

DNA
deoxyribonucleic acid; double helix molecular chains that carry the genetic instructions for growth, development, functioning, and reproduction of an individual – the building blocks of life

dorsal
top line or upper aspect of the body; sometimes refers to the thoracic spine

dorsal flexion
extension of the spine and hyperextension of the spine (bending toward the sky) in quadrupeds

dorsal view
view from above the patient, looking down

dorsolateral
on the dorsal surface moving away from the midline

dorsomedial
on the dorsal surface moving toward the midline

dorsoventral
describes the direction from the dorsal aspect of the body toward its ventral surface

dorsoventral flexion
flexion through the length of the spine in a dorsal and then ventral motion in quadrupeds

EAZA
European Association of Zoos and Aquaria

ecdysis
shedding of the skin

egg binding
where one or more eggs are stuck in the reproductive system or cloaca and are unable to be passed by the female

EHV-1
equid alphaherpesvirus 1, formerly known as equine herpesvirus 1, can cause abortion, respiratory problems, and occasionally neonatal mortality in horses

EHV-4
equid alphaherpesvirus 4, formerly known as equine herpesvirus 4, is the most significant cause of viral respiratory infection in foals

EMG
electromyography used for recording electrical activity produced by skeletal muscles

EOP
endogenous opioid peptides are produced in the hypothalamus

epaxial
axial structures above, or dorsal to, the transverse processes of the vertebral column

EWG
Elephant Welfare Group – a UK-based group of elephant experts

extension
movement of the bones of a joint that increases the joint angle between the bones involved and that usually results in the straightening of these bones

fascia lata
a fascial band on the lateral aspect of the thigh

FCI
Fédération Cynologique Internationale

FeLV
feline leukemia virus

FIV
feline immune deficiency virus

FL
Functional Line; refers to part of the fascial system

flexion
movement of the bones of a joint to reduce the angle between the bones involved, usually resulting in a bending action of a joint or limb

FLPL
Front Limb Protraction Line; refers to part of the fascial system

FLRL
Front Limb Retraction Line; refers to part of the fascial system

fowl
domestic birds of the order of Galliformes, kept for their eggs and flesh

functional release
an osteopathic technique that involves slowly moving joints and soft tissue structures into positions of comfort rather than placing them under further tension

GA
general anesthesia or general anesthetic

GH
glenohumeral

girthiness
term for when a horse repeatedly reacts to the girth being tightened up and there appears to be increased sensitivity around the girth region to touch, brushing or clipping

GI tract
gastrointestinal tract

global
refers to the entire patient, encompassing the whole body

GOLPP
geriatric onset laryngeal paralysis polyneuropathy – a disease affecting the recurrent laryngeal nerve in older dogs

GOsC
General Osteopathic Council – the statutory governing body for all osteopaths practising within the UK

GOT
general osteopathic technique

GSD
German shepherd dog

hallux
the innermost digit of the hind foot

harmonic treatment
a passive form of oscillatory, rhythmic techniques applied to joints and tissues to aid repair and normal function

hemipenes
the male genitalia of Squamata, with one organ on either side of the body

HD
hip dysplasia; high definition (if preceding IRTI, CT, or MRI)

HOD
hypertrophic osteodystrophy, an orthopedic condition

GLOSSARY

HPA pathway
hypothalamic–pituitary–adrenocortical pathway

HPT pathway
hypothalamic–pituitary–testis pathway

HVLA
high velocity, low amplitude

HVLATs
high velocity, low amplitude thrusts

hock
ankle

hypaxial
axial structures below, or ventral to, the transverse processes of the vertebral column

IAAT
International Association of Animal Therapists

IBS
irritable bowel syndrome

IM
intramuscular

IRTI
infrared thermal imaging

IRTS
infrared thermographic scan

ITB
iliotibial band – fascia on the lateral aspect of the thigh attaching to the ilium and tibia, and the muscles of the thigh

IVM
involuntary mechanism – an osteopathic term for the natural expansion and contraction movements of the meninges with the production and flow of cerebral spinal fluid

KC
The Kennel Club of the United Kingdom is the official governing body for activities such as dog shows and operates the national register of pedigree dogs

kissing spines
over-riding dorsal spinous processes – an orthopedic condition affecting the dorsal spinous processes in some horses (see **ORDSP)**

lame
describes difficulty in walking or an altered gait due to a problem affecting one or more limbs

lateral
away from the midline

lateral flexion
bending to one side

LF
the left foreleg in a quadruped

LH
the left hind leg in a quadruped

LL
Lateral Line; refers to part of the fascial system

LPT
lymphatic pump technique

LS junction
lumbosacral junction

lunge
a term used to describe exercising a horse from the ground and in a circle around the handler; it normally involves a lunge line attached to a head collar or bridle with the other end held by the handler

mahout
a traditional name for an elephant handler or a person in charge of an elephant

massotherapy
medical treatment by massage; the term can also be used to describe other forms of bodywork treatment

MBD
metabolic bone disease

medial
toward the midline

MET
muscle energy technique, an osteopathic technique

MF-BIA
multifrequency bioimpedance analysis

MMP-TTA
modified Maquet procedure, tibial tuberosity advancement – orthopedic surgery to alleviate the effects of CCL rupture

MO
metaphyseal osteopathy, an orthopedic condition

motility
the ease with which structures move and articulate with each other

MRI
magnetic resonance imaging

MSc
Master of Science university degree

MSK
musculoskeletal

NMBD
nutritional metabolic bone disease caused by calcium deficiency in the diet

NSAIDs
nonsteroidal anti-inflammatory drugs

OA
occiput–atlas or osteoarthritic

OAA
occiput–atlas–axis

OCD
osteochondritis dissecans

OCF
osteopathy in the cranial field

omothoracic complex
all of the shoulder-to-thorax structures

omothoracic junction
the point at which the shoulder articulates with the thorax

OMT
osteopathic manipulative technique

ORDSP
over-riding dorsal spinous processes, also known as kissing spines, is an orthopedic condition affecting the dorsal spinous processes in some horses

oviparous
describes an egg-laying reptile

ovoviviparous
describes a reptile that produces eggs that develop within the body and hatch within or immediately after release from the parent

PennHIP
Pennsylvania Hip Improvement Program

pentadactyl
having five fingers or toes

per os
orally (on prescriptions)

pes
Latin for "foot" – used to refer to the segment corresponding to the foot in the hind limb

plantar
toward the ground; the under surface of a specific structure

Pleurodira
suborder of turtles that retract their necks by laterally flexing them and tucking them up under the carapace

PNS
peripheral nervous system

posterior
rear view or view from behind

GLOSSARY

RCVS
Royal College of Veterinary Surgeons

PSNS
parasympathetic nervous system

rehab
rehabilitation

RF
the right foreleg in a quadruped

RH
the right hind leg in a quadruped

Rhynchocephalia
tuatara – a lizard-like reptile of which only two species remain in New Zealand

RSH
renal secondary hyperparathyroidism

ROM
range of movement (of a joint or several joints in the body)

rostral
toward the nose and in front of the cranium

rostroventral
from the cranium, toward the nose on the ventral surface

RTA
road traffic accident

ruminant
a type of animal that brings up plant food from its stomach to chew again as part of the digestive process

scintigraphy
a form of orthopedic imaging which uses a scintillation counter and a radioactive tracer within the patient; also known as a gamma scan

scoliosis
a term used to describe any sideways (lateral) curvature of the spine

SCT
synthetic calcitonin

SDL
Superficial Dorsal Line; refers to part of the fascial system

sesamoid bone
a small bone embedded within a tendon or muscle

SI
sacroiliac

sickle-hocked
describes the hock when viewed from the side when the angle is less than 145 degrees

SL
Spiral Line; refers to part of the fascial system

SM
syringomyelia

SNS
sympathetic nervous system

SOAP
Society of Osteopaths in Animal Practice – a UK organization created to support postgraduate development in animal osteopathy

somatic dysfunction
a term used to describe a problem associated with sensory input and motor output to and from the CNS in relation to the body and its surrounding environment that results in an altered state at rest and/or during movement of that individual

spavin
an equine term used to describe a problem in the hock joint

splints
an inflammatory condition in the splint bones usually caused by injury to the interosseous ligament or the periosteum

SPR
sustained positional release, an osteopathic technique

Squamata
lizards and snakes

stifle
a joint in the hind leg of a quadruped (such as a horse or dog) corresponding to the human knee

still point
the moment in time when treating the IVM when all movement ceases in either contraction or expansion of the meninges

straight-hocked
describes the hock when viewed from the side when the angle is greater than 145 degrees

SUV
sport utility vehicle

SVL
Superficial Ventral Line; refers to a part of the fascial system

sway back
ataxic gait which affects the hind quarters in lambs with a copper deficiency; it can lead to long-term altered gait or ataxia

sympathetic dystonia
altered balance within the body which occurs when there is an imbalance between the respective activities of the sympathetic and parasympathetic parts of the ANS, resulting in abnormal function and sensitivity in the MSK

synovitis
inflammation of the synovial membrane

TCWO
tibial closing wedge osteotomy – orthopedic surgery to alleviate the effects of CCL rupture

TFL
tensor fascia latae – the muscle that tenses the fascia lata and rotates the thigh medially

TL junction
thoracolumbar junction, sometimes called the dorsolumbar (DL) junction

TMJ
temporomandibular joint

TPLO
tibial plateau levelling osteotomy – orthopedic surgery to alleviate the effects of CCL rupture

TTA
tibial tuberosity advancement – orthopedic surgery to alleviate the effects of CCL rupture

TTAR
tibial tuberosity advancement rapid – orthopedic surgery to alleviate the effects CCL rupture

TTO
triple tibial osteotomy – orthopedic surgery to alleviate the effects of CCL rupture

u/l
units per liter

ultrasound
can refer to a high frequency scan of internal structures or a form of therapy for the MSK or targeted internal structures

UVB
ultraviolet B – radiation that is in the region of the ultraviolet spectrum

varanid
relating to the Varanidae – a suborder of carnivorous lizards that includes the Komodo dragon and the crocodile monitor

Vari Kennel®
the trade name for a large mobile animal kennel that can be dismantled

ventral
describes areas of the body of a quadruped that face the ground or the underside of the individual

ventral flexion
flexion or bending of the body or spine toward the ground in quadrupeds

ventral view
view from below the patient, looking up

GLOSSARY

ventrodorsal flexion
flexion of the spine ventrally and then dorsally in quadrupeds

vibrissae
long bristles on the muzzle and elbows of otters

viviparous
describes a reptile that produces live young that have developed in the mother's body

V-spread technique
an osteopathic technique that uses gentle forces transmitted along the skull's diameter to facilitate movement in the sutures

WHO
World Health Organization

wobbler syndrome
a term used to describe cervical spine stenosis

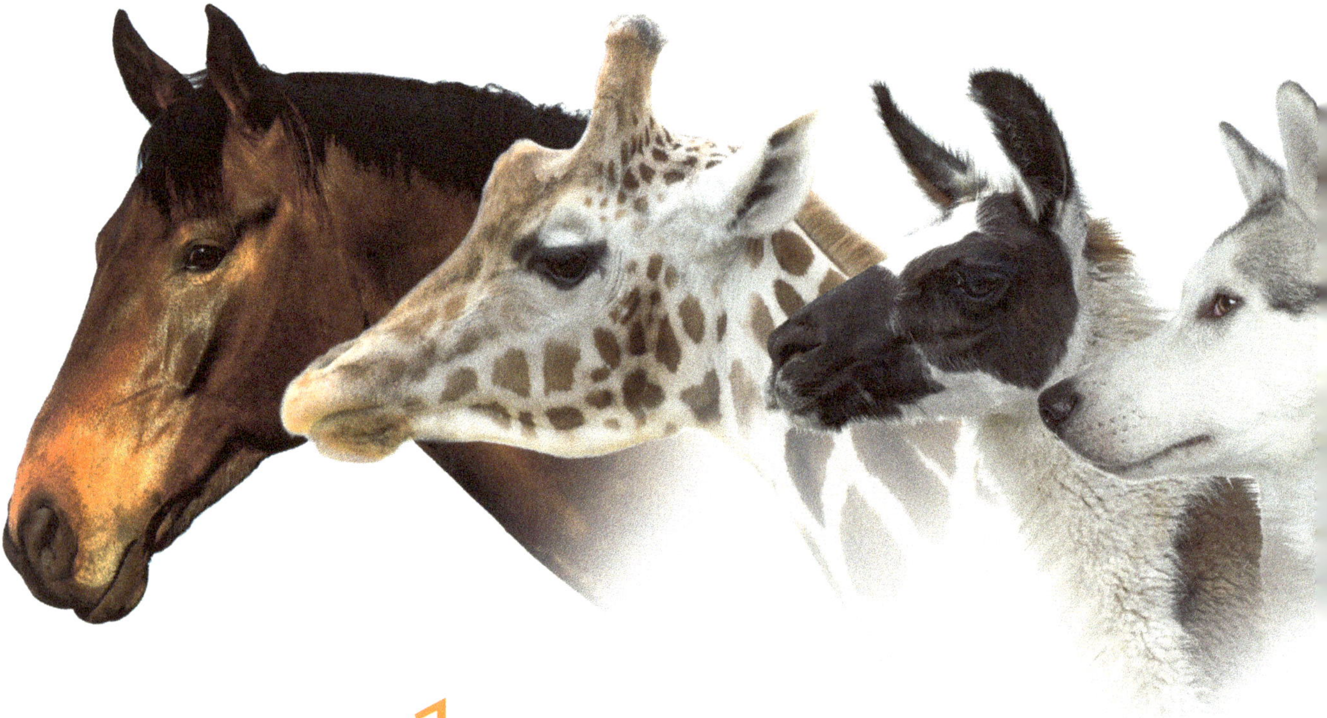

Chapter 1
AN INTRODUCTION TO THE OSTEOPATHIC TREATMENT OF ANIMALS AND BIRDS

Tony Nevin, Julia Brooks, Vibeke Elbrønd, Rikke Schultz, Brendan Atkin, Kate Colles

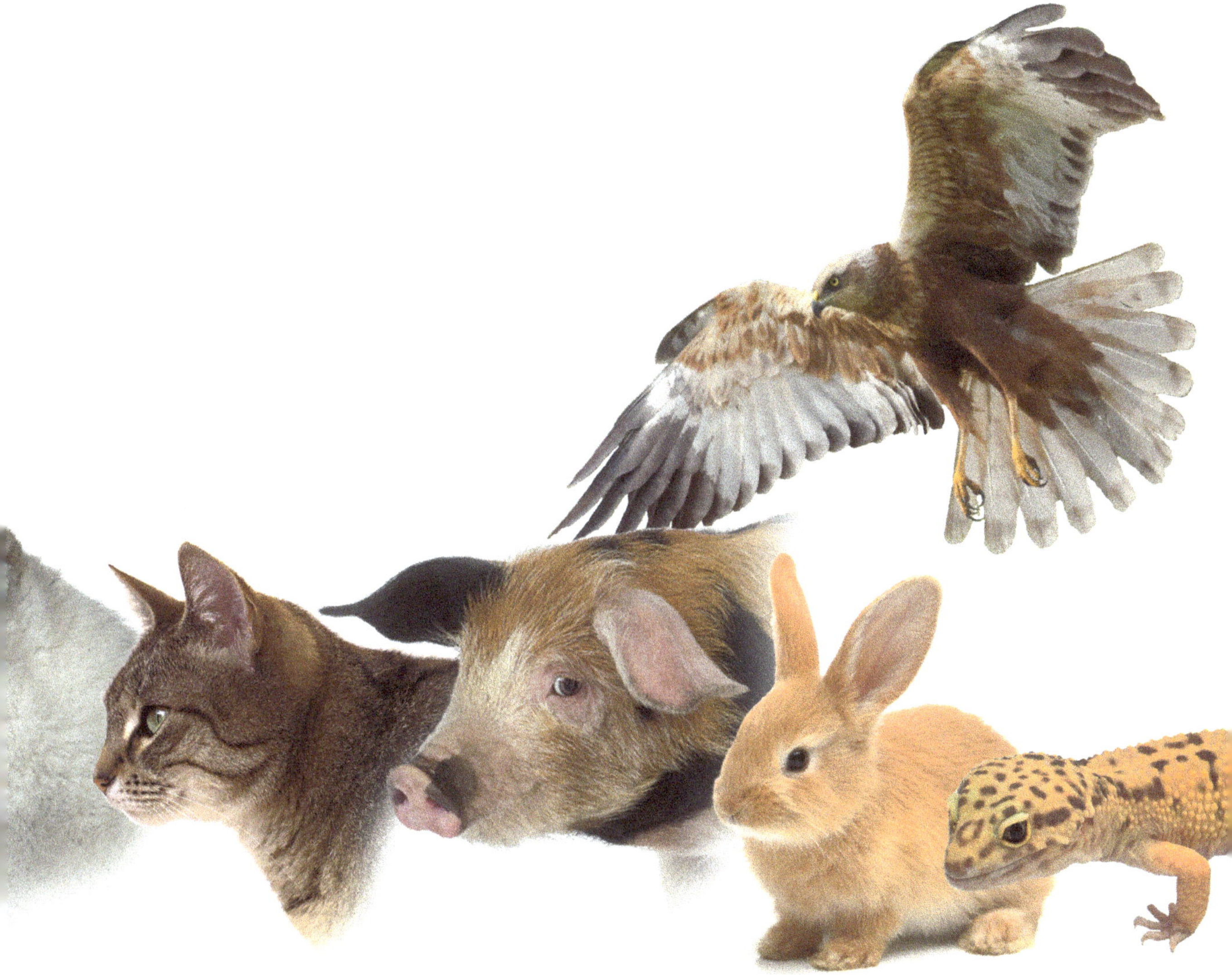

An introduction to the osteopathic treatment of animals and birds

Chapter 1

Introduction

The principles of osteopathy apply to all forms of fauna, and not just humans.

As undergraduates the majority of osteopaths study the examination and treatment of the human patient. Those wishing to expand their practice to include the treatment of animals and birds face many challenges. Not least is the difference in communication and body language between the myriad species and breeds that can be encountered.

In the United Kingdom and some other territories the law states that an osteopath can only treat an animal if it has been referred by a veterinary surgeon (Veterinary Surgeons Act 1966). This also makes the veterinary surgeon legally responsible for that animal's welfare throughout the course of osteopathic treatment.

When following a career in animal osteopathy, there are many differences to working with the human patient; the main ones are listed below:

1. Work is usually only by direct veterinary referral.
2. Case history taking is undertaken via an intermediary such as an animal's owner, the veterinary surgeon, trainer, or keeper. This can result in some lost data or conflicting information if several people are involved.
3. Direct practitioner–patient communication relies primarily on visual body language, with some simple verbal commands when dealing with species such as dogs, horses, and elephants. Observation and reading a patient's body language are essential to safe practice.
4. The chance of contracting a zoonotic disease or parasitic attack is a continual risk, as some of these conditions show few or no signs of infection or infestation in their animal host.
5. There are species and breed-specific anatomical and physiological differences which have a direct bearing on how to apply osteopathic principles when formulating treatment programs.
6. The osteopath must consider their own health and safety in addition to that of the handler and patient, and may therefore decide to treat a patient using sedation or a general anesthetic.
7. Any post-treatment rehabilitation will rely on the full understanding and cooperation of all involved in the patient's care, whether the patient is a top event horse returning to work or an orphaned elephant that will be returned to the wild.
8. Consideration and understanding of the fight-or-flight status of the patients you are likely to treat is essential. Some species may be considered as flight animals, such as equines, but a stallion may behave more like a fight animal if it feels threatened, as can some mares. Similarly, with cats and dogs, it can be difficult to determine what they will do if they feel scared. Primates and some birds can be tricky to handle if the sex of both the practitioner and patient are the same, and the patient is fully conscious during examination and treatment.
9. Species that are kept in collections can pose problems, as they may not behave as one would expect them to in the wild. These need to be considered on a case-by-case basis.
10. There are occasions when the osteopath will be able to effect lasting changes without actually touching their animal patient. This is achieved purely by applying osteopathic principles to active movement training regimens, as well as modified husbandry.

As most osteopaths will have a thorough understanding of the anatomy, physiology, and neurology of the human model they may think that they can simply apply their skills to the treatment of animals and birds. However, just as there are many different aspects to human osteopathy, so there are in this field, with the added complication of many modifications to each of the three systems just mentioned (Dyce et al. 2009).

A study of comparative anatomy is required, along with a working knowledge of the different biomechanics, physiology, and neurological pathways that some species have evolved (Thompson 1996). Without this knowledge, and a genuine desire to work with allied professionals who already know these species, the osteopath will be at a major disadvantage.

A brief history of animal osteopathy

When Andrew Taylor Still developed what we now call osteopathy he based it on the original Native American system of maintaining health. These nations did not only use manual medicine to treat their people - they used it on their animals as well.

From that time onward there are cases mentioned of osteopaths treating animals and birds, usually owned by human patients who could see the benefits of their own treatments; however, it is not until we get well into the twentieth century that we start to see this side of the profession begin to be taken seriously.

Prior to this and the passing of the Veterinary Surgeons Act 1966, osteopaths were working very much on their wits and instinct (RCVS 2018).

Arthur Smith, a graduate of the British School of Osteopathy, was one of the early osteopaths who worked with a veterinary surgeon, again a patient of his. He was, however, unusual in that he not only treated cases for this vet, but also through him saw several hundred referred cases from other vets, thus paving the way for future generations to follow. He pioneered the treatment of horses under general anesthesia, which was much less sophisticated than the techniques used today.

Arthur had originally been posted to the UK to serve in the Royal Air Force during the Second World War. Afterwards he enrolled to study osteopathy and became a resident thereafter. His sons were often involved in assisting with his equine work, unwinding the fascial tension patterns, along with several other strong assistants, and as such they aptly demonstrated the need to treat the whole body and not just a particular point of altered tissue state.

In the 1970s Anthony Pusey started treating animals; again this was initiated by a client asking him to look at their dog. Working with the owner's vet he not only treated the dog, but also built up a thriving referral clinic.

In the 1980s his horse work took off after a meeting with Dr. Chris Colles, a specialist equine orthopedic surgeon. Chris, with a former research background, had noted that many cases referred to him revealed no *apparent* cause for their presentation. These were cases where the horse had gradually lost condition, was finding it difficult to work at a certain level, and generally presented as stiff. However, after thorough veterinary examinations and tests he was unable to discover a cause for the condition.

Chris heard about Anthony's work via two of his own clients who had their horses treated by him. The outcome of the meeting was the creation of a referral clinic, which grew into the largest of its kind for difficult, chronic back cases. Cases seen ranged from Olympic level dressage and event horses through to happy hackers.

Throughout his career Anthony strove to raise the professional standards of animal osteopathy. He created introductory courses and seminars, and was instrumental in getting the first postgraduate master's course validated in the subject. He also wrote and presented several papers, cowrote chapters on animal osteopathy in several veterinary and osteopathic textbooks, and also coproduced the first British animal osteopathy book (Pusey et al. 2010).

His career was sadly cut short when he passed away on March 30th, 2007. His legacy lives on in those he inspired and worked closely with, including his son Rupert who later graduated as an osteopath, and who has begun to dip his toe into animal-based treatment.

Another exponent of animal osteopathy in the UK is Stuart McGregor. Stuart came from an equine science background and combined the two subjects to focus on helping and maintaining the performance horse and dog. He has successfully run his own program of postgraduate studies introducing osteopaths to this fascinating branch of the profession. This has added to the quality of postgraduate study available.

At RMIT University, Melbourne, Australia there has been a master's course in animal osteopathy, which sadly at the time of writing no longer exists. However, one of this book's contributors (Brendan Atkin) has completed the master's course in the UK and is well situated to help resurrect it.

In 1991 the author (TN) was asked to look at an injured badger (*Meles meles*) at a UK wildlife hospital, and thus began a long career applying osteopathic principles to help in the treatment of wild animals and birds that has involved travel, lecturing, and several published papers on the subject (Nevin 1997, 1998, 2005, 2012, 2017; Colles et al. 2004). Since the untimely demise of Anthony Pusey, Tony has been the clinical director of the first British MSc in Animal Osteopathy. This is run in conjunction with the McTimoney College, Oxfordshire, UK. This is in addition to his more mainstream clinics where he treats people, horses, and small domestic pets.

Others who have helped cement animal osteopathy into the fabric of our modern profession are mostly represented as contributors to this book, as authors and proofreaders, as well as content advisors.

Throughout Europe and Scandinavia there are many osteopaths who now regularly treat animals. Some countries have also set up societies and support groups to help steer the development of animal osteopathy, including the Society of Osteopaths in Animal Practice (SOAP) in the UK, which formed the first structured group purely for osteopaths treating animals and offered quality CPD seminars to postgraduate osteopaths.

More recently the UK-based International Association of Animal Therapists (IAAT) has extended its membership to include osteopaths and chiropractors. The IAAT was originally formed to support animal physiotherapy and is part of a growing network for professionals, integrating postgraduate training to further benefit their patients.

As animal osteopathy grows, the need to develop support groups within each economic territory and nation is essential for the profession to grow and strengthen the body of knowledge it is creating.

The need for quality peer-reviewed research is only going to increase, and it is the responsibility of each and every osteopath to contribute to this, even at a basic clinical level. We need only look at other allied professions to see the direction we are all traveling in, and the fact that so little has been proved regarding what we actually do when we treat animals and birds. We assume a lot based on human medical research, or in certain cases animal research, that is often the only data we can use to justify our actions. The authors hope that this book will encourage further advancement of this fascinating branch of osteopathy.

In 2012 the First International Congress of Osteopathy in Animal Practice was held in Rome and highlighted the amount of research that has been produced thus far. The majority of this has been self-funded. Areas of interest were canine, feline, equine, avian, and exotics, with the final day being set aside for practical-based workshops. This was the first time osteopaths from all over the world had met under one roof, and for three days they shared decades of valuable information. This has been followed by the BECAM 2.0 Animal Osteopathy and Wellness congress, again near Rome, Italy, in 2018.

Working with veterinary surgeons and allied professionals

In animal treatment more than in any other branch of osteopathy, the need to work with other professions is paramount to the successful outcome of any treatment program.

At the very least the animal's owner or carer, their veterinary surgeon, and the osteopath should be involved in the treatment. If the patient is a horse then you will need to factor in the farrier, saddler, trainer or riding instructor, and dental technician. If the horse is suffering from a chronic problem then you may also need to liaise with other manual therapists who are already involved in the patient's care.

With regard to zoo and wildlife patients there may well be others involved in addition to those already mentioned. In some cases there can be political interest in a patient, especially if an individual is from a critically endangered species. There may need to be special licenses granted before you are even allowed to touch the patient, and in these cases the professionals involved are then accountable to the body issuing the license, along with any medicolegal implications that this may include.

Being able to work closely with others as an embedded member of a team is vital if osteopathy is to move forward in animal care. It is not an area where isolation can prevail.

Understanding veterinary terminology

For osteopaths to be taken seriously it is essential to get to grips with veterinary terminology. This differs from human medical terminology in certain areas (see Glossary and Fig. 1.5). Vets in particular expect reports to include accurate nomenclature. Use of the correct nomenclature will ensure that they understand what you are saying, and will gain their respect.

When working with farriers and saddlers remember that they often have an established working relationship with a horse's owner and can often influence an owner regarding what you are trying to achieve. They have extensive expertise in areas which affect equine movement - areas where you may only have passing knowledge. By ensuring that you include them in what you are doing you are much more likely to keep them on side, and help them to understand why the horse is suddenly moving differently. In many cases you can encourage them gradually to adjust the work they are doing to help and support your treatment.

Working within the law

Within the United Kingdom all osteopaths must first be registered with the General Osteopathic Council (GOsC), carry professional indemnity cover that includes provision for animal treatment, and only treat animals that are referred by a veterinary surgeon, as laid down in the Veterinary Surgeons Act 1966 (RCVS 2018) and the Osteopaths Act 1993 (GOsC 2019).

The situation in other countries is sometimes different, and within Europe and Scandinavia the profession is still evolving with regard to professional accountability and governance. The authors would strongly advise anyone who is unsure as to their particular situation, with regard to animal osteopathy, to refer to the governing body they are accountable to for the most up-to-date legal requirements.

Research

Many animal osteopathy papers have been written, but only a few have been published in peer-reviewed journals. There are also many undergraduate and postgraduate dissertations which have covered groundbreaking work, yet when compared with other professions, this is an area that has not seen enough work to give that all-important *evidence-based* foundation that is expected today. One stumbling block is the lack of funding available, with all research published to date having been undertaken at the expense of those doing it. As a result, this has restricted research to being mostly retrospective, with some studies involving data collected over two decades. This makes for slower progress than could be achieved with adequate funding.

Diagnostic aids

The osteopath is heavily reliant on the diagnostic and differential diagnosis skills of the veterinary surgeons with whom they are working. The obvious lack of verbal communication directly with animal patients means that all other modes of diagnosis are much more important.

It has already been noted that within the UK, and many other territories, only a veterinary surgeon is legally allowed to "diagnose and treat" a patient. The osteopath, however, may want to have access to the results of any diagnostic investigations. These will include the results of blood analysis, radiographs, ultrasound images, CT and MRI scans, and their accompanying written reports.

Blood samples can be useful in assessing the state of a patient with regard to inflammatory agents and evidence of stress, and also certain types of pathology.

Radiographs can be helpful in ascertaining the preferred resting state of some joints and also for ruling out the presence of any bony pathology or soft tissue masses.

In the case of CT and MRI scans, patients beyond a certain size cannot fit into the scanners, although their limbs, head, and neck often can. In such cases the patient may be heavily sedated or anesthetized.

Infrared thermal imaging

If the osteopath is working on large animals, with a suitable bulk compared to surface area, then the use of infrared thermal imaging (IRTI) is a very good way of assessing musculoskeletal (MSK) problems, and the response to osteopathic treatment. The latest high-definition cameras can help the clinician to evaluate smaller patients, and in much greater detail than was previously possible. IRTI has long been used in many industries, but for some reason has not been widely adopted in human health care or veterinary medicine. It is a noninvasive way to read the heat radiated by an individual and in particular the heat derived from the blood flow directly under the skin, which we know is controlled by the sympathetic nervous system. Alterations in surface temperature will result from altered blood flow, but images must be acquired under carefully controlled conditions to avoid artifactual results. It is important that the patient is in a controlled environment that eliminates reflected heat, and drafts, and only reads radiation given off directly by the patient's body (Holst 2000).

In the acute phase of an MSK problem the affected area will initially show an increase in surface temperature. After a while (usually one to two weeks in larger patients) this will alter if there is increased muscle guarding. Guarding is accompanied by reduced blood flow through the smaller surface capillaries. The temperature measured by a sensitive high-definition IRTI camera will be lower over the whole area supplied by the affected region's sympathetic nervous system (Colles et al. 1994). The resultant images appear to mirror those of dermatomes in human subjects; however, this has not yet been accurately documented in animal models (Vollmer and Möllmann 2013).

A study has been made of data taken from 4,000 horses with chronic long-standing movement issues but no known pathological issues (Colles and Nevin 2015). IRTI scans made throughout their osteopathic treatment programs showed that patterns of temperature differences could be used to locate spinal segments where the reciprocal nerve supply to the MSK system was causing restrictions in normal movement and affecting the overall gait of these horses. The IRTI images were used to chart each horse's progress through their entire treatment program. With horses it was also found that there were no consistently reproducible changes in images acquired less than 14 days apart.

By comparing visual observations of movement with palpation and then looking at the IRTI images these cases were systematically assessed and the commonality of findings was noted over a 25-year period. Some of these findings were used in the first osteopathic paper to be published in a veterinary peer-reviewed journal (Colles et al. 2014).

The author (TN) has found that IRTI also shows similar image results with other large species such as elephant (Colles et al. 2004, 2005), rhino, giraffe, large antelope, deer, lion, and subadult gorillas (which have less dense coats than an adult), and it has helped in the assessment of blood circulation in the limbs of British wild mammal and bird casualties (Nevin 2013).

Modern high-definition digital IRTI cameras will often take a simultaneous digital photograph, allowing an accurate comparison with the thermal image and making report preparation easier (Fig. 1.1).

If using IRTI as part of your clinical or research practice it is important to be aware of some of the physiological adaptations certain species use to thermoregulate their core temperatures. Equids can alter blood flow to their distal limbs (distal to carpus and tarsus), as can many avian species. Elephants use their ears to fan cooler air along their flanks, but also change flow in the ears as part of thermoregulation. These actions can create difficulties when interpreting scan pictures.

Zoonotic disease and parasites

Zoonotic disease needs to be taken seriously. Although most animal and avian parasites and infections are host-specific, many can also cause health issues for humans. The severity ranges from minor aggravations such as lice and ringworm to infectious diseases such as avian influenza, bovine spongiform encephalopathy, and rabies, which may be fatal.

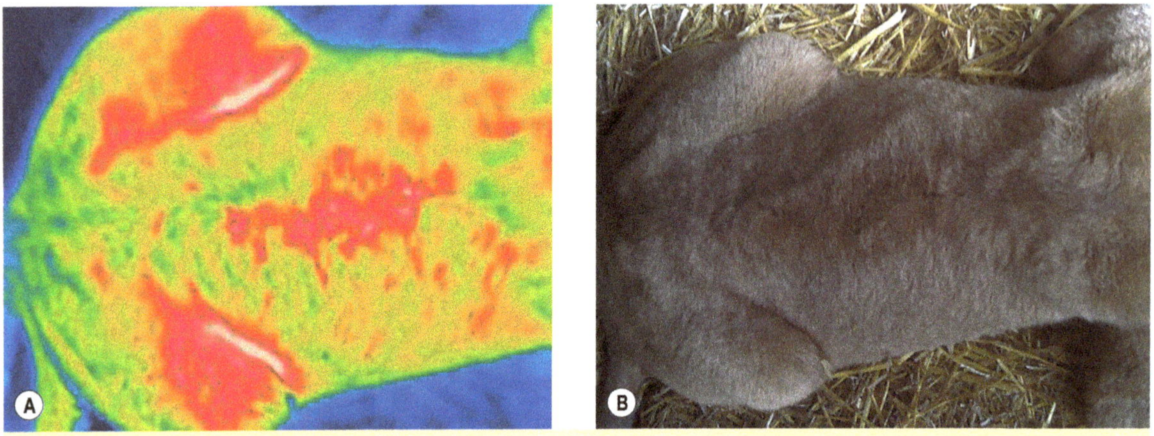

Figure 1.1
(A) An infrared thermal image of the dorsal aspect of a lioness. (B) A digital photo captured at the same moment.

Whatever the law regarding osteopathic treatment of animals is where you are working, the authors would strongly advise you to team up with a veterinary surgeon, especially if you are going to work with birds, wildlife, and livestock. Veterinary surgeons are taught about potential zoonoses as part of their training.

- Infections caused by viruses, bacteria, and fungi can be transferred to a human host. The osteopath can also become a vector for further human and nonhuman infection, and therefore strict personal hygiene during and after every treatment session is essential (Fig. 1.2).
- Internal parasites are those that are ingested and live primarily in the gut, lungs, liver, and bloodstream. Nematodes and flukes can be undetected for quite a while and may only become apparent if the host's health is compromised
- External parasites commonly encountered are fleas, ticks, avian flies, and lice. Although these are mostly host-specific, many will survive and live on humans for varying periods of time. Many external parasites live off their host's blood, and are also vectors for infectious disease (Fig. 1.3).

Appendix A at the end of this chapter lists many of the zoonoses that may be encountered when treating animals. It is not exhaustive, nor should it put you off treating animals.

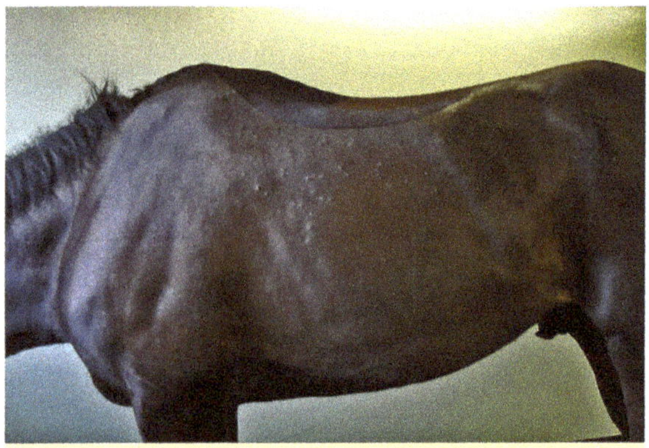

Figure 1.2
A horse with ringworm infection. This is quite obvious in the equine. It may be even more obvious in the bovine, but many other animals, such as cats and hedgehogs, may show almost no clinical signs.

Comparative anatomy

Anatomy varies between species, but generally the differences relate to function. In the long term, beneficial anatomical variations persist, and others are gradually lost. Pretty well all the musculoskeletal features

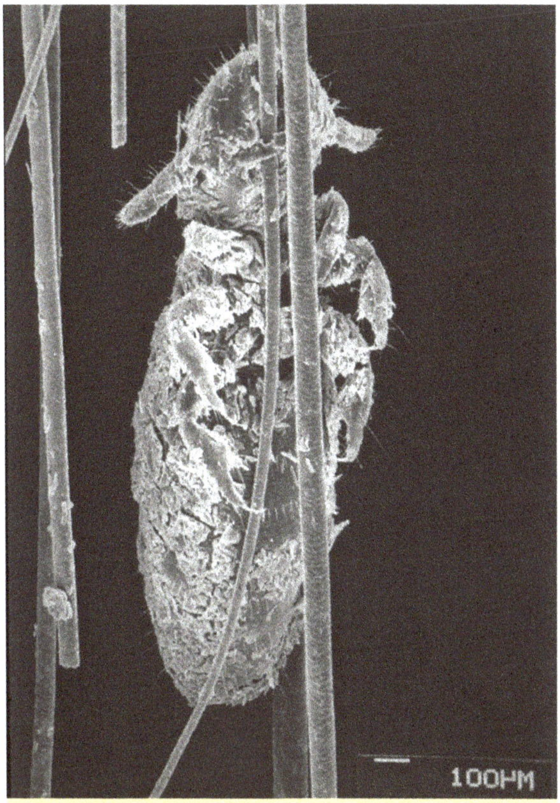

Figure 1.3
An electron micrograph of a louse – one of the ectoparasites commonly passed between animals and humans via physical contact.

that we recognize in ourselves can be identified in other species, particularly of the limbs, once one gets past differences in standing positions and proportion (see Fig 1.4).

The first differences encountered by those used to human anatomy is the terminology used to describe the position and orientation of anatomical structures in what is usually a quadruped stance (Fig. 1.5). The front of the body, or what we would describe as anterior in human anatomy, faces the ground and is referred to as the ventral surface. The surface facing away from the ground is considered to be dorsal. Toward the head, what we would call superior is described as cranial and toward the tail is caudal. In the head, structures toward the nose are described as rostral. As with humans, proximal structures of the limbs are nearer the body and distal structures are furthest away.

The regional anatomy of the musculoskeletal system will vary in form to support the activity of the animal. Some structures are instantly recognizable from human anatomy and others are highly species-specific.

The skull and dentition

The central midline structures of vertebrates are made up of the skull and vertebral column.

The animal skull has a more horizontal orientation compared to that of humans and other primates, and the foramen magnum, by which the spinal cord exits the skull and enters the vertebral canal, opens caudally. The skull bears prominent ridges for the attachment of muscles and ligaments, one of which is the palpable nuchal crest of the occiput providing the site of attachment for strong cervical muscles and the ligamentum nuchae which stabilize and move the head on the neck.

The skull is divided into the cranium, containing the brain, orbits, and ears, and the face, which bears dentition and has an olfactory function. The cranial cavity is not as big as one might think. It houses around 600 g of brain in horses, 30 g in cats and 1 g in a sparrow, largely made up of the primitive hindbrain structures which orchestrate survival and reproductive responses. Of course, the 4,500 g of the whale and elephant beats the 1,300 g of the human organ, but it is the well-developed layers in the forebrain, which are necessary to form the connections and networks required for complex thought, that give humans a cerebral advantage.

The face attached to the cranium is generally elongated, as is the jaw, to give a large dental surface on the maxilla and mandible to grind fodder in the herbivore or to grab, tear, and crush flesh in carnivores. Selective breeding programs may compromise these functions. In dogs, the foreshortened (brachycephalic) face of pugs and boxers can predispose to dental overcrowding and breathing problems, as this shape deviates from the efficient dolichocephalic, wolf-like face structure.

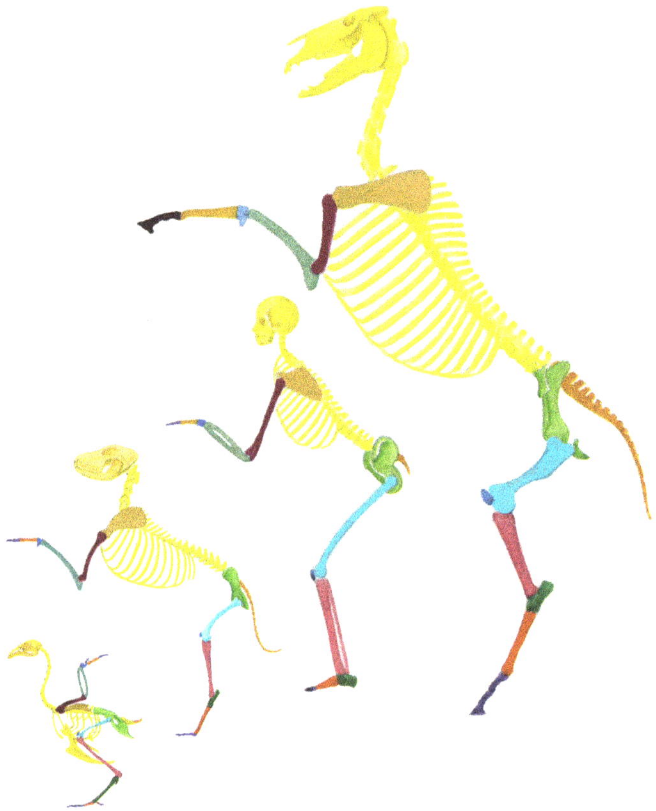

Figure 1.4
The comparative anatomy of the chicken, dog, human, and horse. Adapted from Colles C (2002) *Functional Anatomy*. Kenilworth Press Ltd.

Reproduced with kind permission from Quiller Publishing Ltd.

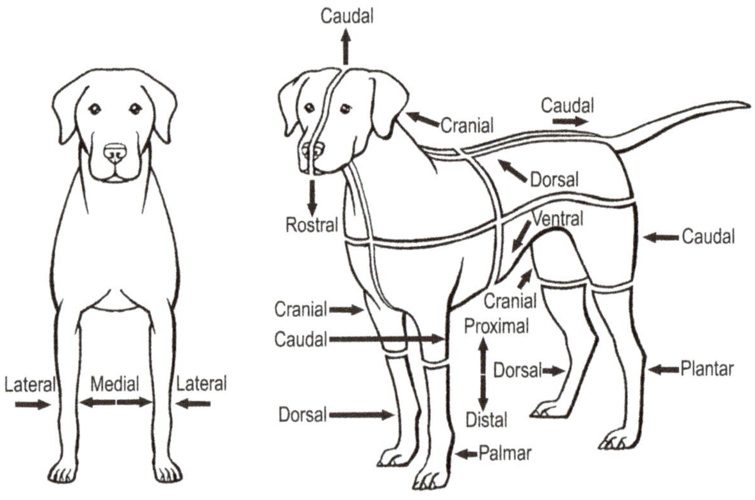

Figure 1.5
The orientational terminology used to refer to quadrupeds.

The nasal passages often form a large part of the face, allowing movement and warming of air, and providing a sensory surface for olfaction. In obligate nasal breathers, such as horses, rabbits, and rodents, the relationship between the epiglottis and the nasopharynx and oropharynx means that, under normal circumstances, air can only be taken into the lungs through the nasal passages.

The maxilla of the face bearing the upper dental arcade is opposed by the dentition of the mandible. The movement of one on the other is controlled by the jaw or temporomandibular joint (TMJ), which is another area where there is adaptation in the interests of function. It is important clinically, as dysfunction here can affect the ability of the animal to feed. It can also influence neck movement by virtue of the strong neurological connections with the suboccipital region. This connection is mediated by the trigeminal nucleus which originates, in part, from the upper cervical cord and whose neuronal projections extend out to innervate the dental surfaces, the skin of the face, the temporomandibular joint (TMJ), and the muscles of mastication. Herbivores have a broad, transversely elongated joint surface allowing side-to-side and rotary movements to facilitate a grinding action. A particular feature of ruminants is the absence of upper incisors which have been replaced by paired dental pads which are pliant but have a cornified surface. Carnivores tend to have a mandibular condyle in the form of a truncated cone which articulates with the base of the skull, to allow mainly flexion and extension for holding and dissecting prey. Some snakes have a complex series of hinges associated with the jaw to allow them to swallow prey of larger diameter than themselves.

Dentition itself is of clinical interest. Herbivores feeding on fibrous material, such as equids (horses, donkeys, and zebras) and ruminants, are hypsodonts, which means that the teeth, fully formed in the mandible and maxilla, are pushed out beyond the gum line throughout life, to compensate for the attrition effect of grinding. In horses, this occurs at a rate of around 3 mm per year and the gradually altering appearance of the incisor cross-section is used as a rough guide to determine age. This constant eruption may cause problems with different types of feeding regimens imposed by domestication. Constant grazing with the head down allows the mandible to fall forward and approximates the grinding surfaces to give even wear of upper and lower arcades. Periodic feeding at raised levels, such as occurs with hay nets and mangers, may result in uneven wear and lead to hooks and sharp edges on the teeth.

Elephant teeth are unique in that they grow as if in a line, from the back of the mouth, with two molars in wear at any one time. As these front molars wear away, grinding the fibrous material in their diet, substitute teeth migrate forward to replace them. They are replaced six times in a lifetime after which starvation is the usual cause of death.

Carnivores, by contrast, have one set of adult teeth. They have characteristically large canines, which are particularly well developed in lions and tigers. Carnassial teeth, a modification of the fourth upper premolar and lower molar, are well developed in the cat family and are specialized to perform a cutting action. The slightly longer upper dental arcade means that there is little opposition of teeth and no capacity for lateral movement, which explains why carnivores bolt, rather than chew, their food.

Reptiles such as snakes may have additional specialized fangs in the maxilla to administer poison. Birds have dispensed with teeth altogether apart from a deciduous egg tooth to facilitate exit from the egg.

The vertebral column

Supporting the skull is a vertebral column of varying length. The essential components are the same for most species and are identified as cervical, thoracic, lumbar, and coccygeal vertebrae, which also support the limb girdles.

Separating the vertebrae are intervertebral discs. They form 25 percent of spinal length in man, 16 percent in the dog and cat, and 10 percent in ungulates, and this corresponds to the degree of flexibility. Disc prolapses like those that occur in human spines are not uncommon in dogs, notably in the long-bodied breeds such as dachshunds, but the fibrous nature of equine and ruminant discs precludes prolapse in these species, although degenerative changes, particularly at the more mobile segments such as the lumbosacral joint, do occur.

Birds tend to have much of their vertebral column fused to provide a stiff, stable structure for muscles of flight. Snakes are one long vertebral column often of over 300 segments with projections locking vertebrae together to give flexibility without the danger of dislocation. Flexibility is further enhanced by the fact that the ribs are not joined ventrally and only a few species have any vestige of thoracic and pelvic girdles.

Mammals, and this includes the giraffe, always have seven cervical vertebrae, with the exception of the manatee (six) and the sloth (eight to 10 depending on species). Their position in the neck may not be immediately obvious if one goes entirely by the body outline, particularly in grazing animals where the top line is given shape by the ligamentum nuchae. In general, elements of the upper two vertebrae are palpable and observable as they lie near the dorsal surface. Caudal to this, however, the vertebrae snake away in an "S" shape to sit low in the neck, the position being identified by the plate-like transverse processes projecting just above the jugular groove. The ligamentum nuchae itself is an elastic ribbon in dogs and absent in cats, but in herbivores it forms a tough elastic sheet which takes some of the weight of the head. It also facilitates the use of the head as a kind of weighted bob in running as, at certain stages in the stride, stretching the fibers of this structure stores potential energy which is then released later in the gait cycle.

In birds the neck is one of the few mobile areas, which is important for a good range of vision, preening, and for the beak to be wielded in nest building, and for a variety of feeding methods. The number of cervical vertebrae ranges from small birds with eight to the long-necked swan with 25 bones (Fig. 1.6).

The first and second cervical vertebrae are specialized for the connection of the neck to the skull and for specific ranges of movement. The atlas is in the form of a ring, which in most large animals has deep cups on the cranial surface to receive the prominent, rounded occipital condyles of the skull. These tend to be more pronounced than in humans where the head balances on top of the neck in a vertical stance. In quadrupeds the head needs to be attached to the neck with a substantial bony structure and well-developed muscles. This arrangement mainly allows flexion and extension at this level. The wings of the atlas are easily palpated behind the ramus of the mandible. Birds and reptiles have only one depression in the ventral arch to receive the single condyle of the occiput - an arrangement that facilitates the kind of rotational movement that we see in the owl.

The need for powerful muscular attachments is reflected in quadruped animals by the large plate-like expanse of the spinous process of the second cervical vertebra, the axis, compared with the rather diminutive primate version. The odontoid peg of the axis which protrudes upwards from the body of the vertebra into the ring of the atlas is rod-like in humans and carnivores and facilitates rotation for an all-round visual capability. The rather spout-like herbivore version allows less rotation but, as the eyes are set on the side of the skull, the field of vision is extensive without the need for head movement.

The more caudal cervical vertebrae have a marked ventral crest and small spinous processes. The transverse

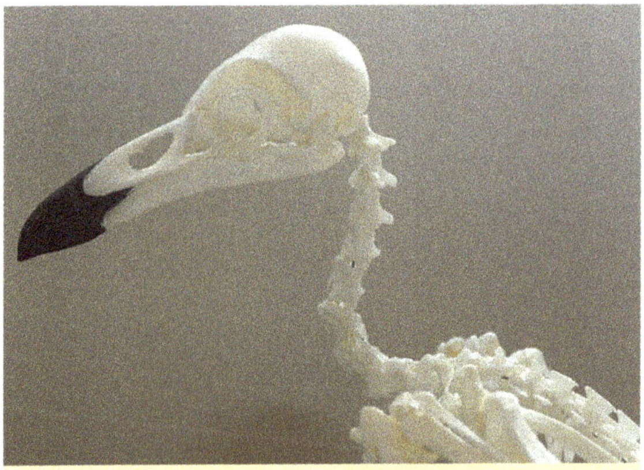

Figure 1.6
Lateral view of the cervical spine of a corvid (crow).

processes are fairly large, allowing for muscle attachments, and have transverse foraminae for conducting blood vessels. This changes at the seventh cervical segment which is the transitional point to the thoracic spine and which has a larger spinous process, no transverse foramen, and also bears a small costal process caudally on its body for articulation with the first rib. Bird cervical vertebrae are uniformly cylindrical with articular processes and rudimentary ribs.

Thoracic vertebrae have short bodies with large spinous processes, particularly over the withers (behind the cervicothoracic (CT) junction), and costal facets for rib articulation. There are 12 thoracic vertebrae in humans, 13 in cattle and dogs, and 18 vertebrae in the horse, which with the ribs that make up the horse's thoracic cage accommodate large lungs. The lungs are in part compressed and released by the movement of the guts against the diaphragm in a pump-like fashion to provide an efficient respiratory mechanism for the horse at speed. The elephant has about 20 pairs of ribs with 20 or 21 thoracic vertebrae.

Birds have a variable number of thoracic vertebrae ranging from three to 10, some of which coalesce. The first two to six fuse to form the notarium (from the Greek *noton* meaning back). This is followed by a single mobile thoracic segment connecting the notarium to the synsacrum, a fusion of the last thoracic vertebrae with the lumbar, sacral, and first caudal vertebrae. This mobility leaves it somewhat vulnerable to trauma. Ribs corresponding to the vertebrae are connected to the sternum, which is a substantial bone to which large flight muscles are attached and from which projects a keel, or carina, that is more prominent in birds that fly well. In common with snakes, they do not have a diaphragm and rely on muscle contraction and elevation of the sternum to draw air into the lungs. Care should be taken not to restrict sternal movement when handling birds.

Lumbar vertebral numbers vary little, with the human having five, dogs and cats seven, and horses six (with the exception of Arab horses, which frequently only have five). The lumbar vertebrae have relatively short, cranially inclined spinous processes and long, flattened transverse processes.

The sacrum is formed from three to five vertebrae which are fused to a variable degree. They have the appropriate number of spinous processes, which can be identified independently in dogs and horses, or form a continuous ridge in ruminants. It connects the trunk to the pelvic girdle.

The synsacrum of the bird is connected to five or six caudal vertebrae and ends in a few fused segments known as the pygostyle, which gives shape to the end of the tail.

The tail of other species is made up of a variable number of simple segments.

In addition to a role in support and movement, the vertebral column provides protection for the spinal cord and a point of exit for the spinal nerves. The vertebral canal is enlarged in regions containing the cervical and lumbar origins of the brachial and lumbosacral plexuses which innervate the limbs. The names of the peripheral nerves forming the plexuses are familiar, for example the ulnar and sciatic nerves supply basically the same structures as they do in the human. Generally, the spinal cord extends much further caudally than in man (where it ends at the level of the second lumbar area). The end point is variable, terminating at L5 or L6 in the pig, L6 in ruminants, L6 or L7 in the dog, S1 in elephants, S2 in the horse, and S3 in the cat.

The muscular system of the back is broadly similar in all species, with the hypaxial muscles lying ventral to the transverse processes and the epaxial muscles lying dorsally. The epaxial muscles are important not only to stabilize and move the vertebral column but they also have a proprioceptive role in establishing the position of the body in space. In particular, the multifidus, lying adjacent to the vertebrae, continues as the sacrocaudalis (sacrococcygeal) dorsalis into the tail, which is a useful handle for treatment of these deeper structures. The hypaxial elements, such as the abdominal muscles, are essential in supporting viscera, and other muscles such as the psoas have a role in limb movement.

The limbs

With some variation, the central structures bear a remarkable resemblance to human anatomy. Limbs, where present, may look less familiar. However, on closer inspection the musculoskeletal elements present in man are also recognizable in birds and vertebrates.

The limbs are connected to the central line by the thoracic and pelvic girdles.

The most notable feature of the thoracic girdle is that, in most animals apart from primates, it has no bony connection with the spine and the clavicles are residual or absent. The ventral thoracic and shoulder muscles, together with the scapulae, form a muscular sling between the forelimbs in which the thorax is suspended. This arrangement facilitates lateral movement of the body as the thorax rotates between the limbs. This compensates for limitations of leg action which are confined to flexion and extension ranges.

Birds have a somewhat different arrangement, although the individual components are still familiar. The scapula is a flat rod running parallel to the spine as far as the synsacrum. It is connected cranially to a large coracoid process, and this junction provides an articular surface for the humerus of the upper limb. The coracoid, rather diminutive in man, extends caudally to attach to the sternum - an arrangement which provides a stable structure from which flight muscles, such as the pectoralis and supracoracoideus, can move the wings. It is also attached at its cranial end to the clavicle. The clavicles are fused together to form the furcula or wishbone.

The main components of the pelvic girdle are the paired innominate bones, formed from fusion of the ilium, ischium, and pubic bones. They have more of the appearance of short, thick appendicular bones than the bowl-shaped human version. Ventrally, they join to form a relatively large symphysis, which involves not only the pubis, as in man, but also the ischial components of the pelvis. Dorsally, they attach to the sacrum. This structure provides an effective springboard by which the substantial muscle and tendon mechanisms of the hind limbs can act to propel the body forward at speed.

Birds have pelvic bones which provide an acetabular surface to articulate with the femur. However, they are not joined ventrally in a symphysis - an arrangement which allows easy passage of eggs.

Quadruped mammals tend to have limbs with the proximal bones, the humerus, and the femur relatively short, compact, and attached to the trunk by powerful muscles. These muscles initiate movement in the long, distal limbs which are interconnected principally by tendinous structures whose potential for storing energy by stretch provides a low energy component to moving limbs across the ground.

In the forelimb, the humerus descends to the elbow whose position is indicated by the prominent, caudally projecting olecranon of the ulna. The ulna lies caudal to the radius at the upper end and lateral in the distal part, holding the foot in a pronated position. In most domestic animals, the firm connections between the two mean that pronation and supination, so important in man to assist in complex manual manipulation, are considerably reduced. These movements are not possible at all in ungulates where they have a fibrous union or in horses where the ulna and radius are fused, the distal ulna being vestigial.

The ulna, if it extends far enough distally, and the radius end in two rows of small carpal bones, often eight in number as in the horse and pig, but with fusion of one or two occurring in other species. Despite its position in the forelimb, this articulation is unhelpfully referred to as the knee in horses and cattle.

In the hind limb, the femur articulates distally with the patella, tibia, and fibula, the latter being residual in the horse, to form the stifle joint. Given that this is the equivalent of the human knee, the joint is found unexpectedly high up, tucked under the skinfold between the trunk and the limb in ruminants and equids. A notable feature in herbivores is the locking mechanism of the stifle where the medial of the three patellar ligaments hooks over the medial trochanter of the femur, fixing the joint in extension. This is particularly effective in horses and is a way of standing with low energy cost, and allows extra weight to be taken on one leg while the other is resting.

Carnivores have a stifle joint more closely related to the human version, with one patellar ligament and located further down the hind limb. Birds are similar, with a tibia and thin fibula familiarly referred to as the "drumstick" at the dining table.

The tibia and fibula of swine and carnivores run distally alongside each other. In ruminants the fibula has regressed, and in the horse it is slender and fades out toward the middle of the adjacent tibia. Distally, the tibia and, where present, the fibula articulate with the tarsal bones to form the hock joint. The tarsals have components recognizable from the human ankle, namely the talus, calcaneus, and tarsal bones, some of which may be fused depending on the species.

Below these structures, things become modified when compared with human anatomy, and the position of the joints is essentially based on what sort of ground contact is necessary to facilitate the activities required. Humans (and bears) have a plantigrade stance meaning that quite a lot of the distal leg is in contact with the ground, starting with the calcaneus (our heel) and ending with the toes. In the dog, the heel has been lifted off the ground to form the "dog leg" of the hock joint, where the calcaneal part of the carpus protrudes caudally. The metacarpals are also not in ground contact and the dog essentially stands on its fingers in what is known as a digitigrade stance. Ruminants, pigs, and horses have taken this to extremes and stand on the distal phalanx with a hoof (ungula) covering in an unguligrade stance.

The distal ends of both forelimbs and hind limbs are similar to the five-digit human hand but modified for traveling at speed. The process involves losing some digits and developing others to take the extra weight. Dogs and cats are down to four digits, with the first not in contact with the ground and lying medially as a nonfunctioning dewclaw. Pigs have no first digit and residual second and fifth digits, leaving functional third and fourth digits. In ruminants, the third and fourth metatarsals have fused, although at the distal end they separate out to provide two rounded articulations for two proximal phalanges. The distal phalanges end in hooves divided by the interdigital cleft.

Equids have just one metatarsal articulating with the proximal phalanx. This third metatarsal is flanked by the residual second and fourth metatarsals, known as splint bones. The distal half of the middle phalanx and the distal phalanx are protected by the circle of keratinized epithelium of the hoof.

The great weight of an elephant requires feet that are adapted for shock absorption. The digits themselves are not in contact with the ground, sitting on and being encased in a tough fatty connective tissue "cushion." Toenails are not attached to the digits but lie in a ring around the foot with four in the front and three at the back in an African elephant, and one more on each foot in its Asian relative. Despite this cushioned pad and considerable bone mass, the sheer size and weight of the elephant means that it cannot leave the ground at faster gaits.

There is of course a marked difference between forelimb and hind-limb arrangements in the bird. The forelimb (wing) has a recognizable humerus and also the ulna and radius forming the midwing. However, the distal wing structure is much reduced with fusion of the carpals with the metacarpal for strength and feather support. A three-digit arrangement forms the end of the wing, with considerable variation in proportions between different species. In the leg, the tibia is fused with the distal tarsals to form the tibiotarsus which gives added length and therefore leverage for running, landing, and taking off. It articulates with the tarsometatarsus, formed from the fusion of the distal tarsals and the metatarsals. The fifth digit is always absent, and most birds have four toes, although this is highly variable.

The common feature of the distal limb is that the muscular arrangement is largely tendinous. This, together with greater length distally, and the heavily muscled shorter proximal limb, permits rapid movement over the ground at reduced energy cost, by using the elastic energy stored and unleashed by the stretching and releasing of these tendinous structures.

When studying the interspecies anatomy, it becomes obvious that musculoskeletal structure, which at first sight seems to show infinite variation, has many common elements. Where divergence does occur it is usually possible to look at functional requirements and find a logical justification for these modifications.

Chapter 1

Identification and treatment of myofascial kinetic lines in animals

Introduction

Myofascial chains in humans have been described by several authors (Richter and Hebgen 2009; Myers 2009). These descriptions were the inspiration for looking for similar chains and functional interactions when carrying out dissections in horses (Elbrønd and Schultz 2014, 2015).

The "chains" have been renamed "myofascial kinetic lines" in order to indicate both their origin and that they are functionally integrated structures. Their main component is fascial tissue, with some muscle involvement. They are involved in the movement of the whole body in flexion, extension, lateral flexion, and rotation. The myofascial lines balance each other in motion and in the standing position. The lines give anatomical evidence of the need for a "whole-body" concept in diagnosing and treating the locomotor system in animals.

The major component of the lines is fascial tissue. The function of this tissue has been neglected for many years. The Western medical world has approached the fascia as an "inert and mechanically stable tissue," which could be cut and replaced in surgery and was not necessarily to be addressed in treatment and rehabilitation of the locomotor system. Recent studies, however, show that the role of the fascia in conjunction with the nervous system, the locomotor system, and other organs is much more complex and significant than previously realized. Research is continually improving our understanding of the fascia as a delicate and well-organized structure, with a high-conforming plasticity in close collaboration and interaction with the nervous system. Fascia has been examined in many ways including: gross dissection; biomechanical, physical, and physiological measurements; specific histological and immunohistochemical techniques; and molecular biological techniques (Schleip et al. 2012a, 2012b; Stecco et al. 2011; Stecco 2015). Stecco's research group has contributed numerous publications to the understanding of human fascia at both the macroscopic and microscopic level, and this has led to the publication of an atlas of human fascial function (Stecco 2015). In 2015 Guimberteau and Armstrong also published a book explaining the structure of human fascia based on endoscopic recordings. These results show the plasticity and activity of this tissue. Importantly, the ongoing results from the fascia research groups support the changing of diagnostic focus from regions to include a whole-body perspective, with the fascia being the element that integrates the body functions. Despite the differences in posture of quadrupeds and bipeds, fascia has been found to be very similar in many ways.

Inspired by Myers (2009), seven myofascial kinetic lines have been dissected and isolated in the equine (Elbrønd and Schultz 2015), and preliminary dissections of the superficial lines in dogs have also been performed (Pedersen 2013). The study and dissection of four deep myofascial kinetic lines in horses is ongoing. Additionally, pilot studies of the histology of equine fascial tissues have been performed. Multifrequency bioimpedance studies of fascia have been carried out on equine clinical cases pre- and post-treatment.

Kinetic myofascial lines

In order to describe and dissect the lines in animals the existing anatomical literature has been studied intensively. No novel anatomy has been discovered, but existing descriptions have been assessed with movement and posture patterns in mind. During dissections it became obvious that when a muscle attachment was released from the bone, the fascial tissue continued into the next muscle, ligament, tendon, or fascial sheet. It was thus possible to isolate the distinct lines from the rest of the body as uninterrupted structures. There are major similarities between the human and equine lines and the three canine lines so far described. It seems reasonable therefore to assume that this system of myofascial kinetic lines may be present in most mammals with modifications to allow for their varying anatomy and movement patterns. The descriptions of the lines in the following section are based on a number of publications and proceedings (Elbrønd and

Schultz, 2013, 2014, 2015; Schultz and Elbrønd 2013, 2014; Elbrønd 2015).

The names of the human lines have been adjusted for quadrupeds. The seven lines, which are described in the following paragraphs, are:

- the Superficial Dorsal Line
- the Superficial Ventral Line
- the Lateral Line
- the Functional Line
- the Spiral Line
- the Front Limb Protraction Line
- the Front Limb Retraction Line.

The Superficial Dorsal Line

The Superficial Dorsal Line (SDL) (Fig. 1.7A–C) is involved with flexion of the hind limbs and extension of the hip, back, and neck. It starts with the flexor tendons of the distal phalanges of the hind limb, the flexor muscles of the thigh to the tuber ischii, and the sacrotuberous ligament of the pelvis. From the ilial wing it continues through the spinalis, longissimus, and iliocostal muscles (the erector spinae muscles) to the neck. Here the cervical part of the muscles continues into the occipital fascia, the temporal muscle, and also attaches to the mandible, with dorsal fibers inserting into the masseter muscle (Fig. 1.7C). A contraction of the SDL (Fig. 1.7A) will leave the animal with an extended back and overly raised neck (as often seen in horses).

The Superficial Ventral Line

The Superficial Ventral Line (SVL) involves the extension of the hind limbs and flexion of the hip, back, and neck (Fig. 1.7B and C). It starts with the extensor tendons and muscles from the dorsal aspect of the distal phalanx, passes to the ilial head of the quadriceps of the thigh, the prepubic ligament, and continues into the straight abdominal muscle, through the straight thoracic muscle, and onto the sternum. From there it runs through the sternomandibular muscle and ventrally into the fascia and masseter muscle to the mandible (Fig.1.7C). A contraction of the SVL creates a flexed back and neck (most often seen in carnivores; see Fig. 1.7B). The SDL and SVL act as antagonists in flexion and extension of the back and neck (Fig. 1.7A and B) and when balanced they allow a correct posture and free movement of the neck and back. They can be seen as an extended version of the "bow and string" theory which was put forward by Slijper in 1946. This theory describes the relationship of the back and abdominal muscles. The SDL and SVL merge at the distal phalanges of the hind limb and in the masseter muscle on the mandible (Fig. 1.7C). This means the temporomandibular joint (TMJ) is very important with regard to movement and balance of the animal (Ros 2011), as is correct trimming and shoeing of the horse.

The Lateral Line

The Lateral Line (LL) (Fig. 1.7A–C) is involved in the lateral flexion of the body. It has a superficial layer and a deep layer. The left and right lines act as antagonists and have to be balanced in order for the animal to stand and move straight. The LL has a superficial layer involved in spinal flexion and a deep layer involved in spinal extension. The line starts with the lateral extensor muscles of the hind limb and continues into the lateral quadriceps muscle. At this point the line splits into the superficial and the deep layers. In the superficial layer the line continues into the tensor fascia latae (TFL), on to the tuber coxae and further into the cutaneous muscle of the trunk, shoulder, and neck, ending in the brachiocephalic muscle. The deep layer involves the superficial gluteal (in the equine) or medial gluteal (in the canine), the oblique abdominal muscles, the intercostal muscles, and the fascia to the splenius muscle. Both layers attach to the mastoid process of the head. A unilateral contraction will cause a scoliosis - a "banana-like" shape of the animal (Fig. 1.7A–C).

The Functional Line

Axial rotation of the body involves both of the helical lines: the Functional Line (FL) and the Spiral Line (SL) (Fig. 1.8).

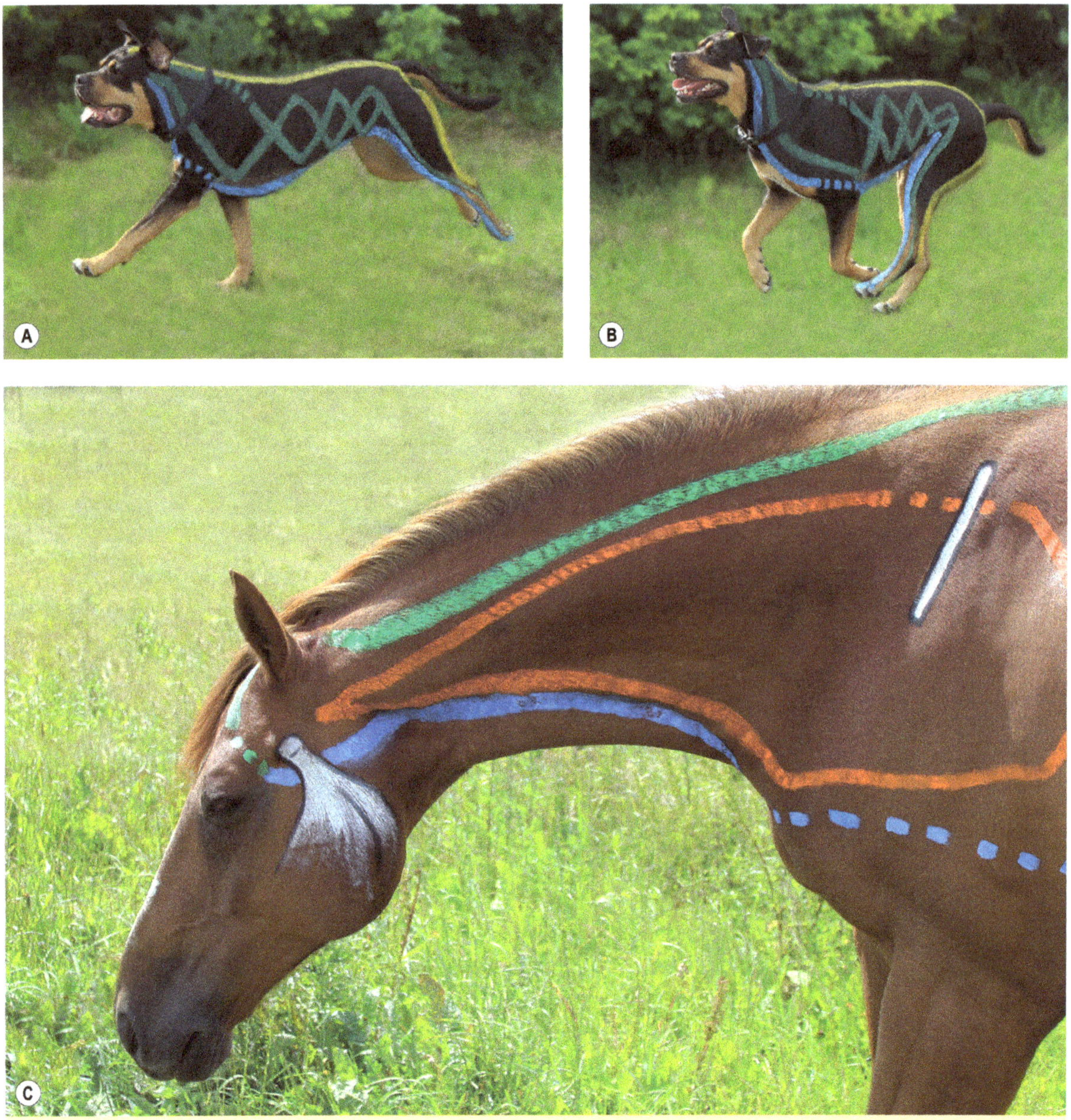

Figure 1.7
(A & B) The Superficial Dorsal Line (SDL, yellow), the Superficial Ventral Line (SVL, blue) and the Lateral Line (LL, green) are shown on a carnivore in motion. Dotted segments of the lines indicate they are running deep to the scapula. During canter a contraction of the SDL occurs in the first part of the locomotor cycle (A), and in the suspension phase the SVL contracts. The LL adjusts to the contraction of the SDL and SVL like an accordion (B). (C) This shows the SDL (green), the SVL (blue), and the LL (orange) outlined on the neck of a horse. The lines merge toward the head and surround and balance the temporomandibular joint.

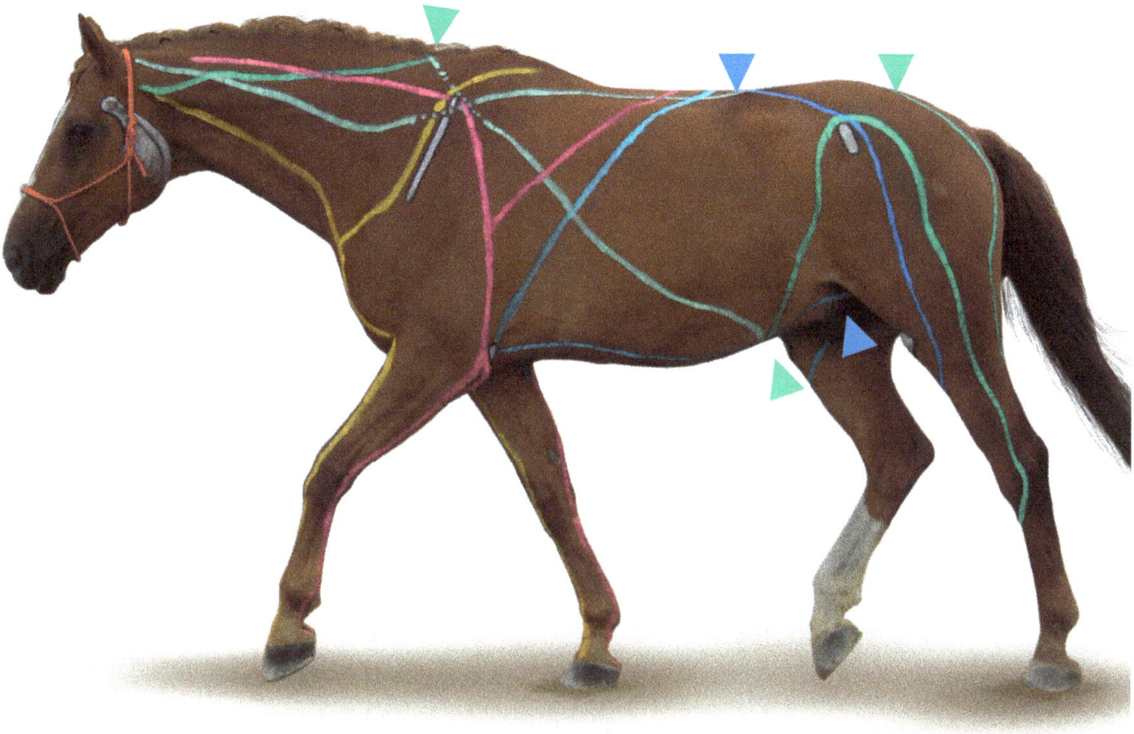

Figure 1.8
This shows the Functional Line (FL, blue and light blue), the Spiral Line (SL, green and light green), the Front Limb Protraction line (yellow), and the Front Limb Retraction Line (pink) outlined on a horse. Crossover points are marked with arrowheads. The Functional Line: the dorsal and the ventral parts of the FL start and end in the axillar region, cross over the midline (blue arrowheads), and meet on the contralateral hind limb, distal to the stifle. The Spiral Line: the spiral part and the straight part of the SL start and end at the head, but on opposite sides. The spiral part rotates around the trunk and crosses the midline twice (green arrowheads), turns around the tuber coxae, runs distally along the extensors of the hind limb to the medial side of the hock. Palmar and distal to the tuber calcis, the spiral part changes into the straight part of the line. This runs on the lateral side of the hock then passes into the deep part of the biceps muscle, running proximal to the sacral fascia (small white rectangle) and ligaments toward the lumbosacral fascia. There it crosses over the midline (green arrow head) before uniting with the SDL and running to the head.

The FL (Fig. 1.8) has a dorsal rotational part, which will also extend the back, and a ventral part balancing it with flexion. It crosses over the midline twice. It starts in the axillary region on the medial side of the humerus with the latissimus dorsi muscle, continues into the strong thoracolumbar fascia, and then crosses over the lumbar midline to the tuber coxae on the opposite side. It continues into the TFL and associated fascia lata to the lateral side of the crural fascia. Just below the patella, and distal to the tibial crest, it crosses over and returns medially into the gracilis muscle. At the ventral surface of the pubic bone, collagenous fibers cross over to the contralateral side, into the straight abdominal muscles and into the ascending pectoral muscle, which has a clear fascial connection to the latissimus dorsi muscle in the axillary region. The FL starts and ends on the same side. There is a right FL and a left FL, which balance each other from side to side.

The Spiral Line

The SL (Fig. 1.8) starts on one side of the head and ends on the contralateral side. It includes three midline crossover points and, as the name suggests, it spirals around the trunk in a three-dimensional pattern. It is the hardest line to follow and understand. The ventral part involves lateral bending of the neck and rotation of the trunk (most marked in flexion of the spine). This is counterbalanced by the dorsal part which involves extension of the spine and the opposite lateral flexion of the neck.

The line starts with the splenius muscle originating from the mastoid process, crossing under the nuchal ligament at the level of C6–T1 to the contralateral side (Fig. 1.8). It passes into the rhomboid muscle, under the scapula, and then into the serratus ventralis muscle. It continues on into the external abdominal oblique muscle and the white line under the abdomen, crossing the midline for the second time (Fig. 1.8), and passing into the internal abdominal oblique muscle which attaches to the tuber coxae. From here it follows the TFL into the peroneus tertius (in the horse) or the peroneus fibularis brevis (in the dog). It returns proximally via the biceps femoris to the sacrum, the dorsal sacral ligaments, and into the third midline crossing at the tuber sacrale region. From here it follows the same pathway as, and connects with, the SDL then into the erector spinae muscles, ending at the mastoid process on the opposite side from the origin. There are left and right SLs (determined by their starting point), which balance each other. The two helical lines may play a significant role in diagonal lameness.

The Front Limb Protraction Line

The Front Limb Protraction Line (FLPL) (Fig. 1.8) starts in the muscles pulling the dorsal part of the scapula in a caudal direction (thoracic part of the trapezius and rhomboid muscle) and the ventral part in a cranial direction (brachiocephalic muscle via its insertion on the humerus). The line continues into the biceps brachii muscle, the lacertus fibrosus, the digital extensor muscles and tendons, to the dorsal surface of the distal phalanges.

The Front Limb Retraction Line

The Front Limb Retraction Line (FLRL) (Fig. 1.8) starts in the muscles and fascia conducting the opposite rotation of the scapula to the protraction line. They cause the dorsal part of the scapula to rotate cranially (rhomboid and cervical trapezius muscles) and its ventral part to rotate caudally (latissimus dorsi muscle). It proceeds into the triceps brachii muscles and the digital flexor muscles and their tendons to the palmar surface of the distal phalanges.

These two lines (FLRL and FLPL) balance the front limb when standing and in motion. If there is an imbalance between them this will result in an abnormal position in protraction or retraction.

Understanding these fascial lines can be helpful in understanding the possible effects of an injury on the rest of the body. They can also lead to the origin of abnormal movement. It is unlikely that any one line can work on its own, rather they interact with other lines. Together they act as a three-dimensional network controlling the posture and locomotion of the whole body.

Treatment

Manual treatment of fascia is different from massage of muscles, as there are different neural receptors in the two tissues (Schleip et al. 2012a). Some of the manual human fascia release or stretch methods are quite painful and therefore not suitable or safe for use in animals. In the authors' (VE and RS) experience indirect functional techniques are very gentle and efficient for fascia treatment. Gentle vibrations from mechanical devices have also proved to be effective (Harrison et al. 2015a) as well as stretches, which work well as long as they are slow and within the patient's comfort zone. Tensions along the entire myofascial kinetic lines (as described) can be released. There are certain anatomical locations where lines overlap, and they become key areas for treatment. These areas include: the atlanto-occipital area (close to the mastoid process of the head); the thoracolumbar fascia; the tuber coxae area; and around the carpal and tarsal joints. Studies show that treating these areas is particularly effective (Harrison et al. 2015a). Certain acupuncture points for each line have also been investigated (Schultz et al., in press 2019).

Bioimpedance

Quantifying and validating the effect of fascial release and its in vivo effect need further investigation. Whether the effects are local or distant, immediate or delayed, or how long-standing they are, are all unknown. In the equine particularly we need to know if there is a "long-distance effect" caused by release of fascial lines as the result of a local treatment.

Although several methods have been used for in vivo measurements in humans (for example, tonometry, ultrasonography, and EMG), fascial release in animals is difficult to track. Anatomical challenges such as the fur, the thickness of the skin, the subcutaneous muscle layer, and the body posture all affect the precision and repeatability of the measurements.

Multifrequency bioimpedance analysis measurements (MF-BIA) have been used to quantify the effect of manual and mechanical fascia release in horses (Riis et al. 2013; Bartels et al. 2015; Elbrønd 2015). Measurements in specifically chosen regions were performed to improve the understanding of the kinetic lines and of the post-treatment reactions in the myofascial structures.

Bioimpedance measurement is a noninvasive and fast technique, which makes it very suitable for use in animals. It provides detailed information about intra- and extracellular physiological conditions in the tissue. The method has been accepted and validated for use in humans and during the last decade in domestic animals (dogs and horses). Even though detailed information is already available, the method probably still has more to offer (Riis et al. 2013; Bartels et al. 2015; Harrison et al. 2015b).

Taking an animal case history

In most cases the osteopath will have access to the case history taken by the animal's own vet. This, however, is often based on annual checkups and inoculations, routine surgical matters, and the prescription of medicines. When an animal has suffered an MSK injury, the vet, unless he or she has a special interest in such cases, is most likely to prescribe anti-inflammatory drugs and/or nerve block and recommend rest. The osteopath will therefore have to work with the vet to gain a more relevant in-depth osteopathic case history.

One of the toughest parts of this is that many animals have several owners. The family dog will be perceived by every member of that family to be "theirs." This is fine except that the practitioner will often hear several versions of a story from them, and deciding what is important is not always easy. A classic response is spouses disagreeing on which leg is the affected one.

If the animal is a horse then there will often be an owner, a trainer, and a rider that all have their own ideas as to what the problem is, or isn't! The practitioner will often be told several differing accounts as to how the horse ended up this way.

With wildlife the case history is usually much shorter, and there are not any actual owners, although there may be important interested parties involved. Never skimp on history taking.

Certain endangered wildlife species require individual licenses to be granted before anyone can attempt treatment, and in these cases the professionals involved are then accountable to the body issuing the license, along with any medicolegal implications that this may include.

Recording the case history

The written case history is arguably the most important aspect of a consultation, with the information obtained crucial to the success of the treatment. Aside from the legal requirements of taking an accurate case history, it is a key part of the osteopathic diagnosis, aligning the principles of osteopathy with striving to determine the etiology or underlying cause of a dysfunction.

Sometimes the etiology can be found in the case history, with owners, handlers and riders providing crucial information that provides the missing piece of the diagnostic puzzle. As with any medical case history, sufficient detail allows the practitioner to differentiate between musculoskeletal dysfunction and pathology, allowing them to recognize their limitations within the appropriate scope of practice. The case history also assists with communicating with other health care practitioners and professionals involved in the care of the animal, such as its veterinary surgeon or farrier.

Although the next sections suggest a case history format, each practitioner should add or modify the questions so that they relate to the individual animal, the type of work or activity required of them, and any pathology present. The following is a suggested format.

1. Identification

The following points should be noted:

- The personal details of the animal's owner, including their address.
- The details of the animal, including the species, name, age, breed, sex, color, or identifiers, and the work or activity desired of the animal.
- Details of the veterinary surgeon, the date of the last consultation, and the nature of the consultation.

2. Case history

A small area for a vet's report on the case history form is a good way to have a clear snapshot of the current health of the animal being treated. This can be similar to a "medical alert" area of a human medical record. There are certain regulations across different countries regarding veterinary permission for the treatment of animals, which makes this section important in certain territories. It is very important to open the lines of communication with the animal's veterinarian to help determine whether there are any details relevant to the case that you need to be aware of before the consultation. This also allows efficient referrals back to the veterinarian if there is a need for further investigation.

In the case of an equine patient it is very important to obtain details of current or proposed work, whether at a racing stable, a showjumping yard, or at a stable that has various disciplines. It is always necessary to clarify what type of work is expected, and the level desired, as this may influence the examination, prognosis, and treatment plan. As an example, an event horse that is required to perform consistently at a very high level may need frequent treatment if it is to be maintained in peak musculoskeletal health, whereas a trail-riding horse may not have the same physical demands placed on it and may only need to be assessed and treated once or twice a year. The animal's daily routine may help determine etiological factors predisposing it to dysfunction and this can guide examination and treatment to the appropriate areas.

This same information should be obtained for the canine patient, whether they are a working dog, racing greyhound, perform agility, are a show dog or the family pet.

3. Clinical signs

Once all of the identifying information has been obtained and documented, the next section of the case history should establish the presenting complaint and current symptoms. This information is absolutely crucial to the success of the examination that follows. The most helpful advice the author (BA) received when considering the symptoms was not just to have a quick checklist of questions but to be very proactive and listen carefully to what the owner, rider, farmer, or groom is describing, in the same way that a practitioner treating a child listens intently to a child's mother before treatment. The connection between rider or owner and the animal is significant and needs to be respected. This innate dialogue, with its subtle yet palpable connection between the two, can often make all the difference clinically.

As a guide, the onset of the clinical symptoms provides an insight into the chronicity of the complaint, giving the practitioner both an expectation for the prognosis and a prediction for the tissue texture underpinning the presenting symptoms. This information is used to help evaluation, comparing what has been said, with the findings of the clinical examination. For instance, if palpation suggests a chronic situation (having the feel of a dehydrated, rope-like or chronically shortened or overstressed tissue) and the onset is reported to be very recent, the two pictures are contradictory. This contrast can be explained to the owner, and further questions may allow an altered diagnosis and a more realistic prognosis to be made. It may also help identify the underlying pathology in cases where the symptomatic picture and palpatory findings are mismatched.

The time of day, daily patterns, and activity levels are also important, allowing for a line of questioning aimed at determining when the complaint is exacerbated. Is it worse in the morning, during the night, or after a day's work? Is it noticeable during the first few steps or does it develop gradually with exercise or during high intensity exercise?

These questions can help to differentiate between an acute or chronic injury, ongoing chronic pathology, or an acute or chronic life-threatening pathology. The following are examples of some typical clinical scenarios:

- A stiffness caused by arthritic change is most often worse in the morning or following inactivity.
- A ligamentous injury is usually more noticeable on a softer surface during higher intensity exercise, as it stresses the checking and bracing capabilities of the joint.
- Dysfunction of the joint surface or capsule may be exacerbated on harder ground, with soft ground surfaces providing a dampening of concussive force.
- A more serious pathological condition may not fit a pattern at all. It may be constant or the symptomatology may come and go and may be unrelated to particular times of day or activities.
- It is important to consider the general health and alertness of the animal in order to rule out systemic conditions, such as an infection which has the potential to manifest as a musculoskeletal problem. A broad series of questions that investigate respiratory fatigue, muscular fatigue, and the animal being "not quite themselves" are all useful indicators for referral.
- Cancerous pathology may cause increased pain during the night, which may be missed in horse or cattle patients, but may be very relevant in a canine patient that lives inside and appears to be unsettled at night.

All of these examples are just a guide and not a specific rule. It is important to use informed clinical judgment and delve further with questioning and examinations to qualify your diagnostic thinking process.

The progression of symptoms is another important factor when considering to what degree the current discomfort is affecting the animal. Has the complaint worsened, fluctuated, improved, or plateaued since the initial onset? Which factors contributed to this change or lack of change, if any? This information will be useful in screening for pathology, raising a high index of suspicion if the complaint is rapidly progressing or is nonresponsive to treatment. If we look at the performance horse, the progression and timing of symptoms can help when formulating a treatment plan. Does the complaint reoccur shortly after the horse is brought back into heavy work following being turned out for a period of time? In this situation, a consultation may be best scheduled as a preseason checkup to ensure the horse is in peak physical shape in order to cope with the sudden increase in workload most effectively.

Further questioning may cover the differences between ridden versus unridden, as the weight of the rider, the skill of the rider, and the tack can make a significant difference and becomes another variable for the osteopath to consider. Useful questions that can be addressed to a rider of any skill level are whether the horse responds to the rider's leg, whether the horse is willing to move forward when asked, whether the horse feels soft and will yield for the rider, and whether the horse provides resistance on one rein or the other. This provides the practitioner with an immediate impression of how supple the horse is in motion and where potential resistance lies, which will be evaluated in the examination that follows. Obviously more specific questions would be asked of a horse and rider at a much higher level.

Additional details that are critical for the complete case history are the details of any current treatment by any health professionals involved in the animal's ongoing care. This includes current veterinary care and, if applicable, the work of the farrier, dental technician, saddle fitter, as well as any other manual therapy.

While the above paragraphs relate more to the examination of domesticated animals, the same basic principles can be applied to most species that may be treated.

Questions specific to horse cases

There are some further questions directed specifically to the care of the equine athlete:

- Information gained from the farrier will include the date of the last shoeing or trim and if the horse has ever had any remedial work (i.e. when the farrier shapes the foot to take pressure off a particular area, such as the heel). The farrier's work is heavily intertwined with osteopathic management, as the changes made on feet can have an enormous impact on biomechanics and limb function. If we take the example of the horse being low in the heel in the hind limbs, the limb will be placed with the foot further forwards, the fetlock, hock, and stifle will straighten, and the load on the deep digital flexor (DDF) tendon will be greater, predisposing the horse to tendon injuries and inclination of the pelvis. This will then have a flow-on effect to the rest of the body. In situations such as this, if the etiology of the dysfunction is from the foot, with resultant changes in biomechanics, remedial shoeing or trimming should be part of the osteopathic plan, and collaboration with the farrier is essential.
- The case history should also include details of dental treatment, including when the last checkup was performed, and any issues that were raised at the time. The health of the teeth affects not only the overall general health and oral health of the animal, but also grazing, chewing, and TMJ function. With the ligamentous and connective tissue connections to the cervical spine, a painful mouth or malocclusion can lead to dysfunction at the cranial aspect of the cervical spine, with the OA and AA articulations most often affected. This can result in the rider feeling resistance to the horse coming onto the bit, and reluctance to form a correct posture, with some owners, riders, and trainers reporting that the horse frequently throws or tosses its head.
- Details of the saddle, the last fitting, and the feel for the rider can be documented, as the seat for the rider is crucial to the soundness of the horse.

Questions specific to avian cases

In relation to birds, further questions might be:

- If captive, then did the owner breed the bird? If not, at what age did the owner purchase it?
- Have there been any problems when molting?
- Is the bird allowed any flight time?

Questions specific to past medical conditions

- The past medical history should pay particular attention to accidents or trauma, as such incidents may be relevant when determining etiology and can potentially leave a memory in the tissues, which may be harnessed in the treatment process.
- Current or previous illnesses and details of any surgical procedures need to be included in the case history. Depending on the condition or surgery reported, this may indicate etiology or may highlight a contraindication to the use of certain techniques.
- A further general health profile can be investigated by asking questions relating to the major systems:
  - For the gastrointestinal screen: has there been vomiting, constipation, or diarrhea recently? Is the animal off its food?
  - For the respiratory and cardiovascular screen: are there signs of unexpected fatigue? Is there shortness of breath? Have there been any episodes of bleeding?
  - For the genitourinary system: are there signs of discomfort with urination or changes in urine color?

- The systemic questioning can also be reinforced by the practitioner's observation of general health, vitality, and the color of the mucous membranes.
- The animal's current list of medications is a crucial part of the case history. It is also important to have a grasp on the main indications and side effects of the most common medications prescribed for an animal.

4. Clinical examination

Once all of the elements of the case history have been obtained from the owner, the examination findings must be recorded. The author (BA) finds it easiest to adapt a common template and tailor it to each species of animal that he regularly examines and treats. The main sections of the examination that are present for every animal are the dynamic and passive motion assessment sections, as most practitioners will request to see the animal in motion or the bird in flight, and every osteopath will perform a hands-on examination of function. Details of the content suggested for the dynamic and passive (palpatory) examination are explored in each chapter of this book and will vary according to the animal or bird being treated.

Depending on the animal being evaluated, additional sections will differ - the equine case history requires a section on the short turn and the backing maneuver. For the canine patient, a section on the symmetry and ease of the "sit" is a useful addition to the case history.

5. Osteopathic assessment

Following on from the evaluation section, an osteopathic assessment will be made. This is not to be confused with a veterinary diagnosis of pathology or musculoskeletal injury. The veterinary and osteopathic findings may be very similar, with the osteopathic assessment detailing more tissue-specific palpatory findings to assist with osteopathic treatment and management. This diagnostic snapshot of the functioning of the animal provides a quick reference for follow-up appointments.

6. Treatment

A treatment section follows this working diagnosis, with all treatment techniques documented in sufficient detail so that they can be understood by other osteopaths or professionals involved in the care of the animal.

It is often helpful to have schematic diagrams of the animal being examined and treated on the case history sheet. This can serve to provide a visual representation for the osteopathic findings and distribution of the dysfunction (such as muscle tightness or areas of tenderness on palpation). Accuracy in this pictorial view of the animal produces another facet for data collection and can also be used in a number of other ways, including as a quick reference guide for the treatment provided.

7. Aftercare

The final aspect to the clinical case history is the aftercare or advice section. This may include stretches, general advice on activity levels following treatment, rehabilitation advice, or exercises. This section will also detail any referral made. Aftercare can also include a treatment plan and/or suggested times for follow-up treatment. Short- and long-term prognoses are also helpful to inform the client, but also to remind the practitioner, serving as a reference for the progression of the presenting complaint. Should the treatment not be as effective as initially expected, further investigations or referral can be sought.

References

Bartels EM, Sørensen ER, Harrison AP (2015) Multi-frequency bioimpedance in human muscle assessment. Physiological Reports. April; 3 (4) e12354.

Colles CM (2005) The use of thermography as a diagnostic tool in assessing musculoskeletal problems in the Asian Elephant, and as a gauge to the effectiveness of osteopathic treatment of such structures, Twycross Zoo. Proceedings of the Seventh Annual Symposium on Zoo Research. BIAZA, Twycross Zoo, Warwickshire, England, p. 67.

Colles CM, Hola G, Pusey A (1994) Thermal imaging as an aid to the diagnosis of back pain in the horse. Proceedings of the 6th European Congress of Thermology, Bath, pp. 164–167.

Colles CM, Nevin A, Brooks J (2014) The osteopathic treatment of somatic dysfunction causing gait abnormality in 51 horses. Equine Veterinary Education. March; 26 (3) 148–155.

Colles CM, Nevin A (2015) unpublished clinical data from 4,000 horses scanned using IRTI.

Colles CM, Nevin T, Coley R, Ray J (2004) Assessing musculoskeletal problems and treatment using osteopathy in a captive Asian Elephant. Proceedings of the Sixth Annual Symposium on Zoo Research. BIAZA, Edinburgh Zoo, Edinburgh, Scotland, pp. 245–246.

Dyce K, Sack W, Wensing C (2009) Textbook of Veterinary Anatomy. 4th edn. Saunders Elsevier.

Elbrønd VS (2015) Myofascial kinetic lines in horses: structure and function: A veterinary aspect. Proceedings of the 2nd EVSO Congress in Veterinary Osteopathy. Berlin, Germany.

Elbrønd VS, Schultz RM (2013) Impact of fascia on performance and general health condition. In: Lindner A (ed.) Applied Equine Nutrition and Training. ENUTRACO 2013, Wageningen Academic Publishers. Available:

https://www.wageningenacademic.com/doi/book/10.3920/978-90-8686-793-6 [April 19, 2019].

Elbrønd VS, Schultz RM (2014) Myofascial kinetic lines in horses. Equine Veterinary Journal. June; 46 (S46) 40.

Elbrønd VS, Schultz RM (2015) Myofascia - the unexplored tissue: myofascial kinetic lines in horses, a model for describing locomotion using comparative dissection studies derived from human lines. Medical Research Archives. May; 3. ISSN 2375-1924. Available at: https://journals.ke-i.org/index.php/mra/article/view/125 [April 19, 2019].

First International Congress of Osteopathy in Animal Practice (2012) Proceedings available: http://www.congressodiosteopatia.it/congresso_osteopatia_veterinaria/eng/index.html [April 18, 2019].

GOsC (General Osteopathic Council) (2019) Osteopaths Act UK 1993. Available: https://www.osteopathy.org.uk/about-us/legislation/ [April 19, 2019].

Guimberteau J-C, Armstrong C (2015) Architecture of Human Living Fascia. The Extracellular Matrix and Cells revealed through Endoscopy. Edinburgh, Scotland: Handspring Publishing.

Harrison AP, Elbrønd VS, Krasnodebska MJ (2015a) Multi-frequency bioimpedance and myofascial release therapy: an equine "AtlasOrange1" validation study. Medical Research Archives. May 2015; no. 3. ISSN 2375-1924. Available: https://journals.ke-i.org/index.php/mra/article/view/124 [April 29, 2019].

Harrison AP, Elbrønd VS, Riis-Olesen K, Bartels EM (2015b) Multi-frequency bioimpedance in equine muscle assessment. Physiological Measurements. March; 36 (3) 453–464.

Holst G C (2000) Common Sense Approach to Thermal Imaging. SPIE Press and JCD Publishing.

Myers T (2009) Anatomy Trains: Myofascial Meridians for Manual and Movement Therapists, 2nd edn. Churchill Livingstone Elsevier.

Nevin T (1997) The osteopathic treatment of British Wildlife casualties to aid rehabilitation. Proceedings of the Wildaid Symposium, Inverness, Scotland.

Nevin A (1998) Osteopathy on wild birds. Proceedings of the Symposium of the British Wildlife Rehabilitation Council, Cheshire.

Nevin T (2005) Using osteopathy to treat musculoskeletal problems in 2 Burmese elephants. Proceedings of the Seventh Annual Symposium on Zoo Research. BIAZA, Twycross Zoo, Warwickshire, England, pp. 68–69.

Nevin T (2012) Osteopathy and exotics – thinking outside of the box; Osteopathy and birds – a global approach; Using infrared thermal imaging to assess osteopathic treatment of 2 Asian elephants. Proceedings of the First International Congress of Osteopathy in Animal Practice, Rome.

Nevin T (2013) Unpublished clinical data from IRTI scans still currently being collected from cases the author has seen at Vale Wildlife Hospital and in UK zoos and safari parks.

Nevin T (2017) Osteopathy as a method of species conservation: zoological osteopathic medicine cases. Proceedings of the VI Fauna International Conference, Lisbon.

Pedersen RW (2013) Verification of the myofascial chains in the canine. Master's thesis. Department of Veterinary and Animal Sciences, University of Copenhagen.

Pusey A, Brooks J, Jenks A (2010) Osteopathy and the Treatment of Horses. Wiley-Blackwell.

RCVS (Royal College of Veterinary Surgeons) (2018) RCVS Code of Professional Conduct for Veterinary Surgeons and supporting guidance. Sections 19.19–19.21. Available: https://www.rcvs.org.uk/setting-standards/advice-and-guidance/code-of-professional-conduct-for-veterinary-surgeons/ [April 18, 2019].

Richter P, Hebgen E (2009) Models of myofascial chains. In: Trigger Points and Muscle Chains in Osteopathy. Stuttgart, Germany: Georg Thieme Verlag, pp.10–26.

Riis KH, Harrison AP, Riis-Olesen K (2013) Non-invasive assessment of equine muscular function: a case study. Open Veterinary Journal. July; 3 (2) 80–84.

Ros K (2011) Zusammenhang zwischen Kiefergelenke-mechanik und Ganzkörperstatik. In: Vogt C (ed.) Lehrbuch der Zahnheilkunde beim Pferd. 1st edn. Stuttgart, Deutschland: Schattauer GmbH, pp. 35–39.

Schleip R, Findley TW, Chaitow L, Huijing PA (2012a) Fascia: The tensional Network of the Human Body. Churchill Livingstone Elsevier.

Schleip R, Jäger H, Klingler W, (2012b) What is 'fascia'? A review of different nomenclatures. Journal of Bodywork and Movement Therapies. October; 16 (4) 496–502.

Schultz RM, Elbrønd VS (2013) Can myofascial kinetic lines be an anatomical foundation for acupuncture meridians? Proceedings of the AAVA/IVAS Joint Conference on Veterinary Acupuncture 2013, New Orleans, Louisiana, USA.

Schultz RM, Elbrønd VS (2014) Can myofascial kinetic lines be an anatomical foundation for acupuncture meridians? Proceedings of the 40th Annual IVAS and 15th Annual ItVAS International Congress on Veterinary Acupuncture 2014, Florence, Italy.

Schultz RM, Elbrønd VS, Due T (in press 2019) Myofascial Kinetic Lines in Dogs and Horses: Anatomy, Function and Treatment.

Slijper EJ (1946) Comparative Biologic-Anatomical Investigations on the Vertebral Column and Spinal Musculature of Mammals. Amsterdam: N.V. Noord-Hollandche Uitdervers Maatschappij, pp. 1–128.

Stahn A, Strobel G, Terblanche E (2008) VO2max prediction from multi-frequency bioelectrical impedance analysis. Physiological Measurements. February; 29 (2) 193–203.

Stecco C (2015) Functional Atlas of the Human Fascial System. Churchill Livingstone Elsevier.

Stecco C, Macchi V, Porzionato A, Duparc F, De Caro R, (2011) The fascia: the forgotten structure. Italian Journal of Anatomy and Embryology. 116 (3) 127–138.

Thompson EE (1996) Anatomy of Animals: Studies in the Forms of Mammals and Birds. Random House UK Ltd. (Bracken Books).

Vollmer M, Möllmann K-P (2013) Infrared Thermal Imaging: Fundamentals, Research and Applications. Chapter 10. Wiley-VCH Verlag GmbH and Co.

Appendix A Known zoonoses

Condition	Agent	Agent type	Animal host or reservoir	Usual mode of transmission to humans	Symptoms in humans
Animal influenzas, including swine and bird flu.	Various influenza viruses	Virus	Livestock, particularly pigs and poultry, humans	Direct contact, aerosols and ingestion. Influenza viruses are highly contagious	Symptoms are similar to human influenza but can be serious and potentially cause pandemics in the human population
Anthrax	Bacillus anthracis	Bacterium	Livestock and wild animals	Contact with infected animals or animal products	Cutaneous and respiratory forms occur. All types have the potential to spread and cause death if untreated. It is often seen as sudden death in animals
Bovine tuberculosis (bTB)	Mycobacterium bovis	Bacterium	Cattle, badgers, deer, opossum, and others	Mainly by ingestion (milk), but can also be by inhalation or wounds in the skin	Similar to human TB, including weight loss, fever, night sweats, and a persistent cough
Brucellosis (undulant fever)	Brucella spp.	Bacterium	Cattle, goats, sheep, pigs, dogs, and occasionally other species	Unpasteurized dairy products in cattle and goats. Direct contact with infected animals	Fever, sweating, and muscle and joint pain
Campylobacteriosis	Campylobacter spp.	Bacterium	Poultry and most animals	Fecal contamination, raw and undercooked meat and poultry, unpasteurized milk	Gastrointestinal symptoms
Cat-scratch fever	Bartonella henselae	Bacterium	Cats	Bites and scratches	Regional lymphadenopathy. There may be transient fever. It may cause malaise, headache, and muscle pain
Cysticercosis	Larval forms of Taenia solium	Internal parasite (tapeworm)	Pigs and occasionally cattle	Ingestion of uncooked infected pork or contaminated food and water in endemic areas	Cysts form in the body tissues including the brain. It can lead to epileptic seizures
Cryptosporidiosis	Cryptosporidium spp.	Protozoan parasite	Cattle, sheep, goats, iguanas, geckos, lizards, tortoises, and snakes	Usually a waterborne disease but occasionally transmitted by feces or ingestion of uncooked meats	Watery diarrhea. It is a serious disease in immunocompromised individuals
Ebola, Crimean–Congo hemorrhagic fever (CCHF), Lassa and Marburg viruses	Ebolavirus group	Virus	Rodents, ticks, livestock, primates, and bats	Direct contact, inoculation, or tick bites. It is extremely contagious	Incubation is 2–5 days. Fever, sore throat, muscle pain, vomiting, and diarrhea. Liver and kidney failure. Hemorrhagic diseases require extensive hospital supportive therapy
Enzootic abortion	Chlamydophila abortus	Bacterium	Sheep	Direct contact or aerosols	Abortion storms in sheep. It can cause abortion in pregnant women. Pregnant women are advised to avoid contact with lambing sheep

Appendix A *continued*

Condition	Agent	Agent type	Animal host or reservoir	Usual mode of transmission to humans	Symptoms in humans
Erysipeloid	Erysipelothrix rhusiopathiae	Bacterium	Fish, mammals, shellfish, and the environment	Direct contact, especially from handling infected fish or raw meat	Local indolent cellulitis
Fish tank granuloma	Mycobacterium marinum	Bacterium	Fish	Direct contact or infected water	Skin lesions about three weeks after contact
Fleas	Various species of flea	Insect	Cats, dogs, small furries, and small wildlife	Direct contact – they can hop several centimeters. In the immature stages they live in the environment	Principally local irritation but fleas can spread other diseases and are famous for spreading bubonic plague. They can also spread catscratch fever
Giardiasis	Giardia lamblia	Protozoan parasite	Humans and wildlife	Waterborne or direct contact	Gastroenteritis and abdominal pain. Irritable bowel syndrome
Glanders	Burkholderia mallei	Bacterium	Equids and occasionally dogs, cats, and goats	Direct contact via skin abrasions	Nodular lesions and ulceration in the lungs. It has been eradicated in most of Europe, Australia, and the Northern United States
Hemorrhagic colitis	E. coli (Escherichia coli)	Bacterium	Mammals	Direct contact or foodborne	Painful, hemorrhagic diarrhea
Hantavirus syndromes	Hantaviridae	Virus	Rodents	Aerosols	Hemorrhagic fever with renal and hepatic symptoms. The virus is fatal in humans
Histoplasmosis	Histoplasma capsulatum	Fungus	Birds and bats	Mainly aerosols from droppings	Symptoms are similar to pneumonia and may develop to weight loss, fatigue, and ocular symptoms. It is mostly found in North America and Central America
Hydatidosis	Echinococcus granulosus (larval form)	Internal parasite (tapeworm)	Dogs act as primary hosts and sheep act as intermediate hosts	Ingestion of eggs excreted by dogs	Humans are occasional aberrant hosts of the intermediate (cystic) form. Cysts may form in any tissues, with various symptoms
Leptospirosis	Leptospira spp.	Bacterium	Rodents	Infected urine or contaminated water	High fever and jaundice
Lice	Various species	External parasite (insect)	All mammals	Direct (close) contact	Lice are generally host-specific and cannot live long on alternative hosts. They cause local irritation and can transmit disease
Listeriosis	Listeria spp.	Bacterium	Cattle, sheep, or soil	Contaminated food products, direct contact especially in immunosuppressed individuals and pregnant women	Gastroenteritis, meningitis, and meningoencephalitis. It can cause abortion

Appendix A *continued*

Condition	Agent	Agent type	Animal host or reservoir	Usual mode of transmission to humans	Symptoms in humans
Louping ill	Louping ill virus	Virus	Sheep and grouse	Direct contact or tick bites	Flu-like symptoms and encephalomyelitis
Louse flies	Hippoboscidae	External parasite (insect)	Mammals and birds	Direct contact	Biting "flies." It is a self-limiting infestation
Lyme disease	Borrelia spp.	Bacterium	Ticks, rodents, sheep, deer, and small mammals	Tick bites	Skin erythema, facial paralysis, arthritis, and meningitis
Lymphocytic choriomeningitis	Arenaviridae	Virus	Rodents	Direct contact	Aseptic meningitis, encephalitis, and meningoencephalitis
Mange	Demodex spp. live in hair follicles; Sarcoptes burrow into skin	External parasite (mites)	Most mammals	Direct contact	Irritating crusty skin lesions
Orf	Parapoxvirus	Virus	Sheep and goats	Direct contact	Pustular dermatitis of the hand, arm, and face. It is usually self-limiting in seven to 10 weeks
Pasteurellosis	Pasteurella spp.	Bacterium	Cats and dogs, but also cattle, sheep, rabbits, other mammals, and chickens	Bite, scratch, and direct contact	Usually pneumonia. It can cause arthritis, meningitis, and acute endocarditis
Plague	Yersinia pestis	Bacterium	Black rats and their fleas	Flea bite	Fever, headache, and respiratory signs. Swollen lymph nodes and death
Psittacosis	Chlamydia psittaci	Bacterium	Birds, poultry, and ducks	Aerosols and direct contact	Five to 19 days' incubation. Mild respiratory signs to severe pneumonia. Joint pain, diarrhea, and conjunctivitis
Q fever	Coxiella burnetii	Bacterium	Cattle, sheep, goats, cats, and dogs	Aerosols, direct contact, milk, and fomites. Abortion tissues and fluids	Incubation is nine to 40 days. Sudden fever, flu-like symptoms, headache, malaise, joint pain, nausea, and vomiting. It can cause abortion in pregnant women
Rabies	Lyssavirus spp.	Virus	All warm-blooded animals including birds and bats	Bite, saliva, and contamination of wounds and mucous membranes	Initial tingling sensation at the site of infection followed by excitement, violent uncontrolled movements, fear of water, and confusion. It is always fatal in humans. Vaccination as soon as possible post contact is essential
Rat bite fever (Haverhill fever)	Spirillum minus, or Streptobacillus moniliformis	Bacterium	Rats	Bite, scratch, milk, and water	Red or purple rash around the injury. Chills, fever, vomiting headache, and back pain

Appendix A *continued*

Condition	Agent	Agent type	Animal host or reservoir	Usual mode of transmission to humans	Symptoms in humans
Rift Valley fever	Phlebovirus	Virus	Cattle, goats, and sheep	Direct contact, mosquito bite	It may be mild or severe. Fever, muscle pain, and headache. Loss of sight, confusion, liver disease, and bleeding
Ringworm (dermatophytosis)	Trichophyton spp. or Microsporum spp.	Fungus	Cats, dogs, cattle, horses, hedgehogs, and other animals	Direct contact	Red, itchy, scaly, circular skin rash. Local hair loss. The rash is usually around the wrist or abdomen
Salmonellosis	Salmonella spp.	Bacterium	Poultry, cattle, pigs, sheep, and terrapins	Feces, contaminated food products, and direct contact	It varies from acute severe gastrointestinal symptoms to septicemia (paratyphoid fever)
Streptoccal sepsis	Streptococcus spp.	Bacterium	Pigs, horses, and many other species	Direct contact and meat	Fever, respiratory and cardiovascular signs, and septicemia. Transmission is rare but can be rapidly fatal
Ticks	Arachnida suborder Acarina	External parasite	Sheep, deer, small wildlife, cats, dogs, and birds	Usually infested from environment	Local irritation. It may transmit diseases such as Lyme disease
Tickborne encephalitis	Flavivirus	Virus	Rodents, small mammals, dogs, ruminants	Tick bite and unpasteurized milk products	Flu-like symptoms, encephalitis, and meningitis. Mortality in 1–2 percent of cases. No specific treatment
Toxocariasis	Toxocara spp.	Internal parasite (nematode)	Dogs, cats, and foxes	Fecal contamination, including dried fecal particles in the coat	It may be asymptomatic infection by immature larvae. Or there may be coughing, fever, abdominal pain, hepatomegaly, lymphadenitis, or ocular lesions, which can be confused with retinoblastosis, particularly in children
Toxoplasmosis	Toxoplasma gondii	Internal protozoan parasite	Cats, ruminants, other mammals, and birds	Ingestion of fecal oocysts (cats) and uncooked meat	Generally asymptomatic. It may cause retinochoroiditis, lymphadenitis, or myocarditis. It can cause abortion in pregant women
Trichinellosis	Trichinella spirosis	Internal parasite (nematode)	Pigs, wild boar	Pork products	Asymptomatic. Or it may cause nausea, heartburn, diarrhea. Edema, periorbital edema, or vasculitis
Tularemia (rabbit fever)	Francisella tularensis	Bacterium	Rabbits, wild animals, the environment, and ticks	Ticks, deer flies, direct contact, aerosols, and inoculation	Incubation is three to 14 days. Fever, lethargy, loss of appetite, reddening of skin, and enlarged or suppurative lymph nodes sepsis. It can be fatal
West Nile fever	Flavivirus	Virus	Wild birds, mosquitoes, and horses	Mosquito bite	Usually asymptomatic. It may cause flu-like symptoms. It is generally self-limiting
Zoonotic diphtheria	Corynebacterium ulcerans	Bacterium	Cattle, livestock, and dogs	Direct contact and milk	Cutaneous diphtheria. It may cause respiratory symptoms

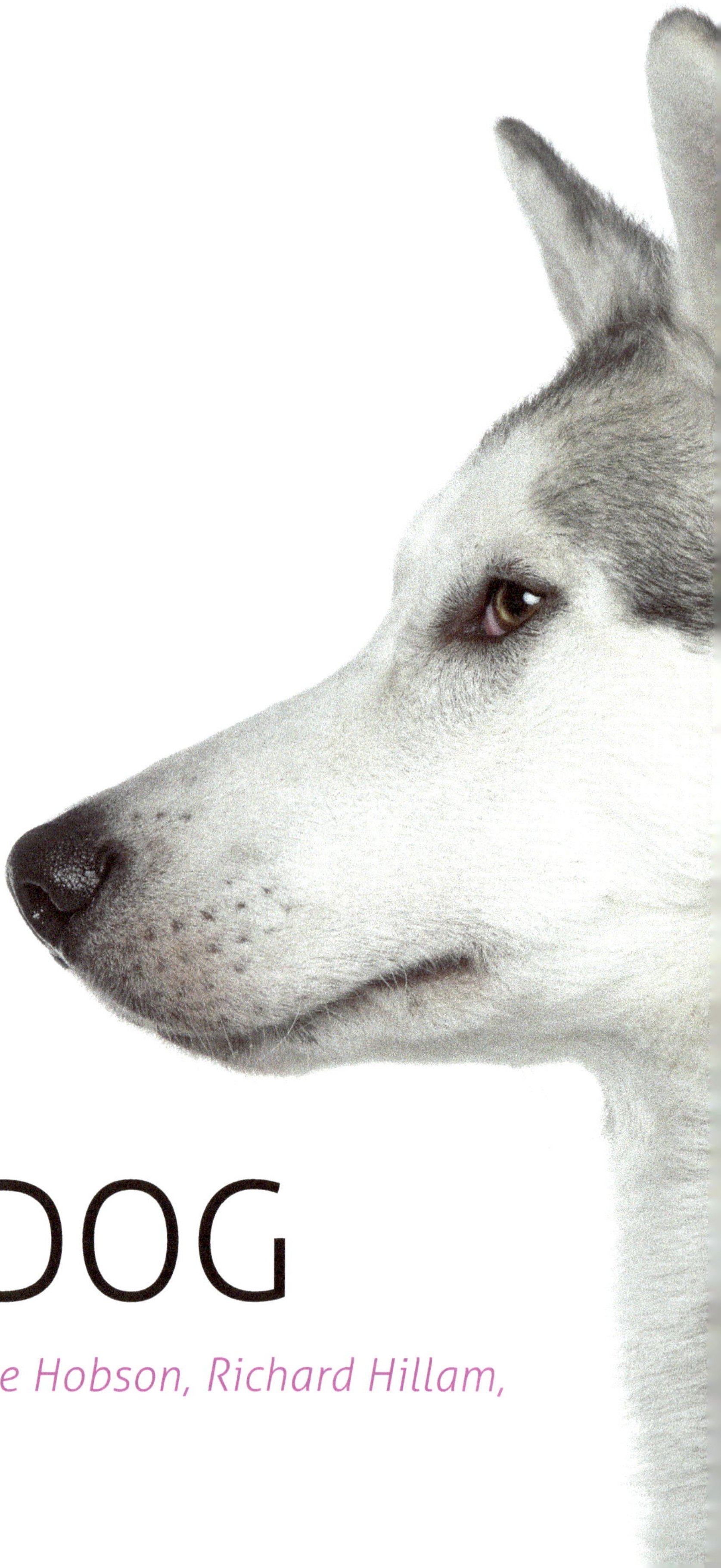

Chapter 2
THE DOG

Tony Nevin, Nadine Hobson, Richard Hillam, Paolo Tozzi

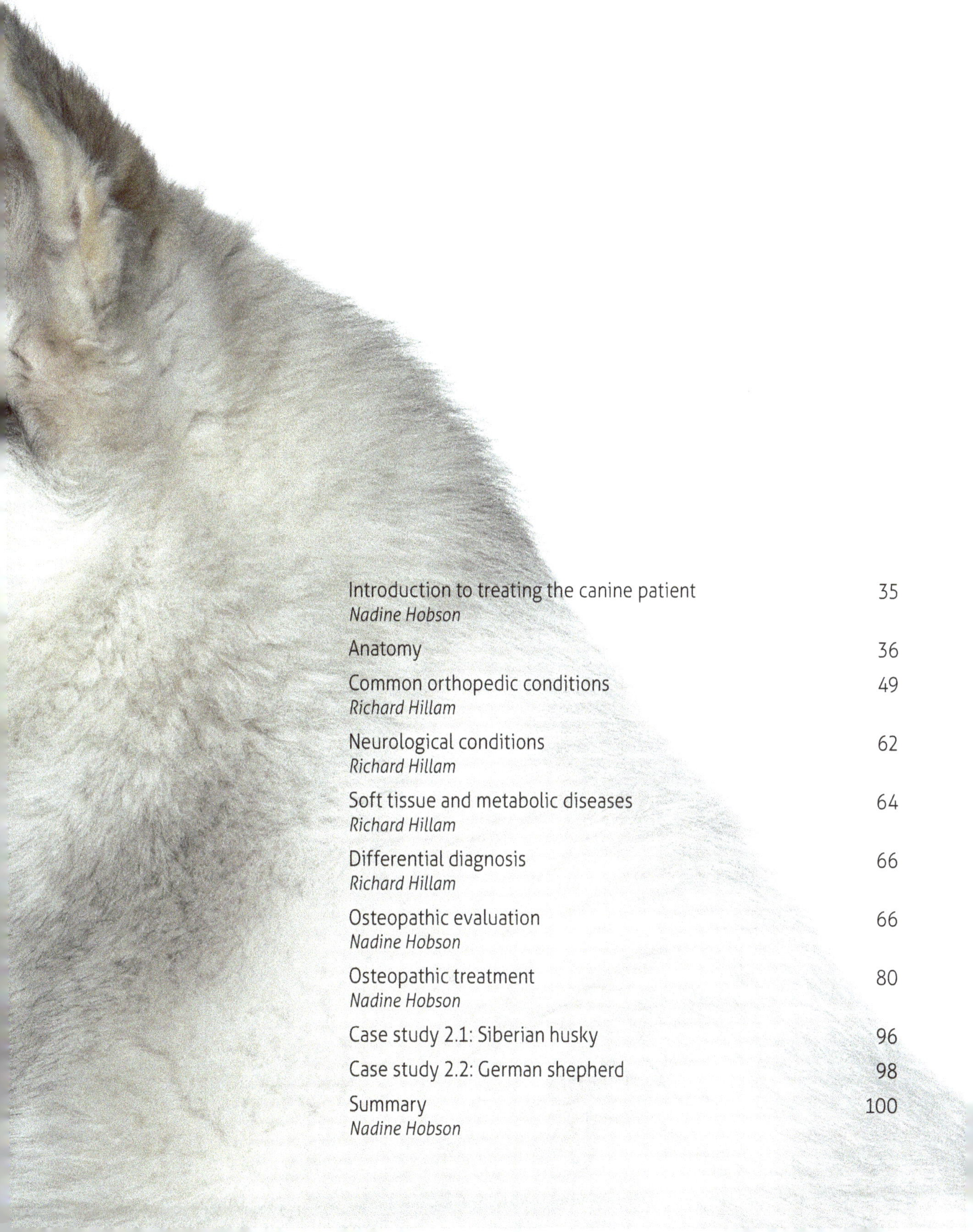

The dog

Chapter 2

Introduction to treating the canine patient

This chapter addresses how the authors work within a system of integrated animal health care rather than providing instructions on how to carry out specific techniques.

The osteopath's ability to differentiate by palpation between tissues subject to inflammatory disease, allergic reaction, the toxicity of renal failure, or hormonal imbalance, to name a few, is an invaluable tool in clinical evaluation. Palpatory findings, in the absence of overt clinical signs, often indicate which veterinary tests may be required to diagnose underlying systemic disease that may coexist with musculoskeletal conditions. In situations where medical tests are inconclusive, an osteopathic opinion offers a different way of looking at a case.

Treatment is case specific and not prescriptive, as are the techniques employed, varying as much with the patient as with the practitioner. Due to the variation in morphology of our canine patients we must apply our osteopathic knowledge and be inventive with our techniques to aid a return to normality.

The majority of referrals are for musculoskeletal (MSK) problems but some other complaints appear to improve after osteopathic treatment. Owners and vets have reported improvements in apparently unrelated conditions due to somatic-visceral interactions. One example of this is the easing of impacted anal gland symptoms after osteopathic treatment for lumbosacral (LS) and sacral or coccygeal problems. This treatment seemed to influence the visceral and somatic pathways and autonomic mechanisms.

Other non-MSK cases seen include recurrent ear infection, blocked tear ducts, sinus congestion, symptoms of laryngeal nerve palsy, breathing-difficulties (of various etiologies), reflux, and symptoms of irritable bowel function. Postoperative input can be useful to assist in the recovery from anesthesia and treatment (not due to any problem in the execution of the surgery, but to enhance the individual reaction and response).

Nonspecific lameness is perhaps the category in which osteopathic input can be most useful to our veterinary colleagues, particularly where there is no peripheral joint or soft tissue pathology detected (Hobson 2012). For example, in cases of forelimb lameness there may be pathophysiological changes in the cervicothoracic (CT) spine, but often nothing is apparent on X-ray. The author (NH) has found that these changes in the spine often present as local pain and sensitivity, with muscle tightness and fascial binding, resulting in a decreased range and quality of movement between T2-T5 and the associated ribs and the scapula. These alterations in function can be classed under the term osteopathic somatic dysfunction (OSD) (Stone 1999). The motion of the scapula in relation to the rib cage at the omothoracic junction (a synsarcosis or muscular joint) is crucial to the mechanics of the forelimb. Differences in the orientation between the scapula, humerus, and thorax across different breeds must be taken into account. The principal muscles influencing scapula motion are the periscapular muscles and the pectoral-thoracic sling ventrally and the trapezius and latissimus dorsi dorsally. The integrated function of these muscles, and the scapula motion, may become disrupted as part of the animal's compensatory mechanisms, causing dyskinesia.

As in cases with identifiable pathology causing forelimb lameness, there can be palpable peripheral joint restrictions secondary to radial and/or humeral shift or torsional patterns.

Consistent osteopathic findings are evident, especially in chronic and episodic cases showing compensatory patterns of dysfunction, for example, muscle hypertonicity and antagonistic hypotonicity, decreased segmental mobility in the cranial or midthoracic spine, and more global ipsilateral or contralateral fascial tethering. These alterations in function contribute to a classic OSD presentation, and frequently interrelated visceral dysfunction, due to autonomic irritation at the correlating spinal segmental levels.

One of the effects of an OSD relative to forelimb lameness is altered gait. Changes will present differently, depending on the location and degree of the pathophysiology. For example, some animals may display a shortened stride while others will avoid weight-bearing through the painful limb. In all cases there will be resultant changes in muscle tone and function. Similarly, in cases of nonspecific hind limb lameness with no discernible pathology, there may be areas of OSD in the thoracolumbar (TL) and/or lumbosacral (LS) spine or pelvis. The associated changes in muscle tone and fascial tethering will prevent a normal quality and range of movement in one or more joints of the pelvic limb, thus affecting the gait.

We must approach our canine patients with sensitivity and care so that they do not feel threatened. We must work with their cooperation. Our body language and a noninvasive touch are vital. Cultivate their trust and they will work with you and indeed guide your treatment.

It is essential to familiarize oneself with the different breeds of dogs and the specific characteristics of build, movement, gait, temperament, disease tendencies, etc. There are variations between breeds that are normal for that breed. It is prudent to spend as much time as possible while out and about observing dogs in a natural environment to help one recognise abnormal or pathological presentations. Normal movement and gait vary enormously, so it is the ease, quality, and length of stride that must be assessed, as should stance and conformation.

A full veterinary history must be obtained when working within UK territories, prior to seeing a patient, and this is advisable in any event. If the osteopath is working within a vet clinic this will be available on site or can be requested from another practice.

After a thorough veterinary and osteopathic history, each case is assessed using observation and clinical examination, before proceeding with the treatment. The dog's temperament, constitution, and their individual symptom patterns are taken into account and will influence your treatment and the expected response.

The advantages of being embedded within a veterinary practice are multifold, whether consulting on or off site.

Anatomy

Most veterinary anatomy is based on the dog, and this chapter covers certain areas in detail. It is assumed that the reader has a good working knowledge of anatomy, but we need to look at specific anatomical features pertaining to the canine patient. The references section at the end of the chapter will allow those needing more clarity the means to attain this (Fig. 2.1).

The head

Pairs of frontal and parietal bones meet temporal, occipital, and basisphenoid bones to form the cranium. Caudally the parietals form a deep sagittal crest along their medial borders. In brachycephalic breeds this is usually replaced by two temporal lines, which extend from the external occipital protuberance to the zygomatic process on the frontal bone.

The posterior aspect of the occiput has a transverse ridge called the nuchal crest. This merges with the sagittal crest at its midpoint.

The orbit comprises the frontal, lacrimal, palatine, zygomatic, and sphenoid bones, the zygomatic process of the temporal bones, and the caudal part of the maxilla.

The cranium occupies about half of the skull's length in mesocephalic breeds. From an osteopathic point of view the position of the jugular foramen between the petrosal part of the temporal and occipital bones is of note. Its opening in the tympano-occipital fissure also carries the glossopharyngeal, vagus, and accessory cranial nerves, along with the sigmoid venous sinus. Very close to these is the hypoglossal canal containing the hypoglossal nerve.

Within the main cranial cavity the tentorium cerebelli has attachments to the tentorium osseum and petrosal crests, creating separate compartments for the cerebrum and cerebellum.

Rostrally the facial part of the head is made up of a pair of incisive bones, which form the nasal openings at the extreme rostrum. Caudolaterally they meet the paired nasal, maxillary, and frontal bones. Caudal to

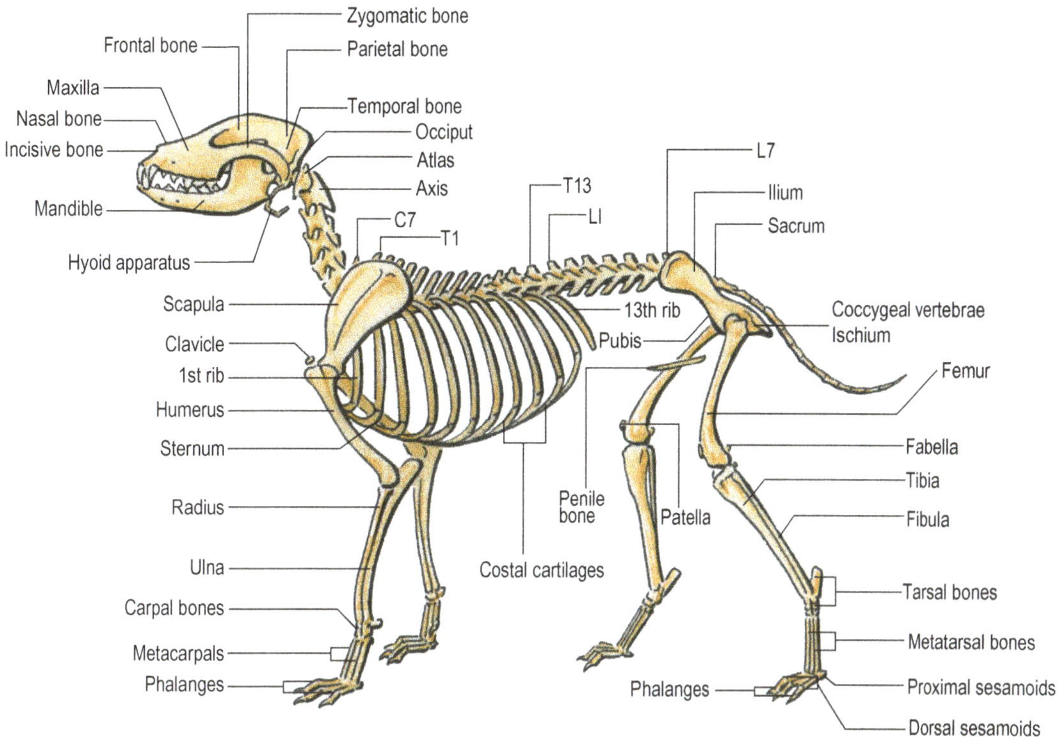

Figure 2.1
Skeleton of the dog.

these the maxilla meets the zygomatic, lacrimal, and frontal bones of the cranium.

Within the presphenoid is the optic canal through which passes the optic nerve.

Within the basisphenoid are the orbital fissure through which passes the oculomotor (CN III), trochlear (CN IV), abducent (CN VI), and ophthalmic (CN V, trigeminal branch) nerves (Fig. 2.2).

The maxillary artery and maxillary branch of the trigeminal nerve (CN V) pass through the rostral alar foramen. The other end of this canal emerges as the caudal alar foramen. Just caudolateral to this is the oval foramen through which passes the mandibular branch of the trigeminal nerve (CN V).

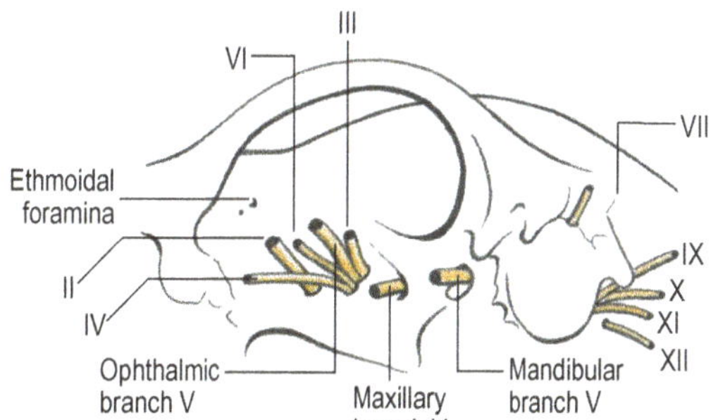

Figure 2.2
Section of the skull showing where the cranial nerves emerge.

The basisphenoid, which is of great importance to osteopaths, sits caudal to the presphenoid and pterygoid bones and rostral to the basiocciput.

The presphenoid bone sits caudal to the vomer, is rostral to the basisphenoid and pterygoid, and has lateral borders with the palatine bones.

The transverse aspect of the occiput has two large occipital condyles situated either side of the foramen magnum for articulation with the atlas.

Nasal cavity

The nasal passages contain the ventral and dorsal conchae - mucosal covered baffles to warm and filter incoming air. Projecting from the cribriform plate is the ethmoidal labyrinth with its ectoturbinates and endoturbinates. The ethmoid structures separate the facial elements from those of the cranium.

The nasal septum rostrally divides left and right nasal cavities.

Sinuses

Dogs have three frontal sinuses sandwiched within the frontal bone layers.

The lateral sinus sits in the rostral part of the maxillary recess, its role being to keep the nasal passages moist during nasal panting.

Mandible

The two halves of the mandible do not fuse completely even in old age, having a permanent symphysis mandibulae. Each mandible is composed of a body and a ramus. On the ramus there is a large masseteric fossa for the masseter muscle insertion above which is the large coronoid process which has attachments for the temporalis muscle. Directly ventral to this is the mandibular canal through which emerges the mandibular branch of the trigeminal nerve (CN V).

Rostrally there are three foramina for the mental nerves. Between the coronoid and condylar processes is the mandibular notch through which passes the motor component of the mandibular nerve.

The most caudal and inferior point is called the angular process, which has attachments for the pterygoid and masseter muscles.

Within the temporomandibular joint are thin cartilaginous articular discs. At their most rostral points the two mandibles meet, creating an interdigitating synchondrosis in adult life.

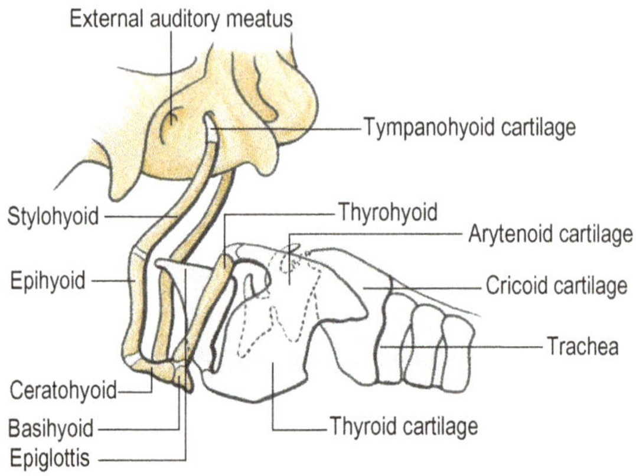

Figure 2.3
The hyoid bone and its relationship with the skull and larynx.

Hyoid structures

The hyoid apparatus is made up of a series of small bones either side, joined by the basihyoid. It extends from the mastoid processes to the thyroid cartilage to create functional support for the tongue and larynx (Fig. 2.3).

Teeth

Adult dogs have 42 teeth, and puppies 28 (Table 2.1).

Vertebral spine

The occipitoatlantoaxial joints are functionally continuous as the dens of the axis passes cranially through the hollow body of the atlas. Here it is held by the transverse, apical, and alar ligaments, the latter attaching to the occiput between the occipital condyles.

The spine of the axis is joined to the arch of the atlas by the dorsal atlantoaxial ligament. Caudally from this point the vertebrae form articulations with intervertebral discs between vertebral bodies and synovial joints between each articular facet joint. Each intervertebral disc has a thick collagenous annulus fibrosus and a gelatinous nucleus pulposus.

The nuchal ligament runs from the axis to T1. It is elastic in nature and is a paired structure (Fig. 2.4).

Table 2.1 The order of teeth in the canine mouth for the adult and the puppy

Adult: upper row x 2	3 incisors	1 canine	4 premolars	2 molars
Adult: lower row x 2	3 incisors	1 canine	4 premolars	3 molars
Puppy: upper row x 2	3 incisors	1 canine	3 premolars	
Puppy: lower row x 2	3 incisors	1 canine	3 premolars	

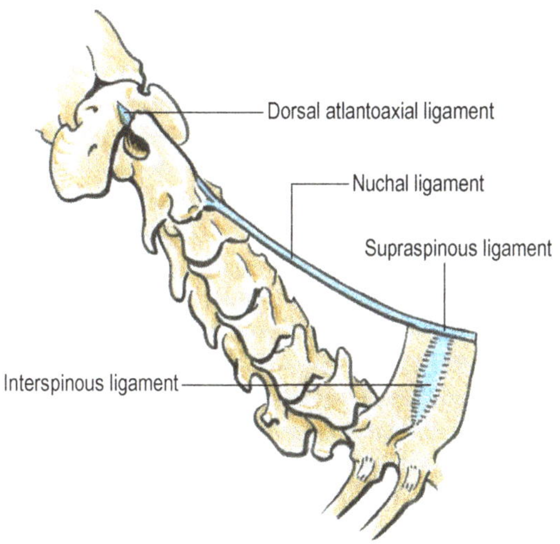

Figure 2.4
The nuchal, dorsal atlantoaxial, and supraspinous ligaments.

The dorsal longitudinal ligament runs along the ventral surface of the vertebral canal, widening at each intervertebral disc.

Musculature

Muscles of the head and neck

The orbicularis oris extends from one lip to the other around the lateral aspects of the mouth. The buccinator forms the main cheek musculature. The platysmus is well developed in the dog and stretches from the orbicularis oris caudally into the raphe of the neck. The levator nasolabialis straddles the nose over the maxillae. It dilates the nostrils and elevates the upper lip.

Just medial to the eyes the lacrimal ducts vent. These connect with the internal lacrimal sac and nasolacrimal duct where the serous fluid enters the nasal meatuses of the nasal cavity. Dogs have a third eyelid, the plica semilunaris, made up of a T-shaped cartilage and conjunctiva.

At the rostral medial juncture of the head and ear is a palpable scutiform cartilage within the auricular muscles. Most of these arise from the median raphe of the neck and then attach into the auricular cartilage.

The root of the tongue lies caudally within the throat structures where it attaches to the hyoid apparatus via the styloglossus, hypoglossus, and genioglossus muscles.

Muscles of mastication

The temporalis and masseter muscles close the mouth, assisted by the medial and lateral pterygoids. The digastricus originates on the paracondylar process of the occiput and attaches onto the body of the mandible. Its innervation is split with the rostral portion supplied by the mandibular branch of the trigeminal nerve and the caudal section by the facial nerve.

The pharyngeal muscles aid swallowing and effectively attach from the cricoid through to the hyoid apparatus and then rostrally into the walls of the pharynx itself. They are all supplied by the glossopharyngeal and vagus nerves.

The larynx is made up of the epiglottic, thyroid, arytenoid, and cricoid cartilages. Muscles controlling this airway include the cricothyroid, cricoarytenoid dorsalis and lateralis, and the thyroarytenoid muscles.

The muscles that create the sling formation with the hyoid are the sternohyoideus, which links to the sternum and first costal cartilage; the thyrohyoideus, which links thyroid cartilage to the thyrohyoid bone; and the mylohyoideus, which form the rostroventral part of the sling.

Innervation is via the hypoglossal nerve (sternohyoideus and thyrohyoideus), and the mandibular branch of the trigeminal nerve (mylohyoideus).

Muscles of the neck and trunk

The superficial fascia of the trunk is continuous with that of the four limbs.

The deep fascia of the trunk attaches to the ends of the spinous processes and transverse processes of all of the thoracic and lumbar vertebrae as well as the supraspinous ligament. From here it passes over the epaxial muscles and wraps around the lateral thoracic and abdominal walls where it forms the origins for several hypaxial muscles, forming the linea alba ventrally (Fig. 2.5A and B).

In the neck the hypaxial muscles are the longus capitis and longus colli.

In the thorax they are the scalenus, serratus ventralis cervicis and thoracis, serratus dorsalis cranialis and caudalis. There are also 12 pairs of external intercostal muscles, whose fibers run caudoventrally from one rib to the next, and the internal intercostal muscles, whose fibers run craniomedially from rib to rib.

The ventral abdominal wall consists of the external and internal abdominal oblique muscles, rectus abdominis, and transversus abdominis. Within the external abdominal oblique is the superficial inguinal ring through which protrudes a sac of the peritoneum, called the vaginal tunic in the male, which envelops the testes and spermatic cord. In females this is referred to as the vaginal process and it envelops the round ligament of the uterus ending blindly near the vulva.

Epaxial muscles. The epaxial muscles (Fig. 2.6) are made up of three main groups: the iliocostalis, longissimus, and transversospinalis.

Within the cervical region the longissimus cervicis is a continuation of the longissimus thoracis. Its four overlapping elements originate from the cervicothoracic (CT) junction and end in the caudal cervical vertebrae.

The longissimus capitis extends from T3–T1 to the mastoid process of the temporal bone, and attaches firmly to the splenius capitis from the wing of the atlas.

The longissimus thoracis and longissimus lumborum originate from the medial aspect of the wing of the ilium and the supraspinous ligament, and then project cranially to attach to the spinous processes of the lumbar and thoracic vertebrae. Their fibers run in a cranioventral direction. At its most cranial point the longissimus has insertions onto the ribs and C7 vertebra.

Transversospinalis group. This is the deepest and most medial group of muscles, extending from the sacrum to the skull. It comprises the spinalis, semispinalis, multifidus, rotatores, interspinales, and intertransversarii.

The splenius sits dorsolaterally from T3 to the skull and lies deep to the serratus dorsalis cranialis and rhomboideus capitis.

The multifidus, interspinales, rotatores, and semispinalis create stability and flexibility to the core.

The iliocostalis arises from the wing of the ilium and attaches to the transverse processes of the vertebrae as well as to the ribs laterally. In its thoracic section it attaches from the 12th rib to the transverse process of C7.

The upper thoracic limb

The thoracic limbs are the main weight-bearing structure (taking 60 percent of the dog's weight). Each has a large scapula caudally inclined from the vertical to which is attached a short humerus which is flexed caudally at its distal end where it articulates with the radius and ulna. These later bones form a pillar with the carpal and metacarpal bones, ending in the digitigrade arrangement of the phalanges of the front paw.

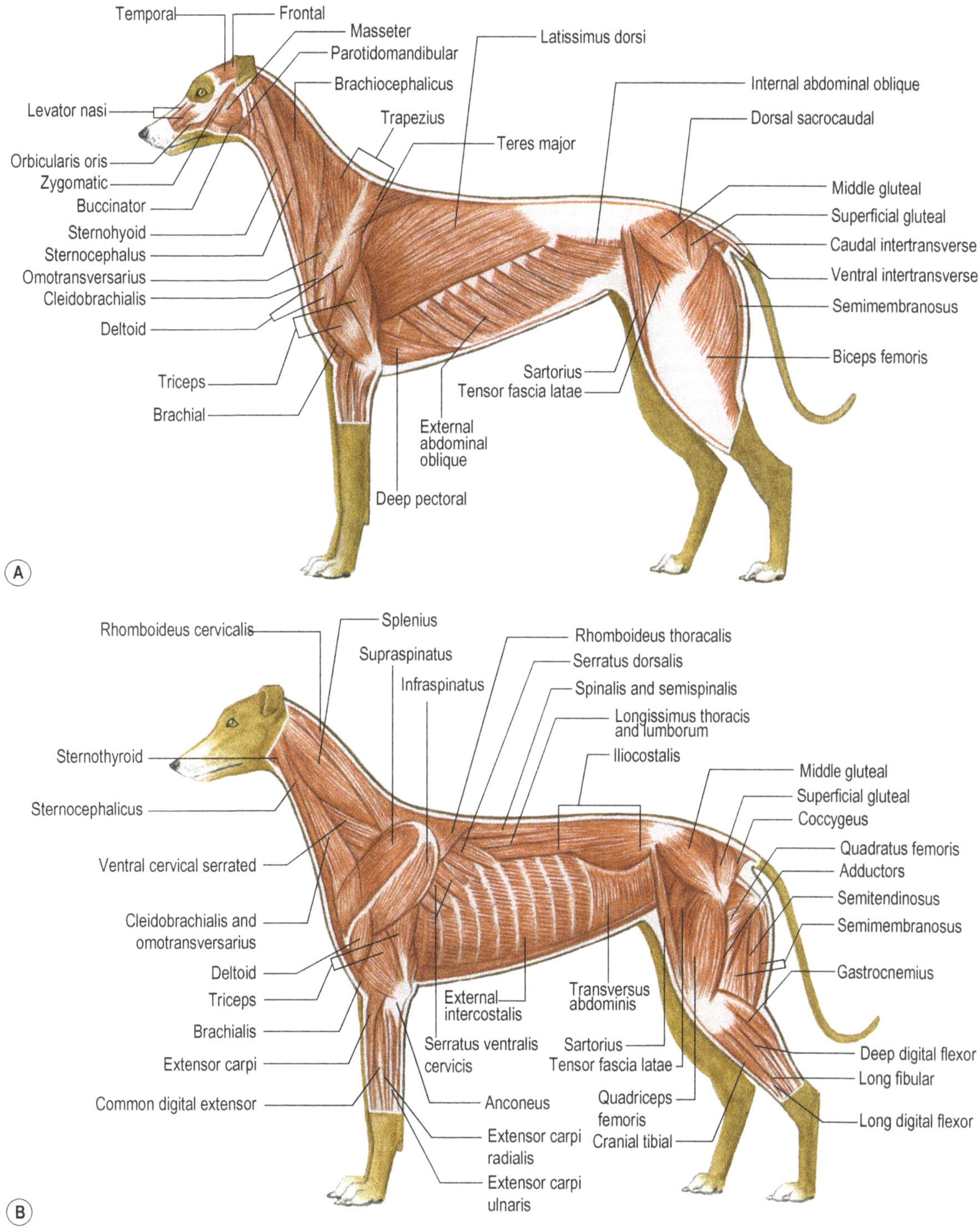

Figure 2.5
(A) The superficial muscles of the dog. (B) The deep muscles of the dog.

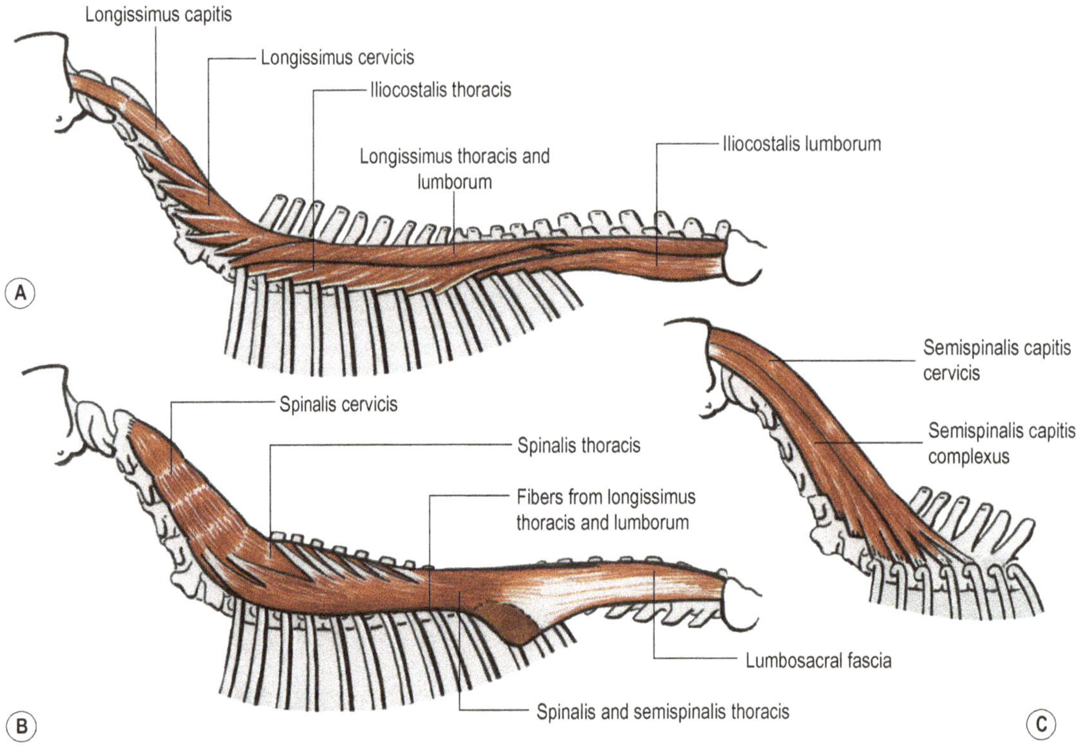

Figure 2.6
The epaxial muscles. (A) Deep layer. (B) Middle layer. (C) Superficial layer.

There is a vestigial clavicle, within the fibrous clavicular intersection of the brachiocephalus muscles, which attaches to the distal third of the humerus and then craniodorsal to the neck and head, crossing over the cranial surface of the glenohumeral joint on its way. The cranial part of this muscle is called the cleidobrachialis. This muscle group has a strong fascial attachment into the axilla.

The sternocephalicus originates on the sternum and runs cranially along the ventral aspect of the throat as a paired structure with linking transverse fibers. It curls laterally and splits to give insertions onto the occiput and mastoid processes.

The omotransversarius is a strap-like muscle extending from the spine of the scapula to the atlas with attachments to the deep cervical fascia medially.

The deep fascia of the neck attaches and separates several muscles already mentioned and envelops the trachea, thyroid gland, larynx, esophagus, the vasosympathetic trunk of the common carotid artery, the internal jugular vein, and the tracheal lymphatic trunk (called the carotid sheath at this point).

The trapezius is thin and is divided into cervical and thoracic portions by a narrow aponeurotic part. It originates from the middle of the dorsal border of the neck, to the ninth or tenth thoracic spine, the left and right muscles meeting on a median fibrous raphe. It inserts onto the entire length of the spine of the scapula.

The rhomboideus holds the dorsal border of the scapula close to the spine and ribs. Its cranial part attaches to the neural crest of the occiput. The dorsal section attaches to the spinous processes of several thoracic vertebrae and most caudally it is covered by the latissimus dorsi. This latter muscle lies caudal to the scapula, attaching into the proximal humerus, wrapping around the ribs, and then tapering caudally until it reaches the ilium and lumbar fascia.

The serratus ventralis forms a major part of the thoracic sling with attachments from the 7th cervical vertebra and the 7th or 8th ribs to the dorsomedial aspect of the scapula. In the dog this muscle supports the thorax and depresses the scapula (Fig. 2.7).

Joints of the forelimb. The glenohumeral (shoulder) joint is a ball and socket arrangement comprising the glenoid cavity of the scapula and the head of the humerus. The main arc of movement is in flexion and extension of the limb. The joint capsule has thickenings either side called the medial and lateral glenohumeral ligaments (Fig. 2.8).

The elbow joint comprises the condyle of the humerus, the head of the radius, and the trochlear notch of the ulna. On each side of the joint are strong medial and lateral co-lateral ligaments. The radioulnar articulation is not load bearing, and the radius and ulna are connected along their length proximally by the interosseus ligament (Fig. 2.9).

The carpus comprises seven carpal bones. There are three in the proximal row (the ulna and radial being weight bearing with the accessory carpal on the palmar aspect of the joint). There are four in the distal row. The joint between the radius and ulna and the proximal row of carpal bones is known as the antebrachiocarpal joint. The joint between the rows of carpal bones is known as the middle carpal joint, and the

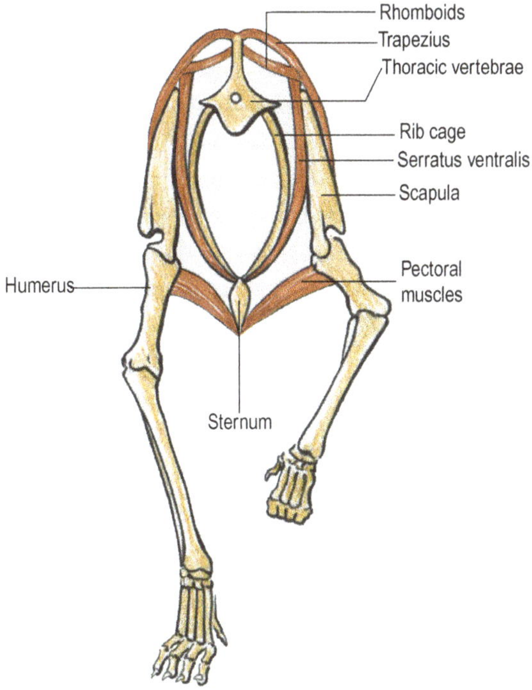

Figure 2.7
The thoracic sling in motion.

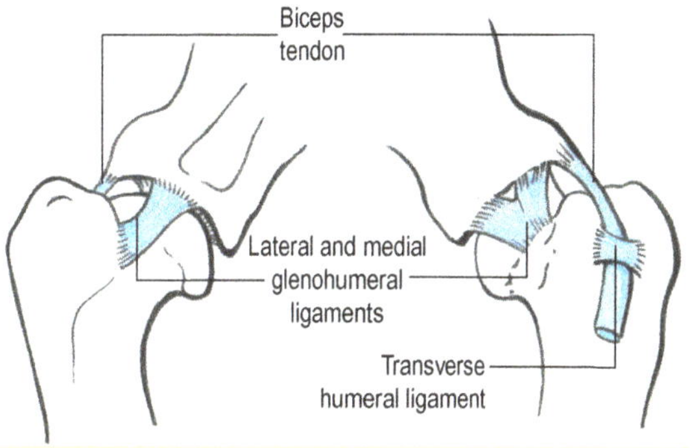

Figure 2.8
The ligaments of the shoulder joint.

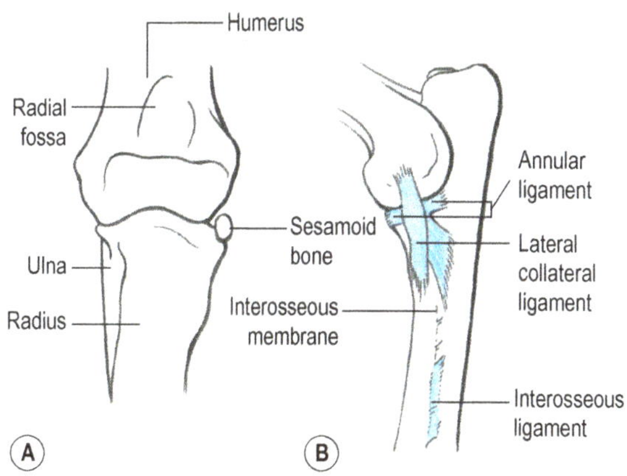

Figure 2.9
The ligaments of the elbow joint. (A) Cranial view of the left elbow. (B) Lateral view of the left elbow.

joint between the distal row of carpal bones and the metacarpal bones is the carpometacarpal joint. On their palmar surface these are all connected by the palmar carpal ligament, which forms a large fibrous sheet.

In the foot itself are the metacarpophalangeal, proximal interphalangeal, and distal interphalangeal joints. Each metacarpophalangeal joint has two sesamoid bones within the tendons that articulate with the flexor surfaces of the metacarpal heads.

Muscles of the forelimb. The shoulder is surrounded by a number of muscles forming a cuff. The deltoideus flexes the glenohumeral joint, and the infraspinatus can flex or extend the shoulder dependent on limb position when it contracts. It also abducts and laterally rotates the limb. When the dog is standing it provides stability by preventing medial rotation of the leg.

The teres minor flexes and laterally rotates the humerus as does the infraspinatus. The supraspinatus provides general extension of the humerus and some lateral limb stabilization. The subscapularis adducts, extends, and medially stabilizes the shoulder, while the teres major flexes, medially rotates, and working with teres minor it can lock the limb in position. The coracobrachialis adducts, extends, and stabilizes the shoulder.

The tensor fasciae antebrachii is a thin strap-like muscle that extends to the elbow. It arises from the lateral surface of the latissimus dorsi, with the caudal half arising from the medial aspect of the triceps brachii, the tendon of which inserts into the olecranon of the ulna. The triceps brachii has four heads: the long, lateral, accessory, and medial heads. All extend the elbow, and the long head can flex the shoulder as well. The anconeus extends the elbow.

The biceps brachii has one head originating on the tuber scapulae. The muscle body is long and fusiform lying on the medial surface of the humerus. Its tendon crosses the glenohumeral joint where it is enveloped in an extension of the synovial membrane. It descends via the intertuberal groove. Between the tubercles on the humerus it is held in place by the transverse humeral retinaculum. At its insertion the tendon splits to attach to the ulnar and radial tuberosities. It extends the shoulder and flexes the elbow.

There is a dense sleeve of fascia on the caudal surface of the antebrachium called the deep antebrachial fascia.

The extensor carpi radialis is held in place on the dorsal aspect of the distal limb by the extensor retinaculum. It originates on the lateral supracondylar crest of the humerus and inserts onto the dorsal surfaces of the second and third metacarpals. This muscle is an extensor of the carpus.

The common digital extensor, along with the lateral digital extensor, ulnaris lateralis, and supinator, originates on the lateral epicondyle of the humerus and inserts onto the extensor processes of the distal phalanges of digits 2, 3, 4, and 5. Within the phalanges the elastic dorsal ligament lies on the left and right of the common digital extensor tendon, attaching to the sides and plantar surface of the middle phalanx and then distally to the dorsal aspect of the distal phalanx. This creates hyperextension of the distal interphalangeal joint causing the claw to retract.

The lateral digital extensor terminates on the extensor processes of the distal phalanges of digits 3, 4, and 5, with attachments also on the proximal phalanges of these same digits. It extends the carpus and digits 3 to 5.

The ulnaris lateralis arises from the lateral epicondyle of the distal humerus and inserts onto the proximal end of the fifth metacarpal and accessory bones. It extends the carpus and provides a small degree of lateral rotation.

The supinator arises from the front of the humerus and inserts onto the cranial surface of the proximal half of the radius. Just proximal to this it contains a sesamoid bone within the tendon. It laterally rotates the distal limb, flexes the elbow, and places the paw medially on its palmar surface.

The abductor digiti longus (abductor carpi obliquus) originates from the lateral border and cranial surface of the shaft of the ulna and interosseus membrane and inserts onto the proximal end of the first metacarpal bone. It abducts the first digit and extends the carpal joints.

The pronator teres originates on the medial epicondyle of the humerus and inserts onto the medial border of the proximal third of the radius. It flexes the elbow and medially rotates the distal limb and paw.

The flexor carpi radialis originates on the medial epicondyle of the humerus and medial border of the radius and inserts on the palmar surface of metacarpals 2 and 3. It flexes the carpus.

The superficial digital flexor also originates from the medial epicondyle of the humerus then takes the form of a long muscle which divides distally into four separate tendons each inserting into the proximal palmar surfaces of the middle phalanges of digits 2 to 5. En route the tendons form the flexor manica (collars around the deep flexor tendon) and both are held in place by the palmar annular ligament at the metacarpophalangeal joints within a common synovial sheath. It flexes the carpal, metacarpal, and proximal interphalangeal joints of these digits.

The flexor carpi ulnaris comprises two heads. The ulnar head originates on the caudal border and medial surface of the olecranon, and the humeral head on the medial epicondyle. They both insert onto the accessory bone and flex the carpus.

The deep digital flexor has three heads. The humeral head originates on the medial epicondyle, the ulnar head on the proximal border of the ulna, and the radial head on the middle part of the medial border of the radius. These tendons fuse and converge at the carpus and are held in place by the flexor retinaculum. They then insert onto the flexor tubercles of the distal phalanx of each digit. The deep digital flexor flexes the carpal and metacarpal joints and the proximal and distal interphalangeal joints.

The pronator quadratus is situated between the shafts of the radius and ulna on their opposing surfaces. It pronates the paw.

Bones and joints of the pelvic limb

The pelvis is formed by the ilium, ischium, and pubis (and acetabular bone in puppies which fuses in adult life). Each pelvic bone is called the os coxae. In the standing dog the sacroiliac joints are situated cranial to the hips. Figure 2.10A and B shows a ventral view and a dorsal view of the pelvis.

The ilium makes up just over half of the os coxae cranially. The cranioventral iliac spine ends with the tuber coxae. The cranial and caudal dorsal iliac spines form the tuber sacrale. The internal surfaces provide attachment for the iliocostalis longissimus and quadratus lumborum muscles. Medially the roughened auricular surfaces form one half of the sacroiliac joints. The medial arcuate line has attachments for psoas minor.

The ischium forms part of the acetabulum, obturator foramen, and the corresponding halves of the symphysis pubis, which in dogs is part of the symphysis pelvis. Caudally it forms the tuber ischii (where the sacrotuberous ligament attaches) and the medial half of the ischiatic arch. Ventrally it has attachments for the origins of the biceps femoris, semitendinosus, and semimembranosus. In males the crus of the penis and associated muscles attach medially to this tuberosity. The ischiatic crest marks the solid joint with the ilium and has attachments for the coccygeus. Caudally the border forms attachments for the obturator muscle tendons creating the lesser ischiatic notch.

The ramus forms the thin middle section and joins medially with the other half, where they fuse with the symphysis pubis caudally. On its dorsal aspect is the ischiatic table, which is the origin for the internal obturator muscle. Its ventral surface serves as origins for the quadratus femoris and external obturator muscles.

The pubis has a body and two rami (cranial and caudal). The iliopubic eminence has attachments for the

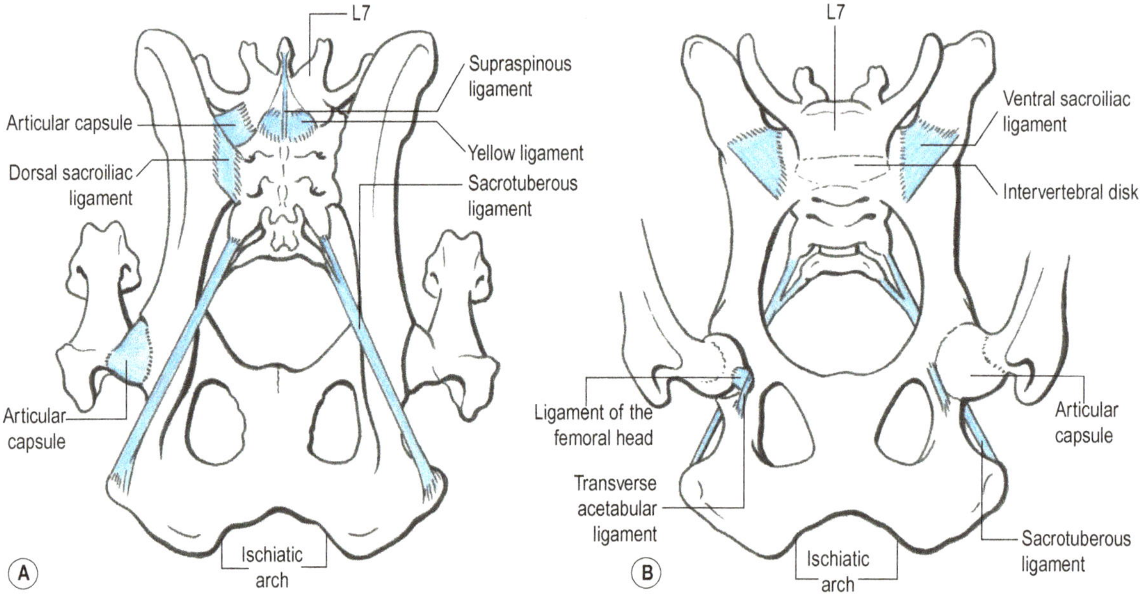

Figure 2.10
(A) Ventral view of the pelvis with ligaments attached. (B) Dorsal view of the pelvis with ligaments attached.

pectineus muscle. At its roughened cranial border it has attachments for the tendons of the rectus abdominis and pectineus via the common prepubic tendon.

The acetabulum is formed from the ilium and ischium (plus the acetabular bone in puppies).

The socket rim is interrupted by the acetabular notch across which passes the transverse acetabular ligament.

Femur. This is the largest bone in the canine skeleton. Beyond the short femoral neck are three protuberances: the greater, lesser, and third trochanters. Between the greater and the third is the intertrochanteric crest where the quadratus femoris attaches (in addition to attaching on the proximal cranial surface of the femur). The greater trochanter also has attachments for the middle and deep gluteal muscles. The lesser trochanter has attachments for the iliopsoas. The third trochanter has attachments for the superficial gluteal.

At the distal end of the femur the trochlea is deep with well-defined vertical ridges either side, with the ridge being larger on the medial side (Fig. 2.11).

Proximal to the large condyles on the caudal surface are facets for articulation with the medial and lateral fabellae (sesamoids that sit within the tendons of the gastrocnemius). Proximal to these facets are the medial and lateral supracondylar tuberosities which mark the origins of the gastrocnemius and those of the superficial digital flexor (lateral side only).

On the extreme medial and lateral aspects of the distal femur are the medial and lateral epicondyles which form the attachment of the co-lateral ligaments of the stifle joint. Laterally there are also attachments for the popliteus and the long digital extensor tendon. On the caudomedial aspect are attachments for the insertion of the semitendinosus.

Tibia. At the proximal end the tibia is wider than its articulation with the femur. Between the two large

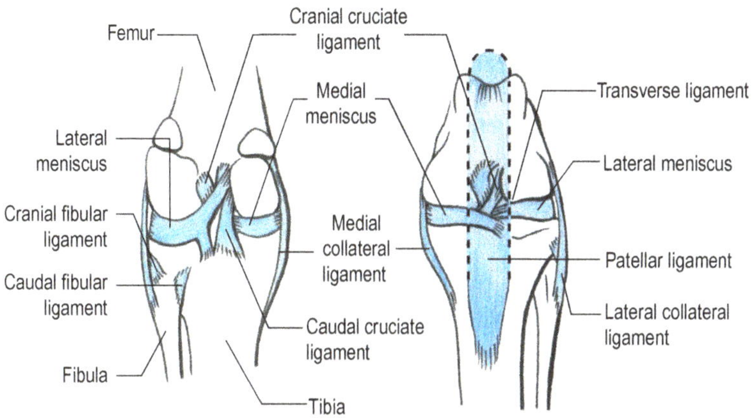

Figure 2.11
The ligaments of the stifle joint.

condyles there is the intercondylar eminence comprising two small tubercles with a shallow dip in between. At the cranial end of this is the attachment for the cranial cruciate ligament (CrCL). The caudal cruciate ligament (CaCL) attaches to the lateral edge of the popliteal notch. This ligament is much heavier and longer than the CrCL.

The tibia has two large cartilaginous menisci separating its articular surfaces from those of the femur.

On the proximal cranial surface of the tibia is the tibial tuberosity on which attaches the patellar ligament. A small, smooth channel, called the extensor groove, sits at the junction of this tuberosity and the lateral condyle, housing the long digital extensor muscle. Distally the tibial trochlea interlocks with the trochlea of the talus forming the tarsocrural joint which allows flexion and extension of the hock. The distal half of the tibia has no muscular attachments.

Fibula. The proximal extremity of the fibula is flattened and articulates with the lateral condyle of the tibia. It extends the full length of the tibia, its distal end articulating medially with the tibia and tibial tarsal bone and forming the lateral malleolus. The distal end of the fibula contains two grooves for the fibularis longus and brevis and lateral digital extensor tendons. The grooves act as deflectors that alter the direction of pull of these muscles.

Tarsal bones. Seven tarsal bones collectively form the hock, in three irregular rows. The proximal row is made up of the calcaneus, which also articulates with the fourth tarsal bone, and the talus. The latter articulates with the tibia, calcaneus, and the central tarsal bone. Posteriorly the calcaneus has a large bony projection for the attachment of the powerful extensor muscles, which attach via the common calcaneal tendon. Medially the lateral digital flexor tendon runs over the bony extension of the sustentaculum tali.

The proximal row is partially separated from the distal row by the central tarsal bone, which articulates with the first three tarsal bones, while the distal end of the calcaneus articulates with the fourth tarsal bone. This latter bone straddles the entire middle row. On the distal part of the lateral surface of this bone is a groove where the fibularis longus tendon runs.

The metatarsals are similar to the metacarpals except that in some breeds of dog the first metatarsal is missing or just a vestige.

The phalanges and their associated sesamoids form the hind paw or pes. They are arranged similarly to those in the manus except that the first digit (hallux) is often missing or just has the terminal phalanx.

Muscles of the pelvis and hip

The TFL tenses the lateral femoral fascia, flexes the hip, and extends the stifle. The superficial gluteal extends the hip and abducts the hind leg. The middle gluteal extends, abducts, and medially rotates the hip, along with the piriformis which is formed from the deep caudal portion of this muscle. The deep gluteal works in conjunction with the middle gluteal. They all originate on the sacrum, ilium, ischial spine, and first caudal vertebra.

The iliopsoas lies on the ventrolateral surface of the lumbar spine and the cranioventral surface of the ilium, inserting into the lesser trochanter of the femur. It flexes the hip and stabilizes the core. The articularis coxae originates on the lateral surface of the ilium, along with the rectus femoris, and attaches to the neck of the femur. This is a hip flexor.

The internal obturator, gemellus, quadratus femoris, and external obturator make up the caudal hip muscle group. They laterally rotate the hip. The quadratus femoris also extends it.

Muscles of the hind limb

The cranial thigh muscles include the quadriceps femoris group. Caudally, the biceps femoris, semitendinosus, and semimembranosus form the hamstrings. All of these flex the stifle, and extend the hip. The sartorius flexes the hip; its cranial part extends the stifle and its caudal part flexes it. The gracilis adducts the hind leg, flexes the stifle, and extends both hip and hock.

Within the medial thigh musculature is the femoral triangle, which is bounded on all sides by the muscle groups already listed. Within this area pass both the femoral artery and vein and it is where the femoral pulse is taken.

The pectineus appears as a defined muscle, however, the adductor magnus brevis and longus often appear as one muscle in certain breeds.

Distally are superficial bands of fascia – the superficial crural, tarsal, metatarsal, and digital fasciae. Within this intricate matrix pass numerous nerve and blood vessels. These fascial bands meet over the stifle and continue in a distal direction as the deep crural fascia, enveloping each muscle and also the tibia and fibula on the way. It also provides direct muscle attachments for the biceps femoris, semitendinosus, and gracilis. Just proximal to the talus it thickens and becomes the extensor retinaculum, holding down the extensor tendons for the hind paw. Over the tarsus the fascia thins and changes its name to the deep tarsal fascia. It attaches to the calcaneum and then wraps around the long digital extensor tendon, where it becomes the tarsal extensor retinaculum.

The cranial tibial, long digital extensor, and fibularis (peroneus) longus muscles flex the tarsus and extend digits 2 to 5 collectively. The popliteus has a sesamoid bone within its distal tendinous portion and provides medial rotation to the distal part of the hind limb. The gastrocnemius has two heads, one on either side of the superficial digital flexor tendon. Within each head is a sesamoid bone called the fabella. The gastrocnemius inserts onto the calcaneum via the common calcaneal tendon. The superficial and deep digital flexor muscles, combined, flex the stifle and phalanges, and extend the tarsus.

Nervous system

The canine central, peripheral, and autonomic nervous systems (CNS, PNS, and ANS) are similar to those of the human in both anatomy and function. The minor differences relate to specific anatomical aspects pertaining to each breed. From an osteopathic viewpoint we are very interested in neurological impact to any altered states within the MSK system. The important structures are illustrated in Figures 2.12 and 2.13.

Circulatory system

The canine circulatory system is also similar to that of the human. The heart is situated between the 3rd

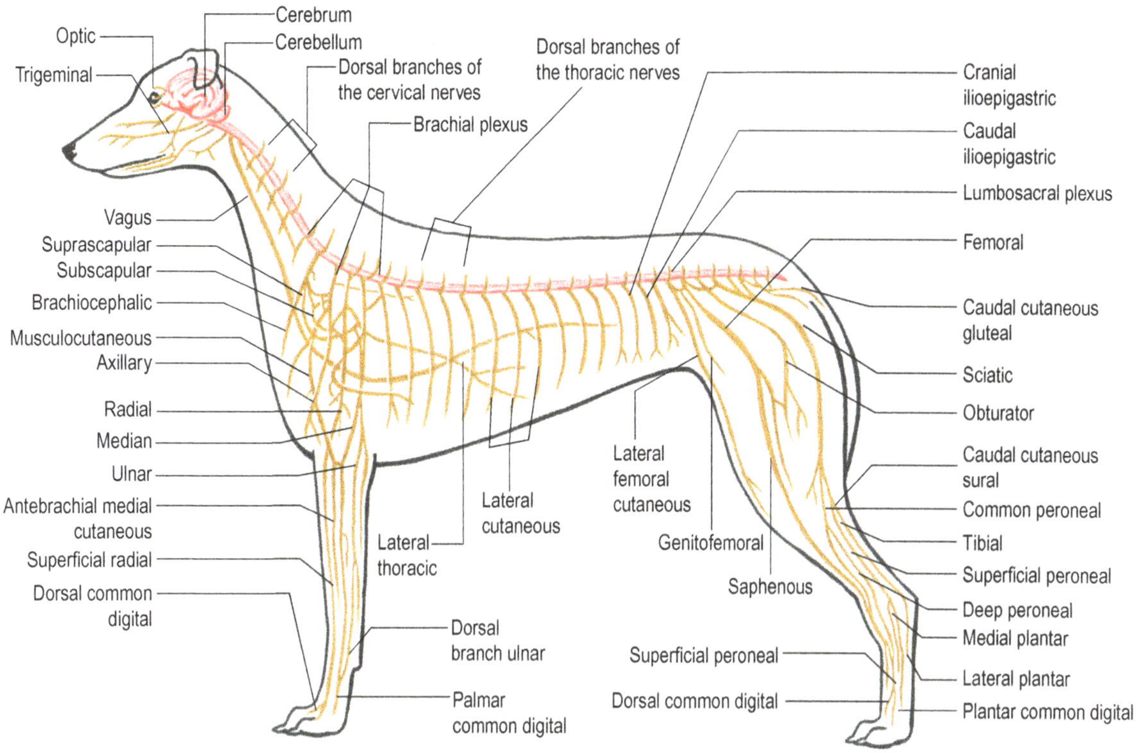

Figure 2.12
Lateral view of the dog showing the central and peripheral nervous systems.

and 6th ribs and sits slightly to the left of the midline. It comprises two separate compartments, each with an atrium to receive blood and a ventricle to pump it out.

The main arteries are the aorta from the heart, the left and right common carotid arteries taking blood to the head, the brachial and femoral arteries taking blood to the forelimbs and hind limbs respectively, and the pulmonary arteries taking blood to the heart itself.

The main veins are the cranial and caudal vena cava taking blood to the heart, the left and right jugular veins returning blood from the head, the cephalic and brachial veins returning blood from the forelimbs, the saphenous and femoral veins returning blood from the hind limbs, and the left and right pulmonary veins returning blood from the heart muscle itself (Figs 2.14 and 2.15).

Common orthopedic conditions

Introduction

Diagnosing and treating an orthopedic condition demands a logical and systematic approach. It is imperative to take into consideration all the soft tissues and nerves as well as the skeleton itself. It is also important to assess the effects of a disease process on the whole body in vivo and resist the temptation to focus solely on

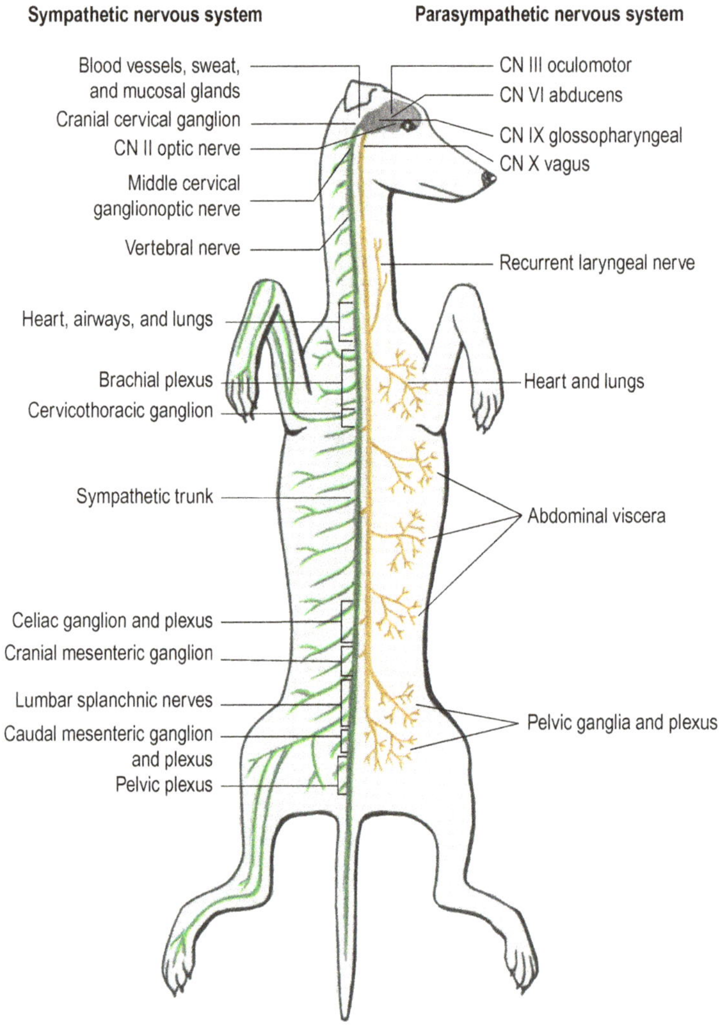

Figure 2.13
Schematic showing the sympathetic and parasympathetic parts of the autonomic nervous system in relation to the spine of the dog.

one specific body area. A primary disorder in one location can lead to secondary problems elsewhere due to compensation for imbalances in load-bearing and subsequent fatigue.

Orthopedic disease can be the result of congenital, developmental, metabolic, traumatic, infectious and neoplastic aetiologies. Sometimes more than one disease process may be implicated in a condition. Patients require a clinical history to be taken, and a thorough clinical examination, before blood tests, radiographs, arthroscopy, CT (computed tomography), and MRI (magnetic resonance imaging) scans are undertaken. Knowledge of clinical histories from the animal's parents and siblings is extremely useful when investigating disease processes that are not traumatic. It is very easy to make assumptions when starting to diagnose an orthopedic condition. A dog that is acutely lame may easily end up undergoing a complex series of investigations if something as simple as a foreign body in a pad or a split toenail is missed.

Certain pedigree pure breeds, or breed types, may be more likely to develop certain orthopedic conditions compared with others. For example, chondrodystrophoid breeds will be more likely to develop

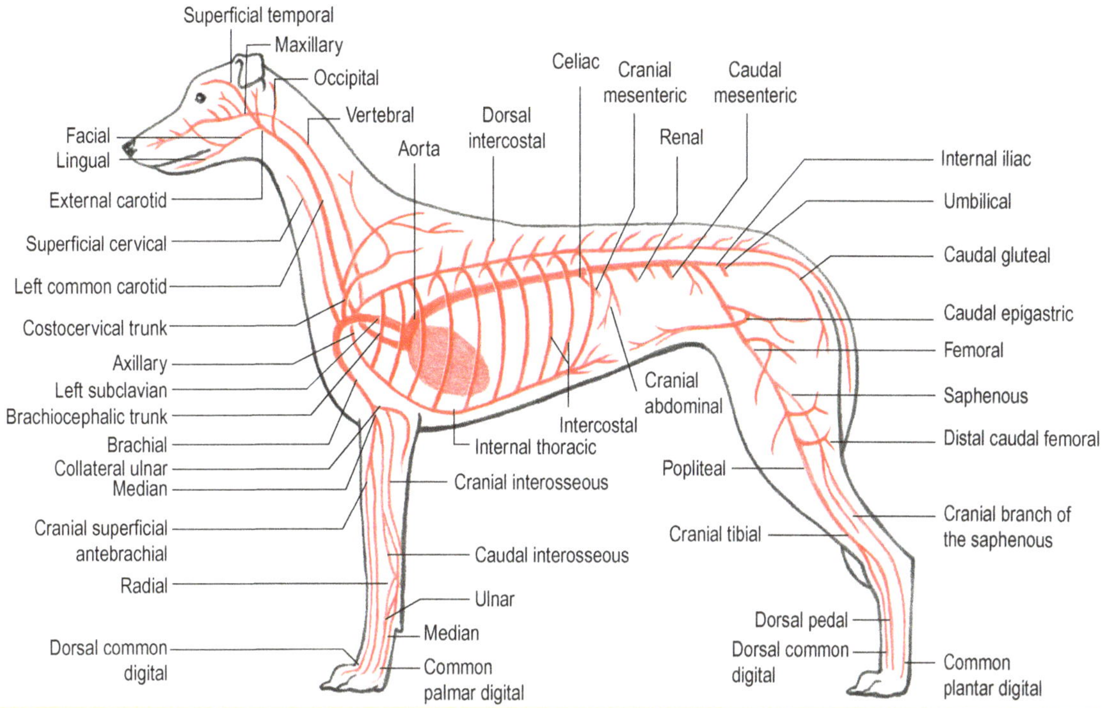

Figure 2.14
The major arteries in the dog.

types of angular limb deformity and degenerative intervertebral disc disease compared with nonchondrodystrophoid breeds. Craniomandibular osteopathy is particularly common in West Highland terriers while the cervical spinal instability condition wobbler syndrome primarily affects large and giant breeds of dogs such as the Doberman Pinscher or Great Dane. Knowledge of breed-specific disorders can prove very useful.

Orthopedic disease can show from a very early age. Obviously trauma can affect any age. Developmental orthopedic disease, which as the name implies affects the growing skeleton, or metabolic disease may produce clinical signs as early as three or four months of age.

You may be working with a team of one or more veterinarians, but it is important that you are provided with a basic core of information relating to your patient. Table 2.2 (p. 53) is a guide that should be useful for your records every time you assess a dog for the first time and during subsequent consultations.

Where possible an attempt should be made to observe the problem. It may be very obvious, intermittent, or particularly mild on the day that you first see the patient. You may have to see the dog walk, circle, reverse, hemiwalk, or wheelbarrow walk outside on a nonslip surface. The author (RH) sometimes asks an owner to video any event so that he can better see the problem they are describing. To make the assessment more objective, the owner should maintain a diary of the condition describing any activity or event that exacerbates or improves its severity. What is going to affect the assessment and treatment of a canine patient profoundly is their temperament. A tense, nervous, or overtly aggressive dog may prove very difficult. You should never put yourself or anyone else at risk. Bites, even from small dogs, can be very dangerous and cause serious injuries. Be careful and sensible!

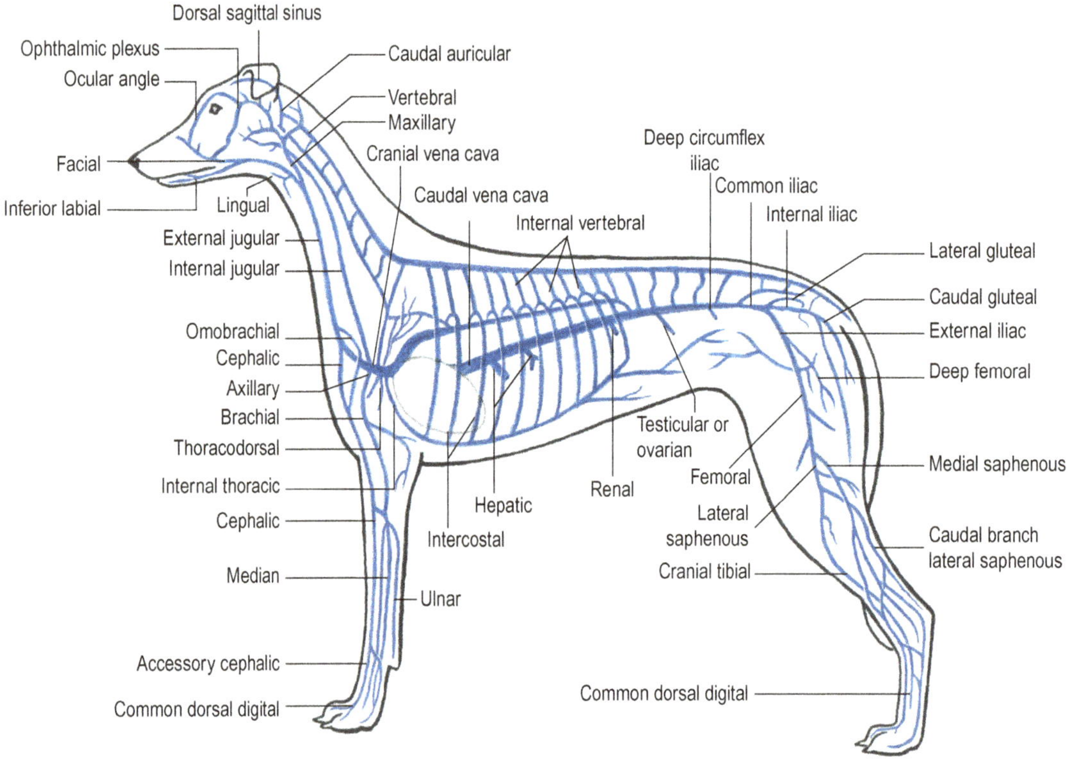

Figure 2.15
The major veins in the dog.

Categories of musculoskeletal conditions

Developmental orthopedic disease

This includes disease that arises in young, growing dogs. The canine skeleton will have finished growing by 11 to 12 months of age in all dogs, with the larger breeds maturing later than the toy breeds. Factors that influence the development and severity of developmental orthopedic disease include genetics, nutrition, and levels of exercise.

Angular deformities. An angular deformity arises in a limb when there is differential rate of growth between two bones that would normally grow at a synchronized rate and/or when there is asymmetric growth across the width of a growth plate. The end result is a limb that develops with abnormal bowing and a deviation to the medial side (varus deformity) or lateral side (valgus deformity). The antebrachium is the only paired bone structure in a dog's limb where the two bones (radius and ulna) weight-bear to a similar extent. Further, both the proximal and distal radial growth plates contribute to longitudinal growth of the radius whereas only the distal ulnar growth plate contributes to longitudinal growth of the ulna. This means it is a complex process for both these bones to elongate in synchrony. Any abnormality in this synchronous growth will result in an angular deformity (Fig. 2.16A). The exact nature and severity of this angular deformity depends on the cause and location of the pathology together with the age of onset in the growing animal. Clinical signs can include carpal valgus, dorsal antebrachial bowing, elbow dysplasia and limb shortening, all of which can produce varying degrees of lameness. The end result is the "Queen Anne" leg conformation. A mild form of this is often considered normal in chondrodystrophic breeds

Table 2.2 Twelve-point guide to the assessment of the canine patient

Find out the dog's age and how long it has been in the owner's possession.	Owners who have owned a dog since a puppy can provide a detailed medical history going back to about eight weeks of age.
If the owner is not the original owner, how many previous owners have there been, and what were the reasons for rehoming?	Sometimes the dog is rehomed because of a pre-existing complaint, which may not be declared. A newly acquired dog that has had multiple previous owners is unlikely to have a reliable medical history.
Assess the body condition score and enquire about the dog's exercise regimen. Find out if the dog undergoes agility training and trials. Does it climb stairs, run half marathons with the owner, etc.? Is it a working dog?	Working dogs and those used for racing and agility may be predisposed to particular injuries. Unfit and overweight dogs may improve simply with weight loss and an increase in fitness. Reweigh regularly and record the readings. Dramatic or persistent changes either way can be the result of a serious underlying disease process such as diabetes mellitus, hypothyroidism, hyperadrenocorticism, or neoplasia.
What type of food is fed to the dog?	This is important especially in dogs under 12 months of age. It is necessary in determining whether the diet is balanced and likely to have contributed to any deficiencies or metabolic disturbances, especially as home-prepared raw diets appear to be increasingly popular. At the same time it is important to note if any vitamin or mineral supplements are fed.
What are the clinical signs?	Obviously this is critical but it is surprising how frequently the owners only know that something nonspecific is wrong. Ask more than one family member and repeat the line of questioning, if necessary, at different times.
When were the signs first noticed?	Often this is not known with certainty especially with slow onset, chronic conditions.
Have the signs been constant or intermittent?	Ideally, you should observe and examine the dog when the condition is obvious. Assessment when the condition is not evident may prove frustratingly fruitless. It will be better to assess the patient again at a later date when you can make a more thorough appraisal.
Have these signs improved, remained static, or deteriorated with time?	It is important to know whether an acute condition is improving or not. If it is then don't interfere!
If lameness is involved, which limbs are affected and what is the grade of lameness (on a scale of 5 or 10)?	Owners may find this difficult when there is a bilateral or mild lameness. Frequently many owners describe a left-sided lameness, for example, as a right-sided problem because they state the side affected when observing their dogs head on. A shifting right or left lameness can balance itself out making an obvious lameness extremely difficult to determine.
Is there any previous history of trauma, surgery, or illness, including infections and pyrexia (fever)?	This is extremely important because of long-term effects on joints, nerves, and soft tissues. Orthopedic implants can break, move, or become infected. Remember, not all implants will show up on radiographs. Young dogs with back pain may have discospondylitis, where the vertebral end plates become infected. In the early disease, radiographs may not demonstrate the pathology. Severely osteoarthritic joints can become infected resulting in osteomyelitis and septic arthritis. Once again this may not be obvious with a quick glance at a radiograph but requires synovial fluid culture for a definitive diagnosis.
What is the breed and is anything known about the medical history of the parents and any siblings?	Family history can help determine whether an individual may be predisposed to a particular condition such as osteochondritis dissecans (OCD) of the proximal humerus.
Is the dog on any current medication?	This can affect the assessment immensely. Many owners treat their own dogs with paracetamol (acetaminophen) or medicines prescribed for other pets. In addition, they often use other products kept in their personal medicine cabinet or those obtained from the Internet.

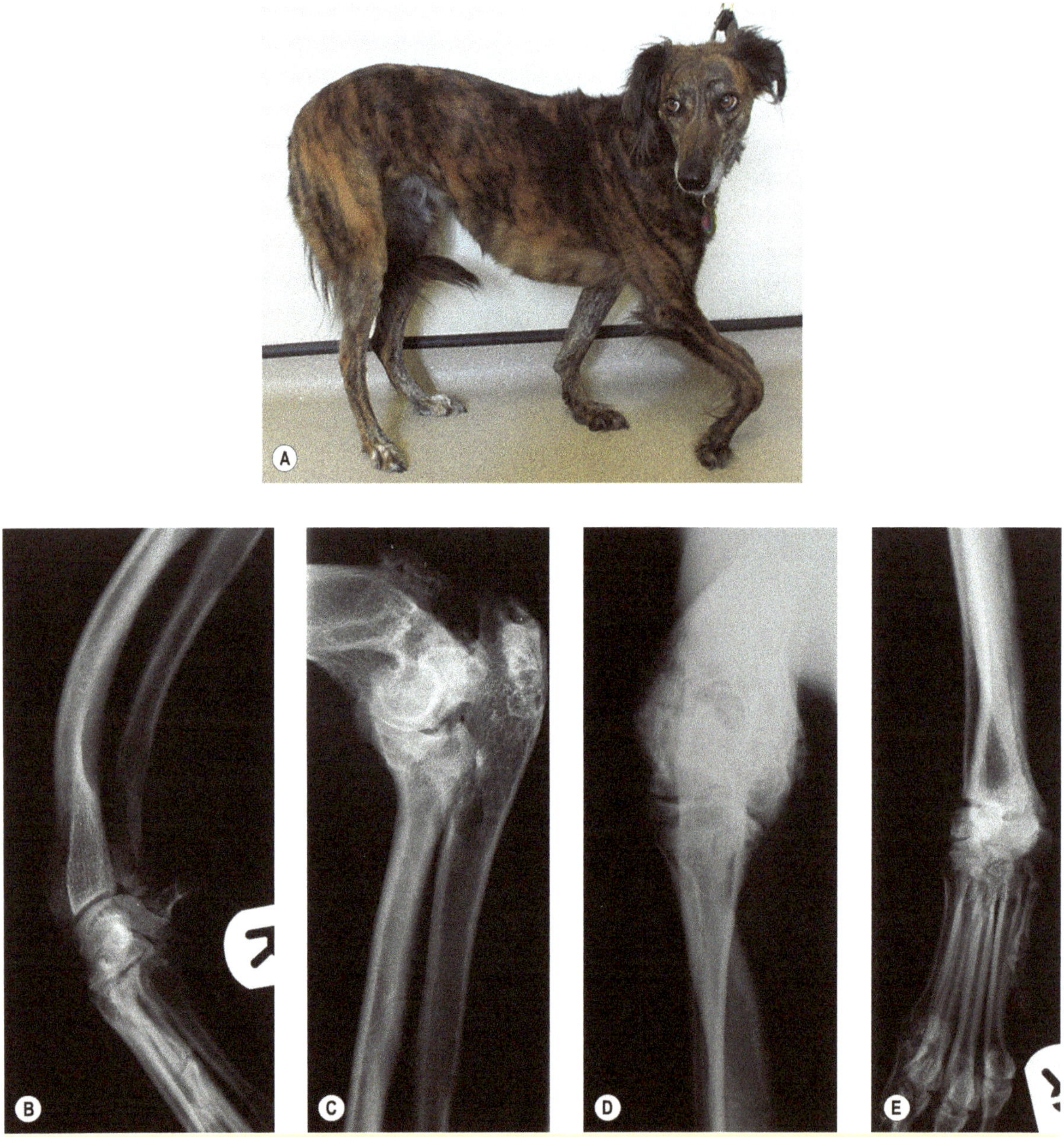

Figure 2.16
(A) Angular limb deformity in a lurcher. (B) Dorsoventral view of a radiograph of a dog showing angular deformity. This rescue dog developed premature closure of the distal ulnar growth plate, possibly having sustained an injury to the right carpus as a youngster, and consequently developed a progressive angular skeletal deformity resulting in a valgus (lateral deviation) (C, D) and outward rotation of the foot (E). There is also dorsal bowing of the distal antebrachium and generalized muscle atrophy of the affected leg. It is clearly evident that the left forelimb is overloaded as it bears most of the weight that should be shared equally between both of the front legs. There is also abnormal loading of the lumbar musculature and back legs in compensation to the abnormal gait and weight-bearing at the front end of the body.

such as the Jack Russell terrier, especially where it is not associated with lameness or elbow pain (Fig. 2.16B–E). It is not just the long bones that are affected in these cases but also the cuboidal bones of the carpus and all of the soft tissues.

Diagnosis is based on the gross appearance of the limbs and radiography. In cases where the degree of angular deviation is minor, and in the absence of lameness, no surgical intervention may be indicated. However, in many cases surgical intervention is required. The prognosis can be quite variable especially when there are surgical complications.

Craniomandibular osteopathy. Craniomandibular osteopathy is often referred to as CMO or "lion jaw." This is a painful, proliferative, non-neoplastic disease of the bones, principally but not exclusively in the skull. It tends to affect young terrier breeds of dog of 4 to 9 months old. Most commonly it affects the skull, temporomandibular joint and mandible; however, long bones may also be affected, namely the ulna. The breeds most commonly affected appear to be the Scottish, West Highland White, Cairn and Boston terriers. It has also been described in the boxer, Labrador, Great Dane, Doberman Pinscher, Shetland sheepdog, the Great Pyrenees (Pyrenean Mountain Dog), bulldog (English bulldog) and bullmastiff. Although it was first described in 1958 its etiology remains unclear. The clinical signs include pain when opening the mouth, decreased appetite, swelling of the skull and jaw, dribbling of saliva and pyrexia. Diagnosis relies on clinical examination, history, breed affected, ruling out metabolic bone disease, X-rays, and occasionally biopsy. Treatment principally consists of providing pain relief and feeding a diet that the patient can manage until the condition resolves by itself.

Elbow dysplasia. This is a developmental disorder of the elbow joint arising from one condition or a number of conditions that result in abnormal load-bearing or instability of this complex hinge joint. The etiology may involve a fragmented medial coronoid process, ununited anconeal process, osteochondrosis of the medial humeral condyle, and joint incongruity arising from abnormal growth rates between the radius and ulna. Elbow dysplasia is usually first noticed in young, active and rapidly growing, medium to giant breeds of dog. Chondrodystrophic breeds are also affected. Clinical signs may develop as early as four months of age with one or both limbs affected. When there is a symmetrical, bilateral condition the lameness can be more difficult to detect than with a unilateral problem. Affected limbs may have the elbow adducted with the carpus abducted. Ultimately the end result will be an osteoarthritic joint that demonstrates thickening, a restricted range of motion, crepitus, and pain.

Diagnosis relies principally on radiography although CT and arthroscopy are being used increasingly and can yield additional information. Treatment may be conservative but open surgery or arthroscopic surgical techniques are often indicated. The long-term prognosis is variable and even in surgical cases osteoarthritis may still develop or progress.

The British Veterinary Association has an elbow scoring scheme for potential breeding stock because the condition has a genetic component to its development.

Hip dysplasia. Hip dysplasia (HD) is a very common condition that is most often associated with certain large to giant breeds such as Labrador retrievers, German shepherds, Rottweilers and Saint Bernards. It can also affect smaller dogs and is frequently seen in border collies. It can affect any breed of dog.

There is a complex mechanism of inheritance with the level of exercise and nutrition affecting the development of this disease.

As the dog grows an incongruity develops between the femoral head and acetabulum. This results in joint instability with abnormal joint surface wear. The consequent pain results in disuse of the affected limb with subsequent muscle atrophy and the development of further joint laxity. This will produce a misshapen femoral head and shallow acetabulum which results in coxofemoral joint subluxation in the short term and ultimately culminates in osteoarthritis (Wardlaw and McLaughlin 2012). One or both coxofemoral joints may be affected and clinical signs can become apparent from around four to 10 months of age.

Diagnosis is dependent on radiography and a clinical assessment performed under general anesthesia. This involves two techniques known as the Ortolani test and Barden's sign.

Many breeders assess the dam and sire prior to mating in an attempt to reduce the probability of the puppies developing the disease. Worldwide there are five particularly widespread and well-established techniques for HD screening. These are run by the British Veterinary Association in conjunction with the The Kennel Club (BVA/KC Hip Dysplasia Scheme), Fédération Cynologique Internationale (FCI), Pennsylvania Hip Improvement Program (PennHIP), The Orthopedic Foundation for Animals, and the dorsolateral subluxation (DLS) score. In addition, there are now DNA tests to assess the genetic predisposition of dogs to developing HD, for example, the Dysgen® test used in Labradors (Idexx Laboratories Ltd.). The management of canine HD ranges from conservative management to a variety of surgical techniques. It depends on the severity of the condition and the age that it becomes apparent. (Smith et al. 2012) (Figs 2.17, 2.18, 2.19, and 2.20).

Legg–Calvé–Perthes disease. This is a condition that principally affects very small breeds, affecting young dogs between the ages of four months to a year. A definitive cause has not been established although it is known to be inherited in Manchester terriers. It is thought that intermittent or temporary disruption of blood supply to the femoral head leads to a delayed death and necrosis of the bone in the femoral head and neck, which effectively crumbles and fails mechanically. The condition may be unilateral or bilateral and may present as gradual onset hind limb weakness or lameness with muscle atrophy and crepitus, however,

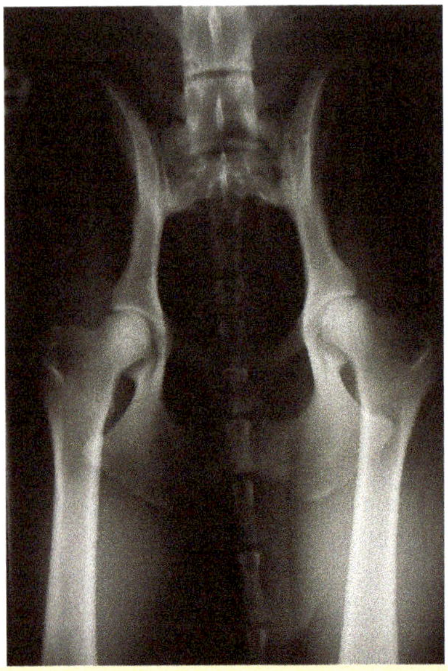

Figure 2.17
Radiograph showing normal hip joints. Taken of a two-and-a-half-year-old German shorthair pointer for official BVA hip scoring. The score assigned for this dog was 8/106, which is below the median score for the breed (9). A perfect score would have been 0.

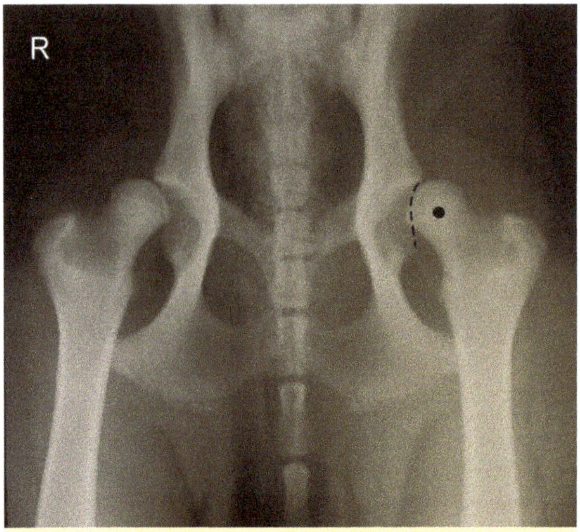

Figure 2.18
Radiograph of hip dysplasia in a nine-month-old, growing male Labrador dog. There are no significant remodeling changes apparent but this dog was extremely painful, weak, and lame on his hind quarters. Unfortunately, he also had bilateral elbow dysplasia with secondary, osteoarthritic changes in both elbow joints. This dog had very obvious hip joint instability in the Ortolani assessment and subluxation of both coxofemoral joints is clearly visible on the ventrodorsal X-ray view. The dot in the center of the left femoral head should lie within (medial to) the black dotted line, which shows the position of the dorsal rim of the acetabulum. This dog required total hip replacement.

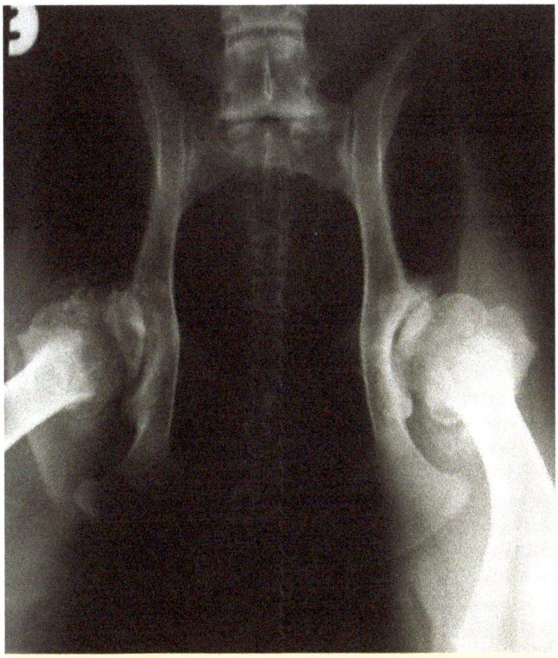

Figure 2.19
Radiograph showing osteoarthritis of the hip. Radiograph of severely osteoarthritic canine hips. Taken of a dog that developed osteoarthritis secondary to hip dysplasia. It is important to realize that the correlation between radiological appearance and clinical discomfort can be difficult to determine.

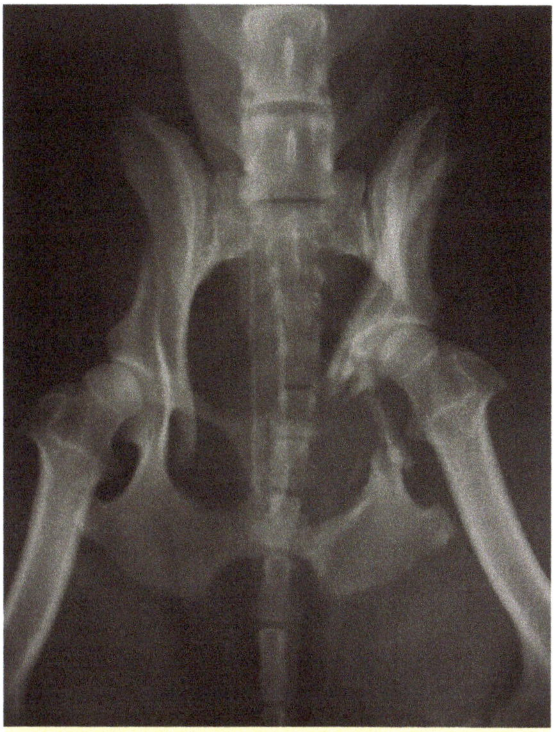

Figure 2.20
Radiograph of the fractured pelvis of a middle-aged male Jack Russell terrier that had been involved in a road traffic accident. There are numerous fractures on both sides of the pelvis. The pelvis forms a box-like structure and it is unusual to find single fractures after such traumatic events. The left and right ilia are both fractured with comminuted fractures of the left ischium and pubis, which has disintegrated. Fortunately the left acetabulum was intact and there was no sacroiliac luxation. Also there was no permanent damage to the obturator or sciatic nerves. Following orthopedic surgery, this little dog progressed very well and was completely sound approximately 10 months later.

it may also present as acute lameness. Diagnosis requires radiography. Treatment is surgical with removal of the necrotic bone of the femoral head and neck, known as a femoral head excision arthroplasty. After this procedure the prognosis for pain-free ambulation is surprisingly good with analgesia and appropriate physical therapy, which strengthens the muscles and helps create a "false-joint" or pseudoarthrosis.

Hypertrophic osteodystrophy. Hypertrophic osteodystrophy (HOD), also known as metaphyseal osteopathy (MO), has an idiopathic etiology. It tends to occur in rapidly growing large and giant breeds between two and eight months of age. In the author's experience, at the time of writing, this is not a very common disease.

Clinically young dogs become depressed, may develop a fever and have painful limbs with very firm, hot, and swollen joints. Primarily the long bones are affected, especially the distal radius, ulna, and tibia; however, other bones may also be involved. The condition tends to produce bilaterally symmetrical disease.

Diagnosis is based on clinical signs and radiological changes consistent with the disease. Treatment involves the use of nonsteroidal anti-inflammatory drugs, which act as analgesics and antipyretics, opiate analgesics, fluid therapy, and antibiotics if blood cultures demonstrate bacteremia (blood-borne infection).

The prognosis depends on the severity of the disease. In some extreme cases dogs have died. Although the disease appears to be self-limiting there may be long-term growth-plate abnormalities that can affect bones and associated joints in the more severe form of the disease.

Osteochondrosis. Osteochondrosis is a developmental orthopedic disease that affects cartilage growth in certain joints of young, actively growing animals. Usually dogs of around five to 10 months of age will be affected. The condition was first reported in dogs in 1939 by Brinker who described shoulder lameness in a Great Dane (Leighton 1998). A manifestation of this disease is osteochondritis dissecans (OCD), where a flap of cartilage detaches partially or completely from a joint surface (Figs 2.21A–D).

The etiology of this disease remains unclear, with certain breeds known to be susceptible and males more frequently affected than females. It is thought to be multifactorial with genetics, nutrition, growth rate, level of exercise, and local mechanical factors all being involved. The etiology may also vary between different susceptible breeds. Often the condition is bilateral (Breur et al. 2012).

Joints commonly affected include the shoulder, elbow, hip, stifle, hock, and LS junction. The disease develops slowly resulting in lameness, which may range from mild to severe. The severity of the lameness is likely to worsen with the duration and intensity of exercise.

Diagnosis requires radiography with possible contrast arthrography, arthroscopy, or CT scans. Not all cases require surgery but in those where it is necessary the prognosis will depend on the joint affected. The outcome of shoulder surgery is good compared with the elbow and the hock where the long-term prognosis is very guarded. Long-term sequelae are osteoarthritis, reduced range of motion of the joint, and muscle atrophy.

Panosteitis. The etiology of panosteitis remains unknown. It tends to affect certain breeds of large dog from two months to five years of age, although most cases are probably aged between four and 18 months. Breeds affected include the GSD, Basset Hound, golden retrievers, Labrador retrievers, Doberman Pinscher, Airedale, Samoyed, Saint Bernard, Irish setter but also the Scottish terrier and miniature schnauzer. The ulna, radius, humerus, femur, and tibia can all be affected with males being more commonly affected than females

The condition is occasionally referred to as canine "growing pains." Digital pressure applied directly onto the affected part of a bone will elicit a pain response. Affected dogs generally respond well to nonsteroidal analgesics or the use of prednisolone corticosteroids.

Patellar luxation. This is a problem in many dogs, with smaller breeds more commonly affected than the larger ones. The condition may be congenital, developmental or less commonly acquired through trauma. In developmental patellar luxation there may be a hereditary component to the condition. In the normal hind limb the patella should be located in a deep trochlear groove on the cranial surface of the distal end of the femur. If there is misalignment of the quadriceps, trochlear groove, and tibial tuberosity there is a resultant "bowstring effect." Consequently, the patella will be displaced either medially or laterally out of the trochlear groove. A patella alta (a patella placed unusually high relative to the femoral trochlea) and shallow trochlear groove may also contribute to the development of this condition. In small dogs medial luxation appears more common. The condition may be unilateral or bilateral. There are four grades of patellar luxation depending on the severity. Grade 1 is mild while grade 4 is very severe with permanent luxation of the patella. Long-term complications of the condition are genu varum (bow-leg), internal rotation of the distal limb, cranial cruciate ligament rupture, and osteoarthritis. Grade 1 cases are often not lame and usually do not require surgery. However, grade 3 and 4 cases require surgery and the sooner it is performed the better the long-term prognosis.

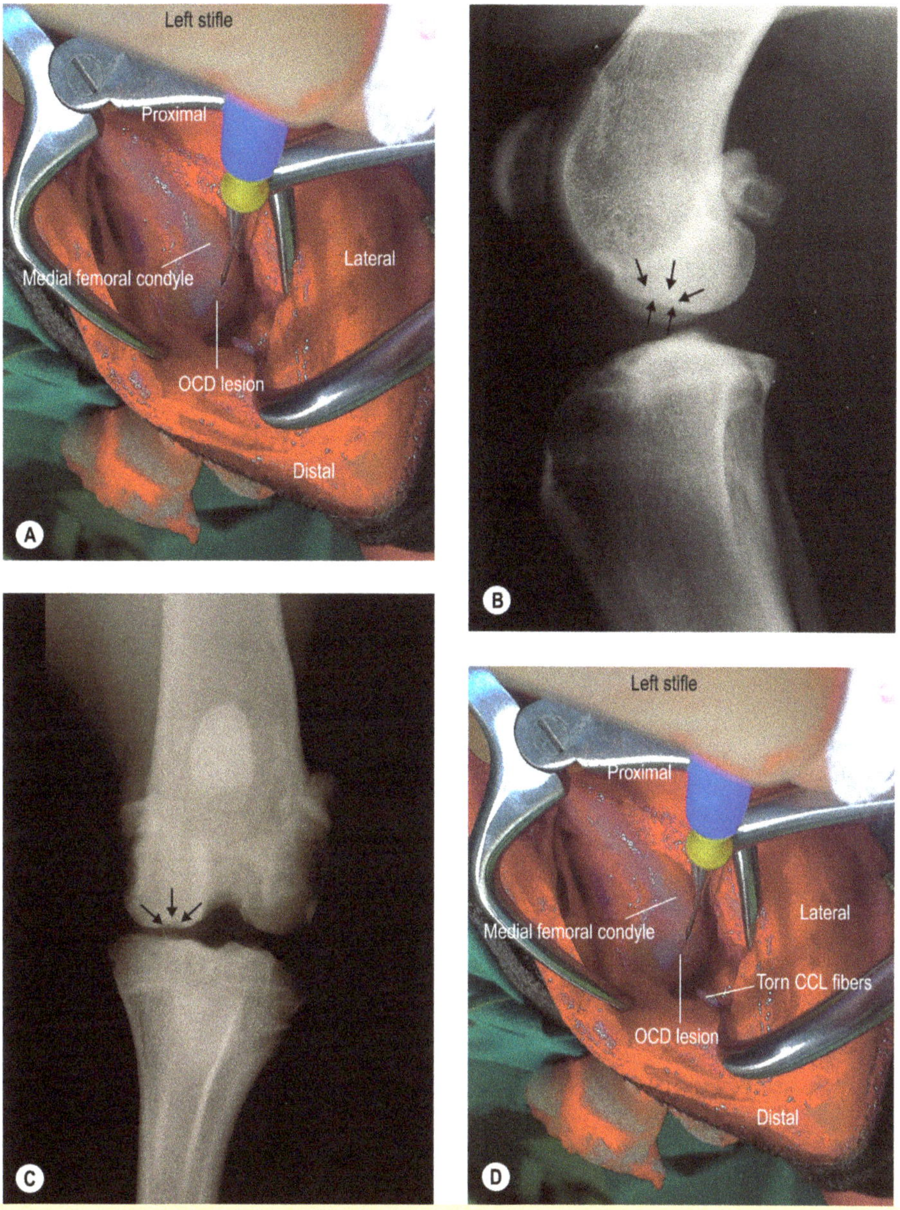

Figure 2.21

Photographs and radiographs of a three-year-old male Labrador with osteochondrosis of the medial femoral condyle with concurrent damage to the cranial cruciate ligament. Radiography confirmed the presence of flattened medial femoral condyles and semicircular radiolucent lesions in the medial femoral condyles. At surgery a defect within the articular cartilage was found that was consistent with osteochondritis dissecans. This was curetted out and left to fill with fibrocartilage. There was also concurrent cranial cruciate ligament damage. Consequently, bilateral TTAs were performed to protect the remains of the cruciate ligaments and menisci. Water treadmill hydrotherapy and osteopathy followed, and 18 months afterwards the dog shows no obvious sign of lameness. (A) Surgical intervention to the stifle showing the OCD lesion. (B) Lateral view radiograph of a stifle with OCD. (C) Radiograph of a dorsoventral view of a stifle with OCD. (D) Surgical intervention to the stifle showing a torn CrCL.

Chapter 2

Traumatic orthopedic disease

The list of possible combinations of trauma sustained by soft and skeletal tissues is infinite. Presentation of the patient to the veterinarian may be immediate, days after the event and sometimes months, or even years later. Late presentation of the patient and the presence of infection associated with open wounds greatly reduce the prognosis for a speedy and complete recovery. Following prompt medical and surgical management, which may necessitate referral to a specialist referral center, appropriate rehabilitation such as hydrotherapy, physiotherapy, and osteopathy can greatly assist the patient in making a quicker recovery. Unless there is specific referral by a veterinarian there should be no intervention by nonveterinary practitioners. They may cause injury and/or expose themselves to potential litigation.

Infectious orthopedic disease

Bone, synovial joints, musculoskeletal soft tissues, and intervertebral discs can all become infected with bacteria and fungus. Infection of bone is known as osteomyelitis, while a joint infection is a septic arthritis and infections of intervertebral discs and their associated vertebral end plates are known as discospondylitis. There are a number of means by which skeletal tissues can become infected. The first is trauma, especially open fractures, while the second is by hematological spread of the micro-organisms in the bloodstream. There are also cases of infection associated with penetrating or migrating foreign bodies, for example, grass seeds, the presence of orthopedic implants, and, in the occasional case, severely osteoarthritic joints.

Bacterial infections appear much more common than those caused by fungus. Whatever the etiology their treatment can often prove challenging, especially in the presence of orthopedic implants. Confirmation of diagnosis requires radiography and the successful culture of samples taken from the infected site. Once identified the clinician must deliver the appropriate antimicrobial in adequate concentration for a sufficient duration, which is usually around four to 12 weeks, to clear up the infection. Often implants must be removed, and the choice of antimicrobials may be made according to laboratory sensitivity tests and potential toxicity of the medication when used systemically. Some drugs are toxic when administered in the high doses required to penetrate the bone, and consequently methods must be employed to deliver the drugs locally to the infected site. Problems arise when certain antibiotic-resistant bacteria are isolated, such as methicillin-resistant *Staphylococcus aureus* or *Pseudomonas aeruginosa* species.

Osteomyelitis. Osteomyelitis refers to an infection of the bone, which is usually bacterial but may be fungal. The commonest causes of the infection are following orthopedic surgery. Infection may arise through contamination in the hospital environment (nosocomial infections), but infections can also result from hematogenous spread of bacteria that settle at the site of the fracture or implants at a later time. Infection is also seen secondary to a migrating or penetrating foreign body. Open fractures involving the bone penetrating through the skin can be contaminated directly by bacteria in the environment. Closed fractures can also become infected, especially if implants are used to reduce and stabilize the fracture site. Implants may develop a glycocalyx carbohydrate coating that enables bacteria to lie dormant and unaffected by antibiotics. These bacteria can subsequently act as a focus for future recurrences of infection and inflammation.

Osteomyelitis usually causes bone pain and lameness if limbs are affected. It will result in heat, pain, and swelling in the area of infection and may also result in a discharging sinus; however, this does not always occur. Diagnosis relies on imaging, which is not always definitive; the radiological appearance of an infected area of bone can be confused with other conditions, such as neoplasia. Definitive diagnosis requires swabs, or tissue, taken for microbiological culture and microscopy. The clinical history, the presence of implants (especially if loose), or the confirmation of foreign bodies are all taken into account when confirming a diagnosis.

Treatment requires that loose implants, and any foreign bodies, are removed and appropriate antibiotics are dispensed for four to six weeks. The patient must have minimal exercise so that the affected part of the bone is not overstressed. For this reason rehabilitation employing osteopathy and hydrotherapy all help to maintain muscle mass and maintain free, full range of motion of the joints.

Discospondylitis. Discospondylitis is an inflammatory reaction in intervertebral discs and the adjacent vertebral body end plates due to infection. Usually the infection is bacterial but it may also be due to a fungal agent. It is usually seen in very young to middle-aged animals.

Clinical signs range from fever and stiffness to back pain. Initial signs can be quite subtle; however, it can progress to severe neurological problems in severe cases that have not been treated.

Diagnosis requires urine and blood cultures plus diagnostic imaging. Radiological changes can take two to six weeks to become apparent. In such cases MRI and CT may prove more useful if this condition is suspected.

Treatment is medical. In cases of bacterial infection, antibiotic courses of up to four months may be required. The prognosis for bacterial discospondylitis is good if appropriate antibiotic therapy is commenced before neurological signs develop; however, it is poor if a fungus is involved.

Arthritis

Arthritis is an inflammatory process affecting synovial joints. There are numerous different types of arthritis. Broadly these can be categorized as osteoarthritis (degenerative joint disease or DJD), traumatic arthritis, infective arthritis (bacterial, protozoal, and fungal infection), and immune-mediated arthritides such as rheumatoid arthritis and systemic lupus erythematosus.

Osteoarthritis. The most common form of arthritis that is diagnosed in the dog is osteoarthritis, although the other forms are also encountered.

Osteoarthritis can develop very early on in a dog's life secondary to hip or elbow dysplasia, osteochondrosis, and trauma. It is a very common condition that can adversely affect the quality of life. There is little doubt that this condition is an extremely common cause for presentation of the canine patient to the veterinarian. Diagnosis can be made by clinical examination, previous clinical history, cytology of synovial fluid aspirates, and radiology. Clinically the patient will present with a combination of the following clinical signs: lameness, joint pain, soft tissue swelling around the joint, joint thickening, crepitus, and a restricted range of motion upon manipulation.

Management may be conservative and rely on weight loss, controlled exercise regimens, osteopathy, hydrotherapy, and acupuncture together with medication using nonsteroidal anti-inflammatory drugs (NSAIDs) and other analgesics such as tramadol, gabapentin and acetaminophen (paracetamol). In addition, pentosan polysulphate sodium is a licensed pharmaceutical that is widely used by veterinarians in the UK and, finally, there are many advocates of unlicensed neutraceuticals, such as various presentations of glucosamine and chondroitin.

There are occasions when arthritis requires surgical intervention. Such measures include arthrodesis, where a joint is fused, and prosthetic joint replacement. Total hip replacement has been performed for many years now in the dog whereas prosthetic elbow replacement and partial replacement of the stifle are relatively new concepts.

Septic arthritis. Joints that are infected with bacteria quickly become very swollen, hot and tender. The dog will be very lame and may have a fever. Septic arthritis is a very serious condition of the joint because it is extremely destructive to the articular cartilage and other joint structures, leading to very significant long-term complications. If suspected, the joint should be radiographed and a sample of synovial fluid or membrane obtained immediately for culture and microscopy. An affected joint is treated by lavage with large volumes of sterile saline, or even surgery, and high-dose antimicrobial therapy with appropriate antibiotics.

An important part of the treatment of this condition is swimming, water-treadmill exercise, and other passive range of motion exercises that ensure full joint mobility because normal weight-bearing is too painful for the patient. Terrestrial exercise must be very limited because of the potential damage to the joint structures and surrounding bone. Prognosis can be variable and depends very much on the severity of the condition at the time of diagnosis, the aggressiveness of the medical therapy, and the successful implementation of the rehabilitation exercises.

In the long term the joint may become severely osteoarthritic and even ankylose naturally. There may also be permanent pain from an immune-mediated response. Salvage surgery may be indicated at a later date to perform ankylosis or possibly to implant a prosthetic joint.

Neoplastic orthopedic disease

Neoplasia is a process of inappropriate tissue development such that its growth is uncoordinated and the rate of growth exceeds that of normal tissue. This growth continues in a similar fashion beyond the time at which the stimuli responsible for its initiation have been removed. Neoplasia results in the formation of neoplasms (tumors or cancers). In the musculoskeletal system neoplasia may develop within the bones, muscles, connective tissue, and nerve tissue. Predisposing factors may include genetics, previous trauma, infection, and the presence of orthopedic implants. In addition, there are a number of predilection sites for bone neoplasms in the dog. These include the proximal humerus, distal radius, skull, ribs, distal femur, and proximal tibia. Treatment options for neoplasms of MSK tissues include radical surgery, limb amputations (with or without chemotherapy), or euthanasia. In most cases the prognosis is extremely guarded to very poor. Life expectancy is often less than a year by the time the diagnosis has been made. This is due to the locally aggressive nature of the neoplasia or secondary metastatic disease where the neoplasia has disseminated to other parts of the body.

Neurological conditions

Intervertebral disc herniation

There are two basic forms of disc herniation. Firstly, there is the Hansen type 1 from where the central nucleus pulposus is explosively ejected out of the annulus fibrosus. This dorsal extrusion of the disc material into the neural canal classically causes very sudden onset incapacity due to acute pain, paresis, or paralysis. It is frequently seen in chondrodystrophoid-type dogs such as the dachshund. Secondly there is the Hansen type 2 form which results in a more chronic, slow and progressive bulging, or protrusion, of the disc material into the neural canal. This tends to occur in non-chondrodystrophoid breeds.

Intervertebral disc herniation occurs in the cervical, thoracolumbar, lumbar, and lumbosacral spine. The presence of the intercapital ligament between the rib heads protects the thoracic spine from injurious disc herniation between T2 and T11.

Clinical signs of disc herniation can vary widely depending on the location of the disc or discs affected and the type and severity of the herniation. Type 2 conditions may be intermittent. Signs range from mild pain and stiffness to complete paralysis. One or all four limbs may be affected.

Diagnosis requires a thorough clinical examination, competent neurological assessment, and imaging via plain radiography, with or without myelography. However, increasingly MRI and CT are becoming widely available.

Treatment for acute or chronic conditions may be conservative with the use of nonsteroidal anti-inflammatories and other analgesics. Specialist surgery, however, may be indicated. In nonambulatory cases, especially where deep pain has been lost from the limbs, surgery is essential. In these situations speed is of the essence because the prognosis will deteriorate with each passing hour that surgery is delayed.

Rehabilitation of spinal conditions should never be contemplated without consulting and working very closely with a spinal surgeon or neurologist.

Cervical spondylomyelopathy

Cervical spondylomyelopathy (CSM) is also very commonly referred to as wobbler syndrome. It tends to affect large to giant breeds of dogs such as the Doberman Pinscher, Weimaraner, Dalmatian, Rottweiler, Great Dane, bullmastiff, and Bernese and Swiss mountain dogs. In general practice it is probably most commonly seen in the Doberman Pinscher and Great Dane.

CSM tends to affect dogs over the age of three years. The mean age for presentation of Doberman Pinschers is seven years and for giant breeds it is four years.

The precise cause of the condition is unknown and there is no proven hereditary basis to date. The most commonly affected region of the spine is C6–C7 and then C5–C6, but other regions can be affected both cranially and caudally. It is possible for multiple anatomical sites to be affected.

Both static and dynamic factors contribute to the development of CSM through stenosis (narrowing of the vertebral canal) which will compress and subject the spinal cord to axial stress.

Clinical signs usually develop gradually, and include an abnormal gait with neurological deficits. In only about 5–10 percent of cases is neck pain apparent. The main neurological deficit is proprioceptive ataxia which tends to affect the hind limbs more, although all four legs may be affected similarly.

Diagnostic imaging is required for confirmation of the diagnosis. This includes plain radiography, myelography, CT scanning, and MRI.

Treatment may be conservative or surgical. Conservative management involves the use of a harness in place of a neck collar, restricted exercise, and employment of medical therapy using NSAIDs or corticosteroids. Careful use of physical therapy may also be of benefit in managing these cases. There is approximately 50 percent improvement following conservative management. Surgery is indicated in certain cases but the specific guidelines are unclear, and what is confusing is that many different surgical techniques have been proposed. Surgery is associated with a significant number of complications including iatrogenic damage to the spinal cord and vasculature. In addition, there is the "domino effect" or adjacent segment syndrome that occurs as a late postoperative complication in around a fifth of surgery cases. The problem is treated at one site which then affects adjacent intervertebral disc spaces several months later. It is reported that improvement is observed in approximately 80 percent of surgical cases; however, complications can be catastrophic.

Degenerative myelopathy or chronic degenerative radiculomyelopathy

Degenerative myelopathy (DM) or chronic degenerative radiculomyelopathy (CDRM) is not an orthopedic condition but it can mimic one and is quite common in middle-aged and older German shepherd dogs. However, the GSD is not the only breed that is affected and increasing numbers of breeds are now recognized as being susceptible. It is a progressive neurological disorder that results in the demyelination and eventual death of neurones in the spinal cord. Clinically it is painless and causes ataxia and paresis in the hind limbs with weakness and scuffing of the toes along the ground in what appears to be a lazy, swaying, "drunken," uncoordinated gait. Eventually the front limbs may also become affected.

Clinically, a tentative diagnosis is made after ruling out any other possible orthopedic (especially hip dysplasia) or neurological condition. However, an unequivocal diagnosis can only be made by postmortem histopathology. Also, CDRM fails to respond to any other form of medical therapy and this feature helps the clinician to confirm the diagnosis. The rate of progression can be quite variable. Osteopathy and hydrotherapy may help but the prognosis is very poor (Tauro and Rusbridge 2015).

Atlantoaxial subluxations

This is a rare condition that may be associated with Chiari-like malformation and syringomyelia (see below).

Chiari-like malformation and syringomyelia

Chiari-like malformation (CM) is an anatomical mismatch between the size of the brain and skull. Put simply, the skull is too small for the brain and this causes a deformation or prolapse of part of the brain (cerebellum) caudally through the foramen magnum. In turn this can affect the flow of the cerebrospinal fluid (CSF) out of the skull down the spinal cord. It can be associated with another condition, syringomyelia (SM), where small fluid-filled cavities, known as syrinxes or syringes, develop within the tissue of the spinal cord. However, not all dogs with Chiari-like malformation develop syringomyelia.

The breeds affected by CM or SM tend to be toy and small brachycephalic breeds. It is well known in the King Charles spaniel, Cavalier King Charles spaniel and Griffon Bruxellois, but these are not the only breeds and it may even be seen in Staffordshire bull terriers.

Clinical signs include head and neck pain, head or ear scratching or phantom scratching, reluctance to exercise, crying out, sleep disturbance, abnormal body posture, scoliosis, bulging eyes, strabismus (eyes that point in different directions), and anxiety.

Diagnosis relies on clinical signs and confirmation using CT scanning and MRI. There is a British Veterinary Association CM and SM assessment and grading scheme available for owners because there is evidence that the condition is genetically inherited in some breeds (Rusbridge 2014).

Treatment may be surgical and/or medical to manage the pain and attempt to reduce the CSF production. It is unlikely that physical therapy is of any benefit. Prognosis is very guarded (BVA and KC 2015).

Soft tissue and metabolic diseases

Cranial cruciate ligament disease

The cranial cruciate ligament (CrCL) is a complex structure. Its function is to resist cranial tibial thrust and limit internal rotation of the limb. Canine cruciate disease was first described in 1926 by Carlin. Later, in 1952, Paatsama stated that "Rupture of the anterior (cranial) cruciate ligament is the most common injury in the stifle joint of the dog" (Arnoczky 1988).

Since the early work of Paatsama, from 1952 onwards, numerous surgical techniques have been developed and described to treat this disabling condition in the dog (Arnoczky 1988; Vaughan 2010; Kowaleski et al. 2012; Innes 2013).

There is little doubt that this is one of the most common reasons for presentation of hind limb lameness in dogs of all age and weight ranges. Rupture of the CrCL can be the result of sudden and excessive force imposed upon it, but it is also thought that the immune system may contribute to a gradual inflammatory degradation of the CrCL collagen fibers, which leads to its ultimate rupture with the perpetuation of synovitis and pain (Bennett et al. 1988; Innes 2013). Sudden complete rupture results in acute lameness with little or no weight-bearing. Examination will reveal craniocaudal joint instability when the stifle joint is flexed, which is known as the cranial tibial drawer sign. There is another assessment used called the tibial thrust test. However, very often the condition has an insidious onset and may be bilateral. In such cases overt lameness is not easy to detect. There is a gradual transfer of load-bearing to the forelimbs with muscle atrophy in the thigh musculature and a compensatory development of the muscles in the chest and forelimbs. Upon palpation of the stifle joints there will be joint thickening with the formation of a medial, knobbly thickening known as a medial tibial buttress. In these chronic cases very little cranial drawer may be evident due to secondary fibrosis and thickening of the joint which partially stabilizes it.

Diagnosis relies on clinical examination, radiology, and, where available, arthroscopic examination.

Treatment ranges from conservative management to a very wide range of surgical techniques.

Small dogs under the weight of 6–7 kg may do well with conservative management, i.e., rest, NSAIDs, and osteopathy. If there is little improvement after six to eight weeks then surgery will be indicated.

Medium-sized dogs (7-20 kg) usually require surgery. Surgery may employ extra-articular stabilization where a synthetic material is used external to the joint to reduce cranial tibial thrust. Alternatively, intra-articular stabilization may be used whereby a graft, typically fashioned from a strip of fascia lata, is passed through the joint in a craniocaudal direction to mimic the torn CrCL. This technique is no longer in vogue because it does not provide long-term stability of the joint.

Large dogs in excess of 20 kg always require surgery. There are many techniques described and employed, each with its own particular indications, pros, cons, and advocates. There is the tibial plateau leveling osteotomy (TPLO), the tibial closing wedge osteotomy (TCWO), the tibial tuberosity advancement (TTA), the tibial tuberosity advancement rapid (TTAR), the modified Maquet procedure, tibial tuberosity advancement (MMP-TTA) and the triple tibial tuberosity (TTO). The surgical procedure usually involves examining the joint for torn menisci, in particular the medial meniscus which is more prone to shearing damage that results in tears. The success rates in experienced hands, appears to be similar with all the different techniques.

In around 40 percent of cases of CrCL rupture the contralateral CrCL will tear within approximately two years. To help prevent this early osteopathic intervention is strongly recommended. Further, late onset meniscal tears can occur months or years after surgery and require secondary arthrotomy. An affected joint will always succumb to progressive osteoarthritis following CrCL rupture, even after prompt surgical intervention. The use of NSAIDs, pentosan polysulfate sodium, osteopathy and hydrotherapy, and ensuring the dog is kept lean and fit all help in maintaining a functioning, pain-free stifle joint for as long as possible following CrCL rupture (see Fig. 2.21D).

Fibrotic myopathy of the gracilis and semitendinosus muscles in German shepherds

Fibrotic myopathy and contracture of these muscles in the GSD is occasionally seen in dogs aged around three to seven years. The cause is unknown, but it has been postulated that the condition may arise as a result of a repetitive strain injury in very active individuals such as police dogs.

There appears to be no pain in affected individuals. The mechanical lameness is initially quite subtle, but gradually progresses to an abnormal and somewhat bizarre gait. The affected hind limb moves in a stilted fashion with some circumflexion and inward rotation of the foot. The stride is usually shorter than usual. The affected muscles can be palpated as a firm and tight fibrous band.

There is no satisfactory means of surgical or medical treatment for this condition. Intensive rehabilitation using osteopathy and hydrotherapy may be of benefit. Working dogs invariably have to be retired.

Greyhound foot pad corns

The cause of foot pad keratomas or corns is not clear. These corns may arise at the site of previous penetrating foreign bodies, have an underlying mechanical etiology, or possibly be secondary to a papilloma virus infection. The lesion is a circular, hard, hyperkeratotic structure 3–4 mm in diameter that develops in one or more pads. It may be raised and visible to the naked eye. It usually causes lameness and a pain response is produced by pressing firmly against the affected pad. Although it can affect different breeds, in general practice it seems to be most common in the greyhound.

Treatment involves surgical excision, but more corns will often develop in the same pad or in the pads of other feet. For that reason, the long-term prognosis for an affected individual is guarded.

Diabetes mellitus, hyperadrenocorticism (Cushing's disease), hypovitaminosis D (rickets), and nutritional secondary hyperparathyroidism

It is likely the osteopath will occasionally see patients where these conditions are involved. However, they are very much a primary veterinary medical condition, and while osteopathy might aid treatment it should not be used solely as an alternative treatment. The scope of this book precludes their detailed consideration.

Differential diagnosis

Table 2.3 summarizes the main points concerning differential diagnosis of orthopedic conditions affecting the canine patient.

Osteopathic evaluation

A full history should be taken and combined with the history from the veterinary surgeon in order to form a working assessment before any examination is carried out. The owner's experience and perception of the problem must be translated into an ordered and coherent body of information. Be alert as serious pathologies can slip through the net, particularly if there has been a time lapse since the referral from the vet. The clinical picture can change and develop in a matter of days. Be vigilant for red flags and contraindications to treatment.

Take time to obtain details and record phrases that may make more sense when looking back at the notes. Owners are often very observant but their recall may not be very well organized. Concentrate on what the owner noticed - not on their diagnosis! For a comprehensive approach to this see the section on Taking an animal case history in Chapter 1. The family history of the dog (sire, dam, siblings) is very relevant, not only for hereditary conditions, but also for temperament tendencies and socializing influences. The owner's own family dynamics (illness, death, divorce, new baby, new partner) are also relevant.

While taking the history, observe the dog's behavior as this is a guide to its temperament. Is it hiding behind the owner or furniture, sitting, lying quietly, panting, yawning, chatting, demanding attention, agitated, or exploring happily?

Veterinary history

Note the details of any surgery or medication, current or previous, and the response to it. Be aware that some owners can allow their personal prejudice regarding drug therapy to prevent administration of medication, and some owners are just not diligent in this regard.

Gender

If the dog has been neutered, note at what age, how recently, and for what reason. Was it for social reasons or due to temperament or pathology?

Breed

For an outline of conditions that affect specific breeds see the section on Common orthopedic conditions earlier in this chapter.

Age

Note the age of the patient. Longevity varies with the breed, as does how quickly a dog ages.

Weight

Sudden weight change (loss or gain) may indicate pathology. Many owners use treats to train their dogs and forget to include these in the overall food allowance, resulting in overweight pets! Obesity predisposes the dog to both mechanical and systemic problems. More rarely the dog may be underfed or overexercised and be overly lean.

Signalment

See Tables 2.1 and 2.2.

Clinical signs of musculoskeletal conditions

The most common presentation is lameness. How it presents may give some indication of pathology. Is there weakness or ataxia?

Some dogs may express pain vocally - whining, yelping, or even screaming. The degree of vocalization is not necessarily representative of the level of pain but can be a personality characteristic.

Is there difficulty rising from sitting or lying, or jumping into a car? There may be reluctance to run or jump, or poor exercise tolerance. The owner may report problems with eating, drinking, and gnawing on

Table 2.3 Differential diagnosis

Age	Condition	Onset	Clinical signs	Duration	Etiology	Veterinary treatment	Prognosis
0–3 months	Fractures	Acute	Lameness	2–3 months	Trauma	External support, surgery, rest	Usually good
3–6 months	Hip dysplasia	Gradual	Bunny-hopping, hind limb weakness, hip pain, lameness	Potentially lifelong	Genetic, diet, overexercise	Limited exercise, controlled and balanced diet, osteopathy, physiotherapy, hydrotherapy, surgery	Very variable
	Luxating patella	Gradual	Intermittent lameness with very brief lifting of the foot off the ground	Potentially lifelong	Complex anatomical conformation abnormalities	Surgery	Usually good
	Elbow dysplasia	Gradual	Lameness and elbow pain	Potentially lifelong	Genetic, diet, overexercise	Limited exercise, controlled and balanced diet, surgery	Guarded with long-term sequelae
	Fractures	Acute	Lameness	2–3 months	Trauma	External support, surgery, rest	Very good
	Salter–Harris growth plate fractures	Acute	Lameness	2–3 months	Trauma or overexertion	External support, surgery, rest	Variable with potential long-term sequelae
	Panosteitis	Gradual	Lameness and pain with pressure on affected areas of long bones	Approximately 3 months	Unknown	NSAID analgesics	Very good
	Nutritional secondary hyperparathyroidism	Gradual	Variable – swollen joints, lameness, stunted growth, pathological fractures	3–4 months	Inappropriate diet	Correction of diet	Usually good
	Craniomandibular osteopathy (CMO)	Gradual	Head and jaw pain	Approximately 6 months	Unknown	Corticosteroids or NSAID analgesics	Very good
6–12 months	Hip dysplasia	Gradual	Bunny-hopping, hind limb weakness, hip pain, lameness	Potentially lifelong	Genetic, diet, overexercise	Limited exercise, controlled and balanced diet, osteopathy, physiotherapy, hydrotherapy, surgery	Very variable
	Luxating patella	Gradual	Intermittent lameness with very brief lifting of the foot off the ground	Potentially lifelong	Complex anatomical conformation abnormalities	Surgery	Usually good

Table 2.3 *Continued*

Age	Condition	Onset	Clinical signs	Duration	Etiology	Veterinary treatment	Prognosis
	Elbow dysplasia	Gradual	Lameness and elbow pain	Potentially lifelong	Genetic, diet, overexercise	Limited exercise, controlled and balanced diet, surgery	Guarded with long-term sequelae
	Fractures	Acute	Bone pain, swelling, lameness	Variable	Trauma	External support or surgery	Very good
	Salter–Harris growth plate fractures	Acute	Lameness	2–3 months	Trauma or overexertion	External support with rest or surgery	Variable with potential long-term sequelae
	Osteochondritis dissecans (OCD)	Gradual	Lameness	Very variable	Genetic, diet, over-exercise	NSAID analgesics, rest, surgery	Very variable depending on which joint is affected
	Panosteitis	Gradual	Lameness and pain with pressure on affected areas of long bones	3 months	Unknown	NSAID analgesics	Very good
	Discospondylitis	Gradual	Back pain and fever	Variable	Unknown but hematological spread of bacteria likely	NSAID analgesics and antibiotics	Good
	Legg–Calvé–Perthes disease	Gradual	Progressive lameness of the affected limb, often unilateral. Pain with internal rotation of the hip and abduction	Lifelong	Unknown	Surgery, osteopathy, physiotherapy, hydrotherapy	Good
	Nutritional secondary hyperparathyroidism	Gradual	Variable – swollen joints, lameness, stunted growth, pathological fractures	Months	Inappropriate diet	Correction of diet	Usually good
	Metaphyseal osteopathy	Gradual	Joint swelling and pain, fever	1–2 months	Various proposed but unknown	Antipyretics	Variable
	Craniomandibular osteopathy (CMO)	Gradual	Head and jaw pain, especially when the mouth is opened. The dog may only be able to open the mouth partially	6 months	Unknown	Corticosteroids or NSAID analgesics	Very good

Table 2.3 *Continued*

Age	Condition	Onset	Clinical signs	Duration	Etiology	Veterinary treatment	Prognosis
1–3 years	Hip dysplasia	Gradual	Bunny-hopping, hind limb weakness, hip pain, lameness	Potentially lifelong	Genetic, diet, overexercise	Limited exercise, controlled and balanced diet, hydrotherapy, surgery	Very variable
	Fractures	Acute	Bone pain, swelling, lameness	Variable	Trauma	External support or surgery	Very variable
	Luxating patella	Gradual	Intermittent lameness with very brief lifting of the foot off the ground	Potentially lifelong	Complex anatomical conformation abnormalities plus trauma plus cranial cruciate disease	Surgery	Variable
	Panosteitis	Gradual	Lameness and pain with pressure on affected areas of long bones	3 months	Unknown	NSAID analgesics	Very good
3–6 years	Cranial cruciate injuries	Variable	Stifle swelling, stiffness or failure to bear weight	Chronic	Trauma and end stage of an inflammatory joint disease	Rest, NSAID analgesics, osteopathy, physiotherapy, hydrotherapy, surgery	Good but there are potential long-term sequelae
	Intervertebral disc disease	Variable	Ranging from mild back stiffness to acute, intense pain and/or paresis or paralysis	Variable	Chondrodystrophoid breeds; overexertion and spontaneous	Rest, NSAID analgesics, osteopathy, physiotherapy, surgery	Very variable
	Fractures	Acute	Bone pain, swelling, lameness	Variable	Trauma	External support or surgery	Very variable
6–12 years	Cranial cruciate injuries	Variable	Stifle swelling, stiffness or failure to bear weight	Chronic	Trauma and end stage of an inflammatory joint disease	Rest, NSAID analgesics, osteopathy, physiotherapy, hydrotherapy, surgery	Very variable
	Osteoarthritis	Gradual	Joint swelling, stiffness, crepitus and failure to bear weight	Lifelong	Joint instability, inflammatory disease processes, infection, trauma, previous surgery	Rest, NSAID analgesics, osteopathy, physiotherapy, hydrotherapy, arthrodesis surgery	Very variable

Table 2.3 Differential diagnosis *continued*

Age	Condition	Onset	Clinical signs	Duration	Etiology	Veterinary treatment	Prognosis
	Intervertebral disc disease	Variable	Ranging from mild back stiffness to acute, intense pain and/or paresis or paralysis	Variable	Chondrodystrophoid breeds, overexertion and spontaneous	Rest, NSAID analgesics, osteopathy, physiotherapy, surgery	Very variable
	Fractures	Acute	Bone pain, swelling, lameness	4–9 months	Trauma	External support or surgery	Very variable
	Neoplasia	Gradual	Bone pain (may be intense), swelling of soft tissues, lameness, possible fever	Usually fatal	Unknown or previous site of a fracture, infection or surgery	NSAID analgesics, opioid analgesics, chemotherapy, radiotherapy, surgery, euthanasia	Very poor
	Wobbler syndrome	Gradual	Variable – neck pain and hind limb and possible forelimb incoordinated and weak gait	Chronic	Genetic predisposition in certain breeds around 7–8 years of age	Rest, NSAID analgesics, osteopathy, physiotherapy, surgery	Poor
Geriatric (12–15 years)	Osteoarthritis	Gradual	Joint swelling, stiffness and failure to bear weight	Lifelong	Joint instability, inflammatory disease processes, infection, trauma, previous surgery	Rest, NSAID analgesics, osteopathy, physiotherapy, hydrotherapy, arthrodesis surgery	Very variable
	Cranial cruciate injuries	Variable	Stifle swelling, stiffness or failure to bear weight	Chronic	Trauma and end stage of an inflammatory joint disease	Rest, NSAID analgesics, osteopathy, physiotherapy, hydrotherapy, surgery	Very variable
	Neoplasia	Gradual	Bone pain (may be intense), swelling of soft tissues, lameness, possible fever	Usually fatal	Unknown or previous site of a fracture, infection or surgery	NSAID analgesics, opioid analgesics, chemotherapy, radiotherapy, surgery, euthanasia	Extremely poor
	Pathological fractures	Acute	Sudden onset, spontaneous fractures that may not be that painful resulting in lameness if limb bones are affected or back pain if vertebrae are affected	Variable	Any disease process that leads to an osteopenia (bone demineralization) and weakening of the bone	Dealing with the primary, underlying disease process	Very poor

bones or chews. Is there localized pain, heat, swelling, or edema?

Puppies

There is a huge variation in growth rates and ossification dates between breeds.

Teething and resultant excessive chewing can cause jaw (TMJ) pain.

Vaccination issues are not within our remit but it is necessary to be aware of the recommended requirements as some owners have negative views similar to those opposing their children's inoculations. Failure to keep up to date with these, and also worming and other parasite prophylactics, can have repercussions on our own health. This latter issue is of extra importance if the dog is being treated in the practitioner's home or within the environs of a human clinic (see Zoonotic disease and parasites in Chapter 1).

The prenatal and parturition history can have a bearing on the health and vitality of the individual. It is worth asking if the owner has any knowledge of the birth of their puppy. The circumstances (reputed breeder or puppy farm), location (e.g., kennel or kitchen), size of the litter, what number within that litter, natural delivery or cesarean section (for dystocia due to a malpresentation or puppy size relative to maternal pelvis size and shape, etc.).

There can also be postnatal issues due to maternal or owner inexperience or infection that cause a failure to thrive and leave a puppy weakened.

Many times the author's (NH) palpatory findings have led to enquiry about the birth history. Palpable tension or compression or inherent sympathetic irritation within a dog's system may relate back to the pregnancy or birth.

The author also believes that if a bitch has had puppies you need to obtain as many details as possible: the number of litters, outcome of each whelping, medical issues, etc. The ligamentous laxity due to the associated hormonal changes can leave the bitch musculoskeletally compromised after the puppies have been weaned.

Geriatrics

Older dogs present with many common and classic pathologies including:

- dental disease causing pain and difficulty chewing
- heart disease and circulatory problems
- renal and hepatic diseases
- degenerative joint disease (DJD).

Comorbidities are obviously more common in older dogs, highlighting the necessity of a comprehensive veterinary history. Osteopathy can augment the dog's overall vitality and health by improving blood and lymphatic circulation, keeping them mobile.

Observation of behavior and temperament

Ideally one should observe the dog arriving at the clinic, getting out of the car, and entering the premises. Does the dog's demeanor change when it realizes it is going to the vet? Many dogs behave completely differently when in a veterinary center especially if they are of a nervous disposition. Notice the dog's interaction with the owner and with other animals.

If the consultation is at a human practice then the owner can bring a blanket or fleece. Safety and hygiene issues must be observed. If the consultation is at the patient's home, then be aware that you are an intruder in their territory!

Allow the dog to assess you, by sight and smell, as this may be the first time you meet. Be aware of your own body language as well as your patient's! Talk quietly to reassure them. Be mindful of the variation in the temperament of different breeds and of every individual dog *on each occasion* you meet them.

Be confident but gentle. Respect the dog's space. Being too invasive is potentially threatening and being overly tentative will imply nervousness. Either can be perceived as a negative signal and thus provoke anxiety in your patient. Use firm, knowing hands to stroke the dog as a means of introduction and *not* as part of the examination, but do not assume full compliance. Spend time introducing yourself, allowing the dog to get used to your close presence and touch (Bradshaw 2011).

Watch the eyes, ears, lips, and teeth, whiskers, tail, hackles, and muscle tone and tension. These are the dog's communicators, expressing fear, aggression, stress, and pain. Ignore them at your peril!

If the dog is in constant pain, ataxic, or very distressed and anxious, be extremely calm and reassuring and make minimal demands of the patient during the assessment.

Osteopathic observation

General impression

"Bright-eyed and bushy-tailed" indicates a happy, healthy dog, feeling confident and unthreatened by the situation.

Look at the dog standing still. Observe the expression and general demeanor - eyes, ears, mouth, head carriage, and tail position and motion. Watch for any nose licking, yawning, panting, or abdominal tension.

Notice the overall body condition (weight, muscle tone, and bulk). Does the coat look healthy? (See Fig. 2.22A.)

Conformation

Knowledge of breed-specific variation is essential.

When checking stance and posture, look for even balance and weight-bearing on all four limbs. Assess from the front, rear, both sides, and above. Take an overview of the vertebral column, checking the head carriage (level of the ears) and relative positions of the neck, CT, TL, and LS junction areas, and the tail.

Are there normal spinal curves or are there hunched (roaching) or dipped areas, or any scoliosis?

Docking of the tail affects the mechanics of balance during locomotion. The author believes there may be remnants of the shock from the procedure within the mechanism and the wagging motion is greatly altered, becoming very rapid. The tail is a major instrument of communication in the canine world. Alterations in its functional capability may affect how the action is interpreted during socializing with other dogs.

In England tail docking is illegal except in certified working gun dogs, and has to be carried out by a licensed vet. (It is illegal in Scotland, and there are no exemptions.)

Check the positioning of the feet. Are they straight or is there rotation or asymmetry? Notice the joint heights and joint angles. There may be angular deformities ("Queen Anne" legs) in the front limbs of chondrodystrophoid breeds (for example, Basset Hounds, bulldogs, and dachshunds) and in the hind limbs in some terriers.

Assess weight distribution in the front quarters versus the hindquarters and between the four limbs. Look at the muscle volume and note any irregularity, tension, increased bulk, or wasting. Check for scuffed nails (excoriation), lick granulomata, and associated discoloration due to salivary staining.

Ensure that there are no wounds or swellings in and around the paws.

Movement

Whenever possible it is advisable to watch the dog in an area that allows freedom of movement, for example, in a car park (Fig. 2.22B). Where space is limited, the pavement area outside the clinic should be sufficient to do a gait assessment. Always be aware of safety factors for the dog, owner, and passing public.

If possible, assess the dog's gait on both hard and soft ground, as some problems will become more apparent on different surfaces.

Ask the owner to move at a speed that allows the dog to walk slowly (on a short lead but with the head loose and free to move) for a sufficient distance to establish a gait pattern. Ask the owner to return toward you and then observe passing from both sides. Slow and fast walking should be observed, and the transition between them. Slow walking can highlight a gait problem that is masked at a faster pace, and often the dog will be reticent to maintain a slow rate.

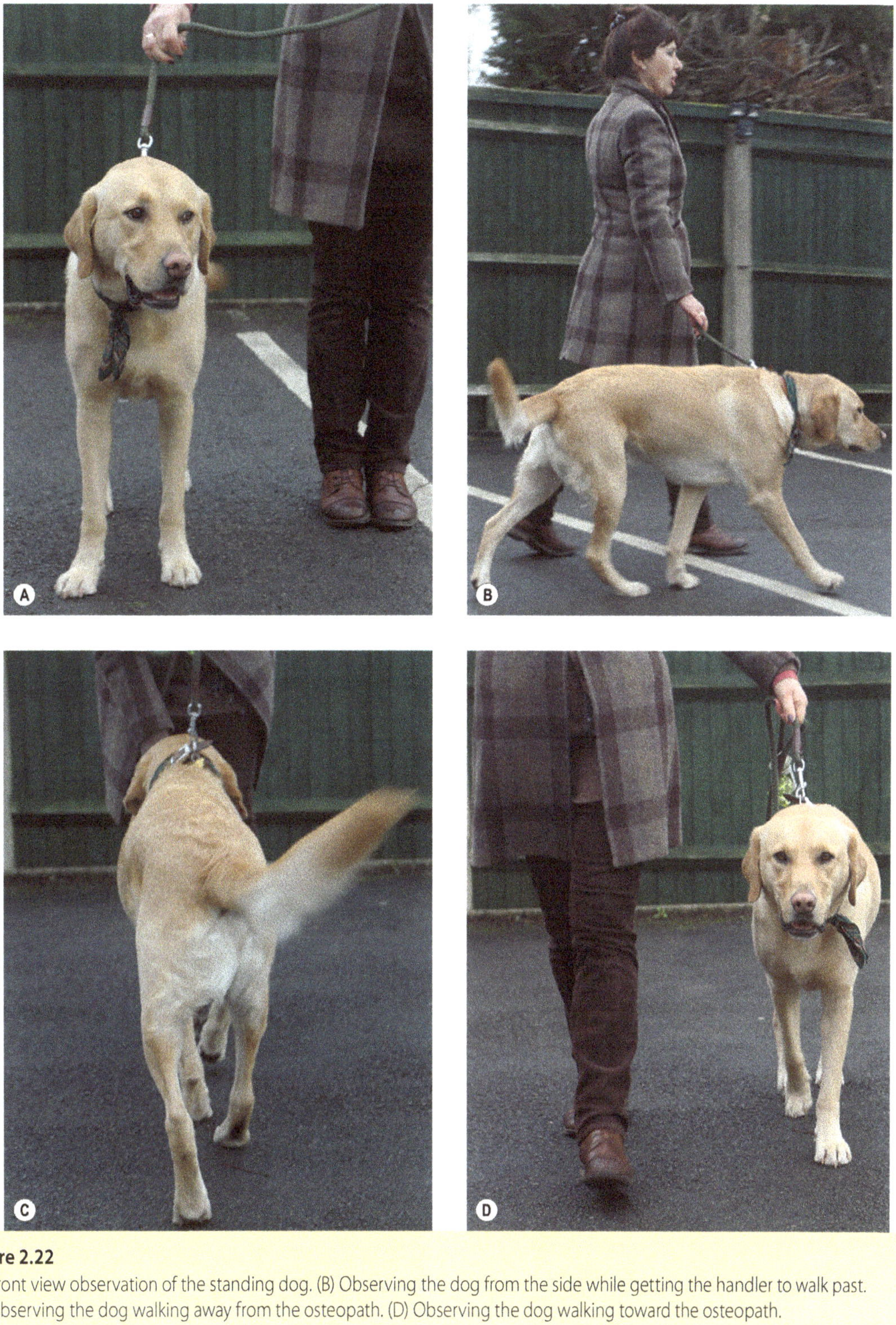

Figure 2.22

(A) Front view observation of the standing dog. (B) Observing the dog from the side while getting the handler to walk past. (C) Observing the dog walking away from the osteopath. (D) Observing the dog walking toward the osteopath.

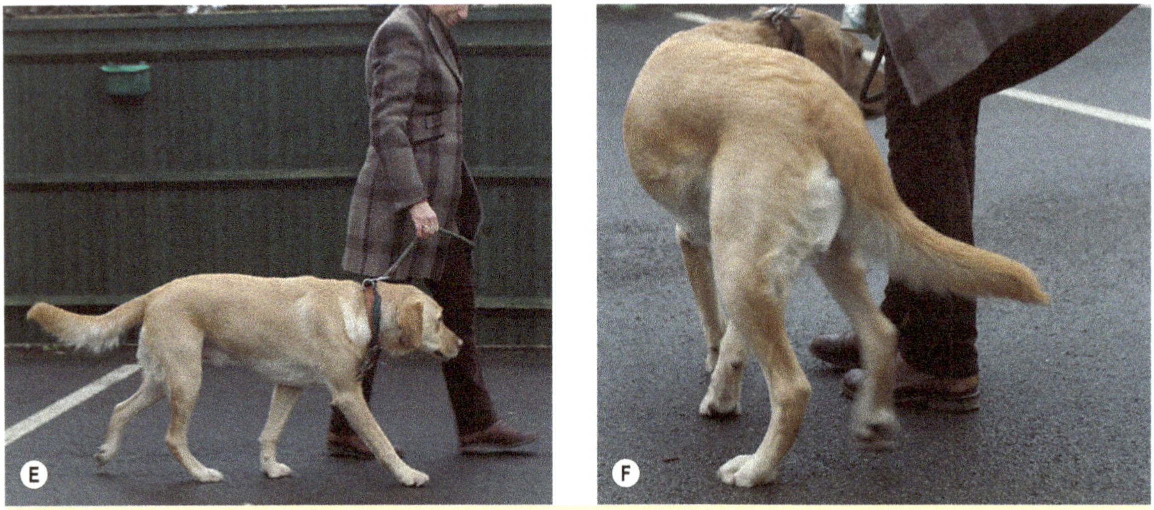

Figure 2.22—*Cont'd*
(E) Observing the dog trotting. (F) Observing the dog turn in a tight circle around the handler. Note that this should be attempted to the left and right.

Ask the owner to repeat at a trot and then run. Observe closely the transition between the speeds. Listen for any uneven foot placement. Is nail drag evident? Look for the flow of movement rather than blocks, and make allowances for the size and breed of the dog.

Observe the legs in sequence, i.e., left hind leg (LH), right hind leg (RH), left foreleg (LF), then right foreleg (RF). Form an impression of the rhythm of motion between them to help identify any abnormalities.

Observing from the behind. Look for symmetry across the hindquarters. There should be an even movement up and down across the ilia. Observe the degree of this movement. Limb movement should ideally be straight forwards and back not to the sides.

A "dishing" motion is accentuated with a loss of spinal flexibility (the limb describes a horizontal arc in the cranial phase).

There should be free movement of the neck and a well-balanced head position. Look at foot placement for tripping, stumbling, and foot or nail dragging.

Observe the height and symmetry of the tail carriage (Fig. 2.22C).

Front view. Look for straight limb movement, even head carriage, levelness across the shoulders, and breadth across the pectorals. Is there even foot placement? If lameness is present how severe is it? (See Fig. 2.22D.)

Lateral view. From the side there should be smooth motion, not in segments, and a flowing movement along the spine.

Compare the amount of weight-bearing through the thoracic and pelvic limbs. Observe head and neck carriage; dipping or nodding indicates lameness. The head nods up when the bad front leg hits the ground (Fig. 2.22E).

Hind limb lameness may also cause head-bobbing: the head goes down to shift weight-bearing further forward and take pressure off the hind legs.

Allowing for breed variations, the tail should be at an easy normal height and able to wag. Low tail carriage and lack of mobility is a sign of an unhappy dog, not just emotionally but due to pain locally in the lumbar or LS spine or pelvis, with either an orthopedic or other condition, for example, cystitis.

Turn the dog in a tight circle in both directions around the owner or handler, following a treat. Assess the ease and angle of turn in both directions (Fig. 2.22F).

Observe the dog walking backwards. Many dogs do not like doing this and are often not cooperative, however, it does highlight pelvic limb weakness and compromised coordination.

Active movements of the head and neck can be assessed using a small treat for the dog to follow into flexion (head lowering), extension (head raising), and lateral flexion in varying degrees and angles to incorporate rotation.

During all locomotion there should be good inter-limb coordination. Assess the quality of movement, fluidity, ease, springiness, and the style of gait: short high steps, long lolloping strides, light-footed, or heavy plod. There are variations with age within and between breeds.

Keep your eye on the dog while you are conversing with the owner. Often they change position demonstrating how they are most comfortable and at ease. In cases of hip, shoulder, or elbow problems they will have discomfort when weight-bearing (sitting or standing) through the affected limb, so they lie down as soon as possible. Spinal pain may well exhibit the opposite with the dog being unwilling to change from standing or move much at all. Transition from lying to standing and vice versa reveals a multitude of coping strategies as the dog avoids exertion through the painful or stiff area.

Osteopathic examination

The osteopathic examination takes into consideration all of the information and observational findings and also tries to ascertain the causation of the symptoms and any predisposing factors and compensatory patterns, leading the practitioner to be able to formulate a treatment program.

Any incidental clinical findings such as enlarged lymph nodes, lumps, swellings, and skin lesions must be reported to the vet.

Palpation

Enhanced palpatory proficiency will ensure that we know when to stop any movement before it is painful. Once the dog understands that we can sense how they feel they noticeably relax. However, there is never room for complacency.

Usually the dog is fully relaxed by the end of the first session and on the next visit comes in more confidently and often presents the offending area for treatment!

Dogs of a nervous disposition may never fully relax but merely tolerate our attentions. Sometimes the owner can help to hold or support the dog for reassurance. Many a small dog is treated while cradled in its owner's arms as if it were a baby.

Some owners, however, can be more of a hindrance than a help if they are anxious or of a worried disposition. On these occasions the assistance of a vet nurse can be invaluable if a second pair of hands is required.

Bribery with treats and chews can be useful as a mode of distraction, especially in cases of benign noncompliance. Overexuberance can be managed in much the same way as when working with undisciplined toddlers!

A muzzle may be advisable when dealing with a temperamentally unpredictable dog. The author has only rarely had to resort to using one, but it is better to be safe than sorry. Chemical restraint is resorted to only when there are insurmountable temperament problems (aggression or total noncompliance due to fear or nerves). Occasionally it is beneficial to use the opportunity of working on a dog that is already under sedation or general anesthesia for radiographs or a minor surgical procedure such as teeth scaling.

The location of the clinical examination depends on the size and temperament of the dog and necessarily the flexibility of the practitioner. Many small dogs are content to be examined and treated on a table. Medium and large breeds are happier on the floor. The use of a small stool or step can make the session less awkward for the practitioner. A large piece of vet bed (fleece) is indispensable for the comfort of both the practitioner and animal.

Most dogs begin the session standing or sitting and may progress to lying either prone, supine or on their side. Labradors and spaniels often collapse into a supine sprawling pose from the outset - not always as convenient to deal with as it may appear!

Some of the small toy breeds are happiest being held and cradled throughout.

Palpate the condition of the soft tissues. Joint mobility can be examined using short or long lever techniques. Toggling and springing are invaluable for analysis of spinal segmental mobility. Depending on the presenting case it may be appropriate to do a head-to-tail toggling exploration, incorporating an overview of rib function within the thoracic cage, before examining the limbs and abdomen.

Consider how these findings may be affecting or reflecting the function of the related visceral organs and their connecting tissues. This is a brief overall assessment and can be used to later aid the treatment.

Forequarters. For convenience, the forequarters are categorized as the combination of the head and neck, cervicothoracic and thoracic spine, ribs and forelimbs.

The musculature of the cervical and cervicothoracic spine is substantial due to its supportive, impact-absorbing and counterbalancing role. These functions are reinforced by the configuration of the underlying ligaments, particularly the ligamentum nuchae, which forms an elasticated bridge with strong recoil capacity.

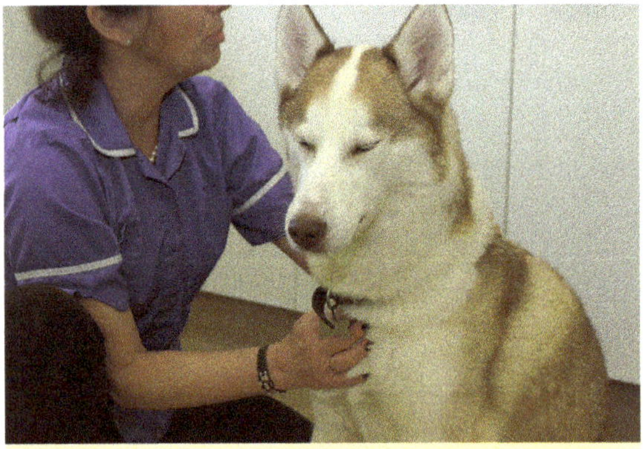

Figure 2.23
Palpating the pectoral sling and pseudo clavicle.

The position of the head and neck influences and reflects the whole body dynamics. The integrated function of all the muscles and the scapular motion can become disrupted as part of the animal's compensatory mechanisms causing dyskinesia. The author finds it useful to imagine a hammock suspended by numerous guy ropes from separate branches of a tree. There is give and take and mobility possible within each structure, and reciprocity between them all. Thus an alteration in the structure or function in any one of the components will dynamically affect all the others (Kardong 2002) (Fig. 2.23). Remember the neurovascular and lymphatic plexuses, which are anatomically related to these musculoskeletal structures and involved in the consequences of OSD. Make sure that you and the dog are suitably balanced and comfortable, then test all the directions of movement of the thoracic limb. Protraction and retraction of the forelimb includes the omothoracic complex. The shoulder joint (glenohumeral joint), can be tested for flexion, extension, and medial and lateral rotation. There is very minimal abduction and adduction as there is no bony clavicular mechanism. Also assess the "give" within the joint itself; this indicates the ability to absorb impact forces in varying degrees of the required ROM during locomotion (Figs 2.24 and 2.25).

The elbow can be guided smoothly into flexion then extension, and accessory mobility can be checked (very slight medial and lateral shift) (Fig. 2.26A and B).

Weight is transmitted through both radius and ulna, and the proximal radioulnar joint allows rotation of the forelimb and supination of the paw. Assess the rotation of the forelimb with the elbow in varying degrees of flexion. Feel for the quality of the interosseous radioulnar ligament and check for any shearing or binding pattern. Holding the antebrachium (forearm) at right angles to the humerus, gently compress and distract the elbow joint to assess its ability to absorb ground pressure transmitted though the limb (Fig. 2.27) (Renberg et al. 1999).

Evaluate the range and quality of flexion, extension, and hyperextension in the carpus, and also medial and lateral deviation. All these movements are crucial for the absorption of concussive forces and subsequent recoil. Unrestricted movement, at the articulations of the intercarpal and metacarpal joints, is fundamental for optimal adjustment to uneven surfaces and a well-sprung gait.

Palpate the ease of mobility between the metacarpals and phalanges and check for the position of the sesamoids (Fig. 2.28A–C).

The tone and texture of the muscles, tendons and ligaments will reflect their ability to stretch and recoil

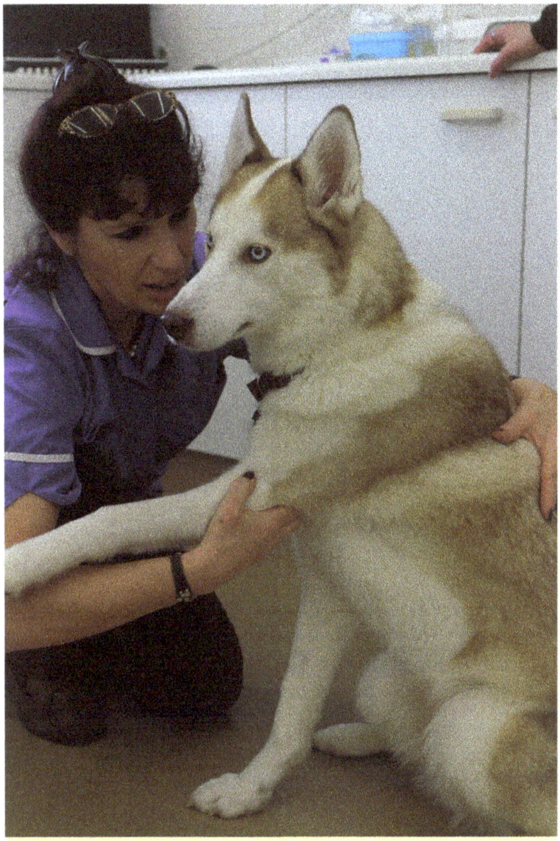

Figure 2.24
Palpating and assessing the quality and range of motion of the shoulder joint.

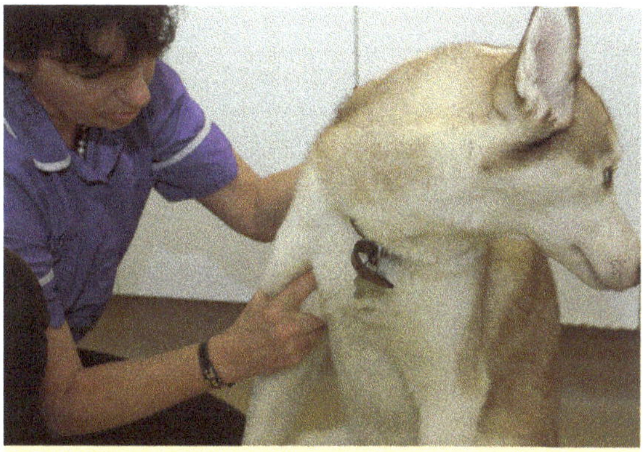

Figure 2.25
Palpating the muscular attachment of the scapula to the thorax.

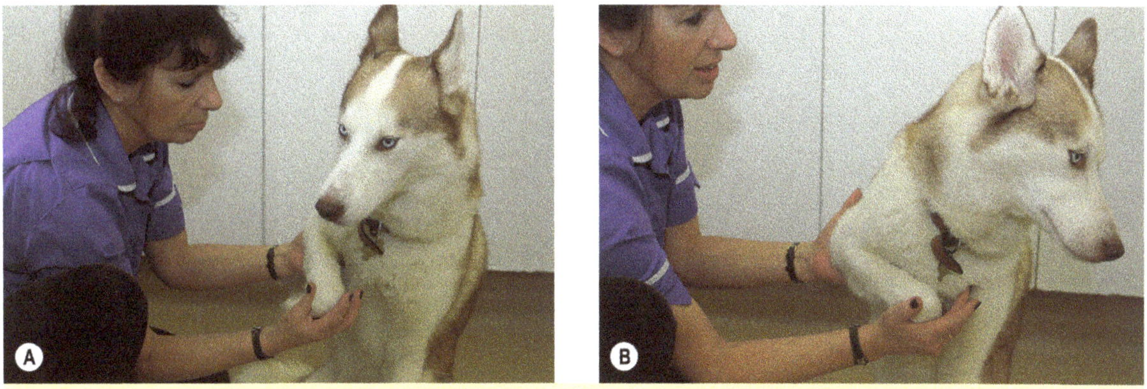

Figure 2.26
(A) Assessing forelimb flexion. (B) With the forelimb flexed, assessing lateral rotation through the shoulder joint.

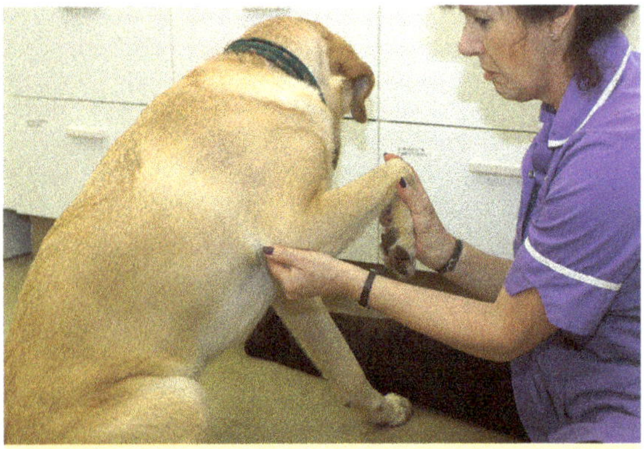

Figure 2.27
Assessing radio-ulnar-humerus articulation and motility.

during locomotion, contributing to shock absorption, weight transmission and also individual joint stability.

Good mobility in the forelimbs is necessary to accommodate stooping or crouching for drinking, eating, playing, and digging.

Overlong nails, on either forepaws or hind paws, will generate an alteration in foot placement, cause painful phalanges, and lead to altered limb mechanics.

Hindquarters. The evaluation of the hind end follows the same rationale as described for the forequarters. The prime function of the hindquarters is propulsion and shock absorption during locomotion. The pelvic

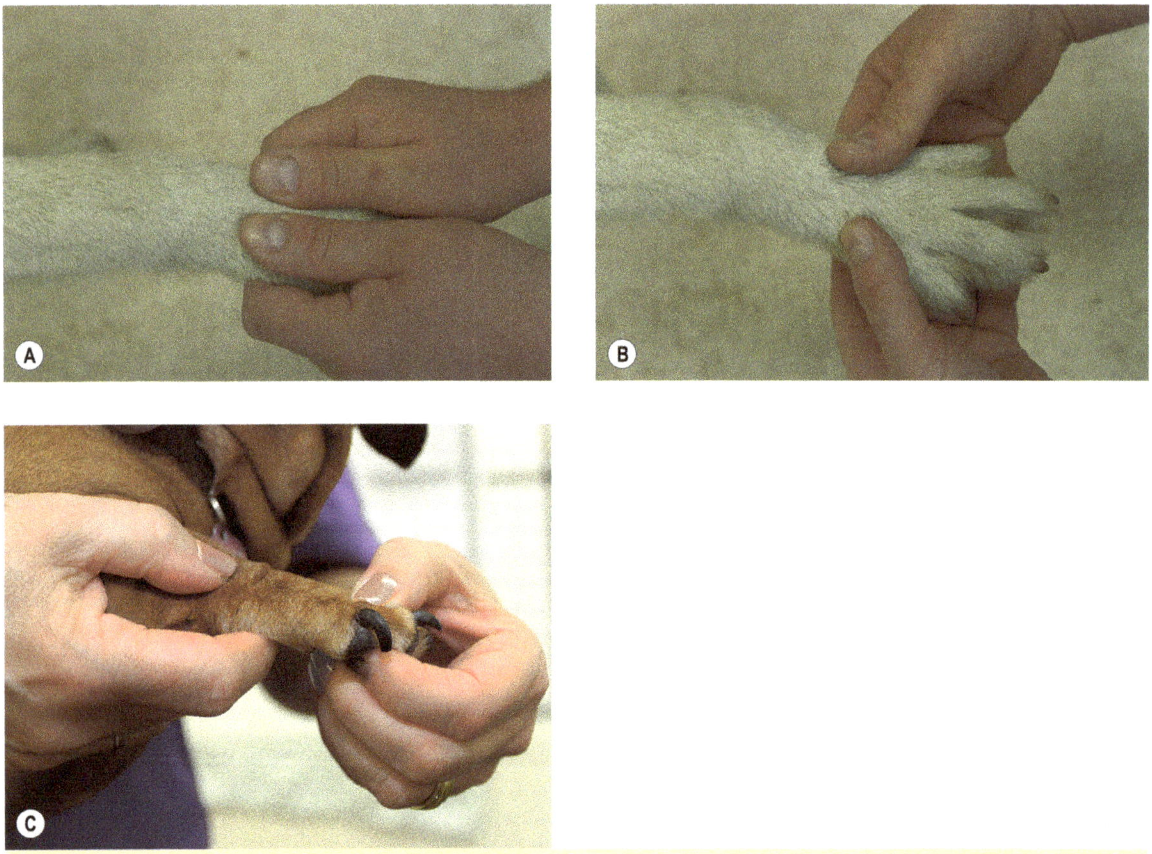

Figure 2.28
(A) Assessing the carpal joints. (B) Assessing the carpometacarpal and metacarpophalangeal joints. (C) Assessing the interphalangeal joints.

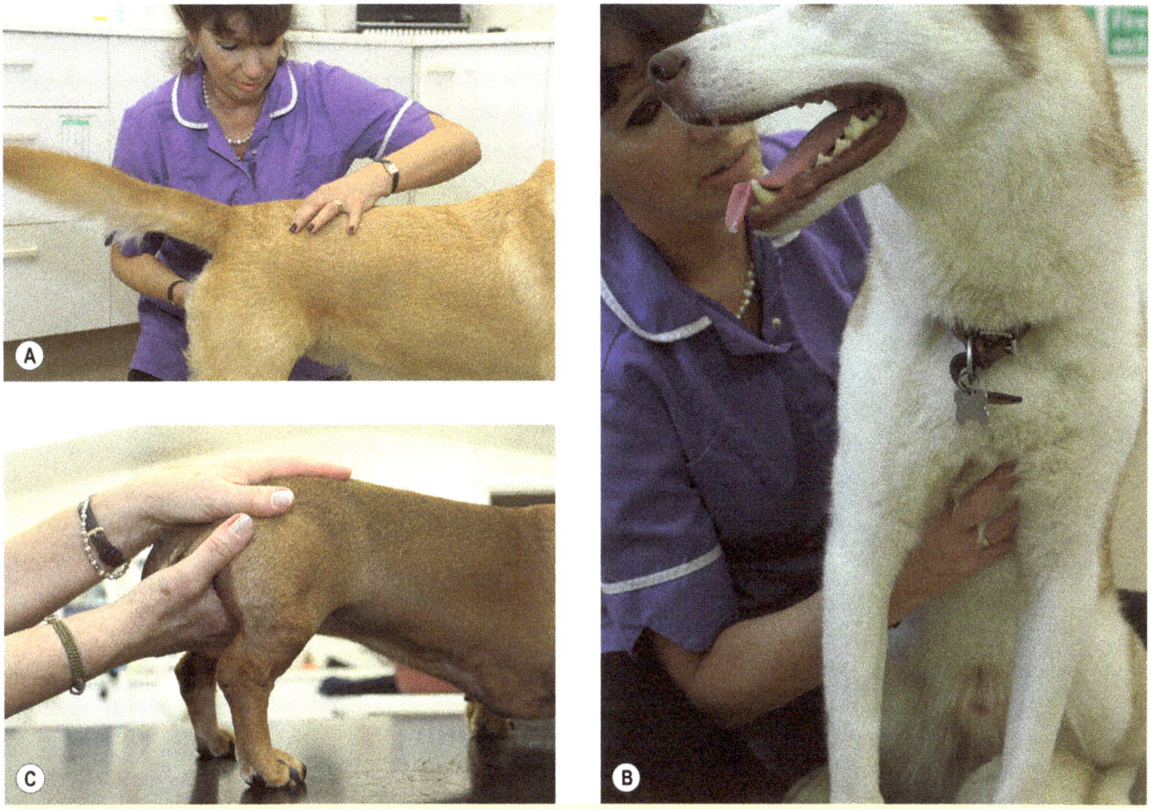

Figure 2.29
(A) Assessing the lumbar epaxial musculature. (B) Assessing the hypaxial muscles. (C) Assessing the weight and fascial directional influence on the abdominal viscera.

limb is firmly attached to the axial skeleton by a strong articular union, the sacroiliac joint, between the wings of the sacrum and ilium. The interlocking articular surfaces and dorsal and ventral sacroiliac ligaments contribute to its stability, supported by the intrinsic muscles of the hip complex.

Check the supportive epaxial muscles of the lumbar spine, the hypaxial muscles, and the weight and directional influence of the viscera (Fig. 2.29A–C).

Palpate the conformation and balance of the pelvis as a whole, dorsally and ventrally, including the tail. The number of coccygeal segments varies greatly between the different breeds, as does the shape and extent of movement. Gauge its overall relationship with the pelvic mechanics (Fig. 2.30).

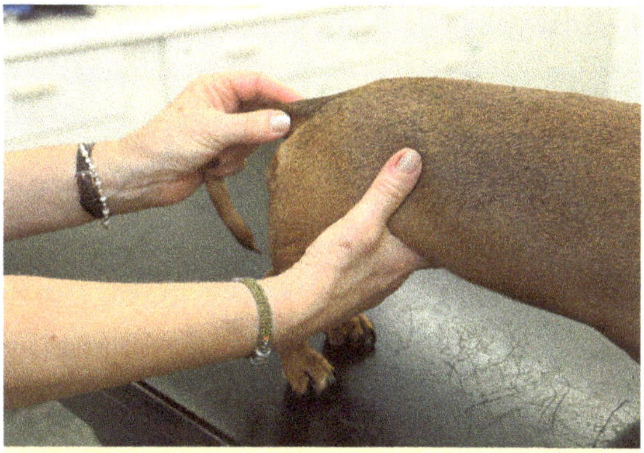

Figure 2.30
Assessing the quality of the pelvic mechanics with the aid of very gentle tail traction.

Hind limbs. The canine hip joint is a deeper ball and socket joint than the shoulder joint, and accordingly it has greater stability and a fuller range of circumduction.

Guide the limb through protraction and retraction, noting the tolerance of the TL spine to the required changes and also the ease of involvement of each peripheral joint (Fig. 2.31A and B).

Support the hind limb from just below the stifle (held in relaxed flexion), check the flexion, extension, abduction, and adduction of the hip, and also the internal and external rotation. The quality of the intra-articular motility of the hip joint can be tested by using a gentle shearing force (translocation) and by direct local application around the proximal femur.

Assessment of the stifle and hock should be carried out individually and in relation to each other, to include the functioning of the tibiofibular interosseus membrane (Fig. 2.32A).

In addition to movements through the main planes, check the accessory motions of rotation (minimal) and crosswise glide. The integrity of the ligamentous and capsular components of these joints is essential for stability. The quality of the associated musculotendinous function dictates the recoil and spring required for propulsion during locomotion (Fig. 2.32B).

Remember that a degree of lateral deviation in the hock is necessary to avoid interference with the front paws when running.

As with the distal joints of the forelimb, the tarsus, metatarsals, phalanges, and associated sesamoids should be examined and assessed in relation to the performance of the whole limb (Fig. 2.32C).

Osteopathic treatment

The therapeutic effect of touch commences immediately on contact with the patient. Remember: *less is more.*

Do not overtreat. Dogs react much more quickly than humans to osteopathic treatment.

Osteopathic treatment may be applied specifically to the site of symptoms (e.g., muscle, tendon or ligament of a peripheral or spinal joint) to alleviate local tissue changes and joint dysfunction. By easing the accessory movements within the joint, the overall ROM in the main planes is improved. Techniques chosen depend on practitioner preference and patient size, temperament, constitution, and individual symptom pattern. Techniques are adapted to allow different operator positions in order to achieve improved motion in the dysfunctional area (tissue or mechanism). The dog dictates its position, which may change several times during a treatment session. They may be standing, sitting

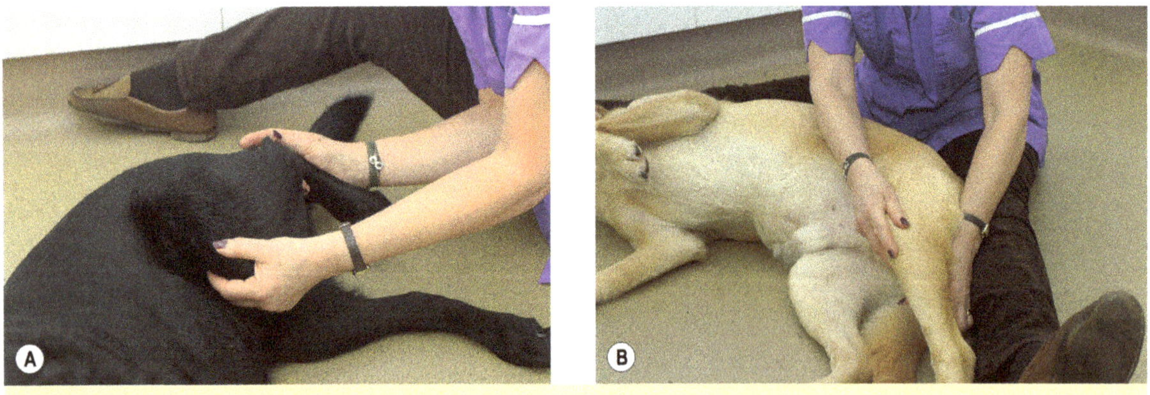

Figure 2.31
(A) Assessing the quality and ROM of the hind limb structures in flexion. (B) Assessing the quality and ROM of the hind limb structures in extension.

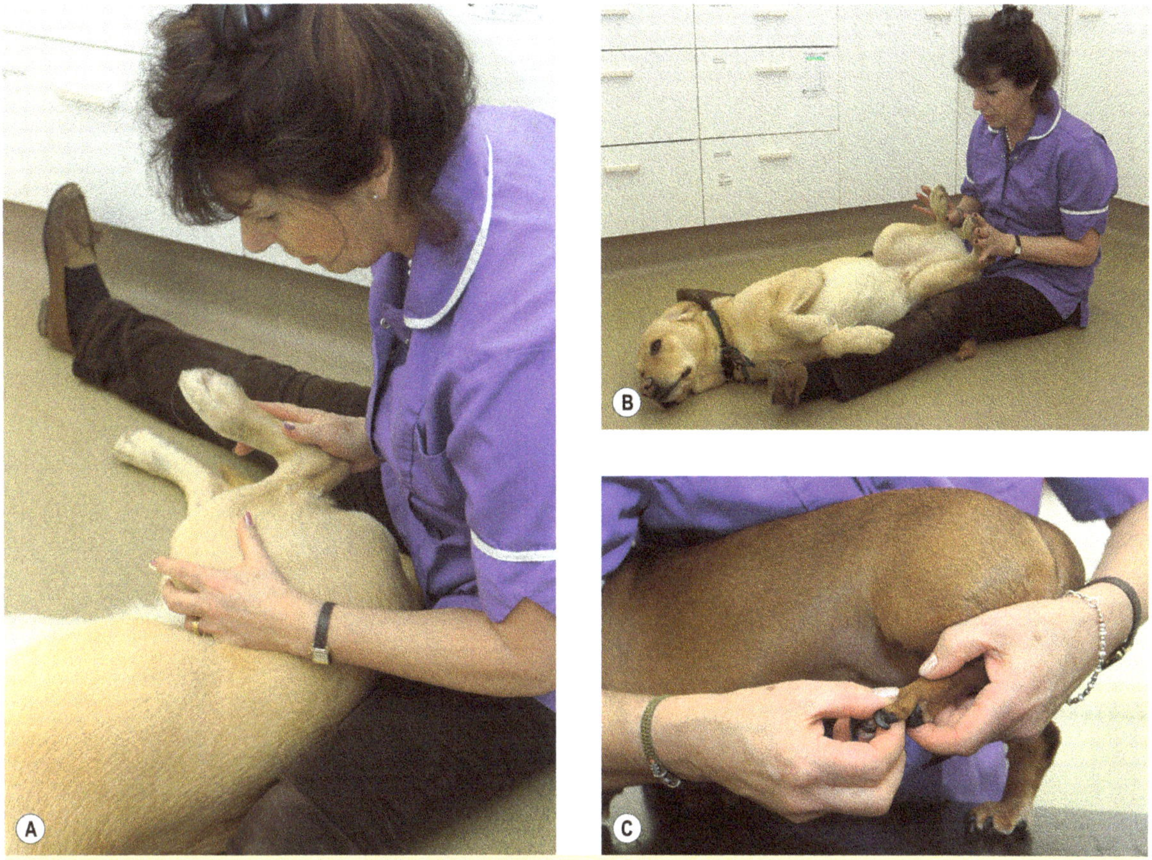

Figure 2.32
(A) Isolating first the stifle and then the hock joints to assess their individual qualities. (B) Assessing the quality of hind limb and lumbar mobility with the dog in a supine position. (C) Assessing the tarsus, metatarsals, and phalangeal articulations.

on the floor (or on the operator's lap), side lying, prone, or supine.

Techniques

Soft tissue. Soft tissue techniques are cross-fiber or longitudinal stretch, inhibition, harmonics, and somatic soft tissue release (Fig. 2.33).

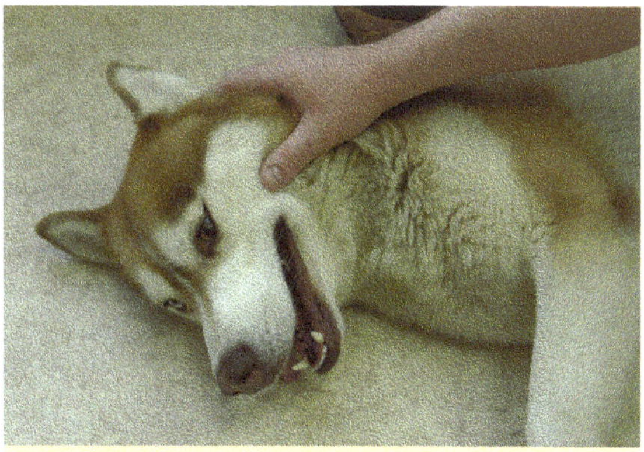

Figure 2.33
Cross-fiber muscle inhibition applied to the masseter muscles.

Articulation and mobilization. The range and direction of movements in the peripheral points have evolved to suit the individual breeds, and treatment must reflect this. The range and rate of articulation has to be considerably modified to the point where we are often testing motility rather than gross mobility.

Translocation (very gentle shearing through all planes of movement) is a particularly valuable action to perform as it highlights precise areas of binding and restriction, both intracapsular and extracapsular.

Articulation of the spinal segments can be very specific using a short lever application, for example, toggle or springing techniques (Fig. 2.34).

Longer lever techniques can be aided by using part of the operator's body as a fulcrum (Fig. 2.35A and B).

Manipulation and high velocity, low amplitude thrust (HVLAT) techniques can be employed in certain cases, but know your facet angles!

Indirect techniques. Positional, fascial, and functional release can all be applied, and spontaneous cavitation sometimes occurs as the dog relaxes into a functional release while being supported in a position of ease. The operator can use their own body as a fulcrum while the pressure can either be gently exaggerated or released depending on the required and desired effect (Fig. 2.36).

Other indirect techniques are balanced ligamentous or membranous tension (Fig. 2.37) and cranial techniques involving the involuntary motion mechanism (Pusey et al. 2010) (Fig. 2.38).

The tail is an invaluable listening tool. Gentle engagement with reciprocal tension via the tail gives the osteopath contact with the total body mechanism of the dog. Treatment can be effected throughout the body from this point of contact using the primary respiratory mechanism and working with the cranial rhythm or involuntary motion. It is often beneficial to utilize your own body as a fulcrum to enhance the efficacy of the process (Fig. 2.39A and B).

Never pull on the tail. By taking a firm grasp of the proximal coccygeal segments, the tail can be utilized for short lever techniques to assess and improve lateral flexion in the lumbar spine, and ventral and lateral flexion of the LS and sacrococcygeal segments. Only perform a few degrees of these movements using this method and do not take the tail into extension. A marginally firmer engagement will allow an element of traction through the caudal spine to reinforce the degree of articulation required (Fig. 2.40).

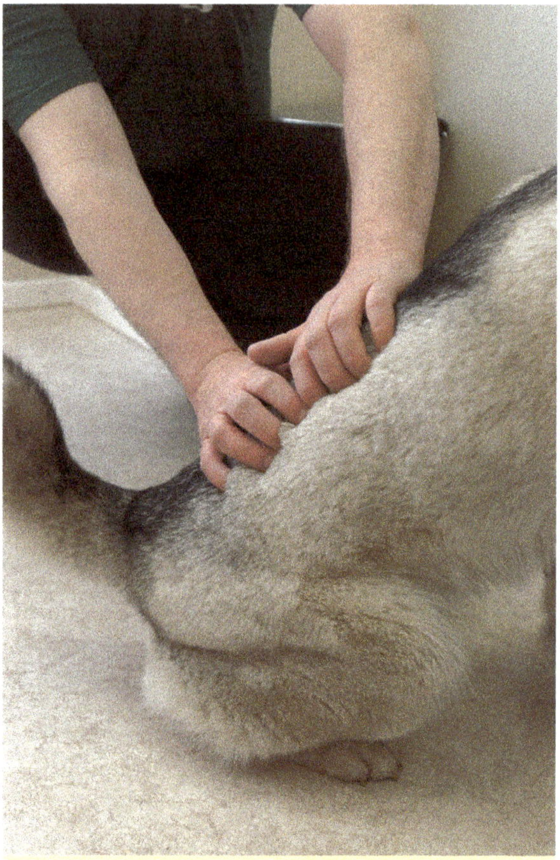

Figure 2.34
Short lever lateral springing of individual spinous processes with the dog sitting.

Treatment of specific areas

The diaphragm. The diaphragm is essential to the health of the patient. It must be able to operate to its full capacity without tightness and asymmetry within its functional pattern. During locomotion it acts as a bellows for the lungs and massages the abdominal viscera caudally.

Apart from the respiratory role, and the mechanical effects on venous drainage, the diaphragm assists,

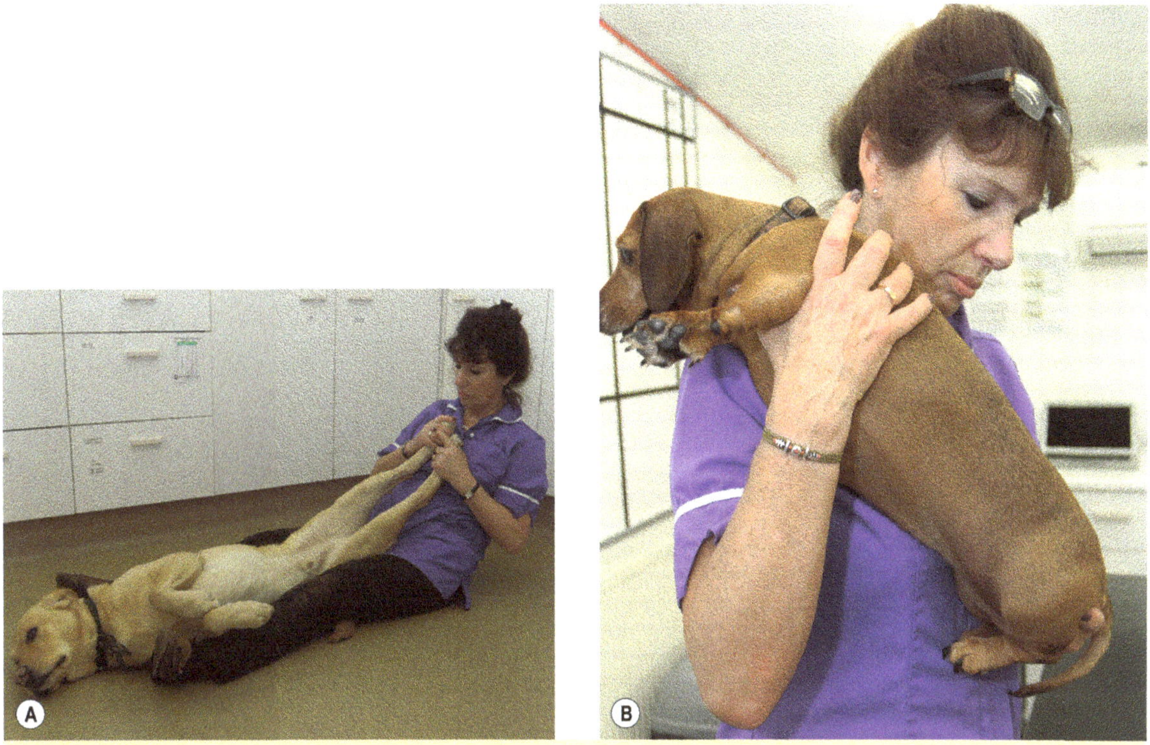

Figure 2.35
The use of long lever articulatory techniques where the practitioner uses their body as a fulcrum (A) seated with the patient supine, and (B) while cradling the patient.

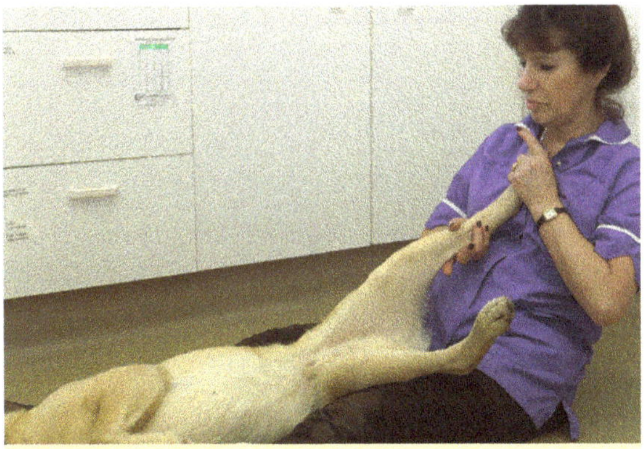

Figure 2.36
Seated technique on the floor with the patient in a supine position and supported by the practitioner's legs allowing a functional release of tension through the hind limbs and axial soft tissues.

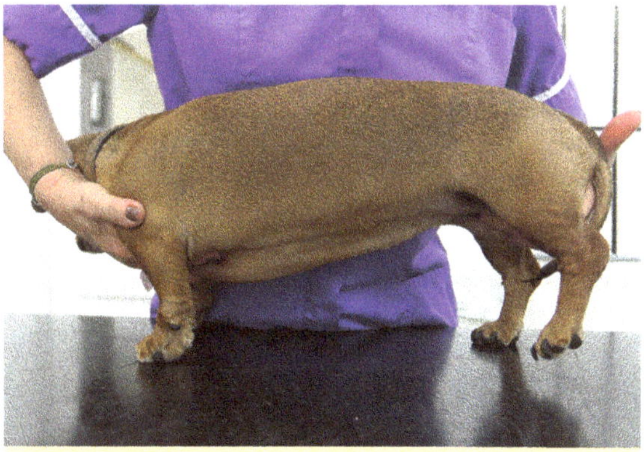

Figure 2.37
Applying a balanced ligamentous release technique.

intrinsically, with lymph transport and thus immune function (Abu-Hijleh et al. 1995).

Autonomic influences, due to the close anatomical relationship with sympathetic ganglia, and osteopathic somatic dysfunction pathways may be widespread.

Digestion may be affected either mechanically (e.g., hiatus insufficiency causing gastric reflux) or due to autonomic involvement of the celiac, splanchnic, and mesenteric ganglia.

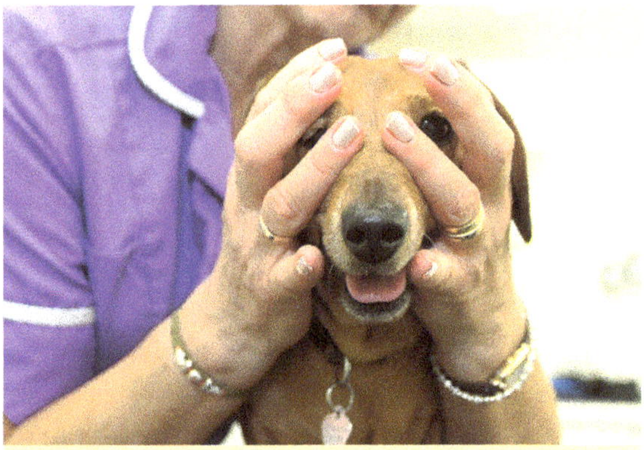

Figure 2.38
Feeling for the involuntary movement of the cranial structures of a daschund.

Tightness of the arcuate ligaments or crura will have local mechanical effects on related muscles and thus their attachments on either the vertebral bodies or caudal ribs and also their distal insertions in the pelvis and hind limb.

The myofascial continuum between the diaphragmatic connections with the pleural and abdominal cavities internally and TL fascia externally is

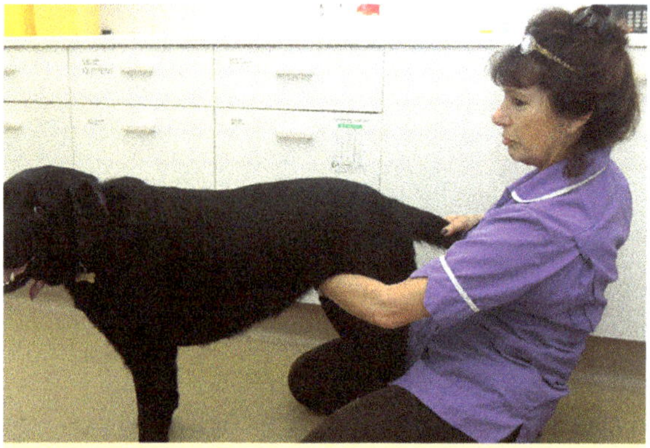

Figure 2.40
With larger dogs the osteopath can cradle around the hind limbs while allowing gentle traction by the dog through the tail. The osteopath can subtly alter the vector of pull to encourage a chain release through the body right up to the nose and mouth.

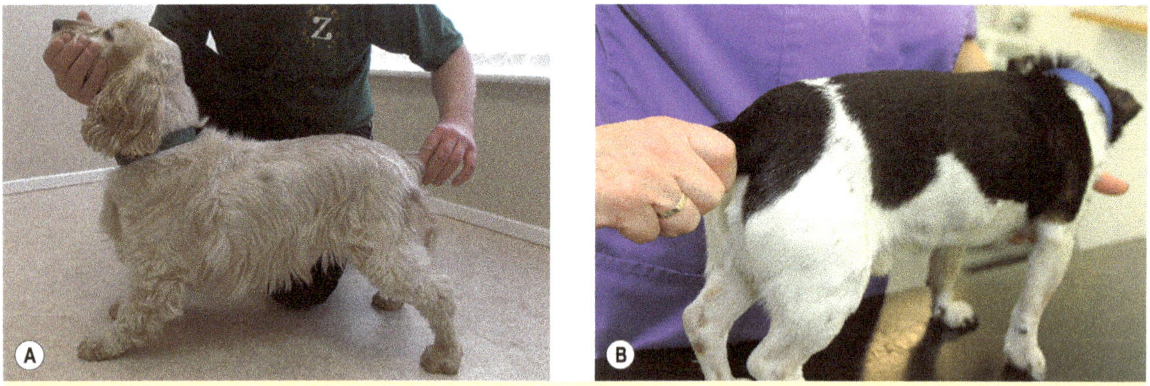

Figure 2.39
Gently using the tail as part of a long lever tool to both (A) assess and (B) assist treatment.

fundamental to the tensegrity of the total body (Fossum 2004).

It is important to consider the function of the diaphragm when treating problems ranging from lameness to visceral dysfunctions. It is also an emotional hub: dogs respond emotionally to their environment. A history of physical abuse, trauma, or upsets in their human family will affect a dog's well-being. The death of a close animal or canine companion can also cause overwhelming distress, which can manifest physically and/or psychologically. The diaphragm appears to reflect these issues. Physical and emotional shock, and the ensuing stress response, profoundly affects its function within the body.

The author (NH) begins each and every treatment session by palpating the diaphragm with one hand dorsally (Fig. 2.41). This initiates a listening communication, and as the patient relaxes, the other hand is placed ventrally to further enhance feedback. The dog does not feel as threatened as when it is being handled around the head and neck or hindquarters. There is palpatory feedback from every level, IVM tide, fascial tethering, muscular tightness, altered visceral mobility, *and* emotional state.

Move on to a head or tail contact with one hand (Fig. 2.42), assessing how to proceed with the treatment, guided by the patient's responses to you. From here it is easy to progress to gentle spinal toggling, then articulatory movements, caudally, cranially, or cephalically and subsequently continue to include the limbs and peripheral joints as necessary. Most dogs enjoy this process, and start to relax and settle into their position of choice, while we receive much palpatory diagnostic feedback. Register the areas of increased sensitivity, the panniculus reflex, muscle hypertonia, inflamed tissues, heat, etc. Tight, irritable thoracic paraspinal musculature is often associated with respiratory problems and digestive disorders (IBS and colitis, and may also accompany diagnosed food intolerances). Which comes first? One may well ask!

Proceed toward the head, through the thoracic spine and interscapular region - always a tricky area to access as it tends to be a narrow channel between the dorsal borders of the scapulae, especially in small to medium breeds. This is frequently the site of mechanical dysfunction (vertebral and costovertebral joint restriction) and associated hypertonia of the intercostal and epaxial musculature contributing to, or maintaining, forelimb lameness. It is very important to bear in mind the differential diagnoses of brachial plexus neoplasia or bony tumors. The clinical presentations are different and the feel of the tissues will be distinctive and characteristic of the pathology (Fig. 2.43).

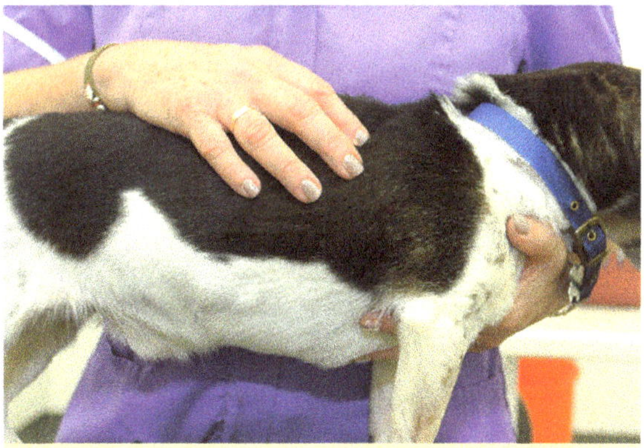

Figure 2.41
Palpating over the attachments for the diaphragm.

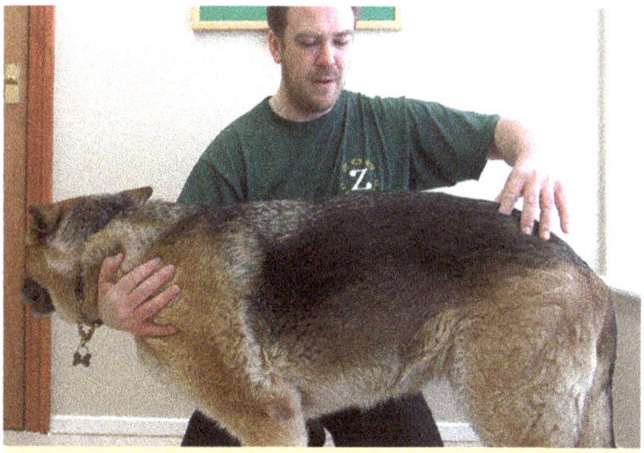

Figure 2.42
Palpating osteoarthritic spinal joints in an elderly GSD. Note the ventroflexed spine.

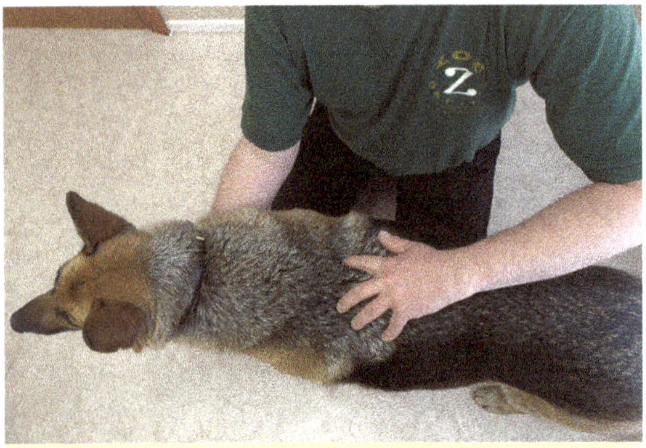

Figure 2.43
Viewed from above, the osteopath assesses tissue quality and general motility in an elderly GSD.

Head. Treatment to the head necessarily involves the temporomandibular joint (TMJ) and occipitoatlantoaxial complex. There can be primary pathology (see Differential diagnosis above) or secondary compensatory dysfunctions arising from problems in the mid-cervical, cervical or thoracic spine, cranial ribs, or forelimbs.

Treatment aims to release tightness, hypertonia, or spasm of the muscles of mastication, dorsal cervical musculature, and the hyoid and laryngeal muscle complexes, and thus also influence local neurovascular lymphatic function. Bony impactions and compression in the cranial bones can be eased using IVM techniques. Alleviate fascial tethering with functional release and unwinding (Figs 2.44A and B).

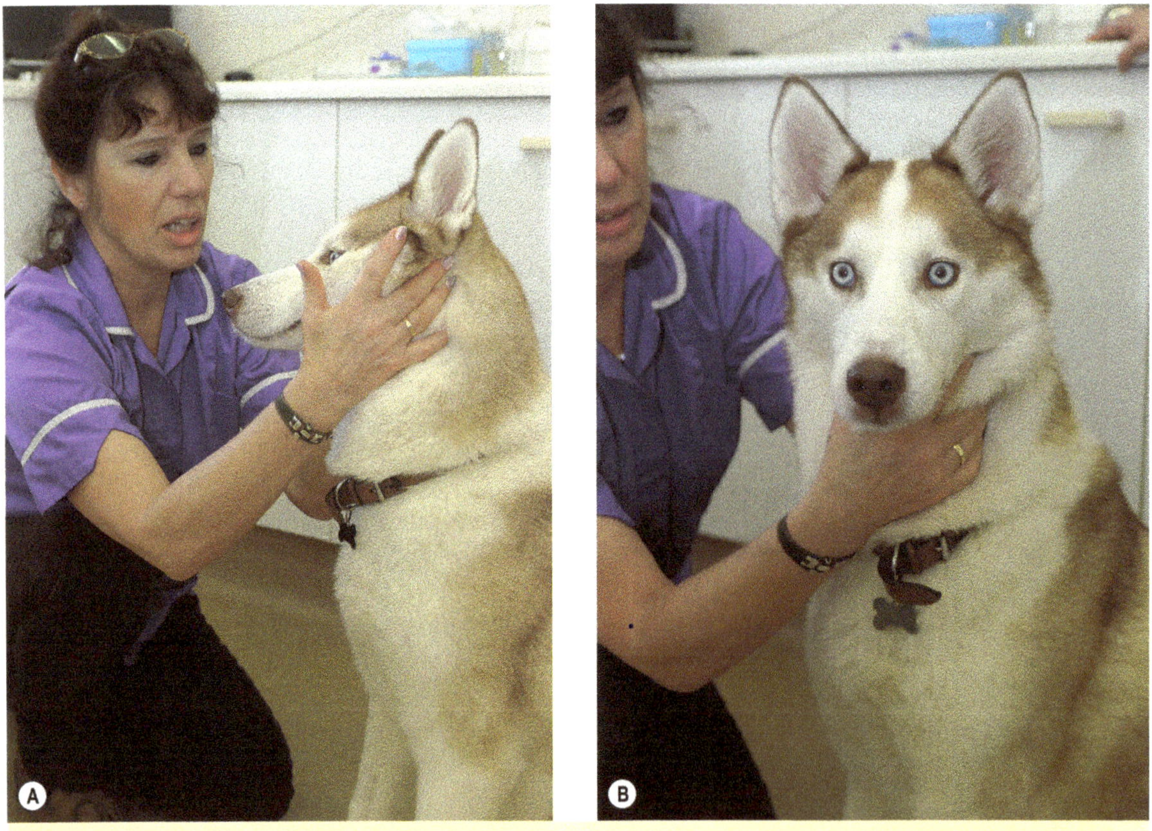

Figure 2.44
(A) Use of both hands to gently hold the dogs cranium allows the osteopath to affect subtle changes to the action of the involuntary mechanism. (B) Alleviating fascial tethering through the ventral throat and thoracic sling structures.

In certain small breeds with a large frontal cranium (Chihuahua or bulldogs) there may be vulnerable open fontanelles, predisposing to consequent problems.

Eyes and ears. The many differing face shapes, with the allied eye and ear positions, have predilections to certain disorders, in particular:

- Dolichocephalic: a long, thin face with deep-set eyes, e.g., rough collies and greyhounds.
- Brachiocephalic: a short-nosed face, e.g., pugs, French bulldogs, and those with protruding eyes (i.e., relative exophthalmos), such as Chihuahua and Cavalier King Charles spaniels.
- Droopy-faced dogs with deep skin folds and long ears, such as spaniels and bloodhounds.

Brachiocephalic breeds are prone to a variety of specific problems, including respiratory issues and spinal deformities such as hemivertebrae. Experience has shown that in some cases, gentle treatment to ease excessive nasofrontal and pharyngeal compression may help to reduce noisy breathing, snorting, and snoring. Also work on the accessory respiratory musculature, and costothoracic function, and encourage a full excursion of the diaphragm (Figs 2.45A and B).

In cases of recurrent eye infections, check for cranial base, vault, and facial bone restrictions. Persistent ear infections often manifest with sensitivity of the occipitoatlantoaxial and temporomandibular complexes.

In ENT-related problems there may be variations of the following musculoskeletal presentations: chronic tightness in the cranial cervical spine, relative hypermobility and facilitation in the midcervical vertebrae, and a complex pattern of tensions within the thoracic outlets, CT junction, cranial ribs, pectoral sling, hyoid complex, and thoracic spine. These palpable findings correspond with the segmental levels of sympathetic or parasympathetic supply to the respective organs, resulting in further disturbances in their lymphatic drainage and vascular supply. This is an example of a viscerosomatic reflex. There can also be adverse autonomic irritation due to an impact injury (e.g., a stick jammed back against the jaw), which can lead to compromised function within the digestive tract - a somatovisceral reflex.

Assess general tissue quality for stasis and edematous tissue as head and neck tightness interferes with the drainage of the local soft tissues of the face, eyes, sinuses, thyroid gland, and throat. This can be reduced by encouraging gentle lymphatic drainage using techniques to restore the expression of normal involuntary motion and release the specific areas and patterns of tension (Fig. 2.46).

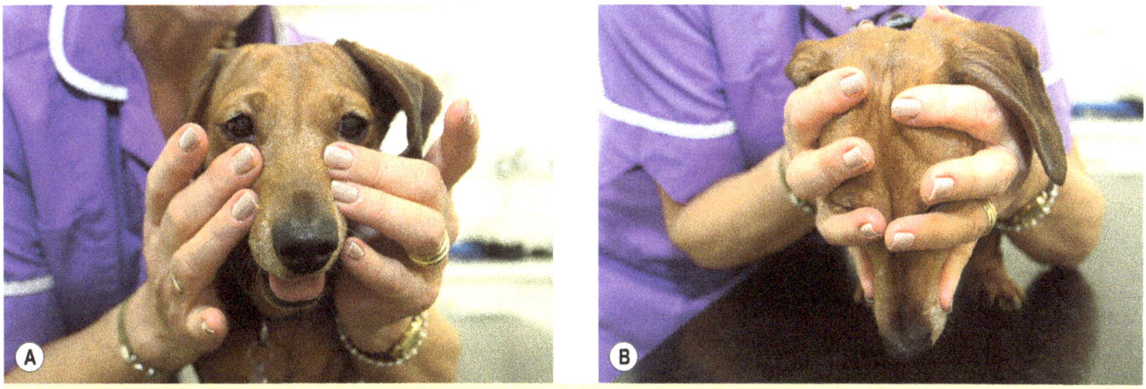

Figure 2.45

(A) Releasing any tension around the facial nerves. (B) Providing a gentle lift to release tension between the parietal and temporal bone articulations to affect changes to the function of the involuntary mechanism.

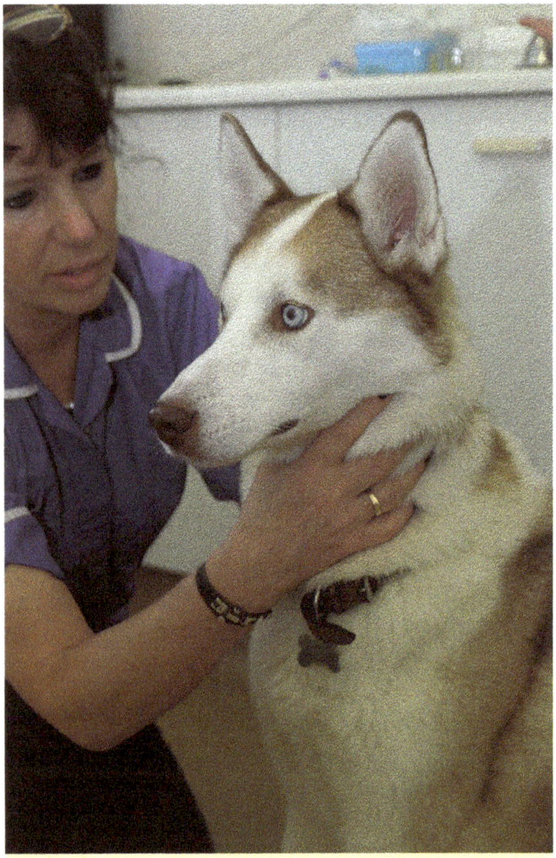

Figure 2.46
Encouraging better blood and lymphatic circulation through the throat structures using the hyoid as a functional lever.

Compromised thoracic outlet function can further compound poor lymphatic drainage. Fascial release and balanced ligamentous tension (BLT) will help the tissues to soften and spread, encouraging textural change as the primary breath engages.

Neck. Specific pathology within the neck will affect the mechanics both locally and in relation to the entire forequarters, so treatment should be commensurate with this. Local pain and dysfunction can be treated symptomatically following osteopathic principles and using apt techniques, while working within the bigger picture to improve the functioning of the whole. The pain caused by acute cervical spondylitis, commonly seen in Cavalier King Charles spaniels (CKCS), sometimes from quite a young age, will be treated differently to the stiffness associated with chronic degenerative disc disease in an older dog.

Laryngeal nerve palsy may be part of geriatric onset laryngeal paralysis polyneuropathy (GOLPP) or as a singular condition, usually unilateral if idiopathic, or due to trauma. Eventually surgery may be required to stabilize the arytenoid laterally and so decrease laryngeal airway resistance. The signs are those of upper respiratory tract obstruction due to dynamic airway collapse (passive closure of the glottis and failure to maintain the arytenoids in abduction, so they rest slightly medially and are sucked across the airway during inspiration). There is local mucosal irritation with edema and swelling due to increased air pressure in the constricted area. There may be coincidental degenerative changes in the cervical spine. In some of these cases the symptoms (a hoarse bark, rasping breath, soft cough to clear the throat, gagging, and regurgitation) have decreased and their progression has been slowed by treating the structures through which the responsible nerves (superior and inferior laryngeal, both branches of the vagus) pass. The symptoms are a mixture of sensory and motor disturbance depending on the individual nerve function.

Cranial base asymmetry and dural tension must be addressed, as should any tightness in the ventral cervical musculature and fascia throughout the thoracic cage. The local congestion around the inflamed larynx can be reduced and any compromised mobility in the cervical spine improved. The diaphragm and ribs should be treated to ensure optimal function, so that exercise intolerance and inspiratory stridor lessen, and any associated esophageal inefficiency is improved (Fig. 2.47).

Forelimb. Treatment of a problem in the forelimb should also involve the whole patient. An injury or pathology in a peripheral structure will have wide-ranging consequences, which must be addressed.

Treatment around the scapula includes soft tissue techniques, periscapular muscular stretch and

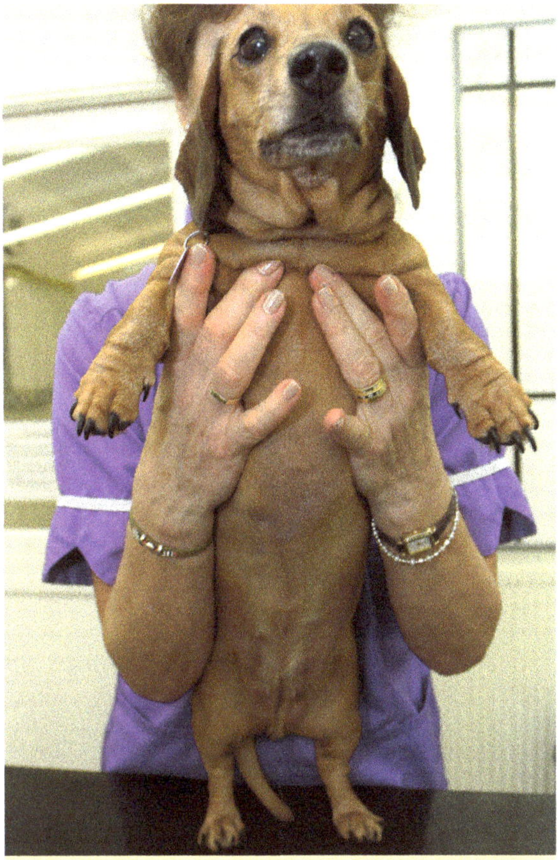

Figure 2.47
Providing a standing lift to allow a decompressive passive stretch through the thoracic and pectoral structures of a small breed dog.

mobilizations. Work generally and specifically to improve the function of the omothoracic complex. Incorporate techniques to address restricted rib function. Support and rebalance the components of the thoracic sling (Fig. 2.48A).

To treat the shoulder joint, use gentle, focused, small amplitude, short lever movements to ease restrictions to the capsule and ligaments. For acute muscle and tendon problems, for example, bicipital and rotator cuff tendonitis, this treatment should reduce inflammation, enhance healing, and facilitate short-term protective compensation mechanisms (Fig. 2.48B). Beware of tendon rupture and avulsion injuries, which require prompt surgical repair. These cases should normally be picked up by the referring vet, but can slip through the net.

It is always advisable to check joints cranial and distal to the symptomatic area and to release associated and compensatory mechanical dysfunctions. Also check the origin and insertion of a muscle where there is an injury either intrinsically or to the tendon.

Work through the structures of the proximal limb to the elbow. Find the position of ease and encourage auxiliary motions within the joints (Fig. 2.48C).

Check for and release radioulnar interosseous membrane strain and any related "pushed or pulled" radius.

Ensure ease of function within the carpus and distal radioulnar joint using gentle articulatory techniques and BLT to ease out strains, shearing, and compression patterns. In a similar fashion, treat the individual digits, releasing any binding of the long and short flexor and extensor tendons along the way and ensuring optimal mobility in the metacarpophalangeal and interphalangeal joints (Fig. 2.48D).

Younger dogs with OCD in the shoulder joint or elbow are very sensitive to movement through these joints due to the inflamed tissues. They may be on prescribed NSAIDs. The treatment aim is to quieten inflamed tissues and reduce mechanical strain through the symptomatic joints by improving the function of the contiguous structures (Fig. 2.49). Understand the pathology and assist the body in accommodating changes that are irreversible.

Thoracic spine and ribs. Common findings in this region are osteoarthritic (OA) changes, costovertebral joint restrictions, and muscular tightness. Remember certain breeds are predisposed to spinal deformities such as hemivertebrae. Short and longer lever techniques can be employed to improve both spinal and rib mobility, restore better muscle function, and improve breathing mechanics. Bear in mind the correlating

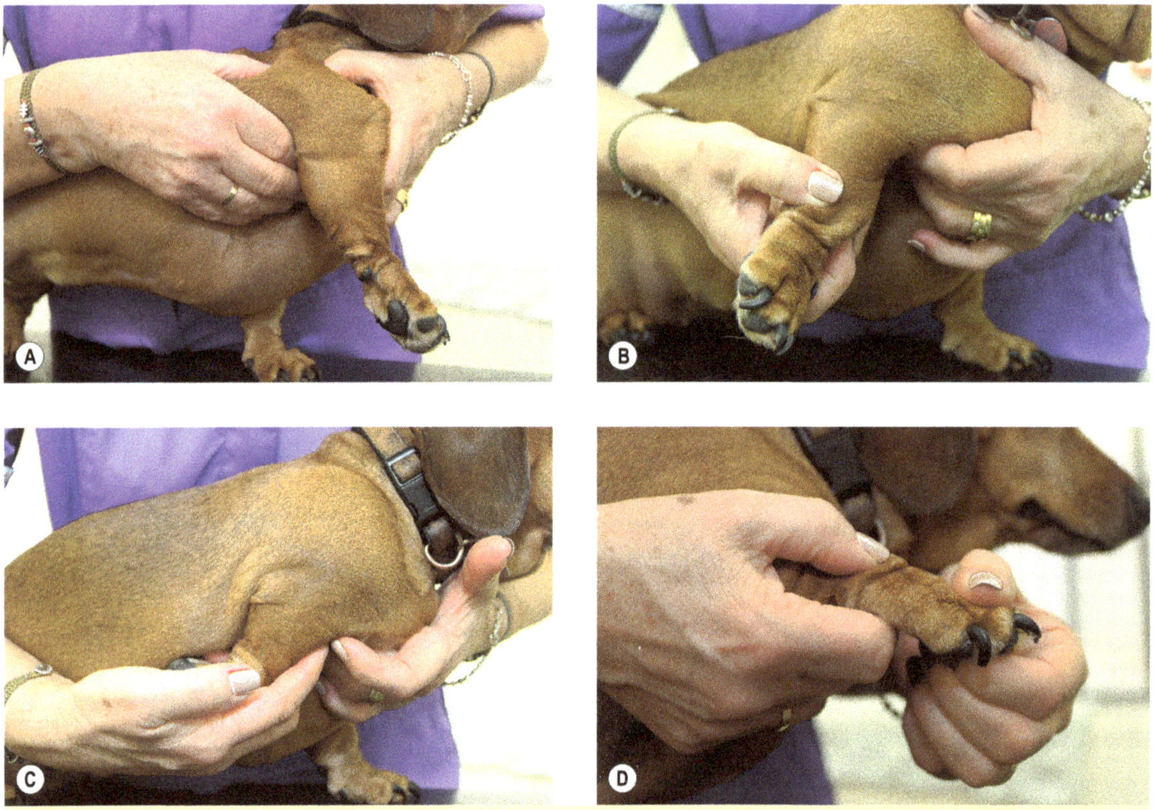

Figure 2.48

(A) Performing a single scapular lift in a small breed dog. (B) Performing specific pectoral muscle inhibition with slight forelimb abduction. (C) Performing shoulder and forelimb retraction with shoulder flexor muscle inhibition. (D) Treating the individual digits of the foot to encourage optimal mobility to this part of the limb.

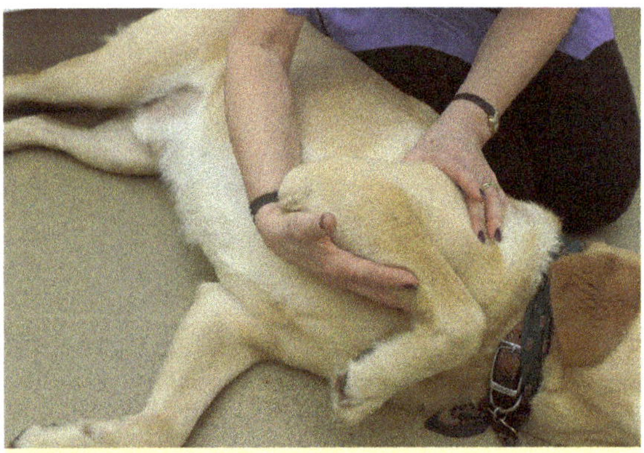

Figure 2.49

Treating a young labrador with OCD of the shoulder joint. The osteopath takes the limb into positions of "ease" to facilitate a normal resting state to these tissues.

levels of spinal and sympathetic nerve supply, and be aware of potential viscerosomatic reflex pathways both within the thorax and the abdomen.

Release any fascial binding within the thoracic cavity that may be causing pleural tethering as this inhibits good lung function and full expansion of the rib cage. With regard to the diaphragm, remember the close relationship to the liver. Palpation sometimes discloses a tightness of the capsule or a feeling of inertia or heaviness of this bulky organ, which can be alleviated using indirect techniques to encourage a restoration of inherent motility and a reciprocal motion with the excursion of the diaphragm (Fig. 2.50A and B).

Abdomen and viscera. Check for tension in the supporting mesentery of the individual viscera within

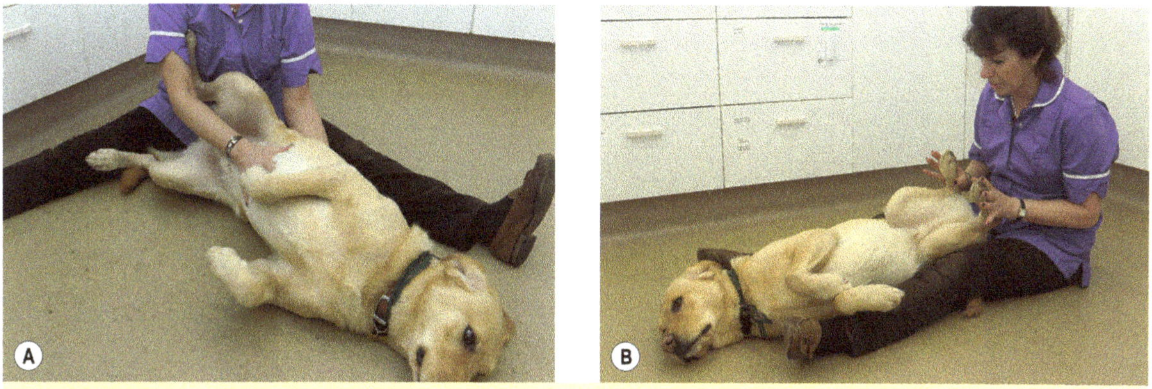

Figure 2.50
(A) Placing the hands dorsally and ventrally over the attachment points of the diaphragm and then performing an inhibitory compression to create a lowering of resting tension within this powerful muscle. (B) Using the hind limbs as long levers to alter tension within the diaphragm.

the peritoneal sac. Locate and release any focal reduction in movement over specific areas and the associated fascia blending with the posterior abdominal wall. The kidneys may be constricted within the deep investing fascia, especially if there is a chronic tightness of psoas or quadratus lumborum on one side, which causes mechanical dysfunction in that region with an allied renal ptosis. Treatment aims to improve organ motility, vascular supply, and lymphatic drainage.

Spondylosis deformans in the thoracic, lumbar, and LS spine presents with rigidity and gross lack of mobility, and tight, fibrous musculature. There is a varying degree of pain or sensitivity. Assess the quality of the bony overgrowth and density, and how each segment relates to the surrounding connective tissues. Gentle treatment aims to increase the fluidity in soft tissues along the full length of the spine, easing the ventral and lateral spinal structures with miniscule lateral amplitude motions, longitudinal release to hydrate the intervertebral discs and BLT.

The TL junction is especially prone to acute and chronic disc problems and is probably the commonest site to require spinal surgery. This condition is especially prevalent in dachshunds. In nonsurgical cases conservative osteopathic treatment may be effective, combined with cage rest and a very gradual return to guided exercise.

Treatment of the lumbar spine follows the same principles as previously discussed, with continuing regard to the degree of pathological changes. In veterinary medicine, LS disease is considered as a separate entity from spondylosis and discospondylitis in the lumbar spine, although the treatment methods are the same (Fig. 2.51A and B).

Pelvis. In cases where there are recurrent anal gland problems assess the lumbosacral, sacral, and sacrococcygeal function. Ease the ligaments and any tightness in the layers of pelvic fascia. Sometimes deep (but gentle!) inhibition techniques on the sacrococcygeal ligaments can be very beneficial for tight tissues in this area. Chronic sacroiliac joint dysfunction due to historic lameness compensation will cause pelvic asymmetry, which may be contributory to unilateral anal gland obstruction (author's own opinion).

Postpartum bitch. Whelping seems to have fewer musculoskeletal aftereffects than in human parturition, possibly due to the comparatively small size of the puppies relative to the maternal pelvis. There are also structural and functional differences due to the vertical orientation of the uterus in women. Elective cesareans are unfortunately the norm for some breeds with

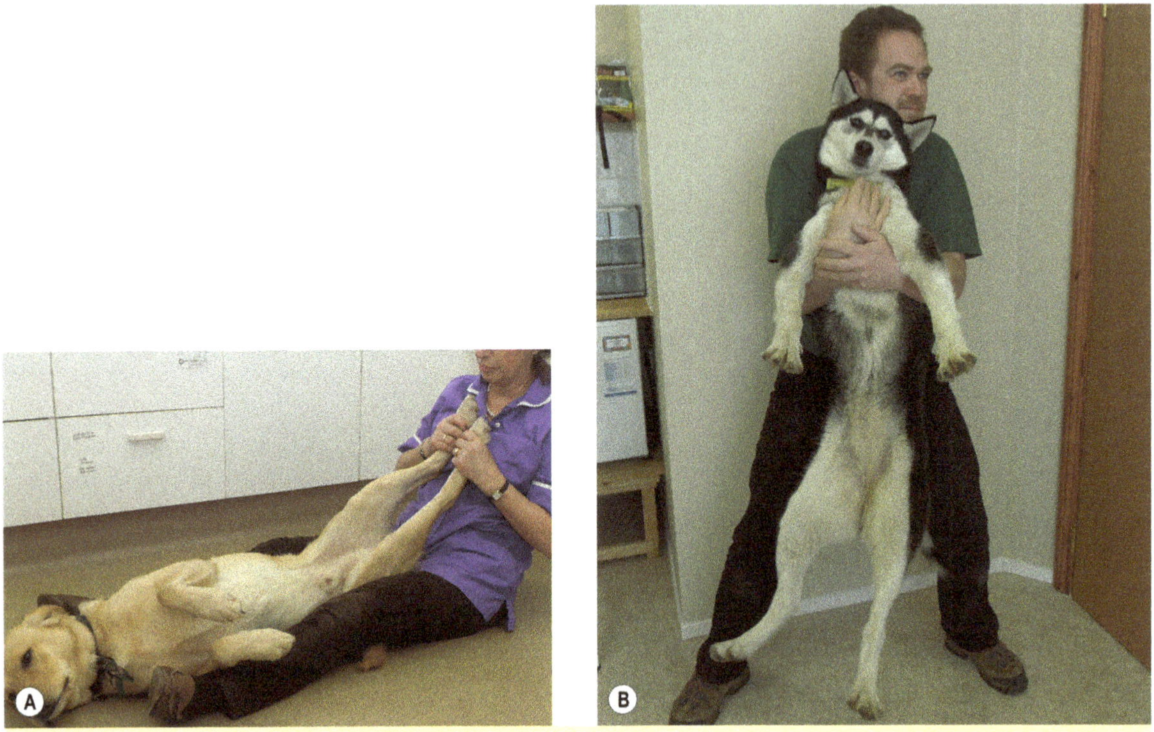

Figure 2.51
(A) Long lever technique using the hind limbs to affect a stretch through the lumbar spine. (B) Performing a standing lift on a large breed dog to create a passive stretch through the thoracic and lumbar spine.

large heads, for example, bulldogs, Boston terriers, and mastiffs.

There are, however, effects from the hormonally induced ligamentous laxity that may cause mechanical dysfunctions sooner or later, especially in the pelvis.

Post spaying. Rather than an ovariohysterectomy some surgeons prefer the option of ovariectomy (Bojrab 1983). There is less internal scarring in the latter operation as the uterus is left intact.

In either procedure the ovarian ligament is pulled not cut. This tears the connecting tissue and blood supply, which promotes a rapid healing response and reduces the risk of hemorrhage. The disruption to the investing fascia and supportive membranous structures, and the postsurgical edematous tissue, will have a palpable effect on the involuntary mechanism and visceral motility.

As with all surgery there is subsequent scarring in both the deep tissues and also superficially at the incision sites. Fibrotic tissues lack stretch and have reduced elasticity. There will be a functional discrepancy in the tensional continuity of the abdominal fascia that can be ameliorated by treatment.

There may be a reduction of sacral motion and LS mobility, with low tail carriage in spayed bitches. Palpation reveals a sensation of cranially inclined fascial drag along the dorsal abdominal wall holding the pelvis in slight flexion and perhaps an accompanying sacral torsion. There may be a slight restriction in the excursion of the diaphragm, often unilaterally as the two sides can be affected differently, demonstrating the functional relationship between pelvic asymmetry and diaphragmatic crural imbalance.

Occasionally bitches suffer some urinary incontinence due to bladder sphincter incompetence secondary to deep fascial tethering, adhesions, and residual scar tissue. There are also hormonal changes as a result of the removal of ovarian influence (Bojrab 1983).

Osteopathic techniques to improve vascular and lymphatic function, and reduce the fibrotic shortening and binding within the connective tissues, may enhance a return to normal function both locally and throughout the areas of protective adaptation postoperatively.

It is the author's experience that there seem to be fewer mechanical consequences of castration, although sometimes there may be evidence of a residual tightness in the caudal lumbar spine and pelvis. Some neutered dogs have a degree of urinary incontinence. It is therefore worthwhile checking for these signs when treating male dogs that have undergone the procedure. Check for pelvic congestion or any perineal fascial tethering and aim to improve the balance between blood supply and venous drainage of the pelvis (Fig. 2.52).

Hind limb

Hip. In cases of degenerative joint disease, for example, hip dyplasia or Legg-Calvé-Perthes disease, there will be stiffness and reduction in the range of movement with unpredictable amounts of pain or discomfort. There may also be swelling and thickening of joint margins due to sclerosis and bony overgrowth associated with osteoarthritis. Gentle treatment can be applied specifically to the hip joint. Use slow, very small amplitude traction release, translocation, gliding motions to encourage synovial fluid production within the joint capsule, and BLT to ease specific strain on musculotendinous or ligamentous tissues around the joint capsule (Fig. 2.53).

Stifle. In an acute presentation due to traumatic injury, for example, ruptured CrCL where the anterior drawer test discloses hyperextension and instability, there will be pain, swelling, laxity, and markedly reduced or no weight-bearing. These cases usually proceed straight to surgery, though gentle osteopathic treatment may help reduce the swelling and pain in the short term.

Intermittent skipping is very often seen, especially in small terriers, due to luxation of the patella. These are often surgical cases, but the associated tight rectus

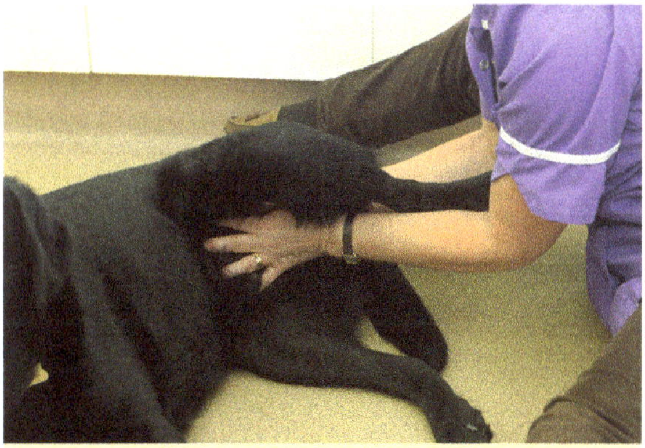

Figure 2.52
Assessing the quality of the abdominal soft tissues and the state of the viscera.

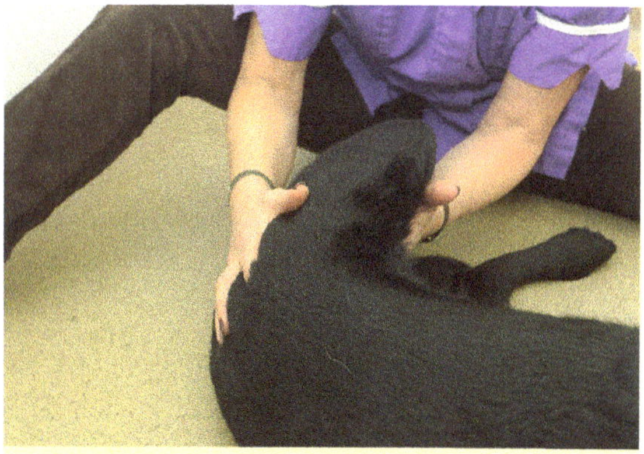

Figure 2.53
Functional release technique applied through the hind limb, and also affecting the hip, pelvis, and lumbar soft tissues.

femoris, apparent decreased mobility of the ipsilateral joint, and shortened quadratus lumborum and iliopsoas respond well to treatment to modify this functional pelvic asymmetry. It is also possible to improve the movement from the thoracolumbar to lumbosacral, sacroiliac, and sacrococcygeal areas. Perform a functional release of any associated rotational strain within the tibia, fibula, and hock. Assess the degree of relative hypotonia of the lateral and caudal thigh muscles, which may also need some rehabilitation treatment. Subsequent to these treatments, there is often a marked reduction in the frequency of the skipping without resorting to surgery.

There are many occasions after surgery when the dog is still lame and not fully weight-bearing through the limb, for example, after cranial crucial ligament repair or procedures to correct patella luxation. In many cases there has been good postoperative recovery and an acceptable range on movement in the stifle. There may, however, be hock or sacroiliac joint issues due to holding patterns within the connective tissues. So despite a good rehabilitation regimen and exercises, it is worthwhile checking if fine-tuning of the limb mechanics is required. "Tweaking" and subtle adjustments within the structural components can make all the difference between slightly compromised actions and 100 percent ease of motion (Fig. 2.54).

Distal hind limb. Treatment to the hock, tarsus, and digits follows the same rationale as for the distal forelimb, to encourage and preserve efficient springy function within the limb (Fig. 2.55).

Management

Rehabilitation

The subject of rehabilitation is too vast to explore fully here. Suffice to say that beyond advice on management and the use of a simple exercise regimen, cases are referred to veterinary centers with the necessary facilities for hydrotherapy (pool and treadmill).

Intensive postorthopedic surgical and neurological rehabilitation is highly specialized. It is most effective if carried out several times daily at the appropriate interval after surgery, while the dog is still an inpatient, and then with regular frequency during the first few weeks.

Care will range from cage rest for a prescribed duration followed by short and then longer controlled walks. It is important to explain to the owner the importance of a slow walking pace to ensure the dog engages the core muscles effectively before progressing to a faster walk and eventually allowing a trot. Do not underestimate the value of slow basic, gentle exercise

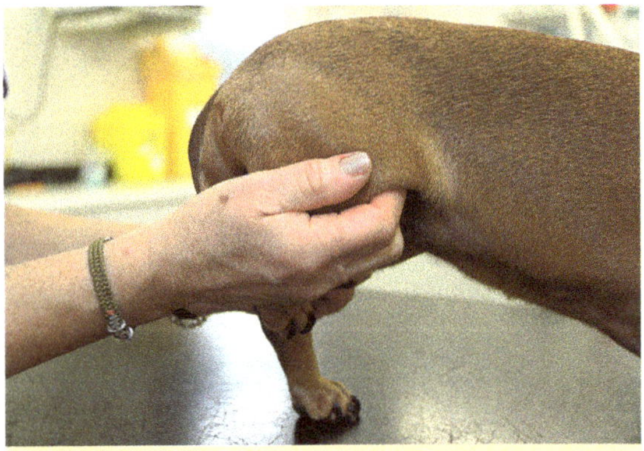

Figure 2.54
Applying a functional release technique through the hind limb to alter weight-bearing and function of that limb.

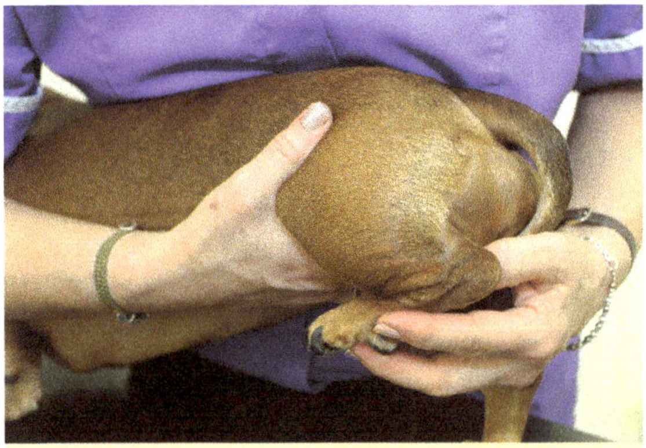

Figure 2.55
Localized treatment to the hock, tarsus, and digits to improve their biomechanical function.

in rehabilitation to establish good, coordinated muscle use from the outset (Sawaya 2007).

Subsequent hydrotherapy and rehabilitation exercises continue to redress functional asymmetry, enhance proprioceptive function, and awaken and strengthen hypotonic muscles. Some of these exercises can be done both during and after treatment sessions. Examples include:

- gently pushing the fore or hindquarters sideways to slightly destabilize the dog, which requires them to readjust their balance;
- folding up one foot at a time, then one front and one hind together (ipsilateral then contralateral), which is a simple but effective way of stimulating balance and coordination.

Owners can be given a wide range of rehabilitation advice depending on their interest, ability, and compliance. It is essential that the owner relay this advice to their household, including spouse, children, housekeeper, and dog walker. Only too frequently the dog is brought back because it shows no improvement or has relapsed. On investigation it is found that someone has decided that it loves chasing a ball or stick, and deserves some fun after having had such a miserable time!

Racing, agility, and working dogs will require an extensive rehab program which the owner or handler should be competent and willing to undertake to ensure full fitness before returning to competition. Failure to fulfil this will compromise their long-term ability.

The most important advice for puppy owners is *do not overexercise*. Rather than running a puppy around the park to exhaust it, arrange structured social interaction with people and other dogs. This will entertain, stimulate, and tire the puppy safely, instilling good socialization skills and positive temperament traits.

The number of treatments required is variable. Financial considerations are an unfortunate reality, and there must be a sensitive compromise and allowances made for cases that would benefit from regular, ongoing therapy when resources are limited.

Experience has shown beyond doubt that creaky geriatric dogs with multiple ailments benefit hugely from regular osteopathic treatment. As well as improved mobility, owners report increased alertness and general well-being.

Advice is often requested on husbandry, living environment, and sleeping arrangements.

Dogs are carnivores with omnivorous tendencies, often grazing on herbage, fruit, and vegetation, but dietary advice is outside the remit of this book.

As with humans, assistance with getting into the car or climbing steps is eventually a necessity for older dogs, both large and small. The range of apparatus and merchandise available to aid the quality of their lives is ever increasing.

Wooden and slippery floors pose problems. Elderly dogs with compromised coordination and degenerative joint disease have difficulty not only with getting up, but also just standing still without their feet slipping. Younger dogs often skid when running around on these surfaces. Nonslip rugs or carpet may not be in vogue but will save on vet fees!

Acupuncture, homeopathic remedies, nutritional supplements, nutraceuticals, and medication must all be prescribed and administered by a vet.

Case study 2.1

Siberian husky

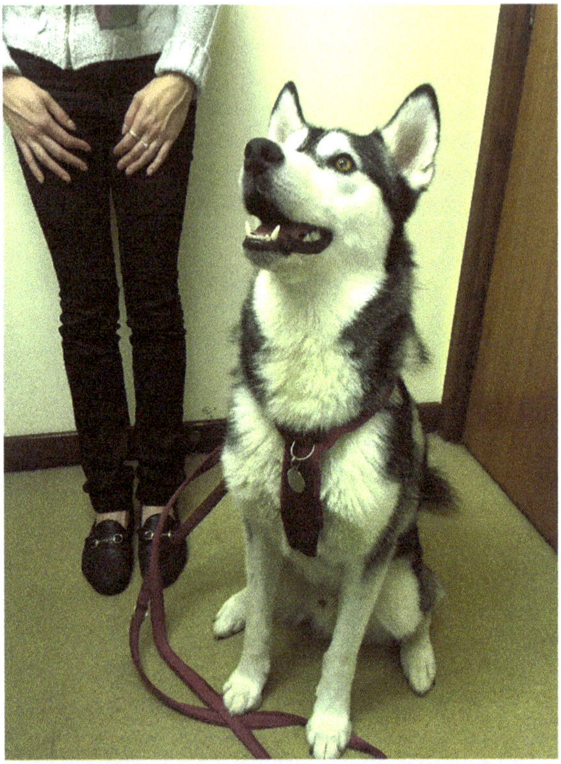

Figure 2.56
Patient S. during one of his early visits. Note the angles and orientation of the hind limbs.

Signalment

Patient S., a male Siberian husky aged two years and weighing 28 kg, was fostered at 18 months old from a UK dog charity by a young couple as their first dog. Prior to this he had lived in a flat without access to a garden or any open spaces. One of his new owners is a physical training instructor and had thought that the dog would make an ideal training companion.

History

Initially the new owners only exercised Patient S. on a lead before progressing to an adapted horse lunge line. It was at this point that they noticed a problem with the way he moved when he transitioned from a walk into a run. Like most huskies he only wanted to move at a run. Instead of a nice smooth ventrodorsal flexion through the spine allowing the hind limbs to swing forward of the forelimbs in the cranial phase, he would arch his back and engage the hind limbs early creating a "bunny-hop" (rabbit-like movement) with both hind limbs together. The hind limbs also appeared more laterally rotated than normal for the breed. Having run a short distance, his owners noticed that he would then keep this mode of movement once he returned to a walking gait. If he stopped to sniff at something then he might walk normally afterwards. They sought advice from their veterinary surgeon who, after examining the patient, decided to refer him to the author (TN) for an osteopathic assessment and, if help could be given, a course of treatment.

Presenting signs

Patient S. presented as a healthy and alert young dog, full of vitality and interest in what was going on around him. The referral notes indicated that all was normal with his main body functions. Visually he presented as a front-heavy dog, with a lack of muscling around the hindquarters and lumbar region (Fig. 2.56). This was confirmed on palpation when he also appeared a little worried about being touched in this area. He was not aggressive, but tried to distract the author from what he was doing.

Observing him move, it was obvious to the author that the patient was not using his primary muscles of locomotion and lacked core stability, which resulted in a less than straight line of movement despite his owner's best efforts. There was, however, no lack of enthusiasm from the patient.

From the case history, visual observations, and palpation the author deduced that the patient had probably never had the opportunity to move correctly. He had developed a restricted gait as a puppy and had never progressed to a more efficient, normal way of locomotion.

Osteopathic treatment

Due to his altered movement there was also a disproportionate resting state to his musculature. The author applied some soft tissue massage to begin with to relax the patient, before centering on a myofascial release technique aimed at redistributing tension and normalizing the resting state of entire muscle chains. Patient S. was compliant and relaxed into the session.

The second part of the program centered on the physical trainer. A program treating Patient S. as if he was a young, unfit human in a sedentary lifestyle was devised.

Patient S. was going to start at the very beginning:

- He would do sets of controlled exercises beginning with rising from the "sit" to the standing position and back again. This would hopefully wake up the gluteal and hind limb muscles.
- He would walk over raised poles to make him lift each limb independently.
- He would stretch up for healthy treats.
- He would be walked up and down steps slowly.
- Finally, he would wear lightweight proprioceptive stimulators around the distal hind limbs to raise his awareness of them.

His new trainer was also going to mix these exercises up to suit his daily moods and then return to see the author again in a month.

On re-examination a month later both posture and gait had improved. There was a definite increase in muscling over the hindquarters and a perceived shift in weight-bearing so that he no longer stood so far over his front limbs. When walked, trotted, and run on the same flat car park surface at the clinic he tracked much better, with very little deviation onto a three-way track.

He felt better on palpation, and had lost the hypersensitivity over his paravertebral and gluteal muscles.

Treatment continued the initial approach with a view to increasing his exercise program to continue the improvement, including hill work to ensure he engaged his hindquarters (Fig. 2.57).

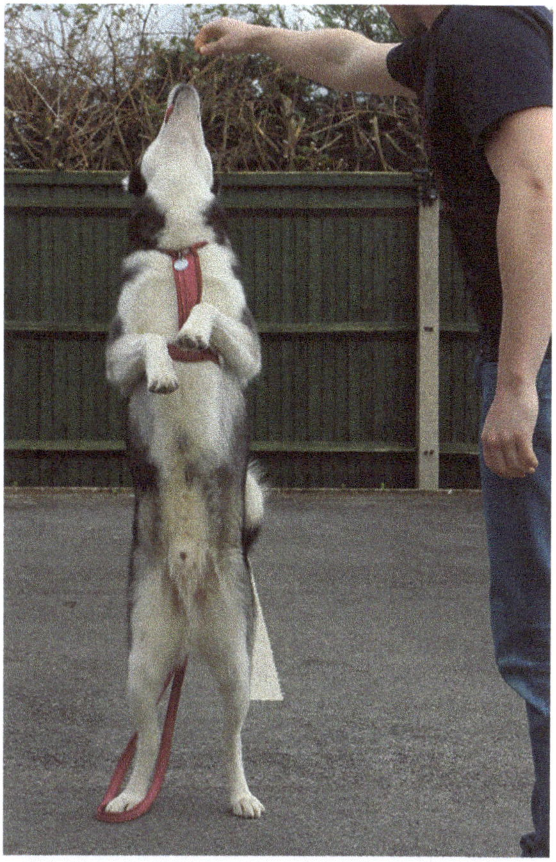

Figure 2.57
Performing hind limb only standing exercise, for several seconds at a time as part of his core strengthening routine.

Outcome

Patient S. responded immediately to osteopathic treatment aimed at normalizing the resting state of the soft tissues throughout his entire body. This was coupled with a very comprehensive exercise program designed to achieve consistent strength and stamina improvements. His progress would have been much slower and probably not as effective without this combined approach. Huskies are a robust breed and so this lent itself well to a positive outcome.

Summary

Patient S. was referred for osteopathic help, but not because he had sustained any particular injury or had a defined condition affecting his overall health. He was suffering from a lack of exercise and general conditioning. In the long term, if this status had remained, then he would probably have developed physical issues due to his asymmetrical way of moving. Because he was already skeletally mature, but was still a young dog, this was the ideal time to treat him and set out a graduated exercise program that would allow him to build up a balanced, healthy MSK system and to retrain him to move in a correct canine manner.

Motivating a younger animal is much easier and this, coupled with one of his new owners being a personal fitness coach, made for a textbook rehabilitation phase of his health care package.

From an osteopathic point of view, it was important to recognize the need to keep the patient mentally occupied while retraining took place. This was also necessary to avoid potential soft tissue and joint injury due to overexuberance (something the breed is known for).

Patient S. responded perfectly throughout and during each osteopathic visit appeared to really enjoy his sessions. Having a veterinary surgeon recognize that this patient would greatly benefit from osteopathy as an integral part of rectifying the gait and muscle function was the single most critical aspect to this case. Left for longer the outcome could have been very different (Fig. 2.58).

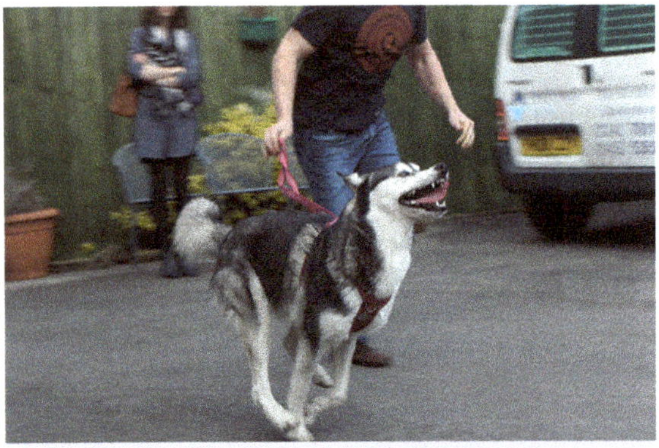

Figure 2.58
Patient S. showing a good turn of speed during a post treatment assessment in the clinic's car park.

Case study 2.2

German shepherd

Signalment

Axel was a 12-year-old male German shepherd dog.

History

Axel presented with a history of cauda equina infection in May 2014, confirmed by hematological and biochemical tests (leukocytes 22 103/mm^3, normal range is 4.9–17.6 103/mm^3). There was also a concomitant hepatic inflammation (ALKP = 325 u/l, normal range is 23–212 u/l; ALT = 210 u/l, normal range is 10–125 u/l). In the following months, the dog developed an altered gait pattern with difficulties in climbing stairs and jumping in and out of the car, together with a loss of sphincter control that led him first to urinary and then bowel incontinence. Administration of an intensive course of antibiotics (clindamycin 30 mg, twice a day for 10 days), anti-inflammatory drugs (meloxicam 0.2 mg/kg for two days, followed by 0.1 mg/kg for eight days), and chondroprotectors (Cosequin® Taste HA for 40 days) produced a remission of symptoms that lasted for a few months. In October 2014 Axel returned with the same clinical presentation. The past clinical investigations had revealed the presence of cataracts, hypoacusia (reduced hearing function), and diffuse degenerative joint disease.

Veterinary evaluation

The neurological evaluation showed impaired proprioception in the hind limbs with a general atrophy of the related muscle tissues, decreased patellar reflexes, and a complete loss of perineal reflexes – a pattern of signs that was compatible with the diagnosis of cauda equina syndrome. In addition, a degenerative disc and vertebral facet disease was suspected from L4 to S1 level.

Osteopathic evaluation

At the first osteopathic assessment, the owner reported no major changes in Axel's behavior, although his general energy levels and vitality had been progressively decreasing in the last few weeks. On observation, the dog showed a shift in weight-bearing, primarily loading the forelimbs, while the hind limbs were kept apart on a wide base of support. There was a loss of muscle bulk over the gluteal region, while mobility testing of the left hip joint indicated a reduction of motion in abduction and extension (the animal was also unable to raise the hind limbs to urinate). On the right side, the hip had limited flexion and the paw dragged on the floor when the animal climbed stairs. One of the most significant changes, in terms of tissue texture and reduction of movement, was felt on palpation over the sacrococcygeal region and in the proximal third of the tail. The base of the tail was held in extension, was sore on palpation, and there was a fibrotic texture to the surrounding soft tissues. Finally, the cranial rhythm showed a poor vitality in particular from the caudal lumbar region below, together with a strong compression of the cranial base.

Osteopathic treatment

Axel underwent osteopathic treatment on a regular basis of two sessions per week for the first month, followed by one session per week in the following two months. The initial aim was to restore vitality and synchrony of the altered cranial rhythm in order to balance dural tension, and promote fluid dynamics where impeded, especially at the most caudal region of the body. This would reduce inflammation and normalize neural and immune function. Techniques such as sacral compression (a technique that follows the same procedure of CV4 but applied to the sacrum) were applied to enhance cranial rhythm transmission into the area, while fascial unwinding and direct myofascial release were chosen to break fibrotic adhesions and restore mobility at the base of the tail and pelvic diaphragm, with an impact on sacral and perineal nerve function. Finally, articulatory and soft tissue techniques were used on the hips to improve the range of motion and blood supply.

Physical therapy

Osteopathic treatment was integrated with a cycle of physical therapy consisting of magnetotherapy (10 sessions of 30 minutes at 10 Hz and 50G), laser therapy (15 sessions of 20 minutes at variable frequency) to hips and sacrum, together with water treadmill sessions (15 minutes). The aim was to reduce inflammation and improve muscle trophism and blood circulation around the pelvis and hips, resulting in balanced weight-bearing through the hind limbs.

Follow-up

After three weeks of treatment, Axel showed an even distribution of weight when standing, an increased gluteal muscle bulk, and regained urinary continence. The owner reported that the hind limbs were also occasionally raised for passing urine. In fact, the range of movement of both hip and sacrococcygeal joints was considerably improved on manual testing. However, the bowel incontinence was still present despite the dog being able to partly raise his tail during defecation. No feces had been passed in the last three days. A dysfunction of the most caudal part of the descending colon was found. It appeared dense, dilated, and sore during external palpation, with the ability to cause a strong fascial drag when feeling for the abdominal connective tissue rhythm. The diaphragm was held in the inspiratory phase, with a reduced range of breathing excursion, while the caudal thoracic spine was held in an extension pattern.

Further investigation and treatment

Having discussed these findings with the veterinary surgeon, a rectal examination was arranged (to rule out the presence of a fecaloma), and a stool analysis was carried out to rule out infection of the lower intestinal tract. The veterinary evaluation concluded that the problem was related to dysfunctional peristalsis only. Treatment with lactulose (1 ml/4.5 kg) was administered twice a day to stimulate evacuation. In addition visceral osteopathic manipulation was applied to the descending colon and related suspensory ligaments with the dog lying on his left side. The aim was to restore balanced tension and normal function to the bowels. A two-handed technique was also applied to improve function of the mesentery with the dog standing and the operator positioned over the patient with one hand under the abdomen and the other contacting over the lumbar spine to functionally balance and release its attachments. Finally, oscillatory techniques to the caudal thoracic spine and functional inhibition of the surrounding soft tissues were applied to normalize somatic function in the area.

Conclusions

After three days the dog passed dry and hard stools. Although he never suffered with this problem again, he also never regained full control of bowel continence. The owner reported, however, that Axel's temperament was much improved, with higher energy levels during the day and a better appetite.

Summary

Osteopaths do not treat "conditions," but a comprehensive knowledge of any pathological process and how it affects the patient determines the therapeutic pathway for each patient. Consider the pathology and how treatment can lessen its consequences and aid the body to accommodate irreversible changes caused by developmental abnormality or chronic conditions. This helps return the secondary dysfunctional areas to normal.

A working diagnosis is essential when cooperating in a health care team as a reference point for communication.

Terminology to describe both qualitative and quantitative function is necessary to relay valuable information to colleagues. Vets are increasingly appreciative of a qualitative appraisal of how the tissues feel in addition to the quantitative assessment of function (ROM). Like osteopaths, they support the entire system while specific areas of pathology return to health.

Tissues affected by infectious inflammation, chronic degeneration, hormonal imbalance, and somaticized emotion (e.g., fear) all have a distinctive palpable feel which will indicate what is required to help redress the health imbalance. In every musculoskeletal case explore the tissue patterns and discover what further help the body may require for deeper support.

Consider all pathways.

Ask the owner if they have noticed any improvement in the general health: more settled digestion, increased energy, ease of anal glands, less scratching or nibbling due to diminished skin irritation, etc. Document these changes and discuss them with the vet to encourage a broader vision and more wide-ranging referrals.

References

Abu-Hijleh MF, Habbal OA, Moqattash ST (1995) The role of the diaphragm in lymphatic absorption from the peritoneal cavity. Journal of Anatomy. June; 186 (Pt 3) 453–467.

Arnoczky SP (1988) The cruciate ligaments: the enigma of the canine stifle. Journal of Small Animal Practice. February; 29 (2) 71–90.

Bennett D, Tennant B, Lewis DG (1988) A reappraisal of anterior cruciate ligament disease in the dog. Journal of Small Animal Practice. May; 29 (5) 275–297.

Bojrab MJ (1983) Current Techniques in Small Animal Surgery. Philadelphia: Lea and Febiger, pp. 334–338.

Bradshaw J (2011) In Defence of Dogs. London: Penguin Books.

Breur GJ, Lambrechts NE, Todhunter RJ (2012) Chapter 7: The genetics of canine orthopaedic traits. In: Ostrander EA, Ruvinsky A (eds.) The Genetics of the Dog. New York: CABI, pp. 136–160. doi: 10.1079/9781845939403.0136.

BVA & KC – British Veterinary Association and The Kennel Club (2015) Canine Health Schemes: Chiari malformation/Syringomyelia scheme. [Online] Available: https://www.bva.co.uk/uploadedFiles/Content/Canine_Health_Schemes/Chiari_Malformation_Syringomyelia_Scheme.pdf [March 27, 2019].

Fossum TW (2007) Small Animal Surgery. 3rd edn. St. Louis, MO: Mosby Elsevier, pp. 702–704; 1316–1356.

Hobson N (2012) A retrospective study of forelimb lameness in canines from an osteopathic viewpoint. First International Congress of Osteopathy in Animal Practice. Rome, 2012.

Innes JF (2013) Role of synovitis in cruciate disease – is this a treatment target? BVOA British Veterinary Orthopaedic Association. The stifle joint. Spring scientific meeting, 03 April 2013, pp. 12–17.

Kardong KV (2002) Chapter 10: The thoracic muscular sling. In: Vertebrates: Comparative Anatomy, Function, Evolution. 3rd edn. McGraw Hill. Washington State University, pp. 380–388.

Kowaleski M, Boudrieau R, Pozzi A (2012) Chapter 62: Stifle joint. In: Tobias K, Johnston S (eds.) Veterinary Surgery: Small Animal. Volume 1. St. Louis, MO: Elsevier Saunders, pp 906–998.

Leighton RL (1998) Historical perspectives of osteochondrosis. Veterinary Clinics of North America: Small Animal Practice. January; 28 (1) 1-16.

Pusey A, Brooks J, Jenks A (2010) Osteopathy and the Treatment of Horses. Wiley-Blackwell, pp. 100–105.

Renberg WC, Johnston SA, Ye K et al. (1999) Comparison of stance time and velocity as control variables in force plate analysis of dogs. American Journal of Veterinary Resources. July; 60 (7) 814–819.

Rusbridge C (2014) Chiari-like malformation and syringomyelia. [Online] Available: http://www.veterinary-neurologist.co.uk/resources/EUROPEAN-J-COMP-AN-PRA-20_7.pdf [March 27, 2019].

Sawaya S (2007) Physical and alternative therapies in the management of arthritic patients. Veterinary Focus. 17 (3) 37–42.

Smith, GK, Karbe GT, Agnello KA, McDonald-Lynch MB (2012) Chapter 59: Pathogenesis, diagnosis and control of canine hip dysplasia. In: Tobias K, Johnston S (eds.) Veterinary Surgery: Small Animal. Volume 1. St. Louis, MO: Elsevier Saunders, pp. 824–864.

Stone C (1999) Science in the Art of Osteopathy: Osteopathic Principles and Practice. Cheltenham: Stanley Thornes Ltd, pp.166–185.

Tauro A, Rusbridge C (2015) Degenerative myelopathy in the Nova Scotia Duck Tolling retriever. [Online] Available: http://www.veterinary-neurologist.co.uk/resources/Canine-degenerative-myelopathy-NSDTRetPK.pdf [March 27, 2019].

Vaughan LC (2010) The history of canine cruciate ligament surgery from 1952 – 2005. Veterinary and Comparative Orthopedics and Traumatology. 23 (6) 379–384.

Wardlaw JL, McLaughlin R (2012) Chapter 58: Coxofemoral luxation. In: Tobias K, Johnston S (eds.) Veterinary Surgery: Small Animal. Volume 1. St. Louis, MO: Elsevier Saunders, pp. 816–823.

Further reading

Bradshaw J (2011) In Defence of Dogs. London: Penguin Books.

Evans HE, de Lahunta A (2012) Miller's Anatomy of the Dog. 4th edn. St. Louis, MO: Elsevier Saunders.

Evans HE, de Lahunta A (2016) Guide to the Dissection of the Dog. 8th edn. St. Louis, MO: Saunders Elsevier.

Levine L, Millis DL, Marcellin-Little DJ, Taylor R (eds.) (2005) Rehabilitation and physical therapy. Veterinary Clinics of North America: Small Animal Practice. November; 35 (6).

Renberg WC, Roush JK (eds.) (2001) Lameness. Veterinary Clinics of North America: Small Animal Practice. January; 31 (1).

Renberg WC (ed.) (2005) General orthopedics. Veterinary Clinics of North America: Small Animal Practice. September; 35 (5).

Schebitz H, Wilkens H (1989) Atlas of Radiographic Anatomy of the Dog and Cat. 5th edn. Berlin and Hamburg: Paul Parey.

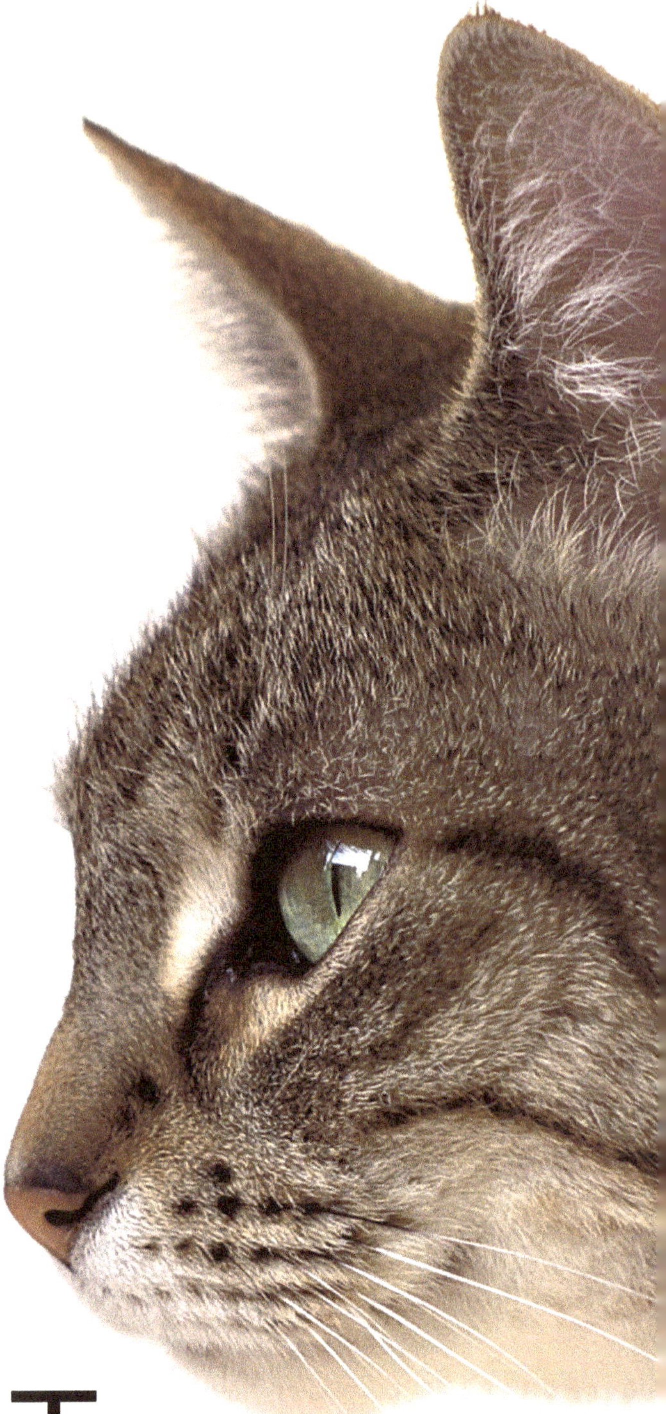

Chapter 3

THE CAT

Paolo Tozzi , Nadine Hobson, Richard Hillam,
Tony Nevin

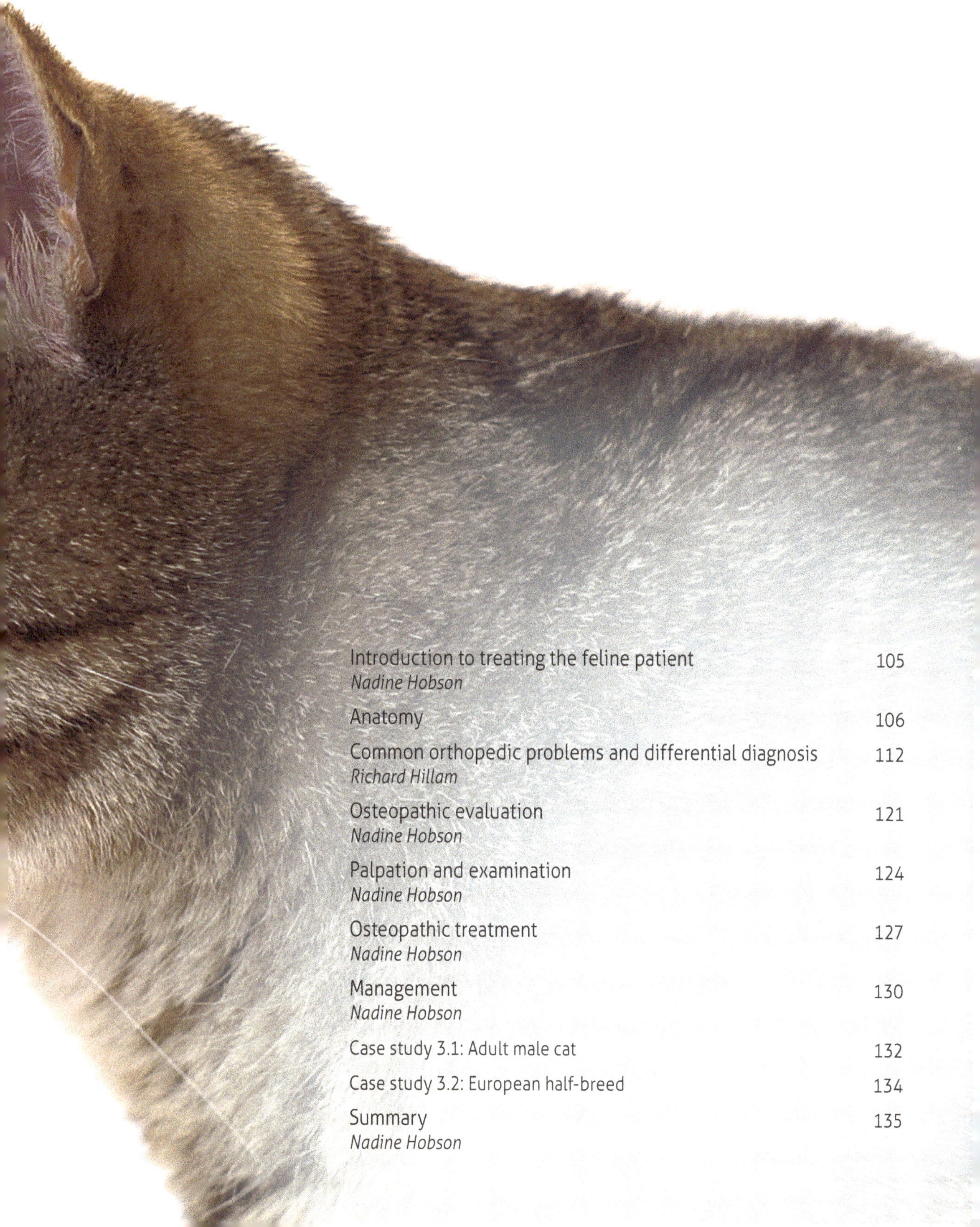

The cat

Chapter 3

Introduction to treating the feline patient

By embracing the philosophy of osteopathy and applying osteopathic principles our role in the health care of these intriguing creatures is extensive. The combination of clinical knowledge, observation, and palpation in the search for dysfunction and disease and then treating appropriately supports the body in its return to health.

In the UK it is preferable that the owner presents a referral letter at the time of the first visit.

If the osteopath is working within a vet clinic a full veterinary history will be available on site or can be requested from another practice.

This is one of the many benefits of being embedded within a veterinary practice along with the ease and convenience of referral by the vets, instant access to a complete case history, and the convenience of adding osteopathic notes directly. The ongoing dialogue and exchange of knowledge and opinions is of mutual benefit to all the professionals involved, offers best practice to the animal patient, and affords kudos to osteopathy as other vet practices will refer outside cases to a center of excellence in integrated health care.

Although cats and dogs are the most common family pets, they are poles apart in their attitude to their human housemates.

Felines are aloof, solitary predators, sure-footed climbers, slight of stature and lithe, fast-moving quadrupeds. The inherent independence of cats predisposes those less socialized to appear as if they have no mind to please their human companions, using them as a convenient source of food and shelter. However, many are docile and affectionate, integrating well into domestic life, and some breeds are especially responsive to human attention making them delightful household pets. Interaction with cats is uniquely fulfilling and emotionally rewarding.

In many ways the approach to osteopathic treatment of domestic cats follows a more similar methodology to the management of small wildlife than to that of dogs because of their innate characteristics. We may not have the indulgence of a leisurely and prolonged time for treatment if the cat is of a nervous or aggressive disposition.

Many veterinary centers have separate dog and cat waiting areas to reduce the stress of having these two potentially confrontational species together. Cats arrive at the vet clinic in an enclosed carrier, and stay there until safely ensconced in a consulting room away from other people and animals. They are often very reticent to emerge under their own steam. Whenever possible it is preferable that the owner lifts the cat out, encouraging them to settle and become accustomed to the strange surroundings. This can be done either on the floor or on the examination table. Likewise, the carrier can be lifted off at an angle, with one end open, to encourage the cat to exit downward with gravity.

It is essential that all escape routes are closed, windows are no more than ajar or covered with secure netting, and doors are firmly shut. Cats are speedy escapologists. Extricating them from the back of a cupboard or a dark corner behind furniture can be challenging.

Treating cats in a human clinic is not advisable on hygiene and health grounds. Many people are allergic to cat fur and there is the risk of parasites, for example, fleas, mites, worms, etc. being left behind with a small but possible chance of zoonosis spread.

Home visits also bring challenges. Some will be accepting of you as a stranger in their space; others may be unpredictable and aggressive toward a perceived threat. Ironically, a cat may often be quieter and more biddable in a vet clinic due to the fact it is not in its own territory.

Temperamentally cats vary enormously, not just according to breed types but as individuals. Many are docile and quite doglike in their compliance and acceptance of handling. Others can exhibit almost feral behavior, snarling, biting, and lashing out with claws extended.

Vet nurses are highly skilled at helping to restrain and contain these feisty felines while the necessary examination and treatment are performed. Never hesitate to request their help and support as the session can then be conducted smoothly and less traumatically for all involved. It may be less intimidating for the cat to be handled when it is facing away from you, the practitioner, and toward the owner or nurse. A hand placed lightly over the eyes prompts a sense of calm, as the cat will relax within the induced darkness. Alternatively, a gentle tapping on the forehead by the owner with a finger distracts the cat as it focuses on that sensation. The use of a Feliway® (cat pheromone) spray or plug-in diffuser in the treatment room may help to appease an anxious feline patient.

As in the field of pediatrics, we should approach these patients with noninvasive body language and sensitivity of touch so that they do not feel vulnerable. If we cultivate their trust they will cooperate and actually guide our treatment.

The majority of referrals for an osteopathic opinion are musculoskeletal cases with the main etiologies being congenital, developmental, due to trauma, or age related, although cases with neoplasia and metabolic disease may slip through the veterinary net.

Trauma is most commonly due to road traffic accidents or fighting with other cats. Occasionally they may be suffering from the injuries sustained in a fall from a tree, roof, or high window ledge and, contrary to common perception, cats do not always land on their feet.

In age-related degenerative conditions there are frequently comorbidities that must be taken into account and indeed many of these associated symptoms have reportedly improved after osteopathic treatment.

Anatomy

Leonardo Da Vinci's quote "The smallest feline is a masterpiece" is never more true than when it comes to feline anatomy. Cats represent the most supremely efficient muscular machines in their ability to jump, twist, and turn. The ratio of their strength to their size is far superior to humans.

Although dogs and cats share the same basic structure, there are some anatomical differences between these two species.

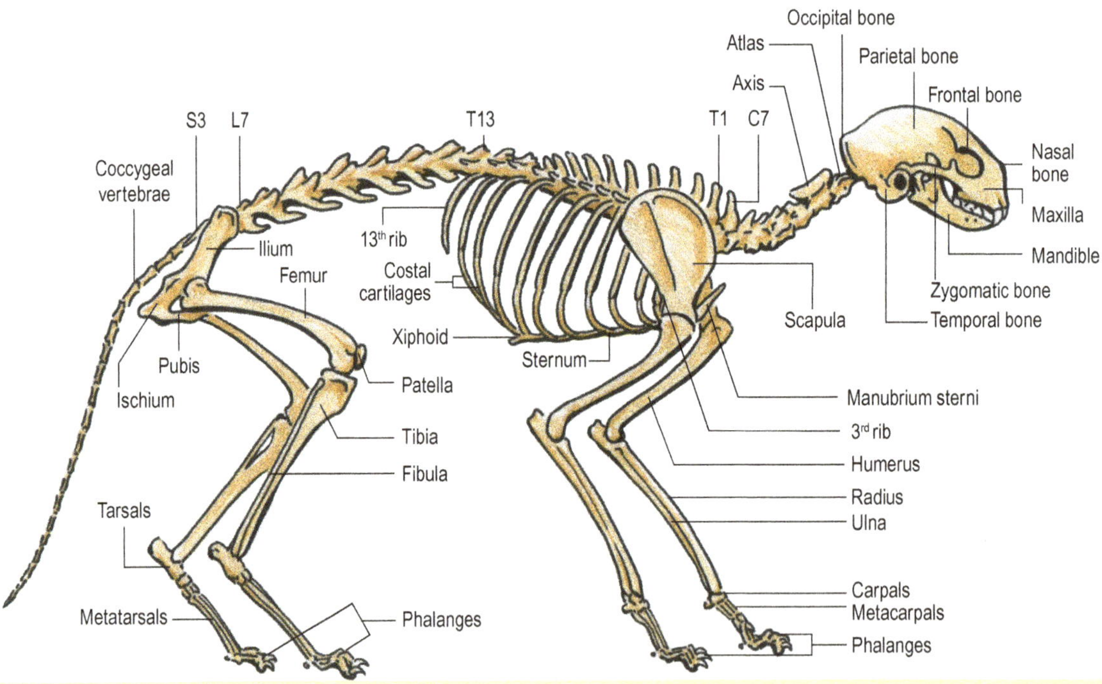

Figure 3.1
Skeleton of the cat.

The cat's skeleton (Fig. 3.1) has 245 bones against the 319 bones in dogs. Furthermore, in cats 517 separate muscles make them very agile animals. Generally speaking, felines are more muscular than canines (Fig. 3.2A–C). The cat's muscles are tough and well-coordinated to make it an agile hunter, and they are basically designed for walking, running, leaping, and twisting. This muscular control and skeletal flexibility enable the cat to right its body in the air during a fall with incredible speed by twisting its head around. A cat's tail, which contains almost 10 percent of its bones, acts as a counterweight in helping it keep its balance.

In a cat there are a total of seven cervical and 13 thoracic vertebrae. The latter are associated with corresponding pairs of ribs. The lumbar area has seven vertebrae and ends at the pelvis, which contains three fused sacral vertebrae. The tail usually consists of 18 to 23 caudal vertebrae.

The cat's skull has large eye sockets and air-filled sinuses in both the frontal and maxillary bones.

The jaw is short and strong with only limited ability to grind food as there is no sideways movement of the jaw (Grandjean and Butterwick 2009). Cats have 26 teeth as kittens and 30 as adults (12 incisors, 4 canines, 10 premolars [6 in the top jaw and 4 in the mandible], and 4 molars) (Fig. 3.3). All of them are sharp and designed for cutting and tearing. Cats have thin enamel that predisposes them to cavities. The teeth also have shallow roots that lead to easy tooth loss if tartar builds up and gingivitis becomes severe.

The neck and chest area of a feline is more muscular and solidly built than that of a canine, with the neck tending to be shorter than in dogs.

In profile (different from canines) the chest appears to be sunken in, with no bones protruding out past the

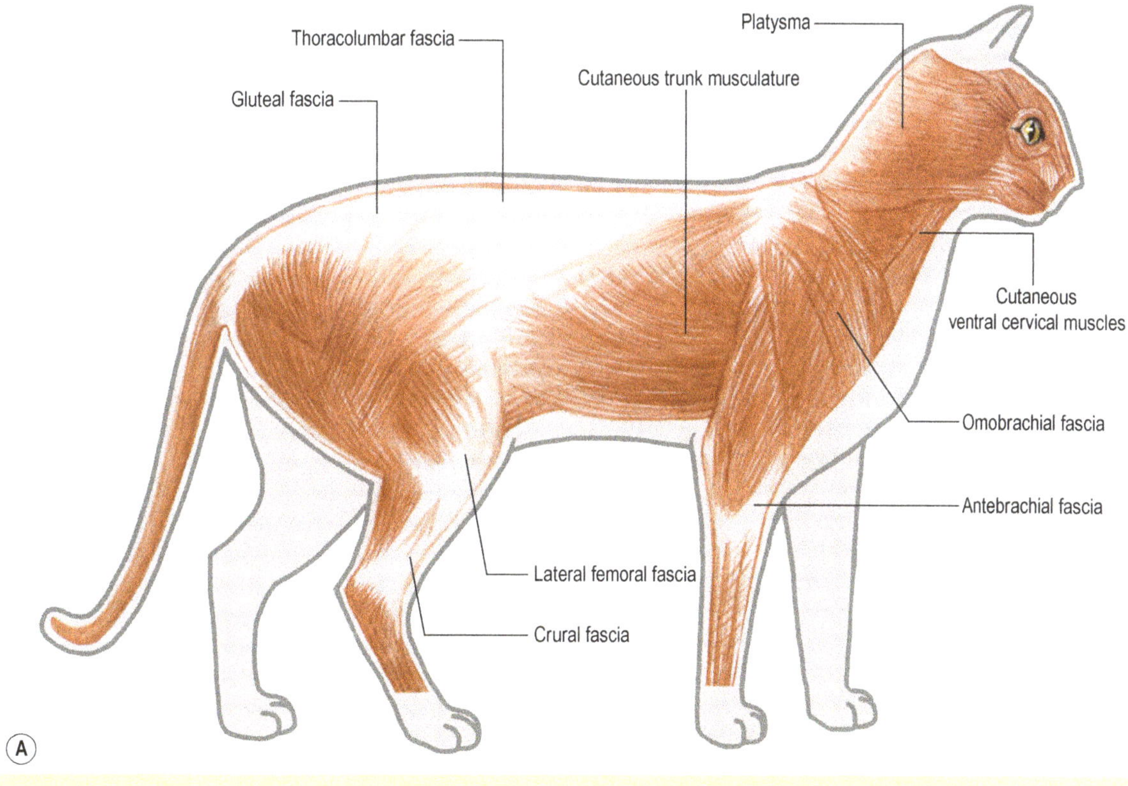

Figure 3.2
Musculature and fascia of the cat. (A) Superficial fascia and cutaneous muscles.

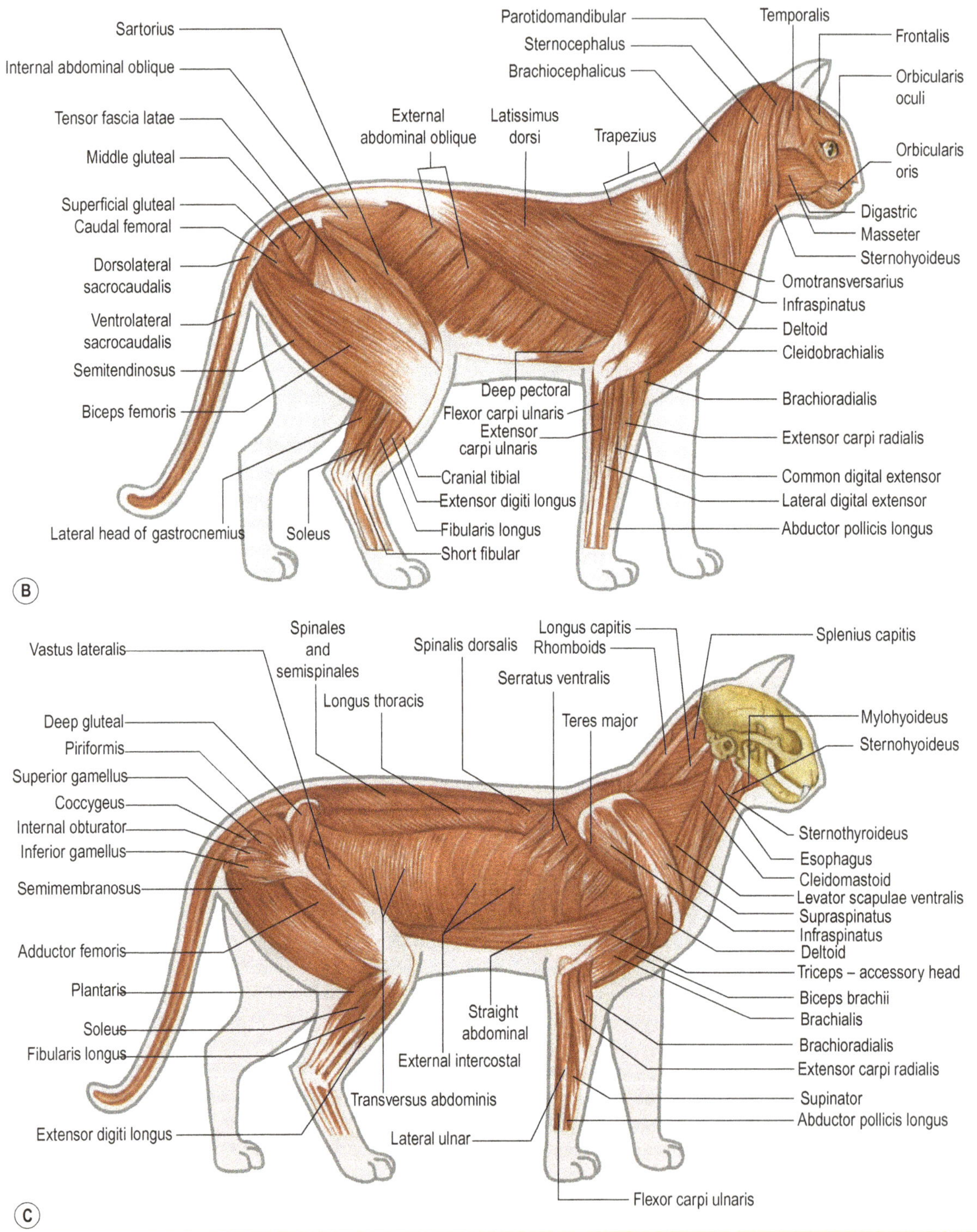

Figure 3.2 ***Continued***
(B) Superficial muscle layer. (C) Middle layer of musculature.

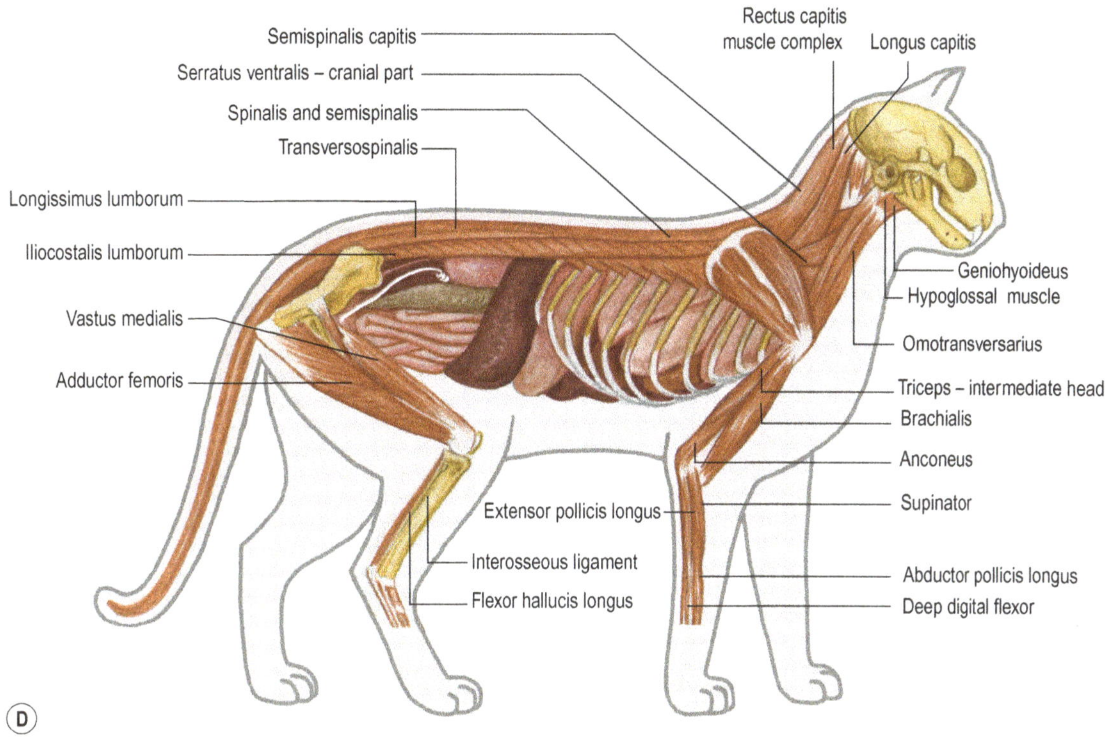

Figure 3.2 ***Continued***
(D) Deep layer of musculature.

shoulders. The rib cage on a feline has a larger cross-section posteriorly than the dog, both in width and depth (Fig. 3.4).

The feline's legs appear thicker, closer, and more connected at the chest than those of canines. The shoulders are larger, and the scapula is attached to the rest of the body only by muscles. This allows the cat freedom to twist and move and to extend the gait for full speed. Small collar bones allow cats to squeeze through tight openings and usually land on their feet from various heights. Cats do have clavicles, but the latter are not attached to other bones, being rod-like, about 20 mm long, and embedded within the brachiocephalic muscles.

The tarsal joint is slightly less defined and toes are fluffier and rounder with less definition. A cat has five toes on each of their front paws (Fig. 3.5) and only four on their back paws. Claws retract into slits and normally do not show. The two dorsal elastic ligaments at

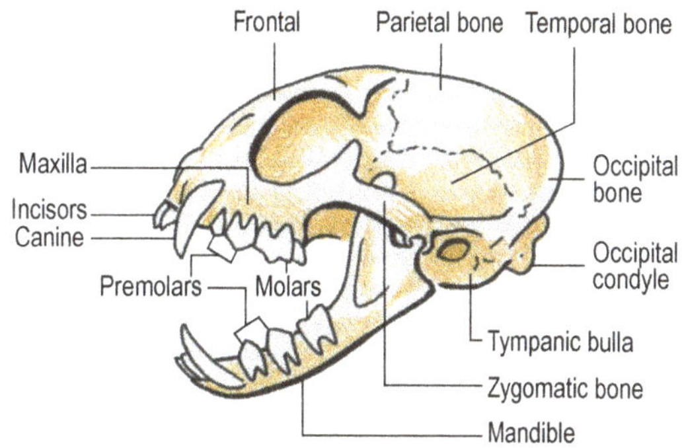

Figure 3.3
Feline skull and dentition.

the end of the distal interphalangeal joints are modified to keep the claws retracted. When the cat unsheathes its claws the deep digital flexor muscle contracts sufficiently to stretch the elastic ligaments.

Cats have exceptional eyesight. Most cats can see wavelengths of light, such as ultraviolet, that are

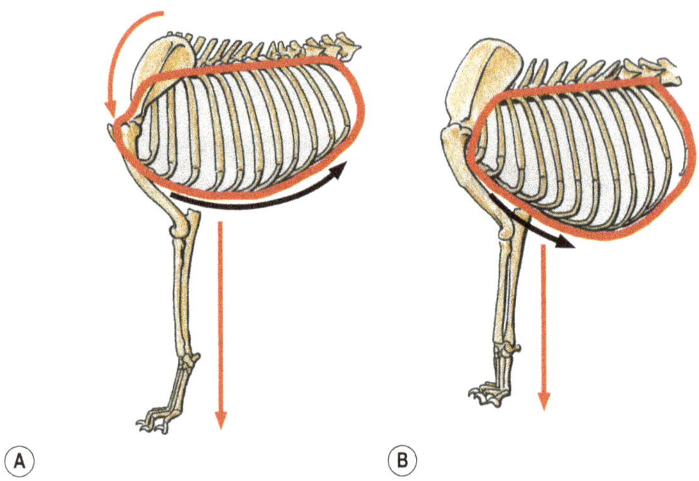

Figure 3.4
Comparison of canine and feline rib cages. (A) Canine rib cage is deeper cranially, and is more forward set. (B) Feline rib cage is larger and deeper caudally than in canines.

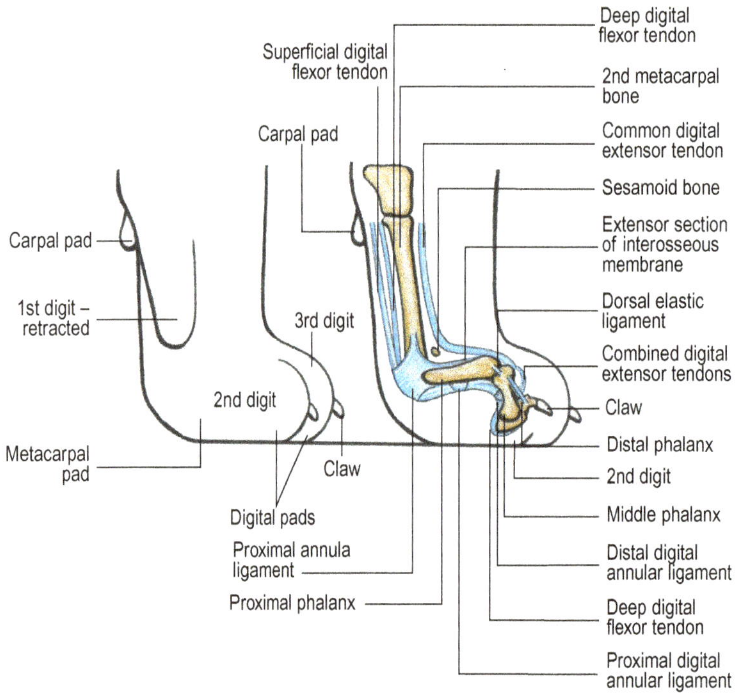

Figure 3.5
A sagittal section showing the ligaments that allow claw retraction.

invisible to humans. In the course of their development the ability to see at night while hunting was more important than the ability to see colors during the day. As far as scientists can tell, cats are probably virtually color-blind.

Cats' eyes are controlled by a pair of shutter-like ciliary muscles, creating the cat's distinctive slit-like pupil in bright light. In darkness, light hitting feline eyes is reflected from a mirror-like membrane behind the retina (causing the glowing of cat's eyes in the dark). This structure is called the tapetum lucidum. It is a layer of iridescent cells at the back of the eyeball which adds to the cat's ability to see at night. In fact, cats need only about one-sixth of the light humans need to function in the dark.

Cats do not have eyelashes, however, in common with many animals they do have a full inner eyelid or third eyelid which is located in the lower part of the cat's eye. This eyelid serves as protection for the eye when fighting or when traveling through brush.

The cat's olfactory nerves are not as sensitive as those of many other animals, and cats do not rely on this sense while hunting as much as other animals do. The cat has an accessory smell organ located in the upper surface of its mouth. This is called the Jacobson's organ and is thought to be used principally to detect pheromones.

The upper surface of the tongue is covered with rasp-like papillae which enable the cat to scrape every piece of meat off a bone or to lick its coat clean. The tongue is covered with taste buds, particularly at the tip and at the back of the throat.

The least important sense in a cat is the sense of touch. First of all, the hair or fur serves as insulation against heat and cold. Hair also protects the cat against various dangers and annoyances. Cats shed their hair according to climatic conditions and their state of health. Hair is shed naturally year round, especially in the spring and autumn. Excessive shedding is a warning signal of possible disease, poor diet, parasites, or overheating.

The skin has many glands. Sweat glands are located only on the foot pads. In fact, sweating is only a small portion of thermoregulation. The cat cools itself primarily by panting. Cats also have sebaceous glands connected with the hair follicles. They secrete an oily substance known as sebum that coats the hairs, thus protecting the fur and making it glossy. In a healthy state the cat's skin is always elastic and pliable, with the ability to regenerate at a rapid pace.

A cat's whiskers are like a radar guidance system, with a large bundle of nerve endings telegraphing details about everything they touch and monitoring shifts in air pressure. Cat's whiskers are the same width as their body, letting them know whether or not they can pass through a narrow opening. Whiskers are also used for navigating. The bristly hairs, found above the eyelids, around the muzzle and on the lower, inside part of the forelegs, help cats move smoothly in darkness. Sensitive to changes in air currents around an unknown object, whiskers enable the cat to avoid the obstacle. A hunting cat uses its whiskers to zero in on the outline of its prey and to let it know where to strike. A cat's facial whiskers are also mood indicators.

The cat's purr has always been something of an enigma. It is thought to result from intermittent contractions of the diaphragmatic and laryngeal muscles at a frequency of 25 to 150 hertz. Research suggests that this sound frequency may promote healing and bone growth.

Cats are fertile animals. A queen, or intact female cat, may produce two or three litters of kittens a year. Female cats are seasonally polyestrous. This means they have many estrous cycles during specific times of the year, triggered by day length. Cats usually come into heat during springtime. Periods of heat last two to 15 days, but if the cat does not mate and conceive the cycle will be repeated in a few weeks.

The uterus consists of a body and two horns. It is in the horns of the uterus that kitten embryos are implanted and develop. The oviduct is a tiny tube that connects the uterus to the ovaries. The oviduct is the actual site where fertilization occurs. The ovaries are a peanut-sized organ located near the kidneys.

Cats are induced ovulators meaning ovulation occurs as the result of mating. The average gestation period is 61 to 63 days. In a normal birth all kittens will be born within two to eight hours after labor begins.

Clinical considerations

- The acromion of a cat's scapula exhibits both a hamate and suprahamate process. The latter projects superficial to the infraspinatus muscle and must be considered during treatment of this area.
- Since the median nerve and brachial artery pass through a supracondylar foramen located distally

and medial to the humerus (Fig. 3.6), they are vulnerable to injury of the distal humerus.

Common orthopedic problems and differential diagnosis

Unlike the dog, in general veterinary practice we see a smaller range of orthopedic conditions in feline patients. They fall into the five main categories: developmental, traumatic, osteoarthritic, neoplastic, and metabolic (Table 3.1). It should be noted that in contrast to the dog, intervertebral disc disease and prolapse appear to be very uncommon, nonetheless, they do occur as does nontraumatic spinal cord disease.

Developmental orthopedic disease

Nutritional osteodystrophies: rickets and nutritional hyperparathyroidism

This category is not very common but is seen occasionally when owners want to prepare the food themselves in preference to buying commercial food – a trend that is becoming more popular in both dog and cat owners. Nutritional osteodystrophies are occasionally seen in young growing cats when they are fed a homemade diet that consists principally of raw or cooked meat, often chicken breast. These diets will mainly consist of muscle with no bone or other added vitamins or minerals. They are extremely unbalanced in their calcium, phosphorus, and vitamin D content compared with the natural wild feline diet and can interfere with normal bone and growth plate development.

Clinical signs are lameness, a hunched appearance, and small stature. Clinical findings, history of diet, radiography, and the biochemistry findings of low serum ionized calcium and high circulating parathyroid hormone levels all confirm the diagnosis (Fig. 3.7A and B, Fig. 3.8A–E).

Treatment consists of changing the diet and the use of analgesics if required. The presence of any

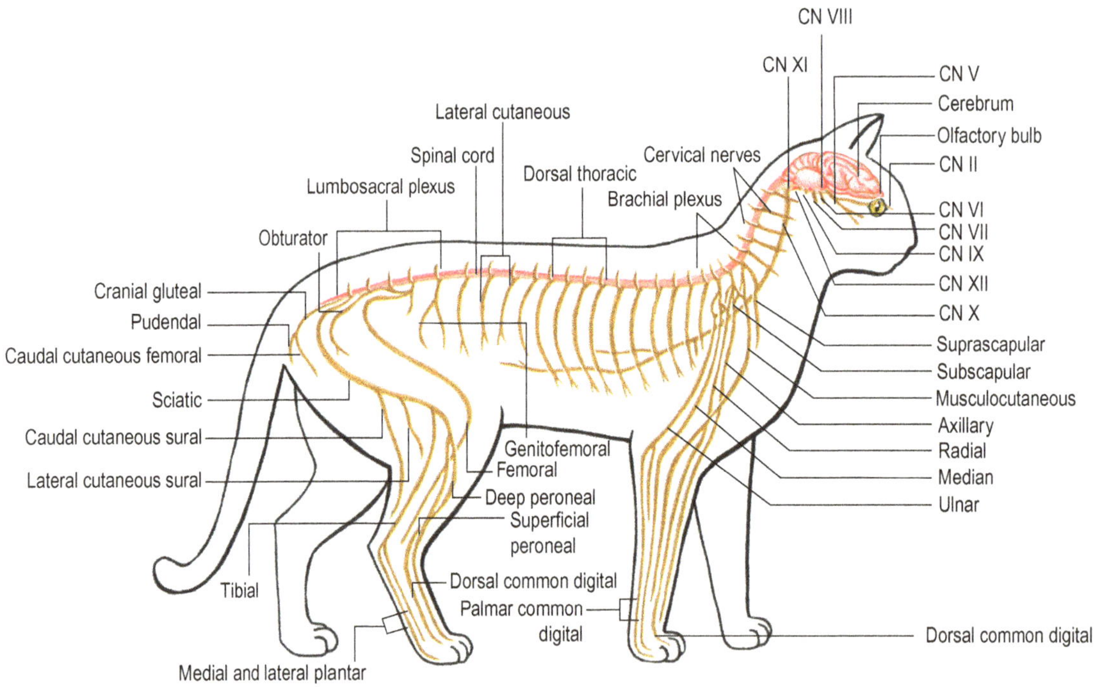

Figure 3.6
The central and peripheral nervous system of the cat.

Table 3.1 Details of feline orthopedic conditions

Age	Condition	Onset	Clinical signs	Duration	Etiology	Veterinary treatment	Prognosis
0 to 3 months	Fractures	Acute	Lameness	2 to 3 months	Trauma	External support, surgery, rest	Usually good
	Osteogenesis imperfecta	Variable	Spontaneous, nontraumatic fractures (often multiple). Joint, rib, spine, and long bone pain	Chronic	Thought to be a genetic defect resulting in abnormal formation of collagen type 1	None	Hopeless
3 to 6 months	Fractures	Acute	Lameness	2 to 3 months	Trauma	External support, surgery, rest	Very good
	Salter–Harris growth plate fractures	Acute	Lameness	2 to 3 months	Trauma or overexertion	External support, surgery, rest	Variable with potential long-term sequelae
	Luxating patella	Gradual	Intermittent lameness with very brief lifting of the foot off the ground. If bilateral the cat may struggle to walk using the back legs	Chronic	Complex anatomical conformation abnormalities	Surgery	Usually good
	Nutritional osteodystrophies	Gradual	Stunted growth, joint pain, swollen joints, angular deformities, pathological fractures	3 to 4 months	Inappropriate diet	Correction of diet	Usually good
	Osteogenesis imperfecta	Variable	Spontaneous, nontraumatic fractures (often multiple). Joint, rib, spine, and long bone pain	Chronic	Thought to be a genetic defect resulting in abnormal formation of collagen type 1.	None	Hopeless
6 to 12 months	Fractures	Acute	Bone pain, swelling, lameness	Variable	Trauma	External support or surgery	Very good
	Salter–Harris growth plate fractures	Acute	Lameness	2 to 3 months	Trauma or overexertion	External support with rest or surgery	Variable with potential long term sequelae
	Luxating patella	Gradual	Intermittent lameness with very brief lifting of the foot off the ground. If bilateral the cat may struggle to walk using the back legs	Chronic	Complex anatomical conformation abnormalities	Surgery	Usually good
	Nutritional osteodystrophies	Gradual	Stunted growth, joint pain, swollen joints, angular deformities, pathological fractures	Months	Inappropriate diet	Correction of diet	Usually good
	Proximal femoral physeal dysplasia	Acute	Hind limb lameness and hip pain	Chronic	Unknown	Surgery	Good after surgery
	Osteogenesis imperfecta	Variable	Spontaneous, nontraumatic fractures (often multiple). Joint, rib, spine, and long bone pain.	Chronic	Thought to be a genetic defect resulting in abnormal formation of collagen type 1	None	Hopeless

Table 3.1 *Continued*

Age	Condition	Onset	Clinical signs	Duration	Etiology	Veterinary treatment	Prognosis
1 to 3 years	Fractures	Acute	Bone pain, swelling, lameness	Variable	Trauma	External support or surgery	Very variable
	Proximal femoral physeal dysplasia	Acute	Hind limb lameness and hip pain	Chronic	Unknown	Surgery	Good after surgery
3 to 6 years	Fractures	Acute	Bone pain, swelling, lameness	Variable	Trauma	External support or surgery	Very variable
	Cranial cruciate injuries	Variable	Stifle swelling, stiffness or failure to bear weight	Chronic	Trauma and end stage of an inflammatory joint disease	Rest, NSAID analgesics, osteopathy, physiotherapy, hydrotherapy, surgery	Good but there are potential long term sequelae
6 to 12 years	Fractures	Acute	Bone pain, swelling, lameness	3 to 6 months	Trauma	External support or surgery	Very variable
	Osteoarthritis	Gradual	Joint swelling, stiffness, crepitus and failure to bear weight	Lifelong	Joint instability, inflammatory disease processes, infection, trauma, previous surgery	Rest, NSAID analgesics, osteopathy, physiotherapy, hydrotherapy, arthrodesis surgery	Very variable
	Cranial cruciate injuries	Variable	Stifle swelling, stiffness or failure to bear weight	Chronic	Trauma and end stage of an inflammatory joint disease	Rest, NSAID analgesics, osteopathy, physiotherapy, hydrotherapy, surgery	Very variable
	Neoplasia	Gradual	Bone pain (may be intense), swelling of soft tissues, lameness, possible fever	Usually fatal	Unknown, previous site of a fracture, infection or surgery	NSAID analgesics, opioid analgesics, chemotherapy, radiotherapy, surgery, euthanasia	Very poor
Geriatric	Osteoarthritis	Gradual	Joint swelling, stiffness and failure to bear weight	Lifelong	Joint instability, inflammatory disease processes, infection, trauma, previous surgery	Rest, NSAID analgesics, osteopathy, physiotherapy, hydrotherapy, arthrodesis surgery	Very variable

Table 3.1 *Continued*

Age	Condition	Onset	Clinical signs	Duration	Etiology	Veterinary treatment	Prognosis
12 to 16 years	Neoplasia	Gradual	Bone pain (may be intense), swelling of soft tissues, lameness, possible fever	Usually fatal	Unknown, previous site of a fracture, infection or surgery	NSAID analgesics, opioid analgesics, chemotherapy, radiotherapy, surgery, euthanasia	Extremely poor
	Pathological fractures	Acute	Sudden onset, spontaneous fractures that may not be that painful resulting in lameness if limb bones are affected or back pain if vertebrae are affected	Variable	Any disease process that leads to an osteopenia (bone demineralization) and weakening of the bone	Dealing with the primary, underlying disease process	Very poor
	Cranial cruciate injuries	Variable	Stifle swelling, stiffness or failure to bear weight	Chronic	Trauma and end stage of an inflammatory joint disease	Rest, NSAID analgesics, osteopathy, physiotherapy, hydrotherapy, surgery	Very variable

pathological fractures may also require specific management.

Osteogenesis imperfecta

This is a very uncommon developmental condition in the cat, and is seen quite rarely in practice, but it does warrant a brief mention despite a dearth of peer-reviewed papers. There is a genetic mutation that leads to abnormal collagen type 1 formation in the bone matrix; consequently the bones develop with thin, weak cortices. These are very susceptible to pathological fractures, which occur during habitual physiological activity, with no history of trauma. The condition may run in families with multiple siblings affected, usually between two to eight months of age.

Clinical signs are usually limb and rib pain with lameness that is related to the formation of spontaneous fractures. Diagnosis is based on history, radiology, and specialist genetic, skin cell culture, and biochemical tests that are not widely available. Radiographs will demonstrate one or, more likely, multiple fractures in different bones with signs of healing in old, previously occurring fractures.

There is no way of treating this condition satisfactorily. The use of vitamin C and bisphosphonates has been tried in the past. Should the osteopath ever encounter a suspected case they are very likely to create more fractures in the process of manipulation. Sadly euthanasia is the only option.

Patellar luxation (Harasen 2006)

Although it is much more common in the dog, patellar luxation is occasionally observed in the cat. As in the dog, the condition may arise suddenly following trauma or develop gradually as the young animal grows. The latter will be less obvious, especially if the condition is bilateral. There may be a predisposition in the Devon Rex and Abyssinian breeds. The grading system used for dogs is also used in cats. There are four grades depending on the severity and whether the patella is occasionally or permanently luxated out of the femoral trochlear groove.

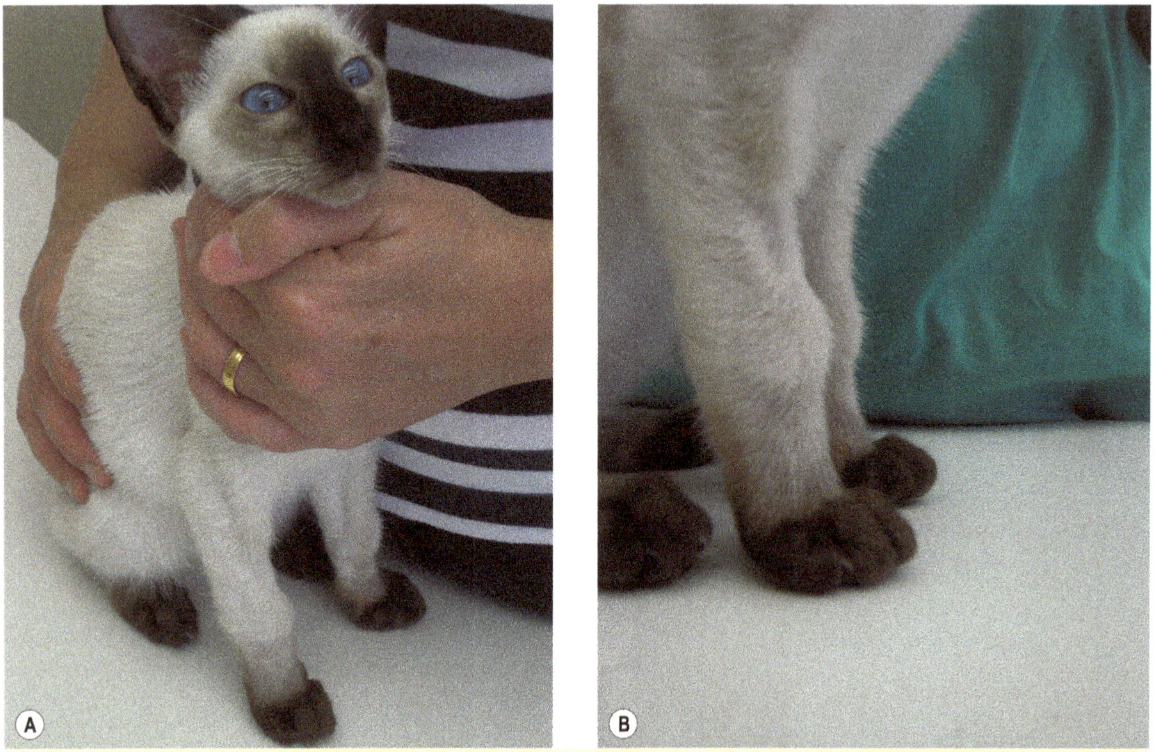

Figure 3.7
(A and B) Feline osteodystrophy.

Clinical findings include the reluctance to jump, an abnormal hind limb gait, holding the affected limb up, a mechanical lameness, quadriceps muscle atrophy, and a possible positive tibial cranial drawer sign.

Confirmation of a diagnosis largely relies on the clinical findings although radiography may be of use (Fig. 3.9).

Grade 1 patellar luxations may well improve without any surgery but the other grades are likely to benefit from some form of surgery. The more chronic the condition the worse the prognosis because of the negative effect this condition is likely to have on hind limb alignment and the normal development of the stifle joint. Adverse effects include cartilage erosion and damage to the cranial cruciate ligament and the menisci.

Proximal femoral physeal dysplasia (Grayton et al. 2014)

This is also known as feline metaphyseal osteopathy of the femoral neck. This is not a common condition but is occasionally seen in cats, including the domestic short hair, Siamese, Maine Coon, and British Blue.

The condition is not well understood. It does not seem to be associated with trauma, with a gradual onset of lameness developing over three weeks or more. It tends to affect overweight males and is bilateral in 50–90 percent of cases. It is thought to be due to abnormal chondrocytes in growth plates that remain "open" (i.e., not mineralized) and that this may be associated with castration at a young age, abnormal blood supply, insulin metabolism disorders, bacterial osteomyelitis, and possible exposure to the feline herpes virus.

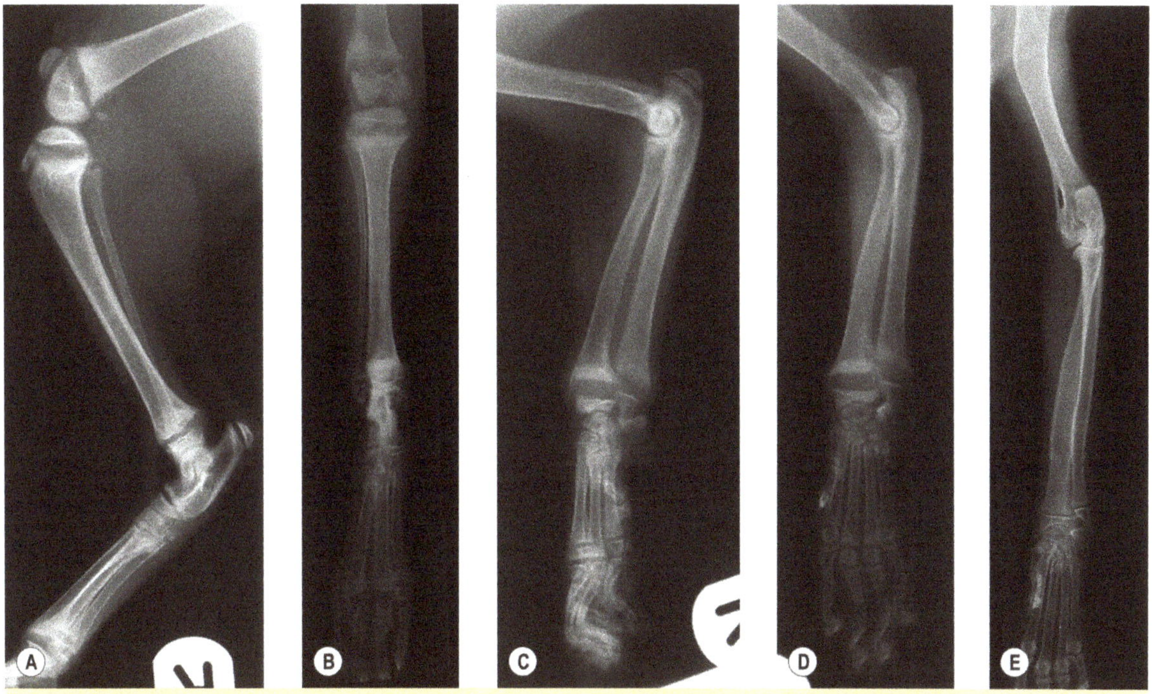

Figure 3.8
(A–E) Radiographs showing bony changes in the presence of nutritional osteodystrophy: rickets and nutritional hyperparathyroidism.

At initial presentation the site of pain may be unclear. Ultimately the cat may be unable to bear weight at all on the affected limb and an examination will reveal pronounced muscle atrophy in the thigh musculature and gluteals over the hips. There is pain on flexion, extension, and lateromedial pressure of the hip joint. Crepitus and asymmetrical limb length may be apparent when the back legs are extended caudally.

Diagnosis relies on radiography of the hips (Fig. 3.10). Treatment requires a femoral head and neck excision osteotomy and the prognosis for an acceptable return to pain-free function is good. Physiotherapy and osteopathy may be of great assistance in rehabilitation following surgery.

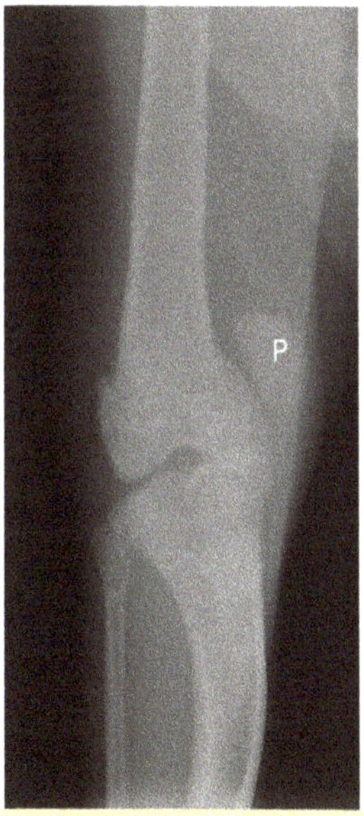

Figure 3.9
Radiograph showing patellar luxation in a cat. P = patella.

Traumatic orthopedic conditions

In the cat this group probably constitutes the most common cause for presentation of the feline orthopedic patient. The array of potential injuries is vast

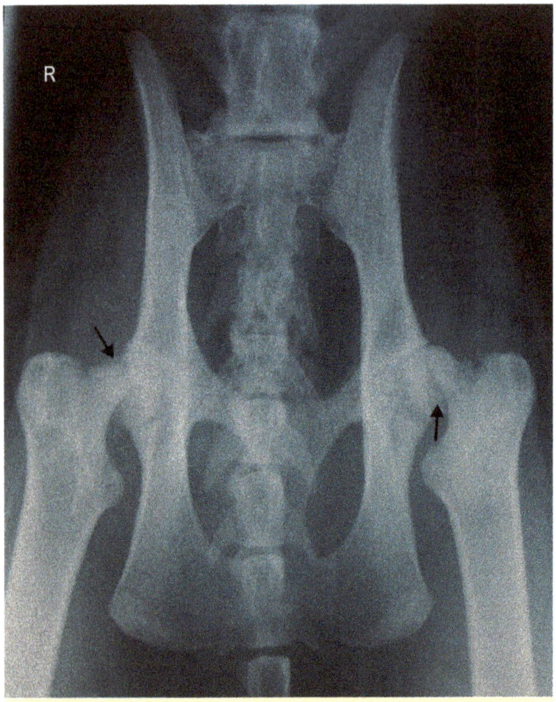

Figure 3.10
Radiograph showing femoral proximal physeal dysplasia in a cat.

with most being the result of road traffic accidents, falls from windows and roofs, gunshot wounds, and dog attacks.

Common fractures are those affecting the humerus, femur, tibia and fibula, mandible, spine, and pelvis, including sacroiliac separations. Fractures range from those that are simple and closed to complex, comminuted open fractures. Joint luxations and subluxations are common including in the hip, stifle, hock (Fig. 3.11A and B), and temporomandibular joint (TMJ). Together with the bony damage there is associated trauma to the soft tissues, which may well be more serious than that to the bones but will not necessarily be evident on radiographs.

Worthy of a mention is quadriceps contracture that occurs in cases of midshaft and distal femoral fractures, especially in young cats, and is quite common. Quadriceps muscle adhesions to the femoral diaphysis, together with muscle contracture, result in partial or rigid extension of the stifle joint. At some point normal physiological activity can result in avulsion of the proximal tibial tuberosity which requires repair with pins and orthopedic wire. The cat is usually left with a permanently stiff and extended hind limb (Fig. 3.12A and B).

Trauma accounts for around 14 percent of spinal cord injuries in cats. Intervertebral disc extrusions can occur but are far less common than in dogs. There are also unrelated cases of nontraumatic spinal cord disease that may be related to infectious agents, tumors, thromboemboli, and other causes. These may or not be painful. There will be neurological deficits affecting areas that vary depending on the site of the cord lesions. Diagnosis relies on a neurological exam, radiology, and MRI scans.

There is little doubt that many of these patients would benefit significantly from rehabilitation in the form of physiotherapy and osteopathy during the recovery from a large number of their traumatic injuries.

Dropped hock

Dropped hock or a plantigrade stance is quite common in the cat. Normally the cat will stand with the weight supported entirely on the toes; however, in the plantigrade stance the distal hind limb from the hock to the toes "sinks" or hyperflexes so that it lies flat against the ground. Rupture of the gastrocnemius tendon or its avulsion (with or without the superficial flexor tendon) from the calcaneus bone may arise through trauma. In addition, the plantigrade stance may be the result of a nontraumatic neuropathy seen in cases of untreated or poorly managed diabetes mellitus. In general practice I have seen this condition far more commonly as a result of a diabetic neuropathy than from cases of trauma but specialist surgical referral centers may observe the opposite finding.

Diagnosis requires a thorough clinical exam with radiographs and blood tests to establish if the etiology

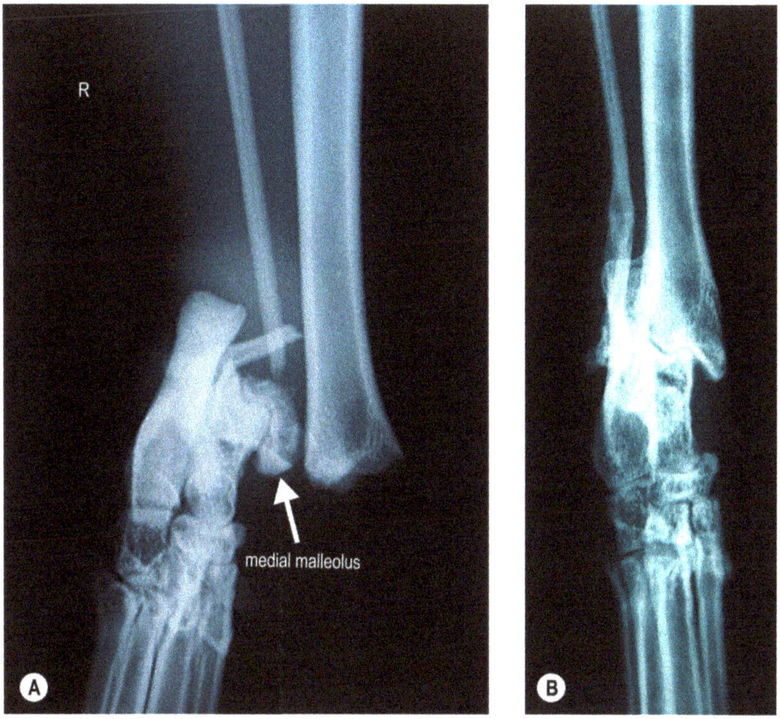

Figure 3.11
(A) Radiograph showing a fracture through the hock of a cat. (B) Radiograph of the same joint, now healed.

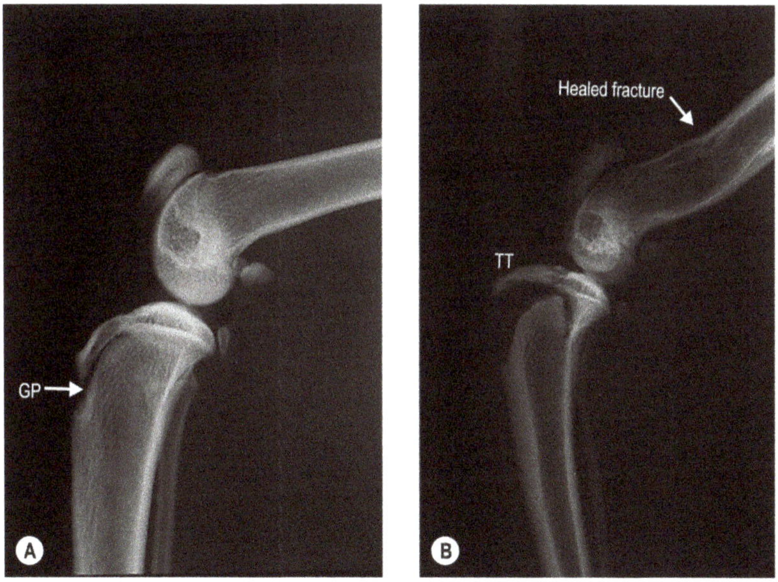

Figure 3.12
(A) Radiograph showing a normal stifle joint in a skeletally immature female cat. (B) Radiograph showing a femoral fracture and tibial tuberosity avulsion in a female cat..

is trauma or diabetes. Treatment of the former requires surgery, cage rest, and then rehabilitation in the form of physiotherapy and osteopathy, whereas diabetes requires precise medical and dietary management with regular monitoring. In both cases the prognosis for return to normal function is good.

Osteoarthritis

Historically arthritides were overlooked in feline patients in general veterinary practice. It was felt that the condition contributed little to feline orthopedic complaints, and if it developed cats could tolerate the discomfort and compensate for it very well. Furthermore, there were very few safe, licensed medical treatment options available for its management that could be administered easily by the owners.

With life expectancy increasing in the cat and obesity becoming more of an issue, osteoarthritis is now accepted as being a significant condition in the older cat and in those patients that have had cranial cruciate injuries and traumatic joint luxations or subluxations.

Diagnosis requires radiography for confirmation. Its management involves weight control and the use of safe, licensed analgesics and anti-inflammatories. Obviously hydrotherapy is not an option here. However, physiotherapy and osteopathy may help significantly in amenable patients.

Neoplasia

Neoplasia or cancer of the musculoskeletal system does not appear to be encountered as frequently in the cat as it is in the dog. Nonetheless it does occur occasionally and can easily be overlooked and left undiagnosed. The most common tumor is the osteosarcoma which affects the appendicular skeleton more frequently than the axial skeleton. Osteosarcomas of hind limbs are more common than those of the forelimbs. However, this tumor may also arise in the spine, skull, scapula, and pelvis. Other tumors can also be encountered such as the fibrosarcoma and squamous cell carcinoma.

Clinical signs include swelling and pain of affected areas, lameness, and muscle loss.

Diagnosis is made by using radiography and histopathology of biopsies. Feline leukemia virus (FeLV) and feline immunodeficiency virus (FIV) infections should be ruled out because some feline tumors can be associated with infection with these immunosuppressive viruses, especially FeLV.

Treatment may involve amputation of affected limbs and chemotherapy or palliative analgesia. Generally, the prognosis is guarded to extremely poor.

Metabolic orthopedic disease

Renal secondary hyperparathyroidism (RSH)

RSH is observed in cats with chronic renal failure which is very common in older cats. In RSH blood phosphorous rises (hyperphosphatemia), calcium falls (hypocalcemia), and vitamin D metabolism is adversely affected. The net result is a reduction of bone calcium which results in bone resorption, osteopenia and, ultimately, reduction in bone strength. Consequently, this can result in pathological nontraumatic fractures, joint and bone pain, and delayed, or nonunion of, fractures.

In any middle-aged or older cat that presents with a fracture or fractures where no traumatic event has been observed bone pain or delayed fracture healing RSH should be ruled out using blood tests and radiology.

This condition requires medical management and constant monitoring.

Hypervitaminosis A

Hypervitaminosis A is not as common as it was 25 years ago, presumably due to better client education. It develops as the result of feeding diets rich in vitamin A. Typically this happens when liver, much loved by cats, is fed in excess or if the owner gives too many supplements with vitamins that contain high levels of vitamin A.

The result is the development of exostoses (new bone) around joints which can eventually lead to ankylosis (fusion). The clinical signs are neck and generalized stiffness which manifests itself as reluctance to jump and climb stairs and lameness. Neurological deficits can also develop in some of the more severe cases.

Diagnosis is based on history of the diet and radiology. The outcome depends very much on the severity of the exostoses and ankyloses at the time of diagnosis. A normal balanced diet must be fed and pain relief provided in the form of nonsteroidal anti-inflammatories. Osteopathy may help in alleviation of the joint stiffness but joint ankylosis cannot be reversed.

Miscellaneous conditions

Ingrowing nails

This is a very common condition in older inactive cats and in those with polydactyly (the presence of additional toes). It develops gradually and results in secondary infection causing pain and lameness.

Clinical findings are obvious together with swollen toes and a very unpleasant smell.

Missing this condition would be negligent, embarrassing, and certainly wouldn't enhance one's professional reputation. Always examine the feet thoroughly in any lame animal irrespective of the species that is being treated.

Cat bite abscesses

Cats frequently fight and consequently they are often presented with very painful bite abscesses that are caused by the *Pasteurella* bacterium. If a limb or the lumbar area is bitten the clinical picture will be one of severe lameness or back pain respectively. More often than not an obvious abscess will be clearly visible, but this is not always the case. Bites to the antebrachium often result in a very diffuse infection with no discrete pocket of pus. Nonetheless they are very painful, cause widespread swelling, and may be confused with a fracture. In addition, a bite to a joint may cause septic arthritis which will cause profound joint swelling, pain, and lameness. The long-term consequences of septic arthritis are very severe so prompt diagnosis and treatment are essential.

Diagnosis requires a thorough clinical exam, the finding of pyrexia, fine needle aspirates of affected areas, and X-rays.

Treatment of bite abscesses involves surgical drainage, antibiotics, and analgesics.

Aortic or arterial thromboembolism (saddle thrombus)

This acute condition is not an orthopedic or spinal problem but may easily be confused with one or a neurological abnormality. The clinical signs can be dramatic with the hind limbs affected. It causes a lot of discomfort or intense pain and paresis or paralysis of the affected limb or limbs, which may also feel cold.

Affected cats usually have an underlying cardiac condition called cardiomyopathy. A thrombus (blood clot) will gradually form in the left side of the heart and at some point it will suddenly detach and pass down the aorta. At some point the thrombus will lodge in the caudal part of the aorta, in the region of the femoral arteries, causing an obstruction to blood circulation. The clinical signs depend on the severity of the blood flow disruption.

Diagnosis relies on the clinical signs, possible previous history of cardiac disease, ultrasonography, and a specialized form of radiography called angiography.

Medical management may help, but even in cases where an improvement is observed recurrences often occur within six months to a year. For this reason, and because the condition can be so dramatic and painful, most cases will be euthanized.

Osteopathic evaluation

Assessment of the cat is reliant on a comprehensive history, including the results of the required clinical tests and a working diagnosis from the vet combined with a detailed description of behavioral changes from the owner. From this overview we can then expand the picture on which to base our osteopathic opinion.

The importance of reported changes in activity, sleeping position or location, and interaction with the household cannot be overemphasized. Is the cat reluctant to go outside, shunning negotiation with the cat flap, with consequent changes in toiletry habits, or no longer sits on raised surfaces (furniture or walls) thus avoiding jumping or climbing? These are typically the only indications of pain or discomfort due to osteoarthritis in the spine or peripheral joints, but are assumed to be normal signs of an aging cat and thus degenerative joint disease (DJD) can to be underdiagnosed. Recent studies show radiographic evidence of DJD (including both spinal and peripheral joints) in up to 90 percent of cats over 12 years of age (International Cat Care 2019).

Osteopaths are exceptionally adept in locating and identifying these problems due to their palpatory skill.

Details of the social history are very helpful to formulate a psychological profile. Is this a rehoming or rescue case with a history of neglect or abuse? Are there other cats or dogs in the household and what are the dynamics between them? Are there any dominant new cats in the neighborhood that might be intruding into your patient's territory? Is this an indoor only cat or free to roam outside?

Be alert, particularly if there has been a time lapse since the referral from the vet, as serious pathologies can progress surprisingly quickly. The clinical picture can change and develop in a matter of days.

Always be vigilant for red flags and contraindications to treatment.

Signalment

Signalment of disease predisposition is considered with regard to the following factors.

Age

The average life expectancy of the domestic cat in the UK is 14.5 years, taking into account the toll of road deaths. Thus it is not unusual to see cats of 16 or 17 years of age (equivalent to the mid-80s in humans).

Degenerative disorders start to take their toll especially when associated with congenital or developmental conditions. The compensatory mechanisms become less efficient, somatic dysfunctions begin to present, and disease becomes evident (see Chapter 1).

Weight

Fat cats are increasingly numerous due to overfeeding or lack of exercise, particularly those that do not have outdoor access. Dry commercial foods, used by many owners due to their convenience, contain up to 40 percent carbohydrate and fat compared to 6 percent in a natural diet, hence the tendency to weight gain.

Underweight cats may be reflecting social issues, such as being a stray or recently rehomed, bullying by dominant housemates, or having their food taken by another cat (or even the dog).

Weight change can also be due to systemic disease. For example, hyperthyroidism is common in cats, causing weight loss, irritability, dry scaly skin, and lackluster fur.

Dietary advice is not within the osteopath's remit so referral back to the vet is necessary to confirm the cause of weight problems.

Gender

There can be issues associated with pregnancy and parturition in queens and also postoperative recovery after spaying. Tomcats are notorious fighters returning home with war wounds of varying degrees of severity. Injuries from bites and scratches are prone to nasty infections so must receive veterinary attention.

Breed

There is a wide range of differing breeds but with less variation in size and fewer breed-specific pathologies than in the canine world. Domestic short-haired cats (commonly known as "moggies") tend to be blessed with remarkable hybrid vigor. Certain breeds are more suited than others to be purely house cats, whereas others thrive on unrestricted outdoor access (e.g., farm cats).

An essential reminder at this juncture is the domestic cat's unique style of locomotion. Unlike other felines and all quadrupeds (except camels, giraffes, and brown bears) which exhibit a diagonal walk using the diagonally opposing limb, the domestic cat walks using the ipsilateral limbs simultaneously in a fluid, pacing motion. These locomotive mechanics, together with the coordinated use of the tail, explain their extraordinary aptitude for balance and agility (Bradshaw et al. 2012). There are three variations in the gallop: transverse, rotatory, and the half-bound They demonstrate differing synchronizations in limb movements adapted to the cat's role as a finely tuned predator. Switching between these three types of motion during high-speed activity is an effective way of minimizing fatigue in the individual limbs.

At best, observation is possible during voluntary movement when the cat is climbing out of the carrier and investigating the surroundings. More typically, the immobility, positioning, and posture are indications of its condition and temperament, particularly if the cat is unwell or in pain. Watch your feline patient out of the corner of your eye while you are reviewing the case notes and talking to the owner. A cat that is not the center of attention is more likely to feel unthreatened and thus curious about its environment.

Is there a stiffness of gait or obvious lameness in either the hind limbs or forelimbs or any degree of ataxia?

Note any asymmetry of the trunk, the position of the head relative to the body, roaching, or scoliosis of the spine. Look for symmetry of the limbs.

Be aware that a reported sudden difficulty in climbing or jumping is *not* definitively the presenting symptom of a musculoskeletal (MSK) problem. Systemic disease due to, for example, endocrine, heart, or kidney disorders, can present with changes in efficiency of mobility.

Notice the overall body condition, weight, muscle tone, and bulk. Does the coat look and feel healthy? A cat that is unwell or in pain for any reason including MSK causes may find eating difficult and also be unable to groom itself effectively. A matted coat can cause considerable discomfort and distress. On occasions this may require general anesthesia while it is disentangled. An isolated patch of knotted fur can indicate a specific mobility problem elsewhere which is preventing overall access for thorough grooming.

Conversely, there can be areas of alopecia caused by overgrooming in response to skin irritation associated with dermatological conditions due to infection, parasite infestation, or endocrine imbalance. Overgrooming is also a soothing displacement activity reflecting the cat's psychological reaction to stress.

A point of interest is that cats follow a grooming routine beginning at the head, using the front paws over the face and around the ears, and then continuing systematically, licking the rest of the body to the tip of the tail (Dodman 1998).

Healthy cats spend about 8–15 percent of their waking time cleaning themselves. In the wild removing the blood of their prey from their fur, the scent of which could in turn attract larger predators, is vital to their survival (Dodman 1998).

Grooming also serves to spread pheromones from scent glands situated around the muzzle and paws, as does the act of rubbing the face and body on a human companion. It is thought that the accompanying chirruping sounds and subtle tail movements have evolved specifically, as a language or communication, in response to human contact. These actions are all characteristic of a cat that is comfortable in its environs.

A cat's whiskers, or vibrissae, are vitally important tactile hairs. They should be the same width as the body for accurate spatial navigation. Intact, undamaged whiskers are especially important in darkness as a guidance system, also assisting in the accuracy of catching and killing prey. The positioning of the whiskers is a reflection of the cat's mood. When they are pointing slightly forward and down from the face, the cat is relaxed and happy. Tense and forward pointing indicates hunting, stalking or aggression, whereas whiskers that are pulled tightly backward against the face signify an angry cat (Cat-World 2019).

Watch the eyes, ears, lips and teeth, whiskers, claws, tail, hackles, and muscle tone and tension. Are the eyes wide open and alert? The ears may flatten, whiskers stiffen, tail twitch or swish, claws extend, the epaxial muscles tense, and hackles rise. These are the communicators of how the cat feels about the situation (fear, aggression, stress, and pain). Ignore them at your peril!

Mouth breathing or panting is a most significant sign of either a very stressed, anxious cat or of respiratory distress, a veterinary emergency, so be vigilant and check with the vet.

Vocalization is also an indication of demeanor and a warning of any potential sudden reactive movement. Take heed of a growling cat - a claws-extended swipe or bite may well follow. Even a purring cat can suddenly strike out with no warning, so constant vigilance is advisable. A vet nurse should trim overgrown claws before the examination or treatment as this reduces the inclination of the cat to extend the claws when lashing out.

This is perhaps a salient time for a reminder to keep up to date with one's tetanus vaccination.

Any incidental clinical findings such as enlarged lymph nodes, lumps, swellings, and skin lesions must be reported to the vet. As we spend so much time with our hands on the patient we are often the first to notice these changes.

Palpation and examination

Broadly speaking it is advisable to palpate a cat using a much lighter touch than for a dog. Experience has shown that for the first engagement during a session placing one hand across the spine at the level of the diaphragm (Fig. 3.13) will give much valuable feedback about the nature of the beast with which you are dealing. As discussed at length in Chapter 2, in the author's (NH's) experience the diaphragm can be affected by, and retain the memory of, both historic and recent shock or trauma.

The other hand can then be placed across the pelvis before progressing to more specific segmental analysis.

Sense the quality of the tissues and assess the nature and degree of response from the individual and from its body. Can you feel heat or swelling, rigidity, tension or spring, and elasticity? Is there bony resistance or soft tissue tightness? Is it protective spasm or lack of give due to fibrotic change? If there is edema, is this due to cardiovascular insufficiency, neoplasia within the related neurovascular plexus, or associated with the toxicity of renal failure? Experience has shown that boggy, pudgy tissues are suggestive of hormonal imbalance.

Moving caudally from the pelvis, the tail can be gently palpated for any signs of abnormality (Fig. 3.14).

Be extremely vigilant as there may be a history of a road traffic accident and one of the most common injuries is sacrococcygeal vertebral separation. This occurs when the cat's rear end sustains a glancing blow as it

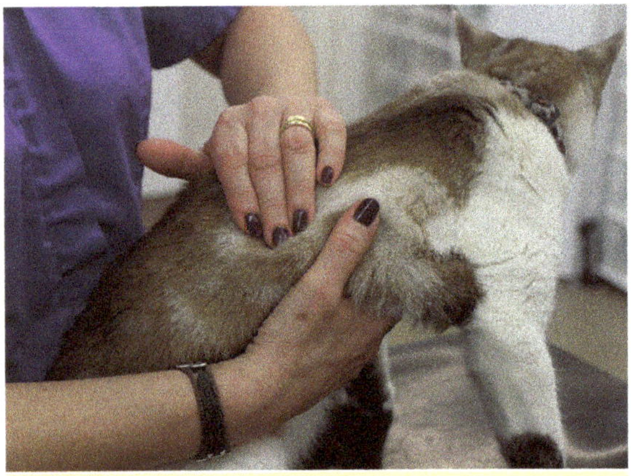

Figure 3.13
Palpation over the diaphragm.

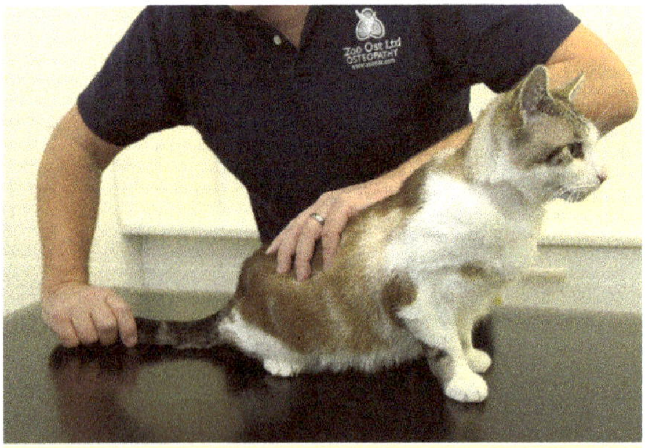

Figure 3.14
Palpation of the caudal coccygeal segments of the spine.

dashes across a road and is hit by a car. Do not be misled; cats can retain a remarkable capability of function despite having severe damage to the pelvic girdle.

The tail is an invaluable listening tool, as with any animal with viable coccygeal vertebrae, but it must be utilized gently and respectfully, both during evaluation and treatment via the involuntary mechanism.

To evaluate the thoracic and cervical spine move the hand cranially from the diaphragm palpating each spinal level up to the occipitoatlantoaxial complex (Fig. 3.15). If the cat is compliant check the temporomandibular joints, anterior cervical structures, hyoid and larynx, and the cranial and facial bones (Fig. 3.16). Notice the large eye sockets which are characteristic of visual predators.

Be aware that short-haired cats are susceptible to sunburn on the exposed skin of the ear pinnae so may be adverse to them being touched.

During this spinal assessment we are testing motility rather than the range of movement. If the cat is easy to handle it may be possible to introduce gentle, slow toggling motions to check the mobility and then to progress as a very small amplitude, articulatory treatment technique if required.

Remember that the therapeutic effect of touch ensures the application of intelligent, knowing hands. Cats are highly responsive creatures. Change occurs fleetingly and will thus commence during the process of evaluation. The experienced practitioner will tend to flow smoothly from assessment to treatment, finding the areas of distorted structure and enhancing the cat's return to normality of function. Do not be tempted to overtreat.

Find it, fix it, and leave it alone.

Assessment of the limbs should commence as purely palpatory, only proceeding to passive movements of the peripheral joints if the cat will permit it. Do not hesitate to ask for the assistance of a vet nurse in holding an unpredictable cat to facilitate a complete examination of the passive range of movements if it is deemed essential to the case.

Some obliging cats will stand, sit, or even lie on their side, which greatly simplifies the process of examination and subsequent treatment. Others refuse to move from a crouched position limiting one to a purely palpatory assessment. Despite this one can usually gently slide two or three fingers of one hand under the pelvis or sternum to gain access to the proximal peripheral joints and related structures.

Then examining the forelimbs, assess the scapular spine in relation to the thoracic spine and ribs, comparing both sides of the thoracic sling musculature.

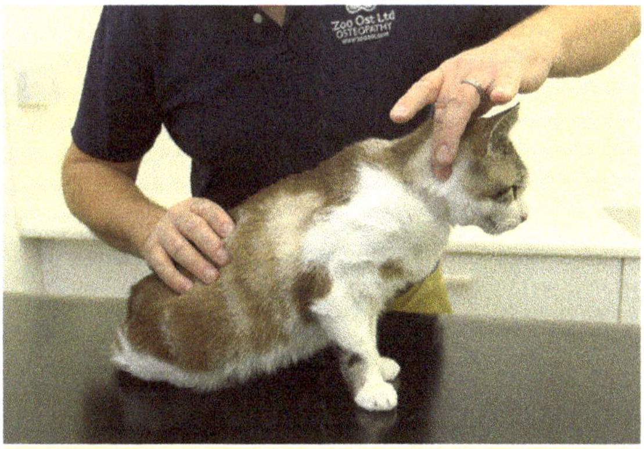

Figure 3.15
Palpating cranially from the diaphragm to the occiput–atlas articulations.

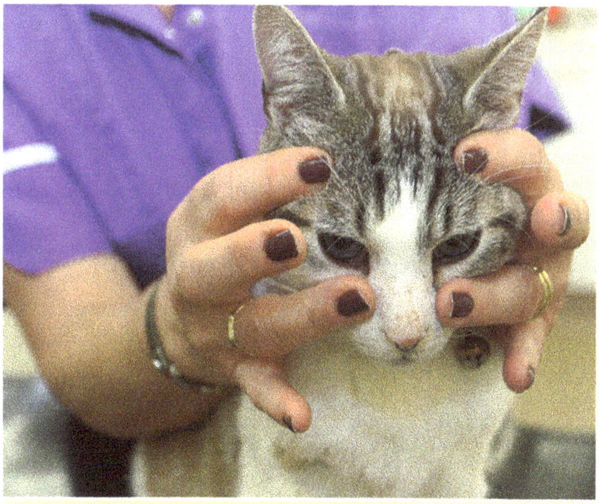

Figure 3.16
Palpating around the temporomandibular joints and the orbits.

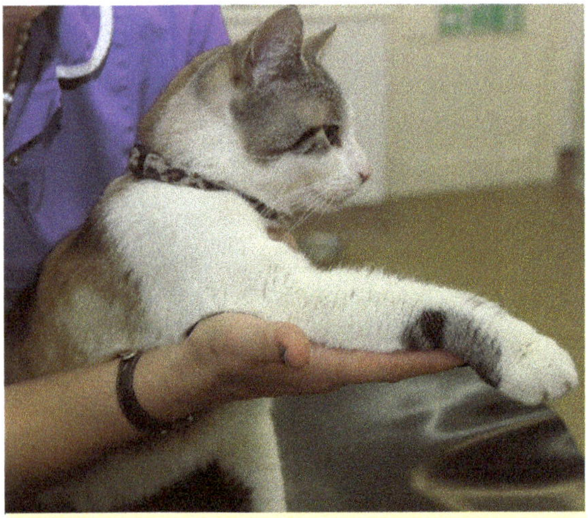

Figure 3.17
Assessing the forelimb structures and range of motion.

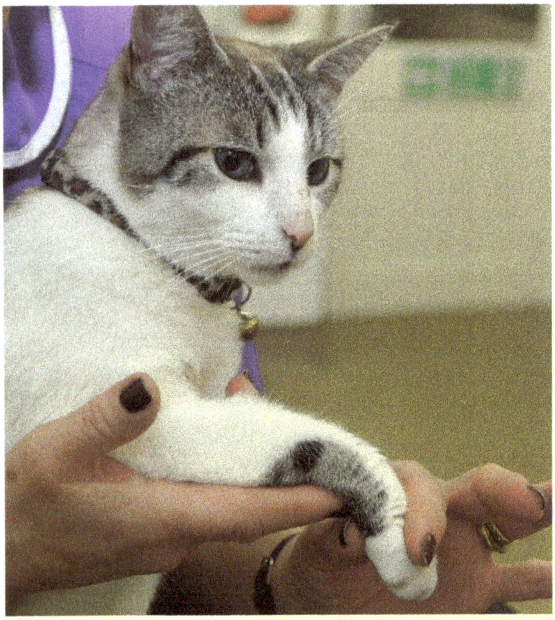

Figure 3.18
Assessing the digits of the foot.

Think globally to ascertain patterns of compensation and locally to find specific tissue discrepancies. Evaluate the movement of the glenohumeral joint, elbow, and carpus individually, the capacity for glide and shock absorption, and their range of movements, including the capacity for accessory pivotal motion

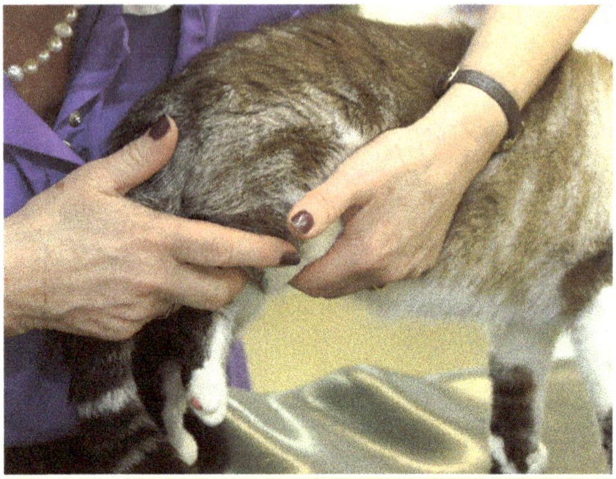

Figure 3.19
Osteopathic evaluation of the hind limb.

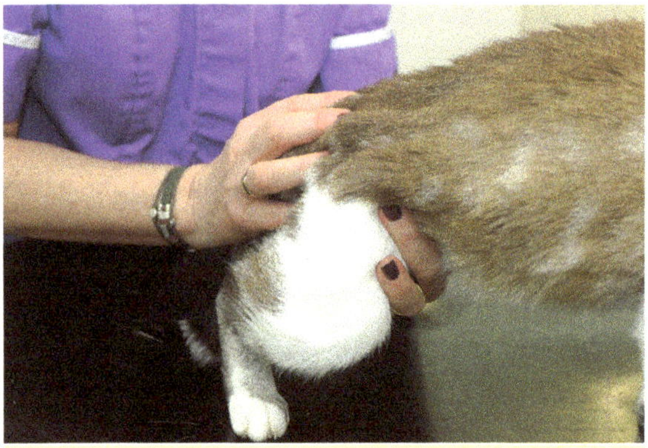

Figure 3.20
Osteopathic evaluation of the pelvis.

within the totality of the assessment. Then guide the limb into protraction and retraction to assess its function as a coordinated unit (Fig. 3.17).

If it is achievable, palpate each foot and the digits (Fig. 3.18), checking the pattern of wear on the paw pads and for any local injury.

Follow the same procedure for the hind limbs (Fig. 3.19): assess the hips, stifles, hocks, tarsi, and feet as separate entities and as part of the synchronized function of the hindquarters.

During the examination take the opportunity to evaluate the thoracic cage, abdomen and pelvis (Fig. 3.20) in relation to the functioning of the whole body.

Osteopathic treatment

Due to both the nature of the feline and also that there is much less size variation in domestic breeds than in the canine population, the selection of techniques appropriate for the treatment of cats is more limited than for dogs. Experience has shown that a predominantly cranial and functional approach is best accepted, also incorporating other indirect techniques such as fascial release, balanced ligamentous tension (BLT), and positional release when expedient.

A gentle engagement with the involuntary motion is recommended. The cranial mechanism of a well cat is light and clear, almost vaporous and phosphorescent rather than fluidic, tending toward the ephemeral and "will-o'-the-wisp." Utilize a light, listening touch as the response and change is rapid, much as for small wildlife (see Chapter 9).

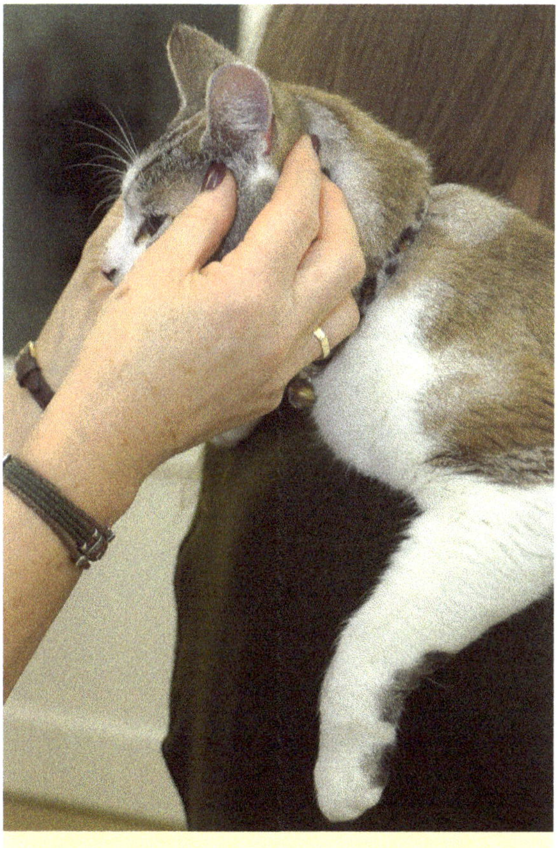

Figure 3.21
Examination and treatment with a cat cradled over the owner's shoulder.

A cat that is happy in the surroundings and relishes human handling will engage well with a sensitive manual therapist and will tolerate a wider range of indirect techniques when it is standing, cradled or even lying over the practitioner's shoulder (Fig. 3.21).

The cat's temperament, constitution, and their individual symptom patterns must be taken into account. All these elements will influence your treatment and also the expected response.

As mentioned above, the therapeutic process begins during our examination of the patient. Be mindful that the most important aspects of the cat's physiology are its flexibility, balance and agility, thus the treatment objective should be to help restore a coordinated, synchronized ease of movement throughout its body (Fig. 3.22).

Head and face

Fractures of the mandible are not uncommon as a result of road accidents. After any necessary surgical procedures there may still be residual problems with the function of the temporomandibular joint and related structures in the head and neck compromised by the vehicular impact and resultant soft tissue impairment, which may be improved by treatment.

As previously mentioned, the cat is a visual predator, relying on a wide range of vision. Thus there must be freedom of movement in the cephalic cervical spine (occipitoatlantoaxial complex) allowing for fine adjustment in the position of the head and neck for both accurate spotting of prey and also for the upright, pricked ears to precisely localize the direction of any auditory signals, either prey-related or threat from potential danger (dogs, other cats, humans, traffic, etc.).

Flat-faced cats such as Persians are prone to breathing difficulties, due to compromised nasal bones, and also tear duct obstruction associated with compressed maxillae.

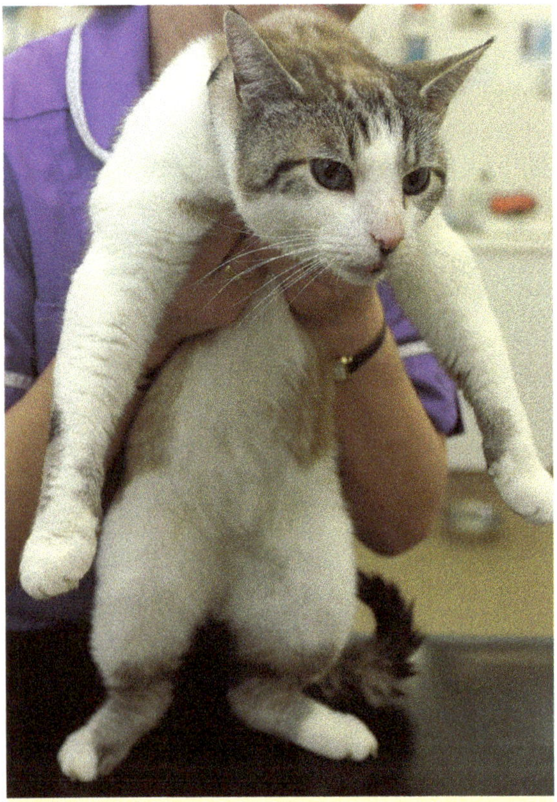

Figure 3.22
Longitudinal whole body supportive release using gravity as an aid to treatment.

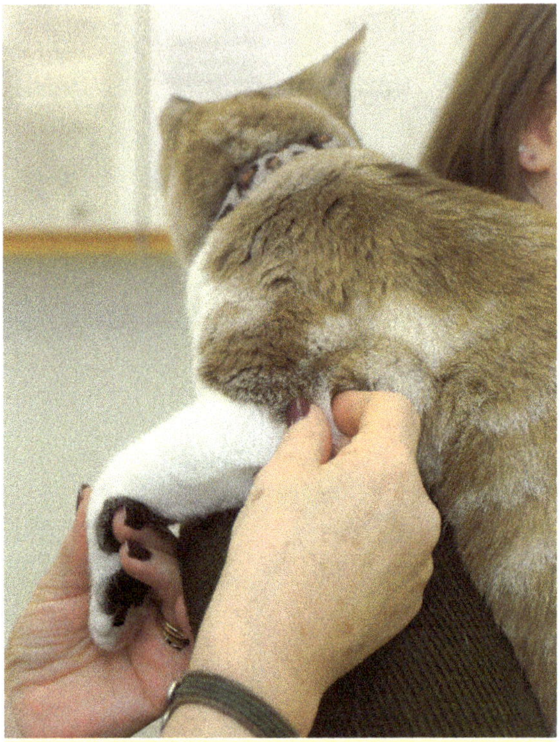

Figure 3.23
Osteopathic treatment of the entire forelimb structures.

Ear infections

Cats are prone to middle and inner ear infections due to the tortuosity of the ear canals. Cranial techniques to free any bony compressive patterns and restore the involuntary motion encourage lymphatic drainage and enhance the blood supply.

Neck

Localized pain or acute sensitivity in the cervical spine tends to be associated with pathology such as a fracture, disc protrusion, discospondylitis or neoplasia. These cases are not suitable for manual therapy so must be referred back to the vet.

Spondylosis is uncommon in this area but mechanical dysfunctions are not unusual, within any global pattern of compensation.

Treatment is to support and balance the length of the cervical spine, ventral and dorsal, in its role as a conduit between the vital sensory organs and the limbs. Ease and release any tethering or tightness within the thoracic sling due to compensatory mechanisms associated with limb or spinal problems.

Shoulders and forelimb

The forelimbs are highly flexible for their use in climbing, pouncing, and grabbing prey in addition to having the strength to support the weight of the comparatively heavy forequarters. Encourage the ease of circumduction within the glenohumeral joint, balancing the muscles of the sling and scapula. Release any shearing between the humerus and radius and ulna at the elbow, ensuring an ability to absorb pivotal compressive forces here and within the carpus and foot while landing and springing (Fig. 3.23).

Having ascertained that any swelling of a joint or joints is not due to infection, fracture, neoplasia, or ligament rupture, all requiring veterinary intervention, then proceed with treatment to alleviate the edematous tissues and address the associated protective mechanisms.

Assess any congestion or tightness within the axillae and treat the causal structures as appropriate.

Areas of reduced mobility and stiffness in the thoracic spine due to spondylotic changes can be gently eased. Locate and free any binding and compromised movement of ribs.

Restriction in the excursion of the diaphragm should be addressed and the holding pattern released (Fig. 3.24).

Lumbar spine, pelvis, and tail

Fibrotic tissues associated with spondylosis and degenerative disc disease in the thoracolumbar and lumbar spine may be ameliorated by gentle techniques to improve the blood and lymph circulation and increase motility at the specific segmental levels as well as providing more global fascial release. Remembering the mechanisms of osteopathic somatic dysfunction and viscerosomatic reflexes, take the opportunity to release any visceral fascial tethering and encourage a healthy functional motion of the abdominal and pelvic organs (Fig. 3.25).

Many female cats and some males have a baggy, sagging belly - the primordial pouch. It serves as insulation, protection during fights, and allows the hind limbs to fully extend when galloping or leaping. The size of this fat-filled skin flap varies in different breeds and as it is also seen in some large cats (lions and tigers) it is thought to be an adaptation for food storage after gorging on a kill. Needless to say if the cat is overweight this pouch can be obstructive to movement and problematic for palpation of the abdomen.

As mentioned in the evaluation section, an avulsion injury to the tail causing sacrococcygeal vertebral separation is a frequent result of a glancing blow across the hind end by a car. Remember that the cat may well still be ambulatory if there are no other injuries which could compromise the locomotor apparatus. There will be tail droop and a varying amount of edema and hematoma around the sacrococcygeal area. Often there is urinary retention requiring manual evacuation by the vet and the owner may have to learn to perform this maneuver if the problem persists.

Experience has shown that heedful, extremely gentle techniques can help alleviate the edematous tissues and encourage lymphatic drainage in the surrounding areas. Treatment should be little and often, ideally a few moments, once or twice daily. Providing the urinary complications are not of neurological origin, it

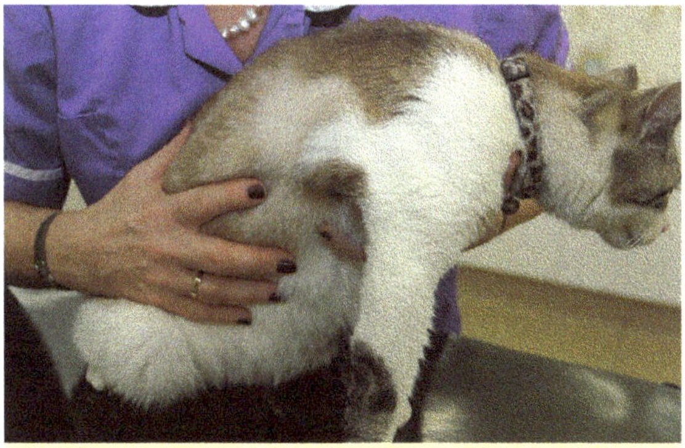

Figure 3.24
Freeing residual tension through the rib cage and diaphragm.

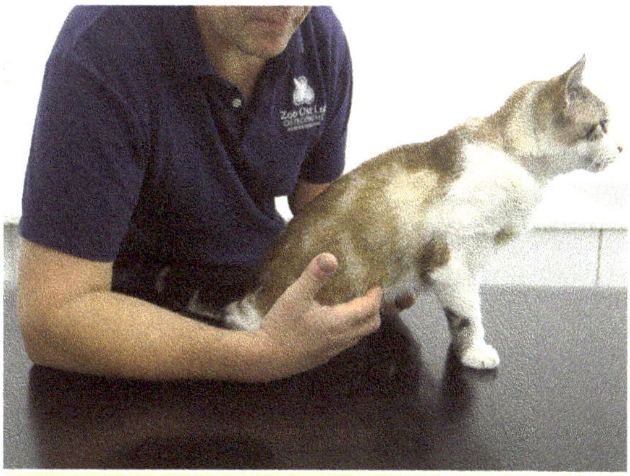

Figure 3.25
Fascial (visceral) release work through the abdominal structures.

appears that osteopathic treatment to decrease swelling and optimize the blood supply, may hasten the return of normal bladder voiding. Also attend to any secondary effects of the force of impact and resultant systemic shock within the myofascial system.

Needless to say, in these circumstances, of sacrococcygeal vertebral separation, do *not* use the tail as a technique applicator.

Traumatic subluxation of the sacroiliac joint and fractures of the pelvic girdle may not require surgical intervention, recovering satisfactorily with cage rest and appropriate medication. Osteopathic input can be beneficial in either situation following the same protocol as discussed above.

The tail is essential for balance, acting as a counterweight. It can be treated as part of the whole spinal mechanism or as individual vertebral segments depending on the problem.

Hind limbs

The bones of the hind legs are stronger, being of a relatively denser build than the front legs, providing the power for acceleration and propulsion in pouncing and springing.

When working around the hip, be watchful for any congestion or swelling in the groin, which may be indicative of pathology in the pelvic viscera or neurovascular plexus.

Treatment of the hind limb follows the same principles as for the forelimb (Fig. 3.26).

Be alert for a fracture of the femoral neck, presenting with an apparent shortening of the hind limb. This requires veterinary attention.

Quadriceps contracture and adhesions subsequent to a fracture in the distal half of the femur will cause compromised movement in both the hip and the stifle. The earlier this is treated the greater the likelihood of a positive result or at least prevention of further deterioration.

Any tightness or binding of the musculoskeletal apparatus of the lumbosacral area will affect the quality of function of the hip and consequently the stifle. Patella luxation is less common in cats than in dogs. Providing there is not a causative femoral trochlear groove problem, a common predisposing factor is misaligned quadriceps action. Experience has shown that it is pertinent to ensure ease and balance within the dynamic relationship of these muscle groups to reduce this predisposition.

DJD in the hip and peripheral joints can be treated using remedial techniques specifically to reduce swelling, ease tight, fibrosed soft tissues to improve joint mobility and calm pain mechanisms (Fig. 3.27). Global techniques will address the compensatory locomotor patterns.

In cases of dropped hock, depending on the etiology (see the section on common orthopedic problems), osteopathic treatment can help in the rehabilitation and maintenance of well-balanced compensatory mechanisms.

Management

Unlike in the management of canine rehabilitation, controlled exercise is difficult to instigate and supervise in cats. It is possible to monitor indoor activity

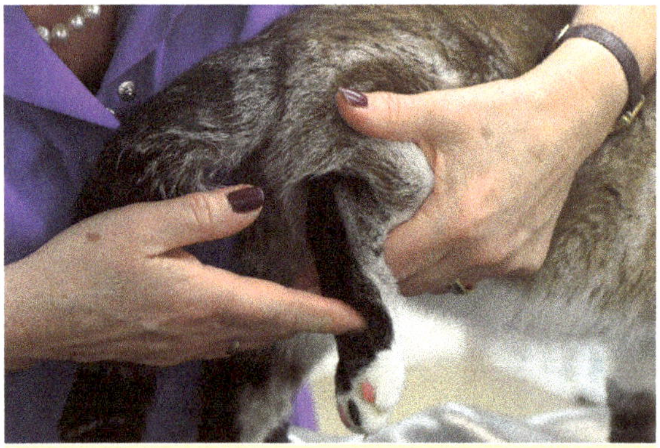

Figure 3.26
Osteopathic treatment of the hind limb.

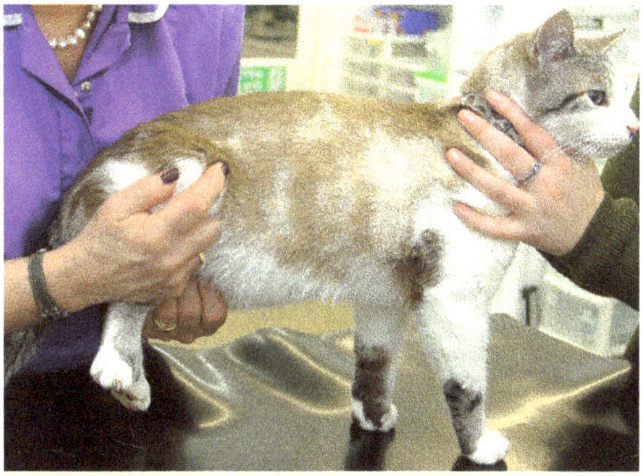

Figure 3.27
Osteopathic treatment of the soft tissues locally around the hip.

while keeping the cat confined after injury or surgery. The natural tendency for a convalescing cat is to remain still and quiet away from noise and disruption.

Any activity requirement is dependent on self-exercise, which can be encouraged by having scratching posts and feline climbing apparatus in the house, to stimulate arboreal tendencies, increase flexibility and help preserve coordination and balance. Games with string and ping-pong balls for example, are also invaluable to improve dexterity in the forelimbs and movement of the head and neck. An aging cat is more reticent to engage in these activities. Mental stimulation is also very important for a housebound cat of any age.

Various aspects of their home care can be modified, for example, heated beds, litter trays, and aids to reach raised perches can be used.

Compliant and capable owners may be keen to do some gentle soft tissue or passive stretch routines to help ease muscle tightness and peripheral joint stiffness.

Some cats will tolerate hydrotherapy if this facility is conveniently located.

It should be remembered that a vet must prescribe any medication, nutraceutical, or special diet.

The administration and tolerance of analgesic and anti-inflammatory medication is more problematic in cats than dogs due to the differences in feline drug metabolism (Caney 2007).

Many cats are notoriously averse to taking oral medication either by hand or hidden in food but can be remarkably accepting of acupuncture (which can only be administered by a vet). This is a very useful adjunct within an integrated approach, helping to support the constitution and reducing pain and muscular tightness.

Chapter 3

Case study 3.1

Adult male cat

Signalment

An adult male cat had been rehomed with the present owner after being found feral in town and ending up at the animal shelter. His age was approximately 8–10 years. The present owner had wormed and treated for fleas and ticks. His overall health was good and he seemed a strong and robust cat that had taken to home life well.

History

Patient D. had settled well with his new owners and over the previous week had been allowed out of the house to roam during the day. Two days earlier he had not returned as usual and when the owner went to look for him she had found him near the road and unable to use his back legs properly. She took him to her veterinary surgery where radiographs showed no bony damage, but it did appear that the sacrum had been shunted cranially within the sacroiliac joints. The surgeon gave Patient D. a nonsteroidal anti-inflammatory injection and advised osteopathy.

Presenting signs

On osteopathic examination the patient was unable to support his weight on his hind limbs, and when placed on the examination table he stood on his forelimbs and allowed his torso and hind limbs to flop on the table (Fig. 3.28). Palpation confirmed the flaccid nature of the limbs and lumbar epaxial musculature, and questioning confirmed that he was having difficulty in controlling defecation although he still had bladder control. He also appeared to have only limited control of his tail with the caudal 10 cm able to move. He was quiet but his eyes and general body language suggested that he wasn't relaxed.

Osteopathic treatment

From palpation the author (TN) decided that he would try to reduce the tension to the sacroiliac joints using muscle inhibition and functional release work using the hind limbs and tail. The owner gently restrained the patient with a hold around his forelimbs and shoulders, such that he couldn't bite her easily, or the author.

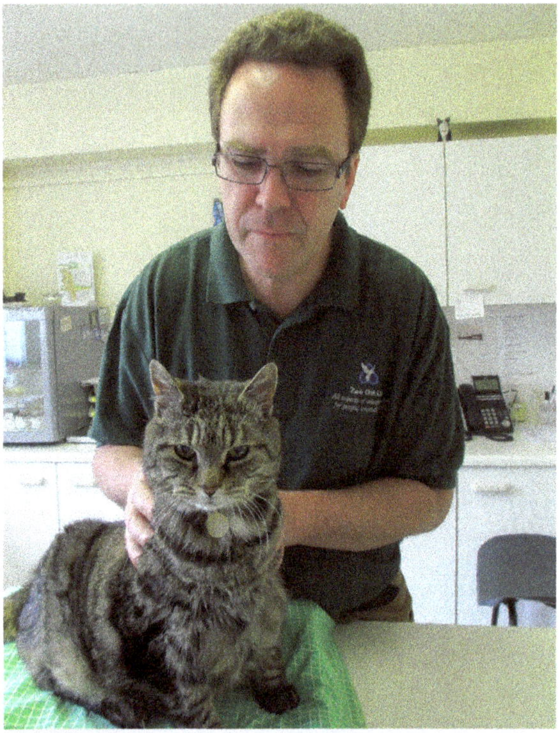

Figure 3.28
Initial examination of the patient.

This first treatment lasted about 10 minutes, after which the patient made it clear verbally and physically that he wanted the session to stop. It was decided to book him back in three days later for a follow-up consultation.

He returned with only a very slight improvement noted by the owner. On examination he still presented with a lot of soft tissue guarding around his sacroiliac joints, and there was still considerable flaccidity to the hind limbs and lumbar region.

The author, in consultation with the veterinary surgeon, decided to try to reduce the cranial shunt of the sacrum using an internal or external mobilization technique, whereby the author would insert a lubricated and gloved digit into the patient's rectum with the pad of the finger gently pressing dorsally along the ventral surface of the sacrum, while the author's thumb was placed over the dorsal aspect of the sacrum externally. With the other hand gently compressing ventrally and medially over the tubera coxae bilaterally, the author applied ventral and posterior vectored pressure to the sacrum while the owner restrained the patient via the forelimb hold.

This was the first time the author had used this technique on a feline patient. Although it was a direct physical manipulation, care was taken to work with the fascia and associated soft tissue structures. The technique was successful (Fig. 3.29) and within 48 hours the patient had full use of his tail, bowel control, and reasonable use of his hind limbs.

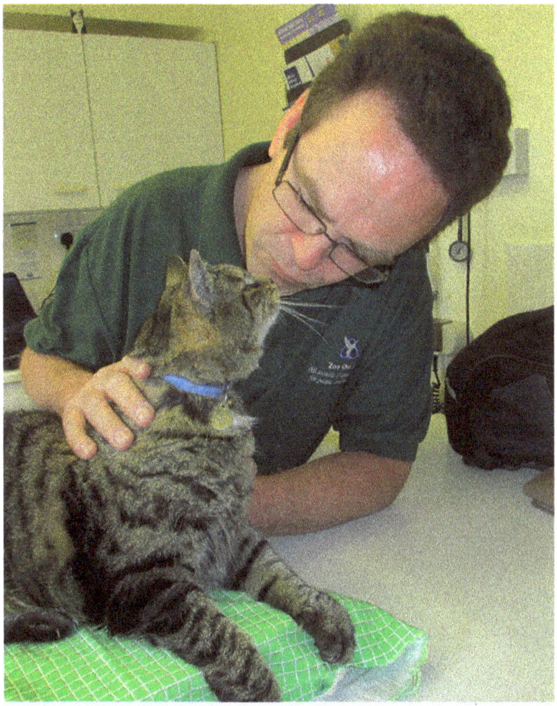

Figure 3.29
Examination given following the previous visit's sacral mobilization technique. Note how much happier the patient appears.

He subsequently received two further osteopathic treatments, which involved functional release work using his tail and hind limbs and work with the involuntary mechanism (IVM).

Outcome

The patient had received physical trauma that had resulted in a dynamic change to the way the spine to pelvis to hind limb mechanics functioned. This had left him with severe neurological deficit to skeletal and visceral motor and sensory input and output. Osteopathic intervention needed to be quick and effective for the prognosis to be good. The decision to use an internal pivotal release to the sacroiliac joint imbalance was vital to the success of this case. When performed successfully, a single application is all that is required, with further work carried out in a more standard external fashion.

Summary

Patient D. had most likely been struck by a motor vehicle. The mild luxation through the sacroiliac joints meant that a NSAID approach alone was not a viable option. Manipulation was going to need to be at the extreme physical range of osteopathy, backed up by softer techniques to ensure that there was no further "shock" to any of the soft tissue structures. With all neurologically impaired cases speed is of the essence. With hindsight the author would have employed the internal manipulation technique on the initial visit; however, it was also the first time he had attempted this on a domestic animal.

As a result of the combination of traditional veterinary NSAIDs and osteopathic treatment Patient D. not only made a quick recovery, but he also became much happier to be handled by his new owners, and by the author and veterinary surgeon. He went on to become completely symptom free having lost one of his nine lives.

Case study 3.2

European half-breed

Signalment

Soni was a four-year-old male European half-breed.

History

Soni was brought to the clinic because of lameness in the left forelimb following a street fight a week previously. The owner reported a lack of appetite and lethargic behavior associated with the loss of mechanical function in the limb. No other relevant elements were present in the clinical history apart from surgical sterilization when the cat was six months old.

Veterinary evaluation

The general clinical examination revealed a warm, swollen, and sore left elbow joint with reduced articular function without neurological impairment. In addition, the animal's temperature was 40°C. The radiological examination revealed only a minimal periarticular swelling without any loss of bony integrity. A cycle of anti-inflammatories (meloxicam 0.2 mg x kg x 1 day, followed by 0.1 mg x kg x 6 days) was prescribed and a blood sample was taken for further biochemical analysis.

Osteopathic evaluation

At the static observation, Soni presented with a slight asymmetrical weight-bearing and the left forelimb flexed at the elbow joint although the foot was still in contact with the floor. During gait, a mild lameness was visible during the stance phase. At palpation, all of the shoulder girdle and elbow muscles were kept in a hypertonic state with signs of discomfort when approaching the elbow complex. Nothing else of major concern was found to be wrong with the limbs, but significant somatic dysfunctions were present at the level of all vertebral junctions (occiput–atlas, cervicothoracic, thoracolumbar, and lumbosacral) together with a severe reduction of mobility and excursion of the upper and middle chest, associated with a sense of compression and heaviness at the manubrium and sternum levels. Furthermore, the amplitude and vitality of the involuntary rhythms were strongly reduced.

Further investigation and treatment

The blood test revealed an increase in white blood cells (27.0 $10^3/mm^3$), a decrease in red blood cells (4 x $10^6/mm^3$), a hemoglobin level of 6 g/dl, and hematocrit at 18%. The SNAP test for FIV (feline immunodeficiency virus) and FeLV (feline leukemia virus) was negative. Following a bone marrow puncture and analysis, the veterinary doctor made the diagnosis of acute lymphoid leukemia. The treatment included a chemotherapeutic cycle of vincristine (0.5 mg/m^2 once a week), prednisone (40 mg/m^2 once a day for one week). This was followed by 20 mg/m^2 once every other day, and cyclophosphamide (50 mg/m^2 every other day). During the first month of treatment, Soni had a mild improvement in his energy levels, although the lameness was still present and his body weight was below the average.

Osteopathic intervention

A combination of the respiratory-circulatory and metabolic models was applied through short (5 to 7 minutes) but frequent (three times a week) osteopathic manipulative treatment (OMT) sessions every other month. Firstly the diaphragmatic system was approached, including the tentorium (using balanced membranous technique through the ears), the thoracic inlet, and the thoraco-abdominal and pelvic diaphragms (by applying functional inhibition of the related myofascial structures). In addition, articulatory techniques were applied to the corresponding vertebral junctions, and a CV4 was delivered during each treatment. Secondly, various pumping maneuvers were administered to the upper and lower chest, abdominal and pelvic cavity, and related organs. At the thoracic level the practitioner made contact by placing a hand on each side of the chest. He then alternated compression and decompression of the thoracic area at different speeds, varying the force and duration (1 pump every 1 to 2 seconds for 2 to 4 minutes) in order to create pressure gradients to improve fluid dynamics, immunity function, and the animal's general response to medication.

Follow-up

Soni responded well to the combination of medical and osteopathic interventions by showing both a resolution of the lameness in the forelimb, a restoration of normal appetite, and a general increase in energy levels (after the third month of combined interventions). However, 13 months after the onset of leukemia, and following an exacerbation of the condition, he died, although most cats with the same pathology that have been treated with chemotherapy do not usually survive beyond six or seven months.

Summary

The treatment of felines, and indeed all animals, requires the osteopath to develop an enhanced physical literacy, as there is no verbal dialogue with these patients, but a dynamic interaction. It is essential that we experience and engage with the event of the treatment, not just sensing the state of the body but also its response to the environment.

References

Bradshaw JWS, Casey RA, Brown SL (2012) The Behaviour of the Domestic Cat. 2nd edn. UK: CABI Publishing.

Caney S (2007) How I approach ... feline arthritis. Veterinary Focus 17 (3) 11–17.

Cat-World (2019) Cat whiskers – everything you need to know. At: http://www.cat-world.com.au [January 16, 2019].

Dodman N (1998) Behaviour problems in cats – etiology, diagnostics, and treatment. Workshop, Tufts University School of Veterinary Medicine.

Ewer RA (1973) The Carnivores. Ithaca, NY: Cornell University Press.

Grayton J, Allen P, Biller D (2014) Case report: proximal femoral physeal dysplasia in a cat and a review of the literature. Israel Journal of Veterinary Medicine. March; 69 (1) 40–44.

Harasen G (2006) Patellar Luxation. Canadian Veterinary Journal. August; 47 (8) 817–818.

Grandjean D, Butterwick R (eds) (2009) Understanding cats. In: Waltham Pocket Book of Essential Nutrition for Cats and Dogs. London: Beyond Design Solutions Ltd, p. 11.

International Cat Care (2019) Arthritis and degenerative joint disease in cats. At: https://icatcare.org/advice/general-care [January 16, 2019].

Schebitz H, Wilkens H (1989) Atlas of Radiographic Anatomy of the Dog and Cat. 5th edn. Berlin and Hamburg: Paul Parey.

Scott HW, McLaughlin R (2007) Feline Orthopedics. London: Manson Publishing.

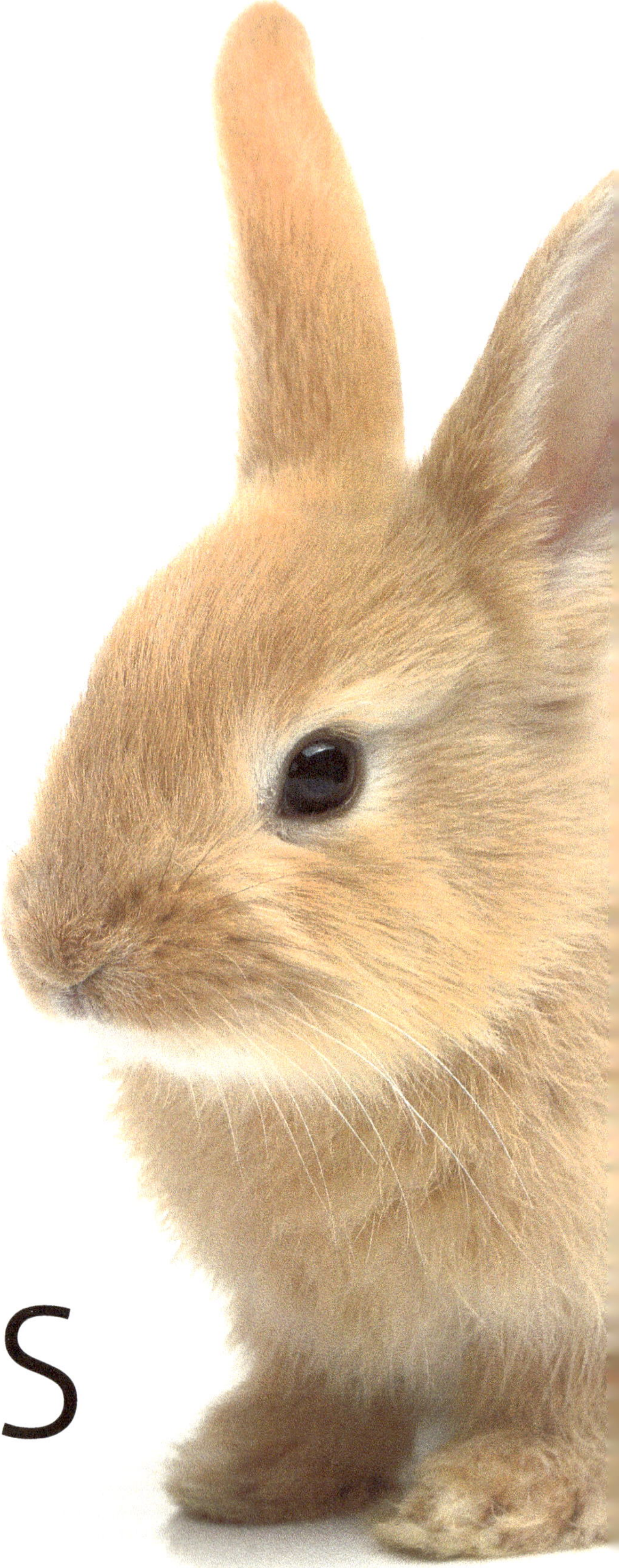

Chapter 4
SMALL FURRIES

Paolo Tozzi, John Hope-Ryan

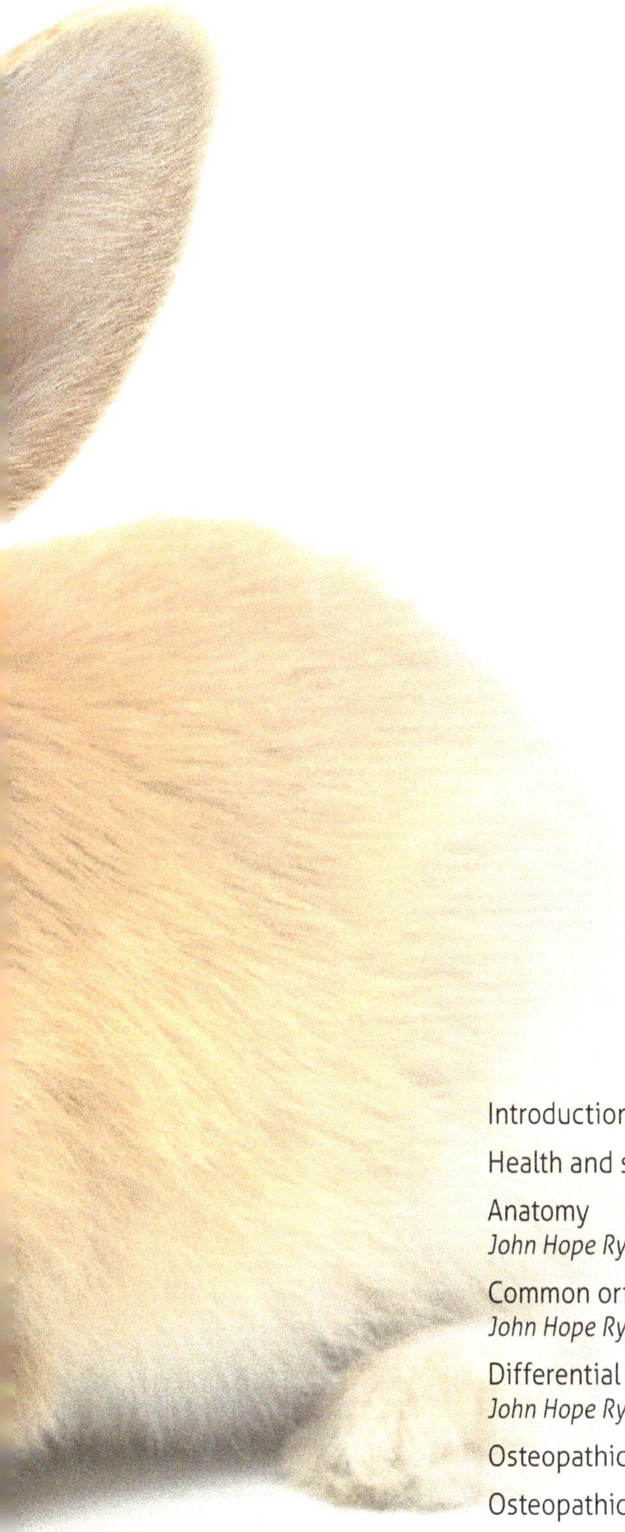

Small furries

Chapter 4

Introduction

Small furry mammals such as rabbits and rodents are lovely creatures to work with and osteopathy is particularly suitable for them due to their small size, docility, sensitivity to touch, and the ease with which they can be handled and manipulated. A comprehensive knowledge of anatomy, good palpatory skills, and clinical experience are essential prerequisites if effective results are to be seen when treating these patients (as with all species). However, with small furries in particular caution and gentleness during handling and treatment are paramount to ensure the safety of both the patient and practitioner.

Nowadays, these animals have become popular as pets, but some are also farmed commercially and used for laboratory research. The ferret, a domesticated polecat, is used for controlling rabbits and rats, but is also kept as a household pet. Rodents (from the Latin *rodere*, which means "to gnaw") can be found in most regions of the globe, from the Arctic to the temperate areas, including the tropics. They comprise the largest mammalian order with over 1,800 species (Hurst 1999). Some rodents, such as the rat and guinea pig, have been part of human life and activity for a long time, while others such as the Syrian hamster have only recently been domesticated (Derrell Clark 1987). This chapter focuses on ferrets and small rodents such as hamsters and mice, but does extend to include rabbits. There are over 70 recognized breeds of rabbit (Batchelor 1999), the majority of which are bred and kept in captivity and have successfully entered into the pet trade.

Health and safety

Most small furries kept as pets receive regular handling from their owners; however, this does not guarantee that any hands-on treatment administered by the osteopath will be straightforward. There are some basic handling guidelines that should always be followed.

Within the main body of text for this chapter are specifics on safe handling, but please remember that there are many zoonotic diseases that these types of patient can and do carry. See the appendix to Chapter 1 for a more complete list of zoonoses.

Most small furries are hard-wired to take flight when anything spooks them. Therefore when handing it is best to ensure you have a firm hold that both restrains and makes them feel secure. This will prevent them from injuring themselves and, once secured, allows them to relax, making examination, assessment, and treatment easier and more effective. Most are easy to treat in your hands; however, make sure that you do carry out treatment over an examination table or suitable platform. If the patient should wriggle free there is less chance of injury from a fall.

Small furries have relatively delicate skeletal frames with large muscle mass, and fractures or luxations to the lumbar spine and hind limbs are relatively common. As with treating wildlife patients, it is best to keep noise and sudden movements to a minimum. Sudden movement can trigger a bite response from mice and hamsters if startled. Ferrets do not like you crowding their faces. Their bite is extremely powerful, and it is often easier to have a trained handler hold the ferret while the osteopath examines and treats. Many small furries are essentially nocturnal, and it is advisable to keep lighting sympathetic to them while still allowing the osteopath a safe working environment.

There is further information regarding safe handling of each type of animal later in this chapter when specific treatments are described.

Anatomy

Introduction

Small furries are generally regarded as any species belonging to the orders Rodentia and Lagomorpha. Rodents make up some 1,800 species and include mice, rats, hamsters, and guinea pigs. Rodentia also includes beavers, chipmunks, squirrels, marmots, chinchillas, voles, lemmings, and many others. The lagomorphs include rabbits and hares.

Digestive system

Rabbits and rodents share a similar dental anatomy with a diastema separating the incisors from the cheek teeth. Most species have elodont teeth, meaning the teeth grow continuously throughout life, hence the need for a correct diet to ensure continuous wear.

The cecum is large in all species and contains most of the ingesta and hence most are hindgut fermenters. Some species will perform coprophagy and produce mucus covered cecotropes which stick to the fur around the anus. These cecotropes are ingested and pass through the gut a second time. This second passage is an important part of digestion, and individuals that leave the sticky pellets around the anus are worth a closer physical examination.

All of these species have a high surface area to body weight ratio, and most have a vegetable-based diet, although some species do ingest meat products. The high metabolic rates required to maintain body heat combined with the low caloric value of the ingesta leave species vulnerable to negative energy balance with even small reductions in food intake. High metabolic rates and a primarily vegetable diet make drug choice and pharmacokinetics difficult to extrapolate from other mammals, as drugs may be cleared quicker than expected. The importance of gut bacteria in digestion means a degree of caution must be exercised when choosing antibiotics, as disturbance of these bacteria can have fatal consequences. Fortunately, for some of the species that are kept as pets vast amounts of biological data are available, as they are commonly used in laboratory studies.

Muscle and bone (Figs 4.1–4.4)

In rabbits, 7-8 percent of body weight is bone, compared to 12 percent in the cat. Muscle mass is high (approximately 50 percent of body weight). A high muscle mass to bone ratio leaves quite a considerable strain on a relatively delicate bone structure. Fracture and trauma from lashing out with the back legs is a

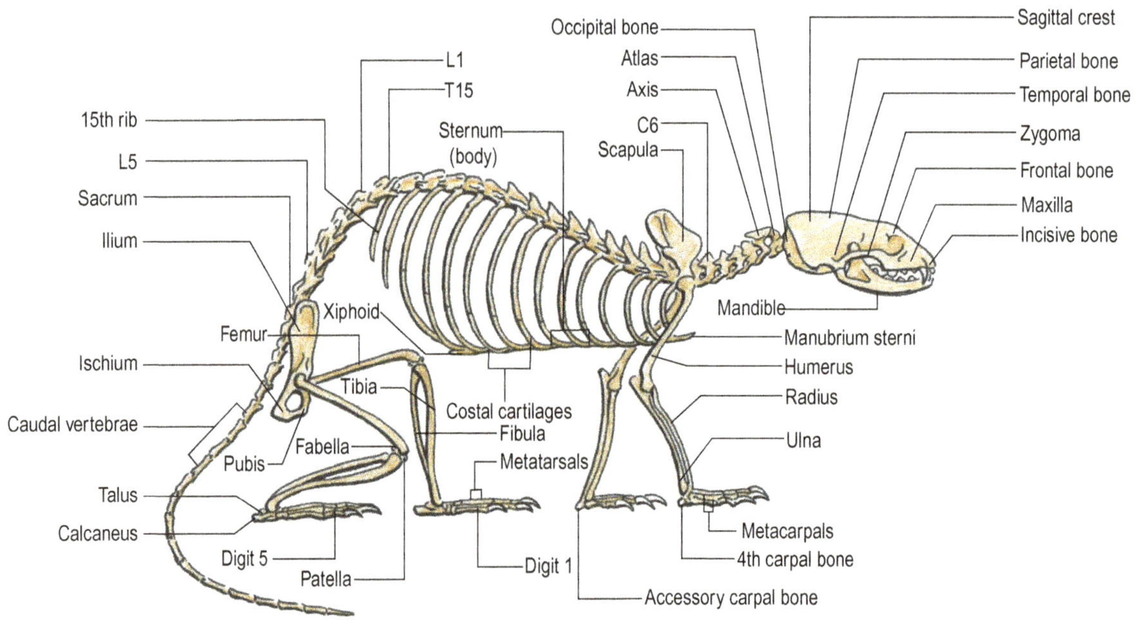

Figure 4.1
Ferret skeleton.

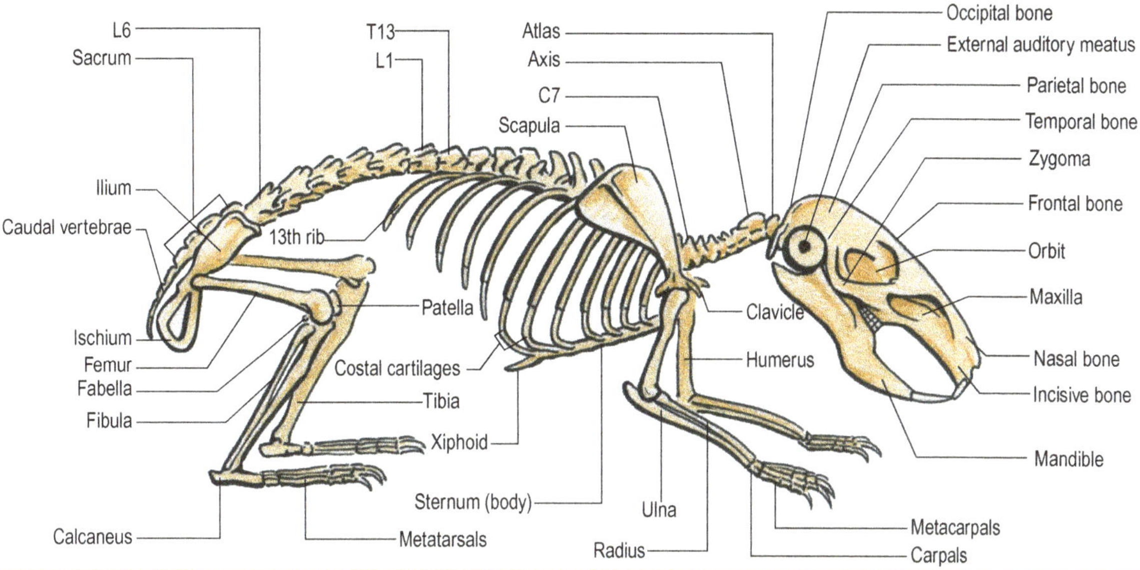

Figure 4.2
Guinea pig skeleton.

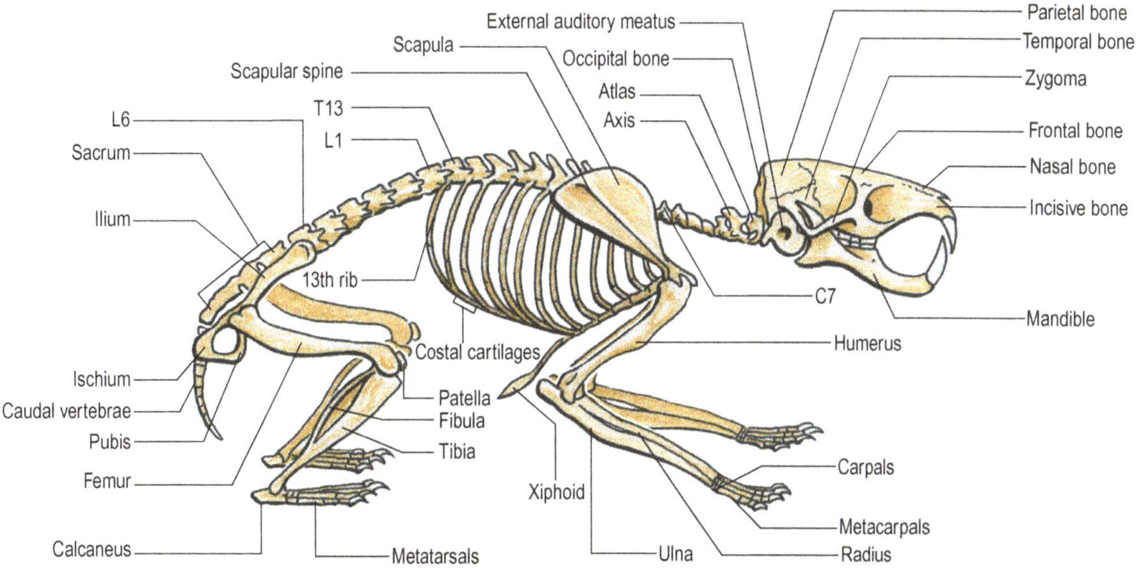

Figure 4.3
Hamster skeleton.

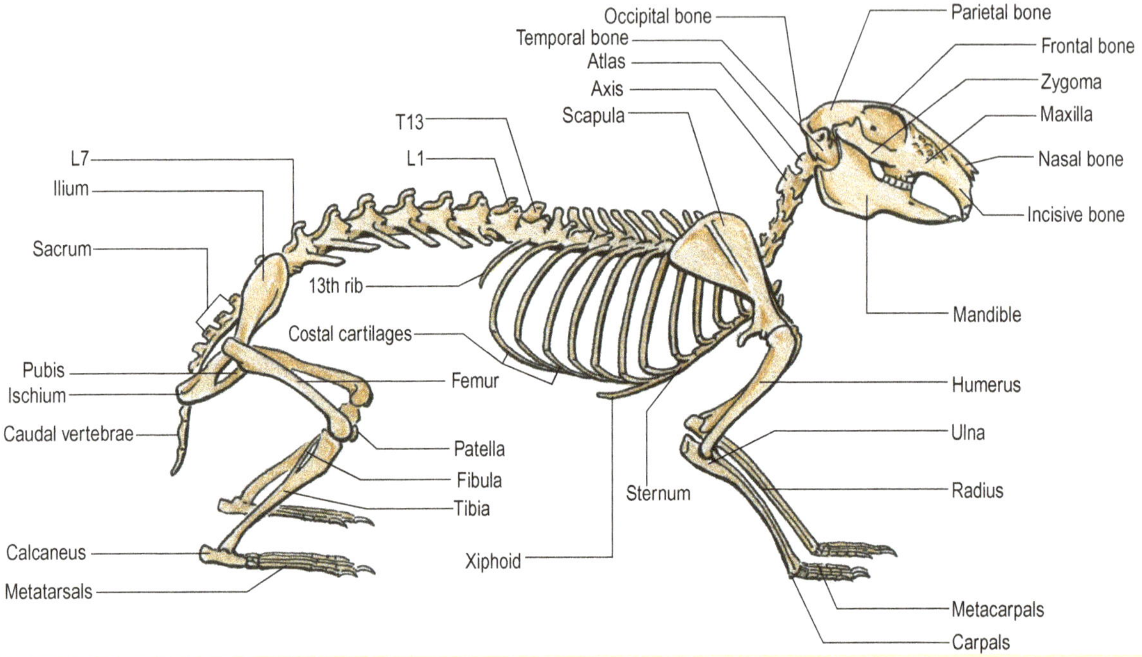

Figure 4.4
Rabbit skeleton.

common complication of insensitive handling of rabbits. Muscle groups and anatomical markers are similar to dogs and cats in all species, although the delicate bone with relative high muscle mass theme is continued through all species.

Cardiorespiratory system

Most species are obligate nasal breathers, as the epiglottis lies dorsal to the soft palate. Mouth breathing is seen as a very poor prognostic indicator and care needs to be taken when handling the nasal areas and mouth. The chest cavity in all species is small compared to dogs, but small alveoli with high surface areas, high chest compliance, and low dead space allow for the high oxygen demands that metabolism requires. Respiratory compromise, however, will quickly lead to hypoxia, and careful evaluation of the respiratory system prior to anesthesia is recommended. The size of the heart is proportional to the size of the animal. The heart rate is high compared to larger mammals due to the low stroke volumes that are available from a small heart.

Sensory system

Most species of small furries are prey in the wild, and hence sensory adaptation is geared toward avoidance of predation and low light activity. The eyes are directed laterally and have panoramic vision with good low light sensitivity. The external ears are well developed and serve a dual purpose of thermoregulation and directional hearing. The tympanic bulla is comparatively large. The olfactory bulb in the brain is large and the vibrissae are very sensitive.

Environmental adaptations

The small furries can be found in almost all environments. Adaptation to extreme cold and heat are achieved through burrowing to escape cold and heat, hibernating during winter, and the use of brown fat for thermogenesis. The high surface area to body weight ratio is energy expensive and requires large amounts of oxygen. Many species have a marked ability to concentrate urine and survive on very small quantities of water.

Hypothermia, hypoxia, dehydration, and negative energy balance are all important considerations when evaluating and rehabilitating compromised individuals.

Common orthopedic conditions

See Table 4.1 at the end of this section for a summary of common orthopedic conditions.

Pododermatitis

All rabbits and rodents have a plantigrade stance when resting, with the hocks placed against the ground. There are no pads in this area to shield against low grade trauma from poor substrates and cage design. Husbandry considerations such as substrate selection and routine cleaning are often overlooked in busy households or breeding establishments. The resultant low grade trauma from placing the hocks on hard and abrasive surfaces, combined with urine and fecal staining, will quickly lead to the development of ulcers, pyoderma, and ultimately infection of the deeper structures of the hock. Obesity and lack of appropriate exercise will contribute to the problem. The tight hair in this region can hide deeper problems until the skin sloughs off as a result of infection. When presented the areas are variably affected with conditions ranging from thickening and hair loss to substantial granulomas, scar tissue, and devitalized areas. Diagnosis is through direct observation of the areas, which are invariably bilateral. Follow-up radiographs and samples for tissue culture to select appropriate antimicrobials can be taken when the wounds are explored and debrided under general anesthesia. As husbandry and housing is the cause of such lesions treatment plans need to focus on this aspect.

Fractures and mishandling trauma

There are two areas to consider involving trauma: the spine and axial skeleton, and the appendicular skeleton. Spinal fractures and trauma are common presentations, often following mishandling by the owner

Table 4.1 A summary of the most common orthopedic conditions together with their main clinical features and interventions

Condition	Symptoms	Diagnosis	Treatment
Pododermatitis	Unwillingness to move Smell or urine staining to rear area Sensitivity to palpation Easy manual depilation of affected areas Erythema and pyoderma	Clinical examination	Change bedding or cage design Routine wound care Pain relief
Fractures and trauma	Lameness Pain evident on palpation Variable swelling	Clinical examination Radiographs	Routine fracture management Pain relief
Splay leg	Gait abnormality Failure to thrive Thrashed bedding Angular limb deformity	Clinical examination	Hobbling Osteopathy Bedding changes Pain management Euthanasia
Spondylitis and osteoarthritis	Failure to thrive Unwillingness to move Weight loss Stiff and curtailed gait Pain on palpation	Clinical examination Radiographs	Osteopathy Pain management Chondroprotectants
Vitamin deficiencies	Neurological deficits Muscle wastage Failure to thrive Other medical complaints, fur abnormalities, poor healing, weight loss	History Clinical examination Exclusion of differential diagnoses (blood tests)	Initially dietary supplementation Dietary changes

or clinician. Luxations will occur, but more often the injury is a fracture in the lower lumbar area, especially in rabbits. The large and powerful rear leg musculature combined with a frail spine and a tendency for some species to panic and thrash out with their hind legs when placed on their back provides an ideal fulcrum in the caudal lumbar area to facilitate fractures. Posterior paralysis or paresis is the presenting clinical sign, with a variable degree of pain in the mid to caudal lumbar area. There is a variable degree of loss of bladder and bowel function. Prognosis is dependent on the extent of the injury and the response to conservative medical management. True paralysis that leaves no bowel or bladder control will almost always result in euthanasia. Less severe cases may respond to supportive treatment such as osteopathy, given time, intensive nursing, and a willing owner.

Fractures to the appendicular skeleton are common and often follow falls or being trampled underfoot. The fine bone structure and minimal soft tissue surrounding the tibia make this a common site. Fractures can often go undiagnosed for some time especially in the nocturnal species. Due to the thin skin of most species, bone fragments will commonly pierce through the skin and open fractures are easily created. Open fractures are commonly missed until examined under anesthesia due to thick fur cover and minimal bleeding. Diagnosis is by radiography, and treatment follows normal orthopedic principles. The very fine bone structure of most species requires careful selection of immobilization techniques, and amputation should be considered for open and complex fractures in the smaller species.

Splay leg

Splay leg is a developmental abnormality of rabbits that is essentially related to hip dysplasia. The affected rabbits are usually young (a few days to a few months old), although it can be seen in older rabbits as a result of osteoarthritis. Splay leg starts with a developmental reduction and flattening of the femoral head which leads to an inappropriate placing of the hind limbs on the ground. If unchecked this leads to subluxation of the hip, valgus deformity, and patella luxation. The loss of hind limb integrity leads to muscle atrophy, loss of adduction, and the back legs splay outward. Urine and fecal contamination of the hind quarters leads to further complications and possible myiasis (maggot infestation). The severity of signs depends on the degree of deformity and time elapsed before presentation, thus symptoms may vary from some degree of poor movement in the hind legs through to complete loss of back leg movement that can mimic a spinal lesion. Diagnosis is achieved through assessment of the history, clinical examination, ruling out spinal lesions, and radiography of the hips. Due to the progressive nature of the condition treatment can be challenging. Advanced cases may respond to hobbling, osteopathy, and supportive treatment. Less severe cases may respond to substrate changes, medical management of pain, and osteopathy.

Spondylosis and osteoarthritis

Most species will experience degenerative joint disease as they age. Symptoms are often confused with other conditions that feature disuse atrophy and urinary staining of the perineum due to lack of movement. Diagnosis is often not made until radiographs of the legs show characteristic joint cartilage thinning and osteophyte formation, or trial therapy with a nonsteroidal anti-inflammatory drug yields better than expected results. Treatment with NSAIDs and osteopathy will often give good results initially but euthanasia is likely to result eventually and many of these animals do have a short lifespan.

Nutritional disorders

Nutritional disorders will affect all species but are becoming increasingly rare due to the wide availability of good complete feeds for all species.

Incorrect calcium to phosphorous ratio in the diet, or lack of calcium in the diet, leads to nutritional hyperparathyroidism. Bone demineralization and possible pathological fractures will result if the imbalance is severe enough. A good example is seen in hamsters fed on a high sunflower-seed-based diet, which has a high phosphorous content. Chinchillas with hypocalcemia will present with cramping of the muscles of the back legs and face, especially prior to feeding.

Hypovitaminosis A leads to neurological symptoms starting with circling and ataxia and leading to convulsions and seizures.

Hypovitaminosis E and selenium deficiency will lead to nutritional muscular dystrophy in all species. It has been implicated in disuse paralysis seen in hamsters and in weakness and atrophy of the hind legs in chipmunks, rabbits, and guinea pigs.

Vitamin C deficiency is unique to guinea pigs, as they cannot synthesize their own endogenously. Lack of vitamin C presents with many symptoms such as lack of hair growth, difficulty eating, teeth grinding, and delayed wound healing. Lameness results from joint swelling and pain as a result of compromised blood vessel integrity and subsequent hemorrhaging into joint spaces, especially the stifle. Pathological lesions can be seen at the costochondral junctions on radiographs, and if there is a history of poor diet a tentative diagnosis can be made.

Differential diagnosis

See Table 4.2 at the end of this section for a summary of the most common differential diagnoses.

Table 4.2 A summary of the most common differential diagnoses

Parasitic	E. cuniculi Toxoplasmosis Cerebral larva migrans
Bacterial	Osteomyelitis Abscess formation Otitis interna or otitis media Suppurative encephalitis
Viral	Rabies Herpes virus
Degenerative	Osteoarthritis Spondylosis Disuse atrophy Degenerative neuropathy
Physical	Trauma Iatrogenic mishandling Pododermatitis
Developmental	Congenital defects Splay leg
Neoplastic	Osteosarcoma Other soft tissue tumors (mammary neoplasia is very common in all species)
Metabolic or nutritional	Hypovitaminosis A Hypovitaminosis E Hypovitaminosis C
Toxic	Exposure to lead paint
Miscellaneous	Hypoxia Vascular vccidents

Parasitic disease

Encephalitozoon cuniculi (E. cuniculi) is a common obligate protozoan parasite of rabbits that has been known to affect rodents as well. It has the potential to be zoonotic in humans that are immunocompromised. The parasite enters the body through ingestion of spores present in the urine and feces of affected animals. Once in the body the parasite divides in blood rich tissues such as the kidneys and liver, eventually moving onto the brain and causing characteristic vestibular symptoms. Treatment with benzimidazoles is successful if instigated promptly and with suitable nursing most rabbits will recover. Careful postinfection preventative measures are required and testing of "in contact" rabbits is advised. The incidence of the disease is now very high in the United Kingdom, and routine treatment of recently acquired rabbits with fenbendazole, for 20 days, is being advised by some practitioners.

Toxoplasmosis can be acquired through the ingestion of feline feces or through vertical transmission. The disease is rarely recorded in rabbits and has similar symptoms to E. cuniculi if infection becomes clinically significant. Differentiation from E. cuniculi is by serological testing, and by the presence of E. cuniculi spores on brain sections on postmortem examination.

Infections have been recorded with baylisascaris (roundworm) causing neurological disease through cerebral larva migrans after exposure to racoon feces. Cuterebra (bot flies) species have also been recorded after the larvae of the species have migrated through ear canals.

Bacterial infections

Multiple bacteria species have been isolated from cases of otitis interna. The preponderance of isolates has been *Pasteurella multocida*. These infections are assumed to follow infections of the upper respiratory tract but can also be acquired through descending otitis externa through tympanic rupture. Symptoms are invariably vestibular in origin. Treatment is through prolonged antibiotics after appropriate culture, sensitivity, and careful antimicrobial selection relevant to the species involved.

Suppurative encephalitis through hematogenous spread of infection to the brain or through the extension of otitis interna has been recorded. Listeriosis has been reported in some species.

Viral infections

Rabies should be considered in any rabbits showing central nervous symptoms in countries where the virus is endemic. Herpes simplex has been reported in rabbits exposed to humans affected with the virus. Affected rabbits suffer from conjunctivitis and central nervous symptoms such as ataxia, circling, and seizures.

Trauma

Fractures of the limbs or spine are common in all species. Careful examination for paresis or paralysis as well as careful palpation of all bones is necessary to rule out injuries. If fracture is possible, radiographs of the suspected areas should be diagnostic. Care should be taken when examining spinal radiographs as the small nature of the bones can lead to misdiagnosis.

Developmental diseases

The young of all species can develop failure of adduction of the hind legs, with a variable degree of inability to walk. The condition varies from mild gait abnormality to severe dragging of the back legs. In growing rabbits this can lead to femoral head flattening, hip subluxation, patella luxation, and valgus deformity.

Degenerative diseases

Osteoarthritis, spondylosis, and disuse atrophy are increasingly seen as a result of the improved husbandry of all species and subsequent improved longevity. Soiling of the perineum and hocks may be the initial presenting signs. Further symptoms are seen as the animals are unable to reach their rear to clean themselves or perform coprophagia. Muscle wastage as a result of disuse and lack of exercise can result in both a forelimb and hind limb splay leg. Rodents are prone to degenerative neuropathies, as seen in canine patients, with a similar spectrum of possible etiologies including diabetic neuropathy.

Toxic conditions

Lead toxicities as the result of ingestion of lead-containing products is now seen less often, as the preponderance of lead-containing paints reduces. The classic case is a house rabbit with a penchant for chewing wood, living in an old house where the wood has been painted with lead-based paint. The commonest signs of toxicity are anemia, anorexia, depression, and gut stasis, but central nervous edema may lead to more global central nervous signs. Blood lead measurements, the presence of radiodense material in the GI tract (on radiographs), and nucleated red blood cells are indicative of this condition.

If used on rabbits and rodents, flea treatments designed for use in dogs and cats may contain sufficient quantities of fipronil, pyrethrin, or permethrin to cause variable degrees of depression and seizures. Standard decontamination and symptomatic treatments are applicable.

Neoplasia

Osteosarcomas are rare in all rodents and rabbits; however, soft tissue tumors affecting tissues adjacent to bone and muscle are common. Lameness may result, related to the bulk of the mass, and associated discomfort and pain. Any malignancy has the ability to metastasize to the central nervous system and cause neurological disturbance.

Other conditions

Strokes have been suspected in some species. Hypoxia as a result of other systemic disease may cause seizures.

Osteopathic evaluation

Generally speaking, small furry patients are prone to becoming stressed. For this reason, during osteopathic evaluation and treatment handling should be kept to minimum, especially if the animal is unused to it. Both domestic and wild rabbits appear to be particularly sensitive to handling by humans if this is performed when they are nursing young, and this can have long term affects (Bilkó and Altbäcker 2000).

Case history

The history should cover routine husbandry practice and any change in the animal's behavior that could point to possible illness. Clinical signs such as loss of appetite, lack of energy, significant weight change over a short period, lethargy, unusual vocalization, or change in eating and drinking habits or bowel and urinary function should all be assessed. Also important is the past medical history and investigations, trauma, and concomitant treatment, including drug therapy. While taking a history it is advisable to cover the cage with a towel to allow the patient to relax before it is assessed. Rats in particular, but also mice, gerbils, and hamsters, are very sensitive to high-frequency noise, and they can hear sounds that are not audible to the human ear (60–80 kHz). These can cause them considerable stress. Care should be taken with high-pitched and ultrasound noises emitted from surrounding equipment like televisions and computers.

Careful assessment of the history will highlight a number of conditions that affect rabbits, rodents, and ferrets; for example:

- Rabbits can easily develop intestinal stasis. Since the gut motility is mainly stimulated by the ingestion of coarse fiber that is rapidly excreted, a lack of fiber in the diet may inhibit gastrointestinal motility (Cheeke 1994). This is particularly likely if the animal is under stress (such as with dietary change or surgery). Intestinal stasis may rapidly lead to dehydration, as there is decreased water and electrolyte absorption from the intestinal tract (O'Malley 2005a).
- Rats and mice are commonly affected with respiratory infections which are usually due to overcrowded or poorly ventilated or poorly cleaned cages. This leads to a buildup of ammonia to which these species are particularly vulnerable.
- Ferrets are commonly affected by adrenal gland neoplasia and insulinoma (Chen 2010). The first leads to progressive alopecia as a primary clinical sign. It is additionally associated with vulvar swelling, prostagomegaly, lethargy, and muscle atrophy. Insulinoma causes hind leg weakness and dullness, as the result of blood-sugar depletion and energy source deprivation.

In general terms, when assessing small furries it should be remembered that, due to their small size, they have a high ratio of surface area to body weight, with a resulting high metabolic rate and energy requirement (Hurst 1999). This makes them susceptible to dehydration and hypothermia as well as to hypoxia and hypoglycemia. In all these species the larynx is placed high in the oropharynx where it can directly access the nasopharynx. This means all are obligate nose breathers, and the integrity of the nares and turbinates are crucial for an efficient respiratory function (Cruise and Nathan 1994).

Observation

Observation is probably the most important phase of the examination. Without causing stress to the patient, it allows fundamental information to be gathered regarding the animal's dysfunctional pattern. This allows the formation of a preliminary diagnosis and treatment plan. Time should be allowed to observe the animal with the least interference possible. First check for the presence of skin conditions (wounds, discharge etc.), bleeding, swelling, runny eyes or nose, and overgrown teeth. All of these commonly affect small furries. Watch how the animal stands. Look for the presence of antalgic posture (a stance adopted to avoid pain), avoidance of weight-bearing, positional asymmetry of the head, spine, pelvis, or tail. Assess the position of the bony landmarks. During movement look for functional asymmetry, limping, altered weight transfer, impaired range or quality of movement, and loss of balance. All of these findings are useful aids to identify any area of restricted movement resulting from a dysfunctional process.

In normal conditions, rabbits should stand plantigrade (as do rats), with the whole area from hock to toe in contact with the ground. They become digitigrade when running. Rabbits have no footpads, only coarse fur on the palmar and plantar surfaces of the limbs, and so they may suffer from pressure sores under the metatarsal regions. This is particularly true if kept on hard flooring or in unhygienic conditions (rex breeds in particular have less coarse hair to protect the thin skin). Finally, look for any damage to the rabbit's nares that may indicate serious respiratory diseases.

Rats and mice are particularly prone to respiratory infections developing into life-threatening conditions such as pneumonia. The presence of runny eyes or nose, difficulty breathing, or snuffling and wheezing should be dealt with promptly. Mammary tumors are also common in rats and tend to develop widespread secondary tumors. Particular attention should be paid to observing the presence of bumps or lumps from the axilla to the groin areas (Komitowski et al. 1982). From a clinical perspective, it is very useful to know that Harderian glands in rats produce reddish brown liquid from their eyes and nose. This secretion is rich in lipids and porphyrin red pigments, and it is copiously produced when the animal is undergoing stressful conditions. These include pain, disease, lack of cage space, noisy environment, poor nutrition, stressful handling, and the close presence of predators such as the family cat.

In rats the lower incisors are usually three times as long as the uppers. At rest the upper incisors usually lie in front of the lower ones.

Ferrets may present with damaged or infected ear pinnae and salivary glands (parotid, mandibular, or sublingual). Typically this follows fights in the mating season. If head tilting and loss of balance are observed, the possibility of otitis interna should be considered (Lewington 2003a).

Hamsters show seasonal variation in testicle size, depending on the natural daylight and temperature. They have the lowest mass in winter and the highest during summer.

Handling

Although there are different techniques for handling small furries, most of the general principles remain basically the same, with only minor variations for different species. In all cases, a firm but gentle approach is needed. The superficial fascia around the neck and shoulders is generally loosely attached in small mammals, allowing for extensive stretching. This feature can be used during scruffing for handling and restraining the animal without causing harm or pain (Fig. 4.5). The practitioner should make the patient aware of his or her presence before approaching, particularly if the animal is asleep, in order to reduce stress of handling and the risk of bite injuries.

Rabbits should always be approached with confidence and calmness. There are blind-spots at the rostral and caudal aspects of the head (especially under the chin), so the animal may be startled if touched in these regions without warning. The operator stands in front of and facing the animal, which is resting on the floor or on the table. This allows maximum control over the patient's movement should it jump to avoid contact. A double-handed hold should then be used to lift the animal with both hands around its chest, before moving it towards the osteopath's abdomen in a secure hold (Fig. 4.6). Position the rabbit at waist height across the practitioner's body. Do not dangle the rabbit in midair or move it away from the ground until it is securely held. If the rabbit's spine is not adequately supported during handling, the heavy hindquarters may twist about the lumbosacral junction and this can cause spinal fractures, commonly at the level of L6-L7, especially in young rabbits (Harkness and Wagner 1995a). Remember the skeleton of these animals is fragile in comparison to their heavy musculature.

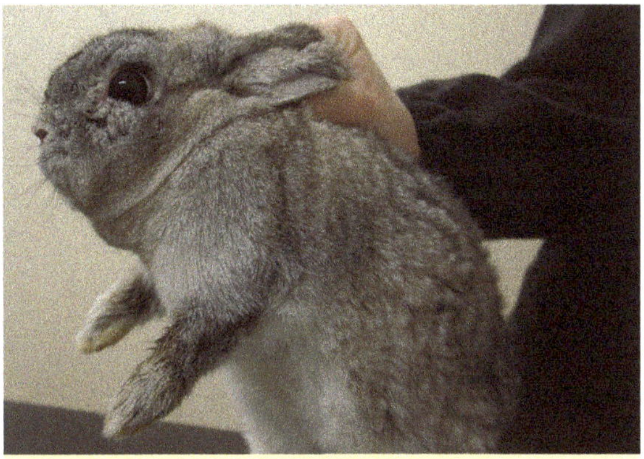

Figure 4.5
Scruffing is generally used to handle and restrain small furries without causing harm or pain. This is possible in these mammals because of the loose attachment of the superficial fascia around their neck and shoulders.

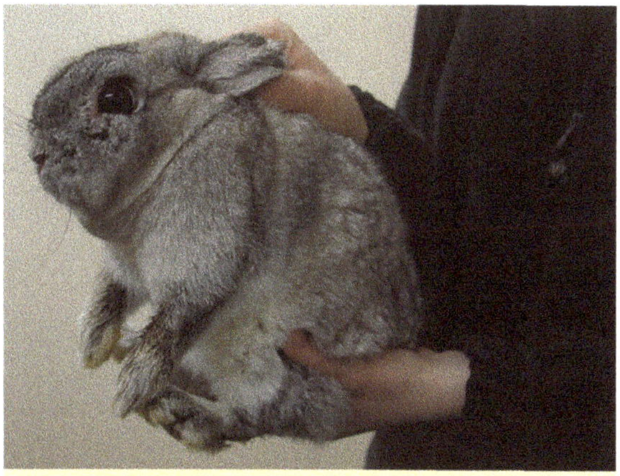

Figure 4.6
Rabbits should be lifted by the scruff, with a second supporting hand underneath the back end.

Gentleness is essential when handling gerbils, mice, and rats. As they will often try to evade capture, it is advisable to remove furnishing from the cage prior to trying to restrain them. While rats rarely bite and are often well habituated to handling, mice tend to be more flighty and less accustomed to human contact, often attempting to jump away from the handler. Both hands may be used as a scoop to hold these small mammals gently but firmly around the thorax (without restricting their breathing). Do not grab them by the tip of the tail as this can cause the tail's skin to separate. Holding the base of the tail is probably the easiest way to pick up a mouse, but for closer inspection it may be necessary to scruff it between the thumb and forefinger. Rats may initially be grasped around the shoulders, then place one of your thumbs under the animal's mandible, to prevent being bitten, while the other hand supports the hind limbs. The same procedure can be safely used with guinea pigs and ferrets. Ferrets are prone to vertebral fractures, particularly heavily-pregnant jills and heavy hobs, so the rump must be well supported when handling. This guards against excessive strain on the vertebral column. A pet ferret is unlikely to bite seriously unless alarmed or in pain.

Hamsters are nocturnal, and if wakened in the day they can become stressed, aggressive, and can bite. Early evening is the best time to handle them, when they are awake and active. Cupping hamsters in both hands is an easy and safe way to handle them, or they can be scruffed starting with the skin near the front of the shoulders, while maintaining a grip on the tail if more restraint is needed. A large amount of skin should be held to avoid the body twisting in your grip. If ambient temperatures are lower than 5°C, hamsters can enter a temporary hibernation, but they still remain sensitive to touch (Lipman and Foltz 1996).

Guinea pigs vary in temperament, and caution should be employed since some can be quite flighty. They can be enclosed in a corner and picked up by supporting both the thorax and abdomen. The latter is weighty and should be well supported at all times. Restraint on a table with the forward hand covering the head can help to calm them down.

Chinchillas can be grasped around the shoulders while supporting the hind feet and/or grasping the tail base.

Once the animal is settled, the osteopath can continue the assessment through palpatory examination.

Palpation

The palpatory routine must be performed in a relatively short time to avoid excessive stress for the animal, but it must be precise and thorough enough to identify any feature of dysfunction at each possible depth of the patient's body. Usually, as the whole animal is palpated, the operator can carry out short-duration mobility testing integrated into the assessment to investigate any region with suspected signs of altered function.

The palpatory routine aims to identify any sign of dysfunction such as sensitivity to touch, increased muscle tone, or bony asymmetry. Also check for abdominal distension, skeletal abnormality, lumps, swellings, loss of tissue integrity, etc. One of the main features that can be noticed when palpating small furries, and rodents in particular, is the large and bulky muscles of mastication, especially the temporal muscles in carnivores and the masseters which in herbivores provide great gnawing power. In all myomorphs a slip of the medial masseter runs through the infraorbital canal to insert on the muzzle, providing more effective gnawing and a strong cranial pull on the lower jaw (O'Malley 2005b). Interestingly, hamsters transport food in their cheek pouches, which are highly distensible invaginations of the lateral buccal epithelium. They extend from the mouth as far as the scapulae (Harkness and Wagner 1995b). All of these structures should be carefully examined during palpation to assess for the presence of pain, spasm, and increased muscle tone. In addition, check for asymmetry of the rest of the cranial, spinal, and appendicular bony landmarks, together with altered tone in the corresponding muscle tissue, all of which can be identified during palpatory examination.

Rabbits and rodents

When palpating rabbits and rodents it should be remembered that they use long hairs - called vibrissae - as tactile organs. These are generally distributed above the upper lip, on the chin, on each side of the nose, and around the upper and lower eyelids, and are extremely sensitive to touch. Because of this, caution and gentleness must be applied when approaching these areas. This is especially important when touching rabbits' nostrils where sensory pads are present making the animal particularly sensitive to pressure around the nose. When palpating the rabbit's thorax intercostal muscles should be fairly relaxed, since rabbits rely mainly on contraction of the diaphragm to breathe (Brewer and Cruise 1994). Compared with rodents, the rabbit presents a large hindgut and abdomen with a relatively small thorax. In fact, the rabbit's cecum is relatively the largest of all animals, with 10 times the capacity of the stomach (Cruise and Nathan 1994). The cecal wall is very thin and can tear easily, so deep and strong pressure should be avoided when palpating this area for any sign of dysfunction. The upper abdomen should also be carefully palpated to check for the presence of any abnormal or dysfunctional organ distension. In particular check the stomach which can get impacted with hair, and the liver which can suffer from torsion around its hilar region (O'Malley 2005a).

Guinea pigs

When palpating guinea pigs particular attention should be paid to assessment of the pelvic region, as cystic ovaries are common in females older than 15 months (Pilny 2014), causing potentially serious uterine disorders. Aged males are prone to develop cystitis due to occlusion of the penile urethra by coagulated seminal secretions or calculi. Cystitis is also frequently found in aged females, associated with bacterial infection, cystic calculi, and diabetes mellitus (Peng et al. 1990).

Hamsters and small rodents

During palpation of hamsters and other small rodents such as rats particular care should be taken with youngsters, since ossification is not complete until one year of age (Fallon 1996).

Rat.s

The sixth cervical vertebra in rats has a modified rib fused to its transverse processes that should not be mistaken with an abnormality. The shoulder joint has a well-developed articular and ligamentous system similar to that of humans. The clavicle articulates with the sternum, and the scapula lies horizontally on the thorax (Fig. 4.7). The rat's tail is very sensitive to painful stimulae and care should be taken when approaching this region.

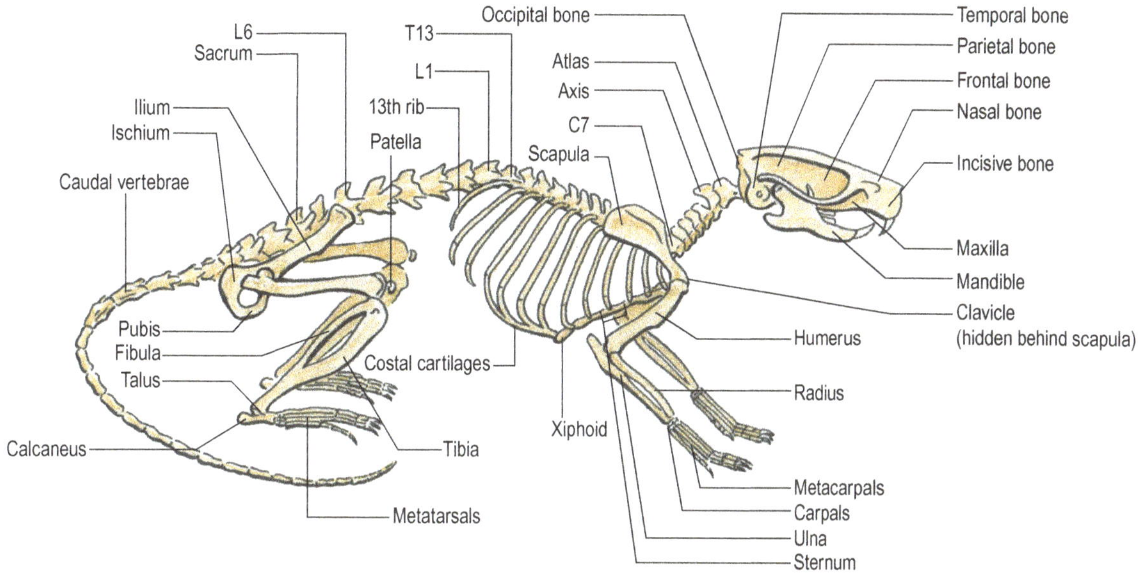

Figure 4.7
Rat skeleton.

Ferrets

When palpating ferrets particular attention should be paid to the abdominal and pelvic areas. Obstruction of the bowels is common (e.g., from ingested plastic toys) and obstruction of the urethra, following prostatic cysts, is a frequent complication of adrenal gland neoplasia.

Mobility testing

Mobility testing is usually integrated with the palpatory routine. It can be quickly performed wherever a dynamic examination of a selected body area is needed, to help formulate a functional diagnosis.

Mobility testing should be gently applied to all the articulations of small furries, including the spine (Fig. 4.8), pelvis (Fig. 4.9), and limbs (Fig. 4.10) to identify any restriction or impaired quality of motion and sensitivity to touch. The skull usually presents a mobile and loose temporomandibular joint (Fig. 4.11), which is capable of rotatory, side-to-side, and forward and backward motion. This is particularly marked in herbivores.

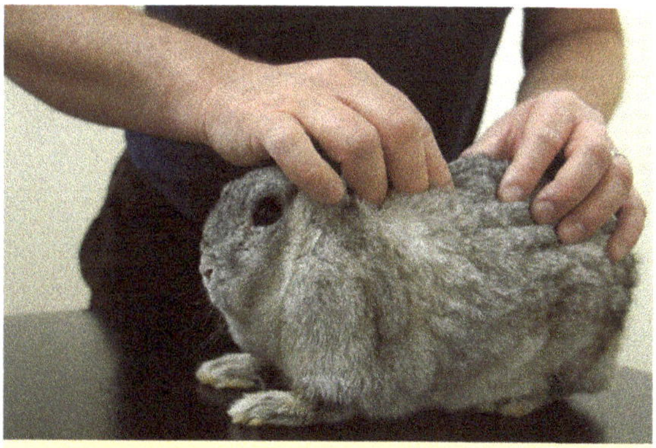

Figure 4.8
Spinal mobility can be assessed by holding the proximal and distal end of the vertebral group being examined and then testing freedom and quality of motion in all planes.

This can be mobility tested by taking hold of the animal's mandible and applying a gentle mobility test with the thumb on the mandibular condyle, while the other hand stabilizes the head using the ipsilateral temporal bone. Bear in mind that molar shearing occurs in all

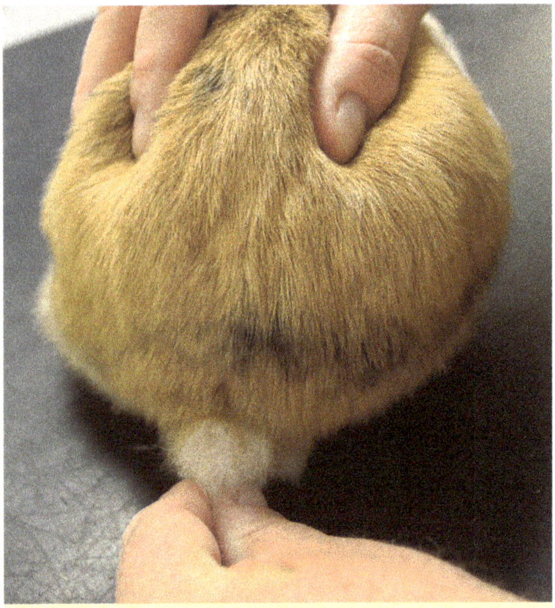

Figure 4.9
The pelvis can be examined by using the tail to test for the mobility of the sacrum and using the limbs as levers to assess motility of the innominate bones.

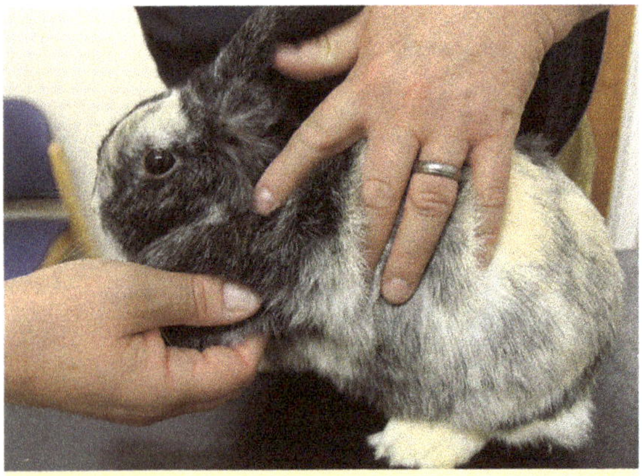

Figure 4.10
The mobility of each joint complex in the limbs can be assessed by holding the bone proximal to the joint, while using the distal bone to test motion in all planes.

three orthogonal directions, whereas molar crushing and incisor biting are predominately directed vertically (Watson et al. 2014).

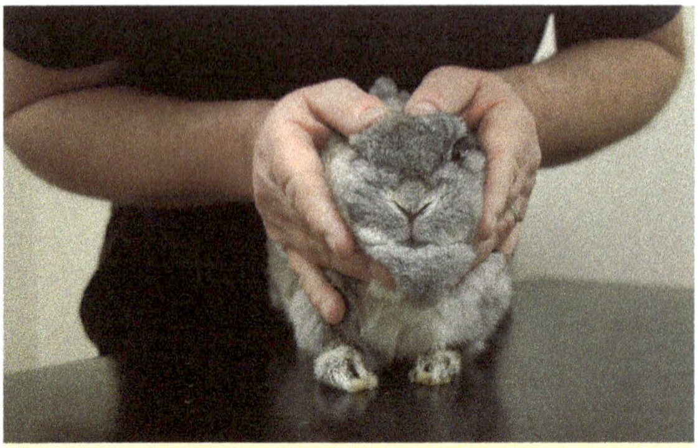

Figure 4.11
The mobility of the temporomandibular joint can be assessed by holding the head and the corresponding temporal area with one hand while the other hand takes a direct contact ventrally on the mandible, to test its motion in all planes.

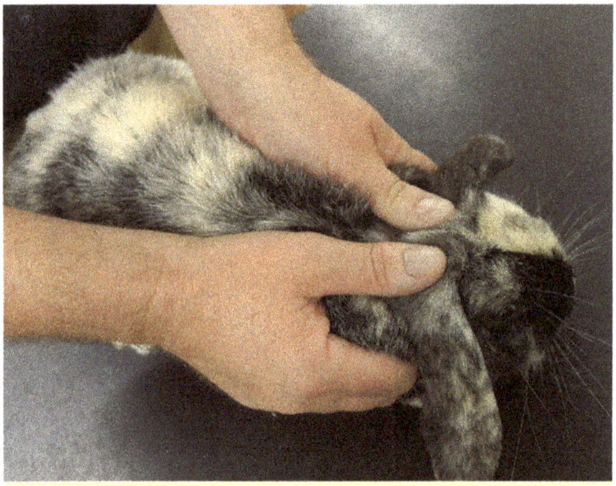

Figure 4.12
The range of movement of the occipitoatlantoaxial complex can be tested in flexion or extension and lateral flexing by stabilizing the trunk and lower cervical vertebrae with one hand while the other hand gently induces motion through an occipitomandibular contact.

The skull also has a large double occipital condyle and a specialized atlantoaxial complex, which provides effective head flexion and extension, as well as lateral flexion. This can be mobility tested by taking an occipitomandibular contact over the head with one hand, while the other hand stabilizes the rest of the body, trunk, and caudal cervical vertebrae

(Fig. 4.12). The same hold can be used to test the rest of the spine by shifting the double-hand contact and the focus of motion over the examined segments. The thorax has a more limited range of motion because of the rib cage, in contrast with the greater mobility found in the lumbar spine, especially in dorsoventral flexion.

In rabbits, the first seven ribs should articulate directly with the sternum; the 7th to 9th ribs show the same attachment but through costal cartilages, while the 10th to 12th ribs are floating (in other species such as guinea pigs the last four to five ribs are floating).

The numbers of vertebrae are variable (Table 4.3).

The guinea pig skeleton is extremely mobile and lightweight. It has long and light appendicular bones (susceptible to fracture), together with a very flexible spine that is consequently subject to fracture and disc injury.

The forefeet of rats, unlike those of the rabbit and guinea pig, are well developed and mobile, being able to flex and grasp food in their palms (Fig. 4.13A and B). This mobility should be tested during examination by stabilizing the proximal segments and using the distal ones as levers to feel for the corresponding joint mobility (Fig. 4.14).

The mobility testing may be concluded with the assessment of the involuntary rhythms like the cranial, fascial, visceral, or fluidic ones, looking for loss of vitality, poor range and quality of motion, asymmetrical expression, and altered frequency. These assessments, however, will often be missed out, since the time available to assess and treat a small furry is usually limited even under sedation.

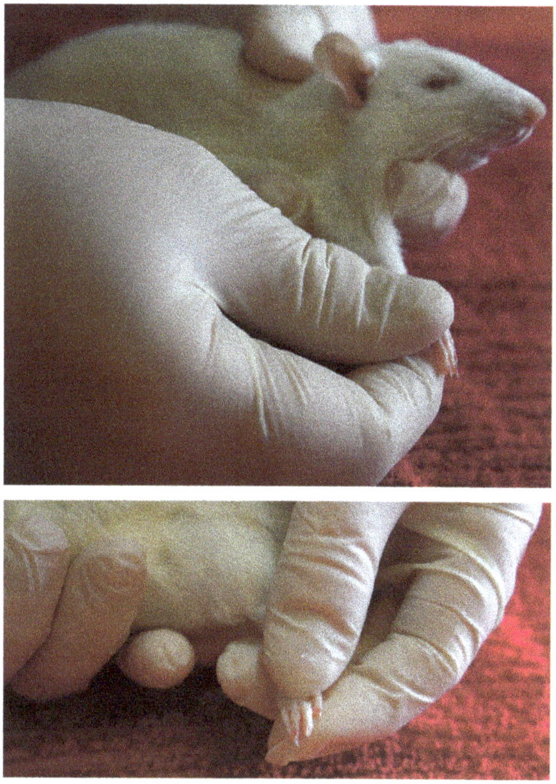

Figure 4.13
The mobile forelimbs in rats can be tested by holding the proximal segments and using the distal ones as levers to feel for the joint mobility, as shown for the shoulder joint (A) and elbow joint (B).

Table 4.3 Number and type of vertebrae in small furries

Species	Cervical vertebrae	Thoracic vertebrae	Lumbar vertebrae	Sacral vertebrae	Coccygeal vertebrae
Rabbit	7	12–13	7	4	15–16
Rat	7	12–13	6	3–4	27–31
Hamster	7	12–13	6	4	13–14
Ferret	7	15	5–6	3	18
Guinea pig	7	13–14	6	2–3	4

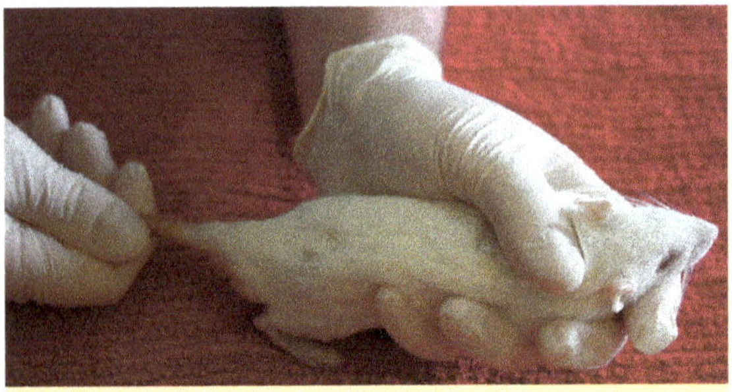

Figure 4.14
Alternating traction or articulatory techniques can be applied along the spine and rib cage by holding the mouse or rat with both hands around the belly and sternum (supporting the head from below the mandible), while using both thumbs to focus the articulatory or tractioning force where needed.

Osteopathic treatment

General considerations

The osteopathic treatment of small furries is mainly based on the findings gathered from good history taking; a long, patient, and acute observation; thorough palpatory examination; and quick but precise mobility testing. The treatment is usually a gradual and progressive shift from the assessment into the correction of the dysfunctions being found. The intervention should be kept to minimum to avoid stressing the animal with prolonged and unnecessary handling. In the experience of the author (PT) a treatment never lasts more than 10 minutes on these small mammals. The effects that can be produced, however, are quite surprising and are often followed by dramatic changes in the animal's behavior.

While applying pressure or traction forces during treatment, always be aware of the tissue and animal response. If any sign of sensitivity, avoidance, or reaction to pressure should become evident, the operator must adapt the intervention accordingly. The hold can be changed or a different technique can be selected to achieve the same objective, with a safer or less invasive intervention. Avoid jerky movements as these may elicit a protective reaction or an aggressive response from the animal. Sedation is rarely needed for treating small furries, due to their generally high tolerance to human contact. Sedation can be useful, however, if the animal shows aggressiveness (as the Syrian hamster might do), hypersensitivity to touch, or excessive reactions to handling and restraint (as may be seen in some species with dysfunctional hormonal cycles). In all cases, the potential benefit and potential risk should always be the primary considerations when planning and applying osteopathic manipulation. If for any reason the risk related to a given intervention would be higher than the benefit that might follow, the practitioner should consider a valid osteopathic alternative or referral to other professions. Different types of treatment such as surgery, drug-therapy, physiotherapy, or acupuncture might offer lower risk or a better chance of recovery in some cases.

Mice, rats, and gerbils

Since mice and rats are quite susceptible to respiratory conditions, the function of the thoracic spine and rib cage, and of the respiratory apparatus, is fundamental for their health. Gentle articulatory techniques, or alternating traction, can be applied in these areas to improve joint mobility and enhance pulmonary function (Fig. 4.15). Light lymphatic pumping techniques can also be administered to these mammals to improve immune function, and increase lymphatic flow and white cell count (Hodge et al. 2007). Although

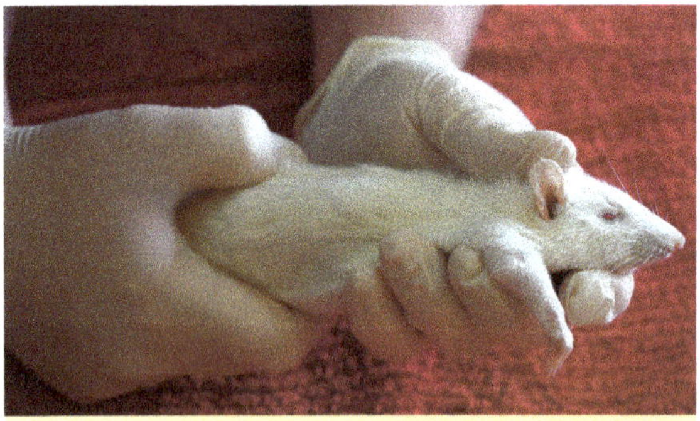

Figure 4.15
By holding the mouse or rat on both sides it is possible to administer gentle and rhythmic pumping pressures along the rib cage.

these effects have only been demonstrated to occur in dogs, it is reasonable to assume that rats and mice may respond in a similar way. Four minutes of pumping techniques for seven consecutive days has been shown to increase leukocyte activity in rats and promote an antitumoral response by the immune system (Hodge et al. 2010). Abdominal visceral mobilization has been demonstrated to prevent and treat postoperative adhesions (Bove and Chapelle 2012), and to reduce postoperative ileus in rats by the attenuation of the related inflammatory processes (Chapelle and Bove 2013).

Rats, mice, and gerbils may also commonly need treatment of limbs that have been trapped in exercise wheels or injured during fighting. Gentle articulation of the related limb joints may help to improve mobility if impaired and restore articular alignment if altered (Fig. 4.16). Particular attention should be addressed to the treatment of the tail in rats and mice, since this plays a large role in thermoregulation (as well as balancing). Together with the ears, the tail is crucial for controlling heat loss by regulating the dilation of blood vessels in these organs (Fallon 1996). Articulatory or fascial unwinding techniques can be applied to free this area if needed (Fig. 4.17), especially in those animals that are distressed by poor environmental temperature control.

Caution should be applied when a rat presents with chromodacryorrhea - the condition where red-brown deposits produced by the Harderian glands appear as tears around the animal's eyes and nose. In this situation, in the author's experience, handling the rat and the treatment should be kept to the minimum essential, or if other pathology, surgery, or drug therapy is present it should be avoided. It might be safer and more effective to improve husbandry practices first. This should have an indirect effect on the rat's homeostatic potential that can be beneficial if treated the following week.

Rabbits

Rabbits are particularly responsive to functional osteopathic work, probably because of the fragility of their skeleton - in contrast to the mass of the surrounding myofascial structures. This appears to make these mammals more prone to respond better to soft tissue and indirect approaches, together with the balancing of the involuntary rhythms. Their docility allows the osteopath to spend enough time to feel and treat such rhythms. It is always important to make sure you have a firm hold of the rabbit throughout examination and treatment as they tend to jump when least expected. When treating the head, the ears can be gently used as levers for various techniques addressing the cranial sutures (Fig. 4.18). The balancing of the splanchnocranial rhythm and tension may be fundamental

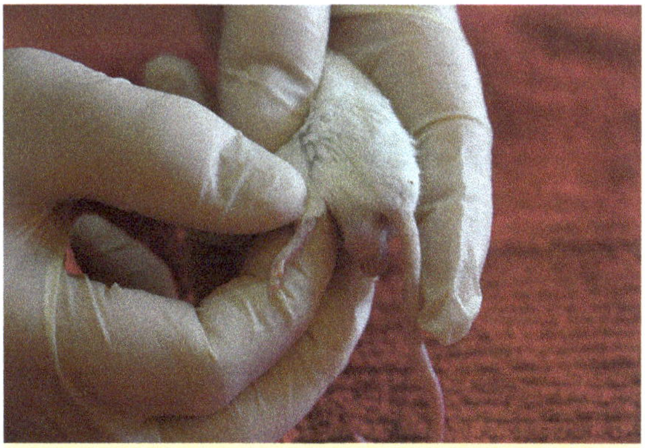

Figure 4.16
The joints of the limb can be mobilized by stabilizing the proximal bone and articulating the distal one.

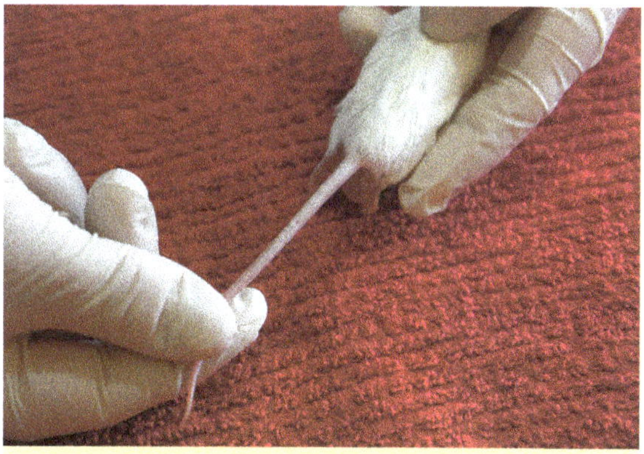

Figure 4.17
Fascial unwinding can be successfully applied along the tail by maintaining a gentle hold and then applying traction to the dysfunctional area. Traction can be maintained or increased following the path of any inherent fascial torsion until release is achieved.

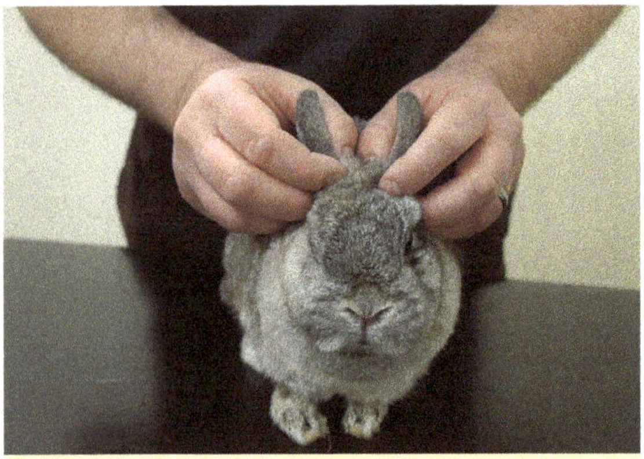

Figure 4.18
Cranial sutures, such as the frontal and parietal, can be released by gentle and rhythmic pressure applied on the restrictive area. The ears can also be used as levers for treating the area. The ears can also be used in cranial holds to assess the primary respiratory mechanism.

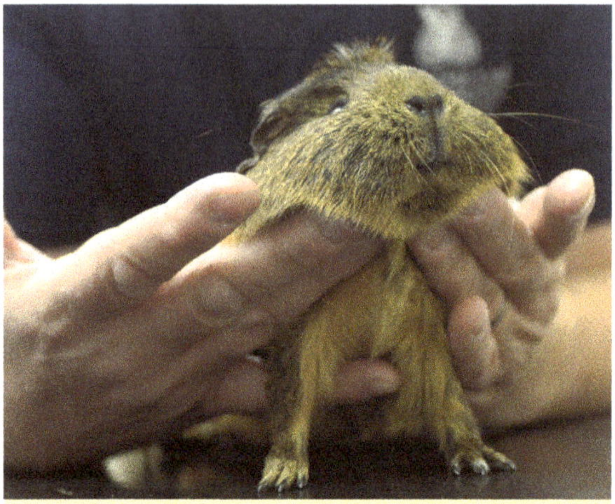

Figure 4.19
Masticatory muscles, such as the masseter and temporalis, may undergo functional inhibition by applying and maintaining a gentle and progressive pressure on the point of major restriction. Articulatory techniques on the TMJ may follow to improve joint mobility.

in rabbits, since the narrow and tortuous nasolacrimal duct makes them vulnerable to duct obstruction (O'Malley 2005a). Maxillary and mandibular correction may help in many tooth conditions that affect rabbits as well as most rodents. Temporomandibular (TMJ) mobility can be improved by applying functional inhibition to the masticatory muscles (Fig. 4.19), followed by gentle side-to-side and back and forward articulatory techniques of the mandible itself through contact on its condyles and ramus.

The ventral cervical structures can be approached with one hand cupping the mandible from below its inferior margin and the other hand gently applying traction via the sternum (Fig. 4.20).

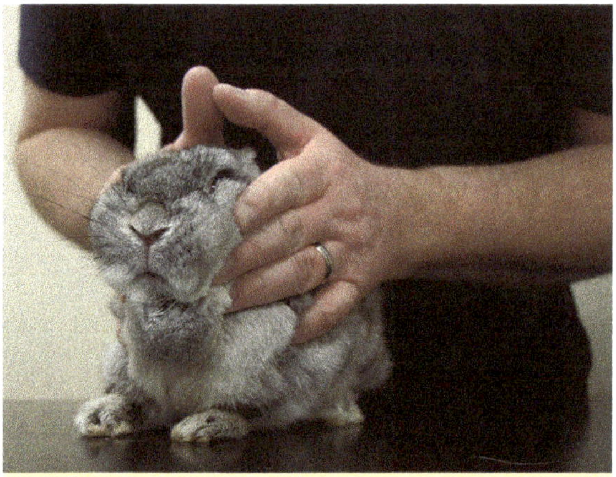

Figure 4.20
Releasing soft tissue tension around the mandible and throat structures in a rabbit.

Because the hindgut plays a major role in the rabbit's health, visceral mobilization of this area may produce profound changes in the general function and behavior of the animal (Fig. 4.21). A double-hand contact on the abdomen may be used to apply opposed traction force in the area of restriction until a release is felt (Fig. 4.22A). Alternatively, the hind limbs can be used as levers to focus the tension in the area of abdominal dysfunction (Fig. 4.22B). Caution must be employed when approaching the cecum, since this is very sensitive to touch, thin, and easy to rupture.

Rabbits are prone to develop restrictions of mobility in the extremities, as they tend to shift rapidly from standing plantigrade to running digitigrade. Balanced ligamentous tension techniques are particularly suitable to treat the joints from hock to toe (Fig. 4.23). When treating the hind limb, bear in mind that the fibula is

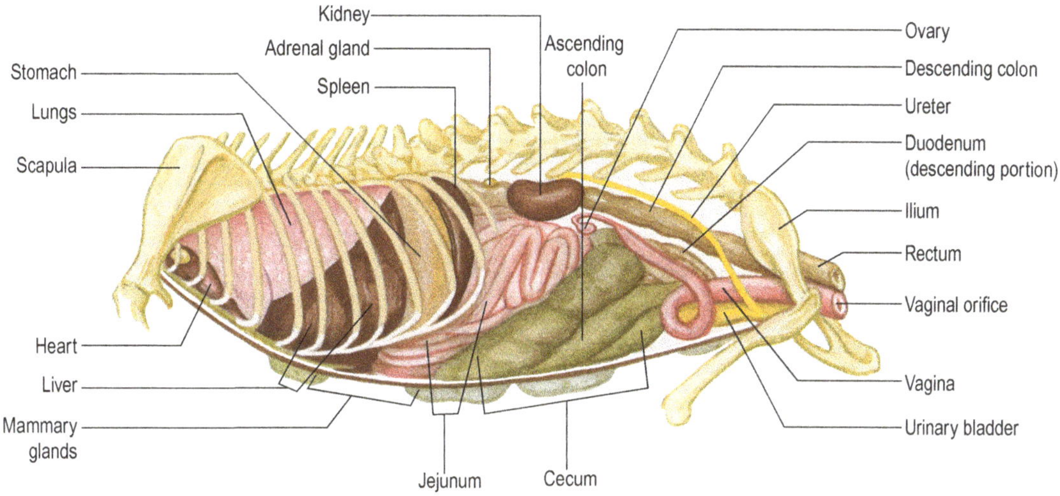

Figure 4.21
Left lateral view of rabbit viscera.

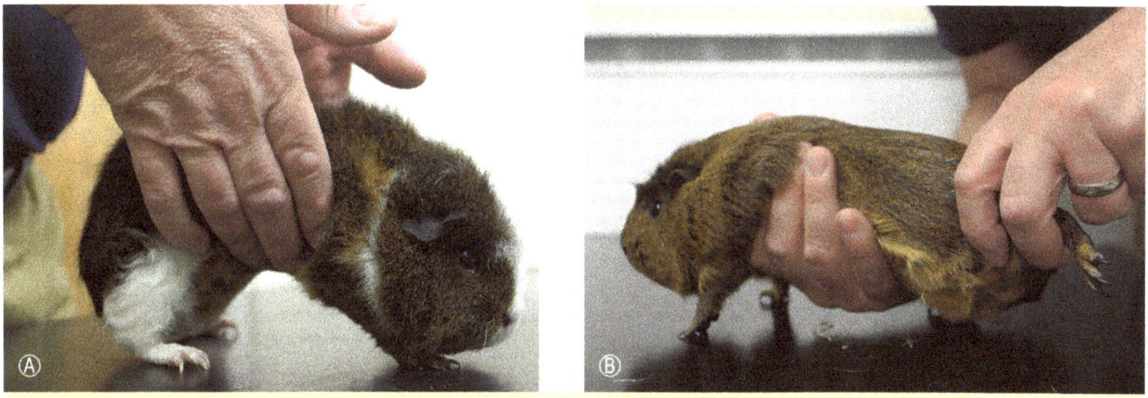

Figure 4.22
(A) An abdominal visceral dysfunction can be approached through a double-hand contact on the point of major density and restriction and applying either a direct or an indirect technique. (B) Lower abdominal and pelvic visceral dysfunction can be treated by using the ipsilateral hind limb to apply pressure against or away from the restrictive barrier.

fused with the tibia for over half its length (Cruise and Nathan 1994).

Ferrets

Ferrets have a thoracic inlet that is narrower than other carnivores, so any abnormalities of even one organ passing through it (e.g., trachea, esophagus, major blood vessels) can seriously interfere with chest function. Because of this a pectoral traction technique can be particularly useful. This can be performed by holding the forelimb in one hand while the other hand applies an intermittent pressure focused at different levels to include the clavicle, scapula, shoulder joint, ventral cervical structures, caudal cervical vertebrae, cranial thoracic vertebrae, and the soft tissue in the thoracic inlet (Fig. 4.24). The aim is to release myofascial tissue tension in those areas in order to enhance

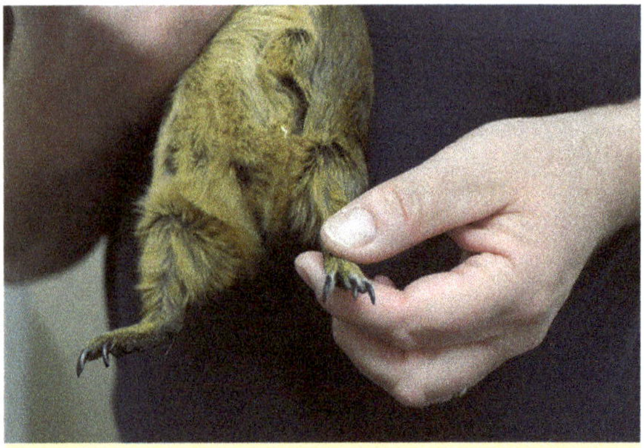

Figure 4.23
The limbs generally respond well to balanced ligamentous tension techniques during which the affected joint is brought to and maintained in a balanced point of tension in all planes of motion until release is felt.

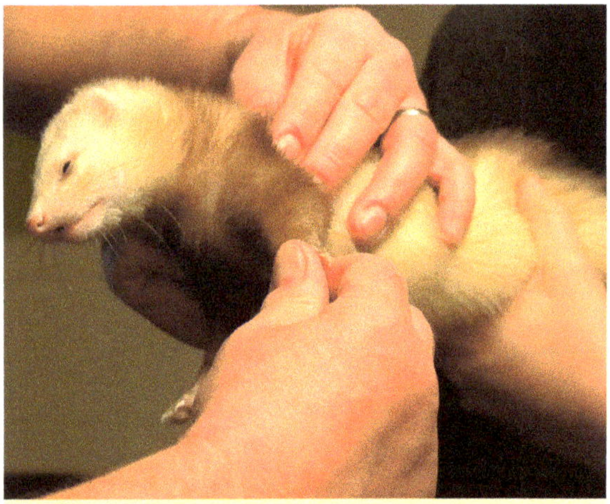

Figure 4.24
A pectoral release, to open the thoracic inlet, can be performed through gentle and rhythmic traction of the forelimb which is held in one hand while intermittent pressure is applied either on the shoulder complex or the cervicothoracic junction with the other hand.

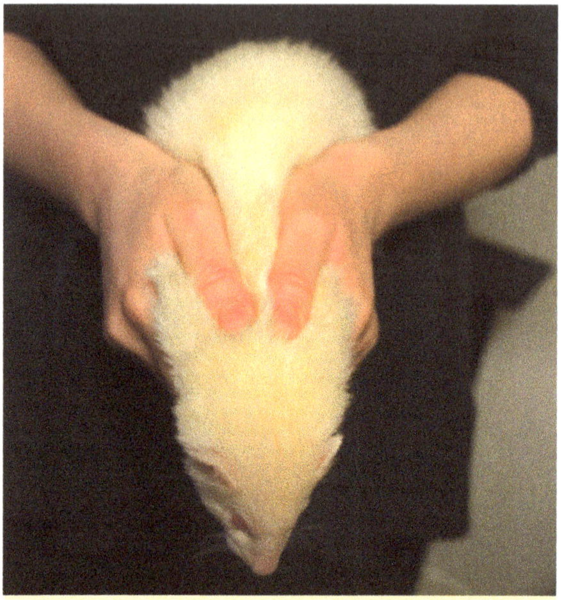

Figure 4.25
Chest pumping techniques are gently applied with a double-hand contact on the thorax, with the thumbs and thenar eminences along the thoracic spine, the second and third fingers on the lateral neck, and the fourth and fifth fingers on the sternum.

related visceral gliding mobility and fluid dynamics. The treatment can continue with gentle chest pumping. Hold the sternum with the fourth and fifth fingers of both hands while both thumbs apply a dorsal counterforce on the thorax, and the second and third fingers control the animal's neck (Fig. 4.25). This procedure can be concluded with a diaphragm release via functional inhibition of its crural attachments (at the TL junction), together with articulation of the lower thoracic and cranial lumbar vertebrae (Fig. 4.26). The spine of ferrets is very flexible and responds well to articulatory techniques, but HVLATs should be restricted as the skeleton is lightweight and susceptible to fracture, and the spine is prone to disc injuries. Pay particular attention to the vertebral junctions (cervicothoracic, thoracolumbar, lumbosacral), as they are frequently dysfunctional due to the highly mobile spine and the quick twisting movements that are made by ferrets.

In female ferrets, ovarian function is crucial to regulate levels of estrogen during estrus. The ovaries are suspended via ligaments attached to the abdominal wall, with the left ovary lying caudal to the middle of the 14th rib and the right ovary lying caudal to the middle of the 15th rib (Lewington 2005). These points can be approached with gentle inhibitory pressure if needed.

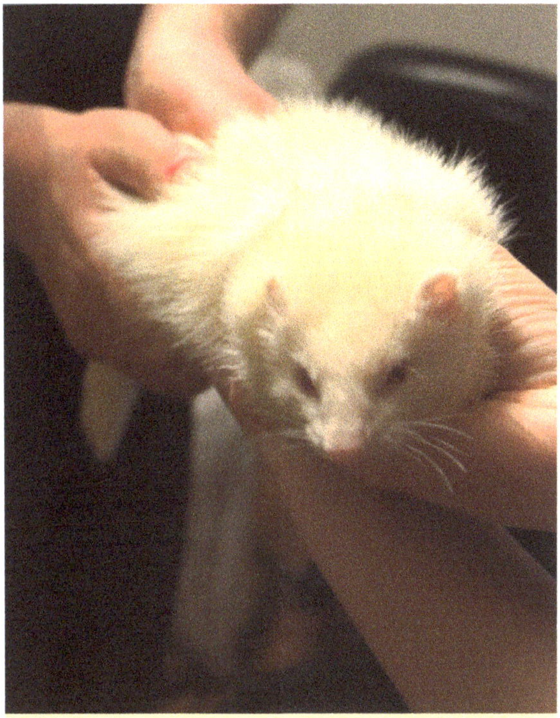

Figure 4.26
Functional inhibition is applied with both thumbs to the diaphragmatic attachments to the thoracolumbar junction.

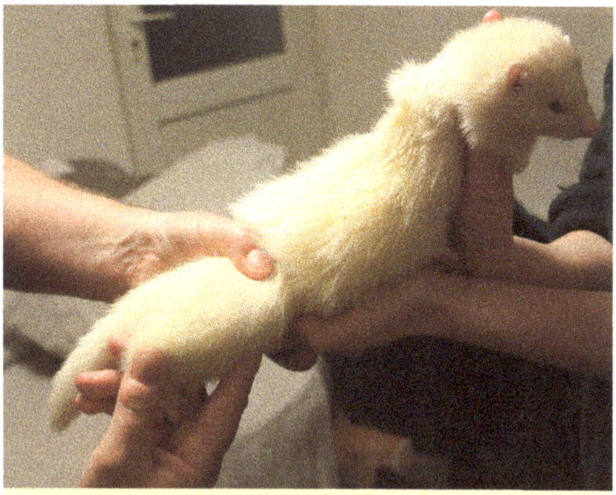

Figure 4.27
Pelvic viscera and related suspensory ligaments may be treated with one hand ventrally on the dysfunctional area and the other hand holding the corresponding hind limb, to apply forces either toward or away from the restrictive barrier.

The pelvic area is another region for osteopathic intervention, as it is the common site of conditions such as vaginitis, prostatomegaly, and prostatic cysts, mostly associated with adrenal gland neoplasia. The dorsal aspect of the pelvis and the sacrum can be treated through a direct contact with one hand, and indirect gentle traction through the tail held with the other hand. If the ventral part of the pelvis needs treatment, the hind limb can be used as a lever instead of the tail, while the other hand can approach the pelvic viscera and related suspensory apparatus ventrally (Fig. 4.27).

Guinea pigs

The pelvic techniques described for the ferret can also be performed on guinea pigs, as they are also likely to develop cystitis. Freeing pelvic and hip mobility, together with a balanced fascial and visceral tension, can enhance fluid dynamics and immunity function in these mammals, which helps to prevent or treat this condition.

Hamsters and chinchilla

Hamsters and chinchilla (as well as ferrets) generally respond well to fascial treatments. A full body release can be achieved by approaching the cranial and caudal ends simultaneously with a double-hand contact (keep at least one finger below the mandible to protect yourself from being bitten). The operator can follow the tissue dysfunctional vectors, or approach the restrictive barrier, until release is achieved (Fig. 4.28). The cranial hand can focus, for instance, on any tension felt along the hamster's pouches up to the scapula, while the caudal hand can approach any dysfunction found in the abdominopelvic region. With chinchilla in particular, the tail can be used as a further lever to reinforce the maneuver. The same hold can be employed with a focus on the dorsal part of the body to perform articular techniques on the spine and inhibitory pressure on the paraspinal muscles where needed. Pumping techniques are also beneficial and applicable to the chest and abdomen of these mammals,

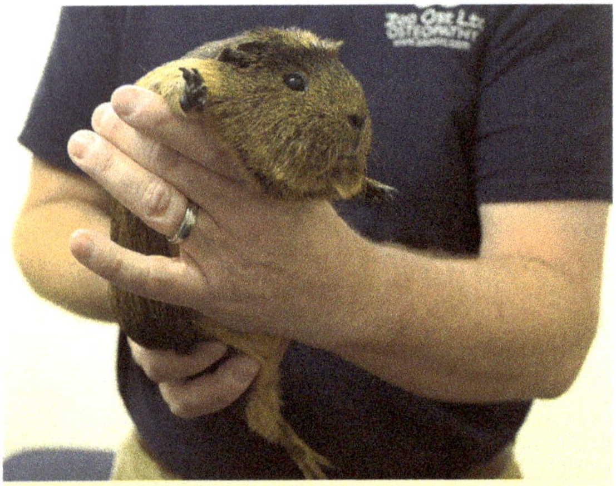

Figure 4.28
Fascial unwinding can be performed with a two-hand contact supporting the whole animal from cranial to caudal aspect. A gentle traction or compression is then applied to start the untwisting maneuver until an inherent fascial dysfunctional pattern is fully released. The technique is being demonstrated on a guinea pig here.

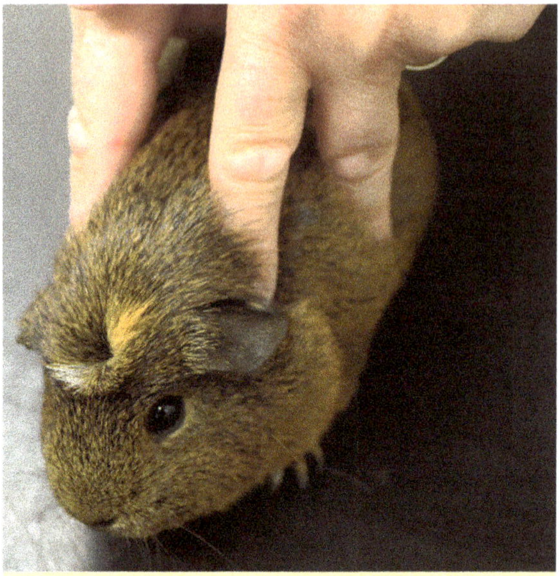

Figure 4.29
Pumping techniques can be gently applied to the thorax of hamsters and chinchillas through a double-hand contact on both sides of their chest. Then administer rhythmic pressure at variable speed and duration as dictated by the tissue response. The technique is being demonstrated on a guinea pig here.

using both hands in a lateral-lateral hold (Fig. 4.29). The author has found a good response when pumping is kept to a rate of one pump per second for about 30 seconds.

Facilitated positional release techniques are certainly among the most effective approaches for treating these small animals. As the tissues are brought toward ease, and a balanced tension point is achieved and maintained, a rapid overall relaxation is likely to occur in the animal as release is achieved.

Management

Husbandry considerations are often paramount for a successful treatment of small furries. Ensuring low lighting, quiet surroundings, small and warm bedding, a regularly cleaned cage, and distance from predator species are all ways to keep stress to a minimum and encourage a swift recovery. The housing should maximize insulation and allow ventilation. Clean, non-dusty materials, such as shredded paper, are the best form of bedding, since they retain heat and allow air to circulate, as well as being absorbent. This can help prevent rats and mice from developing upper and lower respiratory diseases. The recommended temperature range is between 18–22°C for mice, rats, gerbils and hamsters; between 10–15°C for chinchillas; and between 15–21°C for rabbits (Batchelor 1999). Most small furries are sensitive to extremes of temperature and can get stressed when it is over 27°C (over 21°C for chinchillas). High temperatures may also inhibit drinking in some species, which can hasten dehydration and be fatal. Fluid therapy is therefore essential in these cases.

A large hutch should usually be provided, since these animals need lots of space to run around and play, especially ferrets. Adequate furnishing, such as ramps and cloth tunnels, cardboard rolls, and exercise wheels should allow small furries to climb and explore the cage, as they are usually very active. Being prey animals, many small mammals are shy, so somewhere to hide should always be available. Nesting material (e.g., soft paper or soft wood) should also be provided for comfort, to help regulate temperature and light levels, and to provide somewhere to retreat and hide from cage mates or threatening stimuli. A gnawing block will also help them to wear their teeth down. Keep the cage indoors, out of direct sunlight and strong winds and away from busy or noisy areas (e.g., away from TV or music systems), as noises and vibration stress these animals. Small furries need constant access to fresh clean drinking water from a suitable water bottle with a metal spout or a bowl that needs to be clean at all times. Minimizing human-to-patient scent transfer can be achieved by wearing examination gloves when handling the animal or its bedding and hutch. Some mammals like guinea pigs, chinchillas, mice, and rats need to stay with others of their species to have a good quality of life, since they are very social animals and used to huddling together for warmth and reassurance. If left on their own, they are likely to get lonely and stressed. In contrast, the Syrian hamster is unique among pet rodents, as they need to be kept singly because the female will attack the male except when in estrus. Dwarf hamsters will often live happily in pairs. The female ferret, unlike other mammals, must be mated (or she will die from postestrus anemia) or she must have chemical suppression of estrus (Proháczik et al. 2010).

The amount of food needed depends on age, body weight, level of activity, reproductive status, health status, and the type of food given. Sudden changes in diet may lead to digestive disturbances. Therefore, any diet changes should be made gradually. Rabbit diets should be high in fiber, low in carbohydrate, and without added sugar. A low fiber, high starch diet may predispose rabbits to malocclusion and proliferation of intestinal pathogens. High fiber diets are also essential for coprophagia (consumption of cecal pellets), which is crucial for rabbit health (providing the necessary intake of protein, vitamin B, and potassium). A low fiber diet leads to hypomotility of the gut, with an increased cecal retention time and a consequent reduction in the formation of cecotropes (the pellets ingested in coprophagia) (O'Malley 2005a).

Like humans, guinea pigs cannot synthesize their own vitamin C because they lack the enzyme L-gulonolactone oxidase which synthesizes ascorbic acid. For this reason, about a teacupful of food such as leafy greens, peppers, tomatoes, spinach, asparagus, etc., which are all high in vitamin C, should be provided each day. This is vital to keep their teeth and digestive system healthy.

Food restriction, rather than ad libitum feeding, has been found to increase longevity (Turturro et al. 1999) and preserve neuronal activity (Lin et al. 2014) in aging rats. The latter can get obese if they eat too many calories and cannot exercise enough. Rats can be fed twice a day with pellets, but mice, gerbils, and hamsters need mixed seeds and nuts. In most species it is valuable for the diet to be augmented with small amounts of fresh fruit and vegetables. Hamsters are omnivorous and coprophagic.

Ferrets should have a high protein and fat but low carbohydrate and fiber diet, and should be fed no more than twice a day (Lewington 2003b). They are carnivores and cannot survive on a vegetarian diet.

Chinchillas need day and night access to good quality hay or grass. This is vital to keep their teeth and digestive system healthy.

Case study 4.1

European rabbit

Signalment

The patient was a 10-year-old female European rabbit.

History

The patient, named Polly, presented with a history of ovariectomy performed through a suprapubic laparoscopic access in November 2003. Eight years later, in December 2011, the owner found Polly temporarily unconscious on the floor. After having ruled out the most common metabolic and infective diseases, the veterinary surgeon formulated a diagnosis of diffuse degenerative osteoarticular disease on the basis of radiological findings (Fig. 4.30). The most significant osteoarthritic changes were found at the cervicothoracic junction, T9–T10 segments, L6–S1 levels, and left SI joint, and were associated with vertebral osteophytosis, subchondral bone sclerosis, and joint space narrowing.

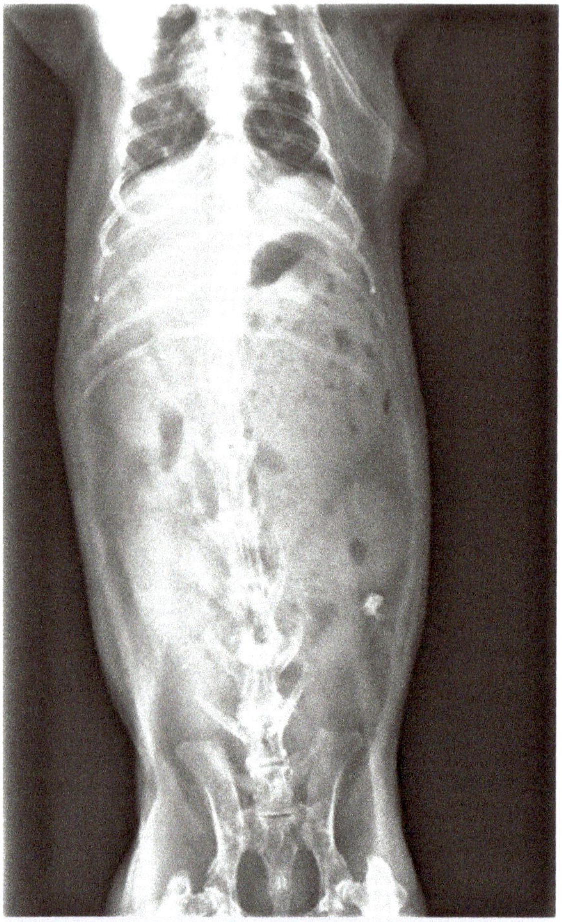

Figure 4.30
Dorsoventral radiological imaging. The X-ray investigation showed diffuse osteoarthritic changes associated with subchondral bone sclerosis and osteophytosis, particularly involving the vertebrae of the CT junction, and the middle thoracic and pelvic regions.

Diagnosis

The working hypothesis was a hyperalgesic state caused by an acute osteoarthritic presentation that induced the rabbit to pass out (faint).

Veterinary and physiotherapy treatments

As a result of the diagnosis, Polly underwent treatment with anti-inflammatory drugs (Metacam 0.2 mg per day for 7 days), physiologic solution (administered subcutaneously every 3 days), and dietary supplements (Ribes Pet® each day). This was followed by seven days of physiotherapy treatment consisting of laser therapy (15 sessions of 8 minutes at variable frequency), massotherapy, and joint mobilization. The aim was to reduce pain and inflammation, and to improve the general articular range of motion.

Osteopathic evaluation

At the first osteopathic assessment, the rabbit was awake, active, and apparently in good health. When standing, however, there was visible avoidance of weight-bearing on the left hind limb, and this worsened considerably during the propulsive phase of the gait. Close observation showed the left gluteal muscles were reduced in bulk, while palpation indicated that the surrounding soft tissues showed chronic fibrotic changes, thought to be associated with an internal rotational dysfunction of the corresponding hip. The owner reported that Polly used to urinate on her own back legs, probably because she was unable to shift her weight sufficiently posteriorly to pass urine normally.

Mobility testing of the spine revealed a significant dysfunction with increased muscle tone around C1 on the left side, while the left temporal bone was relatively "fixed" in internal rotation during cranial "listening" and the ipsilateral TMJ presented with compression and restriction of motion. Finally, the myofascial assessment indicated a strong fascial drag toward the suprapubic scar, together with a general restriction of sliding motion of the surrounding soft tissues, which is typical of postoperative adhesion formation. The bladder mobility was also found to be impaired during manual testing, with chronic changes to its fascial suspensory apparatus, particularly on the left side.

In terms of dysfunctional potency and severity of tissue changes, the pelvic pattern was thought to be primary, and the cranial changes were considered secondary.

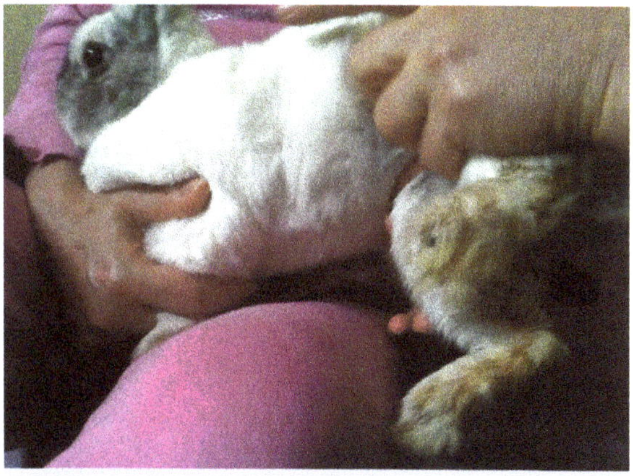

Figure 4.31
Myofascial release of the scar tissue. A direct myofascial release technique was applied to correct dysfunctional scar tissues above the pubis. One hand holds and stabilizes the rabbit from the dorsum, while the other hand gently takes a contact around the scar tissue, holding tension against any restrictive barrier until tension yields.

Osteopathic treatment

Polly underwent osteopathic treatment on a regular basis of one session per week for the first month, followed by one session every other week in the following month. The aim was first to restore function in the pelvis and hip joints, then to balance the cranial and cervical compensatory pattern. Techniques such as myofascial release were used to break down the fibrotic tissues in and around the scar above the pubis (Fig. 4.31). On more than one occasion the left hind limb was engaged as a lever to unwind the tension pattern in the pelvic fascial system. Finally a "lift" of the bladder was applied to normalize tension in the surrounding suspensory apparatus. (This is a technique that applies a gentle and progressive cranial traction of the bladder until a balance point is found and maintained, in all directions, before release is gained.) At the end of the maneuver the rabbit quite often urinated spontaneously, emptying the bladder following the release. Once mobility and functional symmetry was re-established in the pelvis, the osteopathic intervention addressed the cranial pattern, first by correcting the resting orientation to C1 with gentle articulatory techniques and cervical traction, then by approaching the left TMJ with functional inhibition of the surrounding soft tissues (Fig. 4.32). This culminated in releasing tension around the ipsilateral temporal bone, and balancing the craniosacral rhythm with cranial

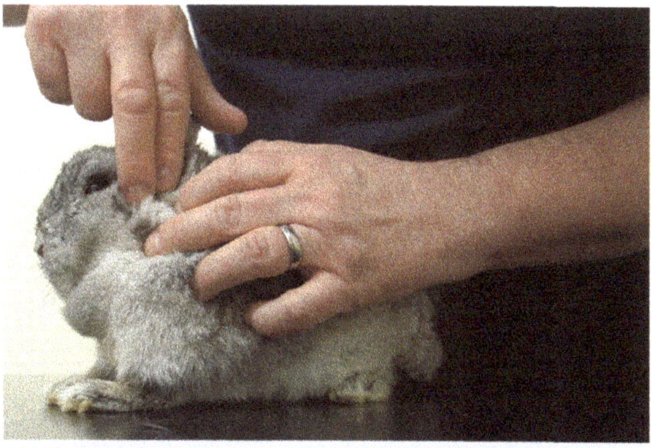

Figure 4.32
TMJ functional inhibition. This image demonstrates the technique that was used on the patient. The operator applies a gentle constant pressure perpendicular to the dysfunctional tissue layers surrounding the TMJ. The technique may be integrated with a functional or cranial treatment around the mandibular and temporal bones, which are maintained in a position of ease until release is felt.

techniques. Oscillation was commonly used to integrate most of the aforementioned techniques and also to induce a state of relaxation in the animal.

Follow-up

After four weeks of treatment, Polly showed an equal distribution through her hind limbs when standing and in motion. No limitations of movement were found in the hip and pelvic regions, although the scar tissue above the pubis was still maintaining a dysfunctional pattern. The left gluteal muscles were still showing reduced bulk, and the rabbit was still passing urine on her own hind limbs. Having discussed these findings with the veterinary surgeon, Polly was sent for a second course of physiotherapy, consisting of stretching and proprioceptive exercise, hip joint mobilization, and massotherapy. The owner was also advised to allow Polly to spend time each day in the backyard (rather than on the slippery house floor) to stimulate the use of the hind limbs.

Conclusion

At the end of the second and last month of osteopathic and physiotherapy treatment, the effects of the dysfunctional scar tissue were negated, as was the cranial compensatory pattern (left temporal/TMJ/C1 asymmetrical patterns). The gluteal muscles had regained their normal bulk, bringing weight-bearing back to normal when standing or moving. Polly continued to urinate on her own legs, however, although she never "fainted" again after the first episode.

References

Batchelor GR (1999) The laboratory rabbit. In: Poole T (ed.) UFAW Handbook on the Care and Management of Laboratory Animals, Volume 1. 7th edn. Oxford: Blackwell Science, pp. 395–409.

Bilkó A, Altbäcker V (2000) Regular handling early in the nursing period eliminates fear responses toward human beings in wild and domestic rabbits. Developmental Psychobiology. December; 36 (1) 78–87.

Bove GM, Chapelle SL (2012) Visceral mobilization can lyse and prevent peritoneal adhesions in a rat model. Journal of Bodywork and Movement Therapy. January; 16 (1) 76–82.

Brewer NR, Cruise LJ (1994) Physiology. In: Manning PJ, Ringler DH, Newcomer CE (eds.) The Biology of the Laboratory Rabbit. 2nd edn. London: Academic Press, pp. 63–70.

Chapelle SL, Bove GM (2013) Visceral massage reduces postoperative ileus in a rat model. Journal of Bodywork and Movement Therapy. January; 17 (1) 83–88.

Cheeke PR (1994) Nutrition and nutritional diseases. In: Manning PJ, Ringler DH, Newcomer CE (eds.) The Biology of the Laboratory Rabbit. 2nd edn. London: Academic Press, pp. 321–331.

Chen S (2010) Advanced diagnostic approaches and current medical management of insulinomas and adrenocortical disease in ferrets (Mustela putorius furo). Veterinary Clinics of North America: Exotic Animal Practice. September; 13 (3) 439–452.

Cruise JL, Nathan RB (1994) Anatomy. In: Manning PJ, Ringler DH, Newcomer CE (eds.) The Biology of the Laboratory Rabbit. 2nd edn. London: Academic Press, pp. 47–61.

Derrell Clark J (1987) Historical perspectives and taxonomy. In: Van Hoosier GL, McPherson CAW (eds.) Laboratory Hamsters. Orlando, FL: Academic Press, pp. 3–6.

Fallon MT (1996) Rats and mice. In: Laber-Laird K, Swindle MM, Flecknell P (eds.) Handbook of Rodent and Rabbit Medicine. Oxford: Pergamon, pp. 1–39.

Harkness JE, Wagner JE (1995a) The Biology and Medicine of Rabbits and Rodents. 4th edn. Baltimore: Williams & Wilkins, pp. 40–49.

Harkness JE, Wagner JE (1995b) The Biology and Medicine of Rabbits and Rodents. 4th edn. Baltimore: Williams & Wilkins, pp. 13–30.

Hodge LM, King HH, Williams AG Jr., Reder SJ, Belavadi T, Simecka JW, Stoll ST, Downey HF (2007) Abdominal lymphatic pump treatment increases leukocyte count and flux in thoracic duct lymph. Lymphatic Research and Biology. June; 5 (2) 127–133.

Hodge L, Harden L, Pedrueza M, Zhang X, Jones H, Minotti DE (2010) Lymphatic pump treatment increases leukocyte trafficking and inhibits tumor formation in the lungs of rats. Journal of the American Osteopathic Association. August; 110 (8) 478.B41

Hurst JL (1999) Introduction to rodents. In: Poole T (ed.) The UFAW Handbook on the Care and Management of Laboratory Animals, Volume 1. 7th edn. Oxford: Blackwell Science, pp. 262–274.

Komitowski D, Sass B, Laub W (1982) Rat mammary tumor classification: notes on comparative aspects. Journal of the National Cancer Institute. 68 (1) 147–156.

Lewington JH (2003a) Ferret Husbandry, Medicine and Surgery. Oxford: Butterworth-Heinemann, pp. 177–198.

Lewington JH (2003b) Ferret Husbandry, Medicine and Surgery. Oxford: Butterworth-Heinemann, pp. 54–74.

Lewington JH (2005). Ferrets. In: O'Malley B (ed.) Clinical Anatomy and Physiology of Exotic Species: Structure and Function of Mammals, Birds, Reptiles and Amphibians. London: Elsevier Saunders, pp. 226–250.

Lin AL, Coman D, Jiang L, Rothman DL, Hyder F (2014) Caloric restriction impedes age-related decline of mitochondrial function and neuronal activity. Journal of Cerebral Blood Flow & Metabolism. September; 34 (9) 1440–1443.

Lipman NS, Foltz C (1996). Hamsters. In: Laber-Laird K, Swindle MM, Flecknell P (eds.) Handbook of Rodent and Rabbit Medicine. Oxford: Pergamon, pp. 59–91.

O'Malley B (ed.) (2005a) Clinical Anatomy and Physiology of Exotic Species: Structure and Function of Mammals, Birds, Reptiles and Amphibians. London: Elsevier Saunders, pp. 164–86.

O'Malley B (ed.) (2005b) Clinical Anatomy and Physiology of Exotic Species: Structure and Function of Mammals, Birds, Reptiles and Amphibians. London: Elsevier Saunders, pp. 199–215.

Peng X, Griffith JW, Lang CM (1990) Cystitis, urolithiasis and cystic calculi in ageing guineapigs [sic]. Laboratory Animals. April; 24 (2) 159–163.

Pilny A (2014) Ovarian cystic disease in guinea pigs. Veterinary Clinics of North America: Exotic Animal Practice. 17 (1) 69–75.

Proháczik A, Kulcsár M, Trigg T, Driancourt MA, Huszenicza G (2010) Comparison of four treatments to suppress ovarian activity in ferrets (Mustela putorius furo). Vetrecord. January; 166 (3) 74–78.

Turturro A, Witt WW, Lewis S, Hass BS, Lipman RD, Hart RW (1999) Growth curves and survival characteristics of the animals used in the Biomarkers of Aging Program. The Journals of Gerontology. Series A, Biological Sciences and Medical Sciences. November; 54 (11) B492–501.

Watson PJ, Gröning F, Curtis N, Fitton LC, Herrel A, McCormack SW, Fagan MJ (2014) Masticatory biomechanics in the rabbit: a multi-body dynamics analysis. Journal of the Royal Society Interface. October;11 (99).

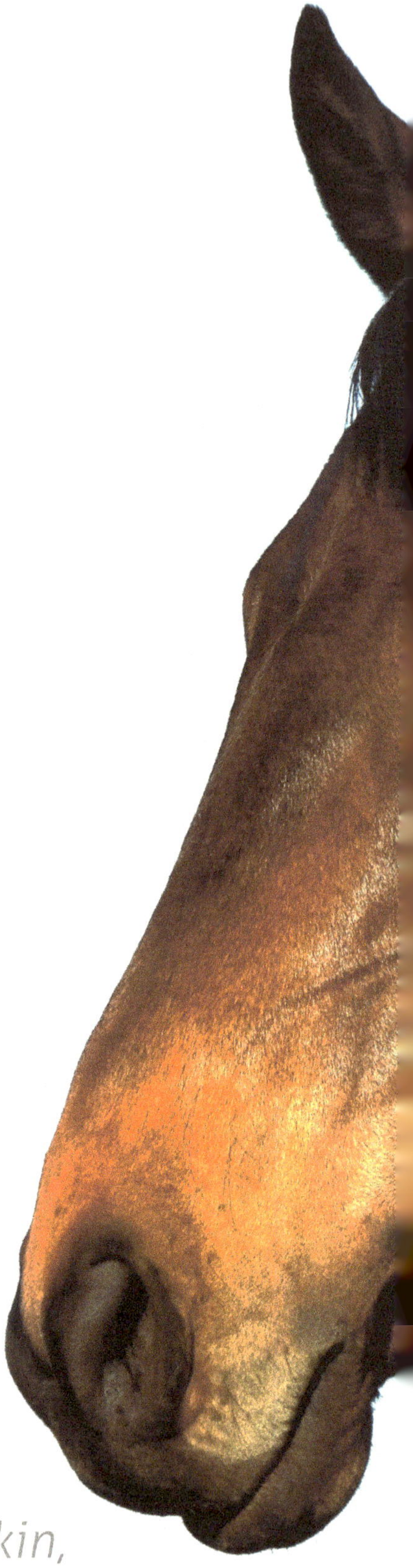

Chapter 5

THE HORSE

Chris Colles, Tony Nevin, Brendan Atkin,
Julia Brooks, David Gutteridge

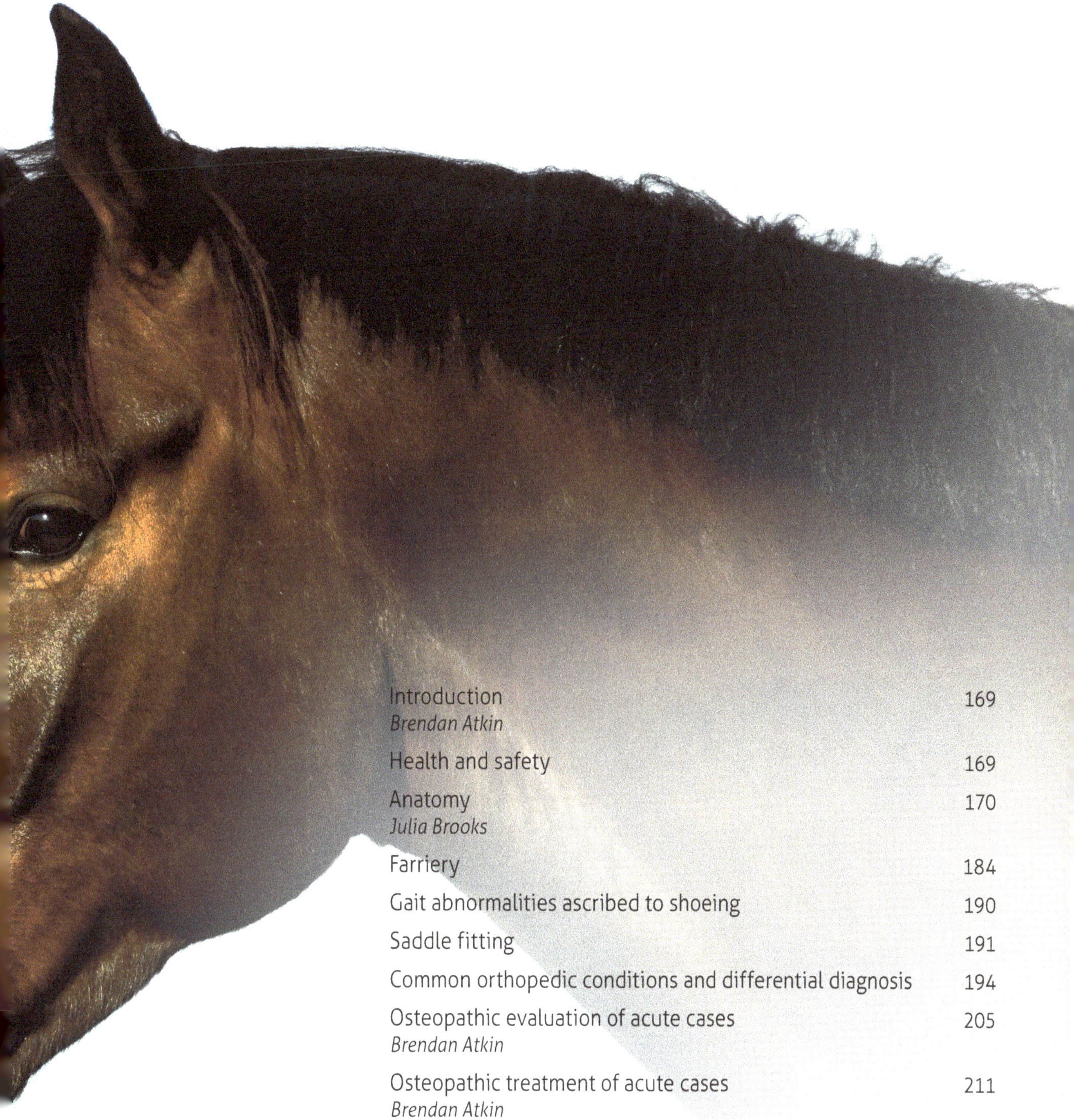

Introduction

The horse is unusual amongst our patients, as it is normally kept in order to be ridden or driven. It is its athletic ability that is its prime reason for domestication, and also probably its prime reason for injury. A number of surveys of disease have suggested that 60 percent of lameness is centered in the front foot or fetlock, and 60 percent of hind limb lameness is in the hock joint. There may currently be a tendency to underestimate the incidence and significance of back problems in the horse. This is partly because the horse is very good at compensating for back dysfunction and hiding obvious signs of pain. It is also very difficult to make an objective diagnosis of back pain using imaging or other investigative techniques, the diagnosis of many cases relying on subjective observation, which can be a difficult skill to acquire.

The horse is unique amongst animals, in routinely being shod. The practice of shoeing can in itself introduce lameness, but more importantly from the osteopathic practitioner's point of view it can cause changes in action and limb flight. A basic understanding of farriery and anatomy and function of the foot is necessary when treating horses, and for this reason the section under lameness in this chapter outlines basic principles of foot balance and how it affects limb function. Farriery is an extensive subject, however, and for a fuller understanding of shoeing, and how it can assist treatment of disease or correction of limb flight, the reader is referred to Colles and Ware (2010). Better still, spend some time with an accomplished farrier who is used to carrying out work in conjunction with veterinary surgeons. In many cases it will be found that treatment of back conditions is greatly aided by simultaneous attention to shoeing.

A further complication with horses is the presence of a rider and saddle. Once again saddlery is a complex subject, but a brief outline of how to check for problems has been included below.

When to refer

Recognizing one's limitations, and electing to refer a horse, is a sign of a good osteopath. Asking for an opinion from another professional should not be considered a failure of approach or diagnostic skills, but evidence of patient care. The practice of equine osteopathy can become dangerous when a practitioner works in total isolation and does not involve allied professionals in the overall care.

There are many triggers that initiate referrals. All cases resulting from pathological lesions should be presented to a veterinarian first (bear in mind that in the UK, and some other countries, initial diagnosis may only be made legally by a veterinary surgeon). Some cases with specific pathology may appear as musculoskeletal dysfunction and initially be presented to an osteopath. It is essential for the osteopath to recognize red flags and always refer cases that are not clear-cut. This can be a case where the history and findings from the examination do not appear to correlate, or where a horse with a complaint that you expect to improve with treatment does not do so. In such cases referral is often in the best interests of the horse.

Health and safety

The horse is a domesticated animal, but it should never be taken for granted. It is large and easily spooked. Its primary defense mechanism is to kick or bite first, and then run away, rather than assessing any suspected threat. Even well-handled and good-mannered horses can panic for the slightest reason, and because of their size and speed of reaction you can easily be injured. A horse moving about in a stable can easily stand on your foot or squeeze you against a wall - not always unintentionally! Remember even the smallest of Shetland ponies weighs more than you, reacts faster, and is far stronger. It is probably sensible to wear steel toe-capped footwear, and many people handling horses routinely wear hard hats for protection, not just when riding the horse.

Handling the horse is an art in itself. Quiet movement and confidence, coupled with lack of fear, will bluff a horse into behaving, but this is a skill that has to be learnt or acquired over time. Although some chronic cases will benefit from treatment under sedation, or even general anesthetic (GA), routinely osteopathic treatment is carried out on conscious horses.

The osteopath will normally rely on the owner to hold and manage the horse, but should be aware that not all owners have as much control over the patient as one might like. Routinely treatment will take place in a stable or loose box. The treatment area should be quiet and away from any other animals or places where sudden noise or movement may startle the patient. It is best if the patient is familiar with the environment in which it is treated. As with all animal treatment, be aware of your own position, and make sure that if the horse is suddenly startled you have a clear escape route and will not be trapped in a corner with no escape possible. The horse should be presented in a halter, and the owner should hold the animal throughout treatment. Be aware that owners are inclined to drop the rope and move away in order to get a better view of how treatment is progressing. Do not treat the horse if it is not being held at all times. A bridle may give the owner more control, but the extra leather work and the bit limit palpatory examination and treatment around the head area quite considerably. You may also want to consider why a bridle is necessary for the horse to be managed and whether or not you want to treat such an animal.

Treatment of chronic cases or difficult horses may be carried out under sedation. Correct sedatives do in fact have a beneficial chemical effect in aiding treatment and helping to make the horse more easily managed. Many injuries to personnel, however, have occurred with sedated patients. The sedated horse can be more aware of its surroundings than you anticipate, and a sudden adrenalin release may allow it to wake up and kick or bite. Do not relax your guard, and be aware a sedated horse does not give the usual warnings you expect from a fully conscious horse before it kicks you.

Anatomy

The review of comparative anatomy in Chapter 1 highlights the similarity in the basic structure of animals and humans (see Fig. 1.4). Where there is divergence, it usually reflects the way an animal stands and functions.

Horse anatomy has evolved for an herbivorous lifestyle, with running away as a defense mechanism. When this locomotor system fails, a detailed knowledge of structural anatomy is undoubtedly necessary when considering treatment. One should, however, resist the temptation to assume a particular structure or tissue is the sole source of a problem. As clinicians, we frequently have clinical cases where the diagnosis is inconclusive and a broader perspective is needed, incorporating alterations in neural control systems (see Chapter 1).

The horse has a quadrupedal stance with a center of gravity considered to be around the 13th rib. Approximately 60 percent of the horse's weight is taken through the forelimbs. The limbs are designed for a low-energy, long-lever system of flight. They are elongated so that the horse stands on its 3rd finger and toe, the distal limb movements being controlled by elongated tendons arising from the upper leg musculature.

The following anatomical descriptions use positional terms appropriate for quadrupedal stance and are included in Chapter 1 (see Fig. 1.5).

The head

The head is large and the nose elongated (Figs 5.1 and 5.2). It acts as a weighted bob to assist in forward movement. It can be divided into the cranium, which houses the brain, and the face, which provides a surface for dentition and the passage of air.

Surface anatomy

Starting at the high point of the head, the poll (the highest point) is formed by the nuchal crest of the occipital bone, a marked ridge to which the ligamentum nuchae is attached. From here, the interparietal crest runs in a sagittal line splitting to form the two external sagittal crests of the frontal bone, running toward the upper part of the orbit. On either side lie the temporal muscles, which insert on the coronoid processes of the mandible. From the side, the facial crest is a continuation of the zygomatic arch onto the maxilla and extends the line of attachment for the well-developed masseter muscle. From the front, the nasal bones run rostrally to form the nasal peak. Either side of the peak, the nasoincisive notch forms the bony opening of the nasal passages.

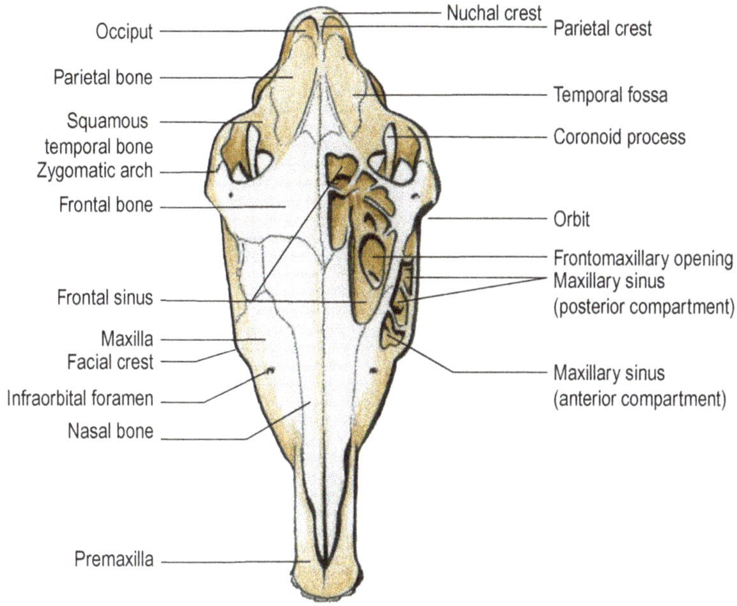

Figure 5.1
A dorsal view of the horse's skull showing the bones of the skull and the position of the sinuses.

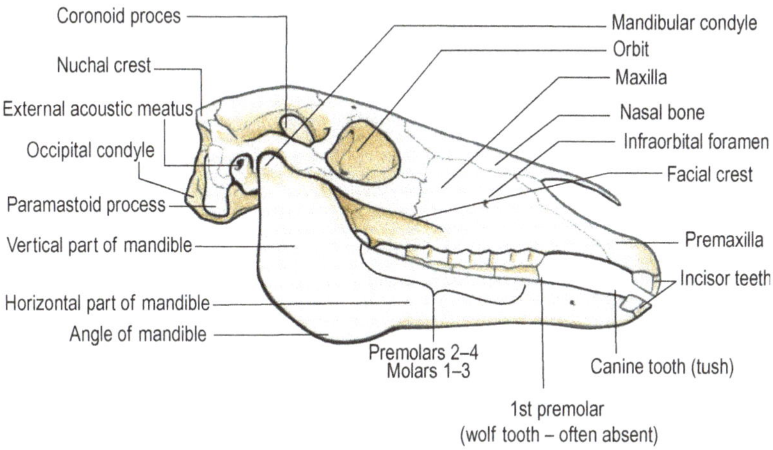

Figure 5.2
A lateral view of the horse's skull showing the bones of the skull.

The ramus of the mandible descends from the temporomandibular joint and turns sharply at the angle to run rostrally to form the body of the mandible. Rostral and medial to the angle lies a vascular notch which conducts the facial artery and nerve and the parotid duct. The pulse may be monitored at this point.

The cranium

The cranium, extending from the nuchal crest to the temporal fossa, is small compared to that of the human and contains only about 600g of brain tissue. The cavity is divided into a larger section housing the cerebrum, which is separated by the tentorium cerebelli from a smaller area containing the cerebellum. The bones of the vault are relatively thin. Rostrally, they are overlaid by the thin bones of the sinuses.

The eye has good all-round vision with 215 degrees largely monocular vision. There is a "blind spot" for approximately 1.2m immediately in front, caused by the expanse of the nose, which is a good reason to approach the horse from the side. Another limitation in equine vision is restricted scope for accommodation, which is compensated for by a nonuniform, craniocaudal flattening of the globe, which gives the eye a varifocal capacity. The upper part of the retina is further from the lens and gives near vision, whereas the bottom can focus on distant objects. The horse therefore needs to be able to move its neck to adjust head position for changing focus, particularly in activities such as jumping.

The eye has a protective third eyelid which moves across the cornea when the eyeball is depressed and the fat behind the eye is displaced. The same effect occurs in spasticity of the extraocular muscles which occurs in tetanus and is a diagnostic sign of this disease, especially if the nose is raised.

Caudally, the occiput has large occipital condyles. These articulate with depressions in the ring of the atlas. It is an area susceptible to compression injuries when falling, which can influence flexion and extension movements.

The auricular cartilages form the outline of the ears and extend down to attach around the external auditory meatus of the temporal bone. The cartilages are freely mobile to allow multidirectional hearing, their movements being controlled by numerous muscles radiating from the scutiform cartilage (a small quadrilateral plate in front of the auricular cartilage). Functional osteopathic techniques using the ears as "handles" work on the fascia and musculature of the skull and subocciput.

The face

The face is made up of the maxilla, premaxilla, nasal, lachrymal and zygomatic (malar) bones, turbinates, vomer, mandible, and hyoid. These form the elongated oral and nasal cavities and also contain a number of sinuses.

The sinuses have a functional role which is to lighten the large skull. They have a clinical significance in that they can become infected. The sphenoidal part of the sphenopalatine sinus is difficult to access and may be a site of continuing infection. Some of the inhibitory and cranial techniques may be used to assist with sinus drainage.

Horses are obligate nasal breathers. The nasal passage is divided by a septum and is roofed over by the nasal bones, which taper rostrally to form the nasal peak. The walls are formed by the maxillary bone and the floor by the hard and soft palates.

Below the nasal passages lies the oral cavity with the palates above and the geniohyoid and mylohyoid muscles slung under the mandible, forming the floor. The hard palate and its musculomembranous extension, the soft palate, run back to encircle the epiglottis and arytenoid cartilages, closing off the oral cavities during breathing.

The oral cavity contains the tongue, the multidirectional intrinsic and extrinsic fibers of which blend with the muscles running from the hyoid to the mandible to form the floor of the oral cavity. The hyoid itself is an important part of the framework of the larynx and airways, and the tongue may be used under general anesthetic as a handle for testing and treating fascia and musculature in the suprahyoid region. The intermandibular space also contains lymph nodes, swelling of which can indicate the presence of upper respiratory tract infection. The sides of the oral cavity are formed by the buccinator muscles. Rostrally are the highly innervated sensitive and mobile lips.

Equine dentition is an important subject. The state of the teeth may affect the horse's nutritional status and may also affect the function of the temporomandibular joint, which can compromise upper cervical function. Permanent teeth replace the deciduous teeth between the ages of two-and-a-half and five years.

On each side in the upper and lower jaw are:

- three incisors
- usually in the male a canine (or tush), which is often absent in the female
- four premolars, the first being absent or represented by a vestigial tooth (wolf tooth)
- three molars.

Rostral to the premolars is a gap known as the diastema where the bit sits. Wolf teeth, if present, may affect the comfort of the bit in the mouth, and so they are usually removed.

The mandible is narrower than the maxilla, so the grinding action of the molars may result in the formation of sharp edges on the inside of the lower teeth and outside edges of upper teeth. Hooks may also form at the front of the premolars or back edges of the molars, and so a six-monthly check-up for these problems is generally recommended.

The temporomandibular joint is formed from the transversely elongated mandibular condyle and the glenoid cavity of the temporal bone with an intervening fibrous disc. It allows movements around transverse and vertical axes as well as forward and backward glide. It facilitates grinding movements, and is controlled principally by the masseter and temporalis muscles. It is controlled by the trigeminal nerve, fibers of which supply the articular structures and the muscles of mastication. It has a central nucleus extending from the brain stem to the upper cervical cord where it merges with the dorsal horn of the upper cervical spine, and so compromise in one region will often influence function of the other.

The vertebral column

The vertebral column is relatively mobile in the cervical region, with relatively rigid thoracic and lumbar regions. The bony structure of the individual vertebrae reflects their function, with a substantial vertebral body through which propulsive forces from the limbs can be transmitted. There is a neural arch, through which the spinal cord runs, and dorsal and transverse spinal processes for the attachment of powerful ligaments and muscles. These basic structures are modified according to the requirements of each particular region. The column is made up of seven cervical and 18 thoracic vertebrae. There are six (or sometimes five) lumbar vertebrae, and the sacrum is formed of five fused vertebrae. There are approximately 18 coccygeal vertebrae (Fig. 5.3). Each vertebra is separated by a fibrocartilaginous intervertebral disc, which absorbs concussion and permits movement between the segments, but there is no nucleus pulposus.

Cervical spine

The cervical spine is one of the most mobile parts of the spine, and it has an important proprioceptive function in determining the position of the body in space.

Surface anatomy. Observable and palpable points are determined by the position of the vertebrae in the neck. The 1st to 3rd vertebrae are near the dorsal surface of the neck. The large wings of the atlas are easily identified caudal to the temporomandibular region. Between the angle of the jaw and the transverse process of the atlas, the largest of the salivary glands, the parotid,

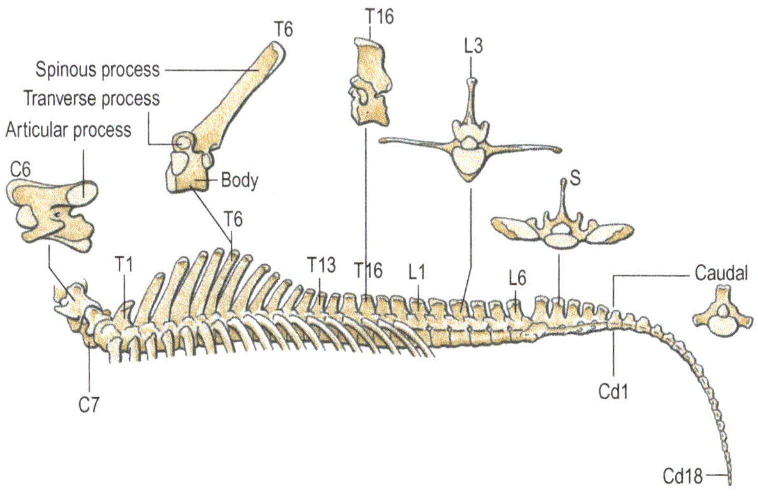

Figure 5.3
The horse's spine showing how the vertebrae change shape in different parts of the spine. Redrawn with permission from Pusey A, Brooks, J, Jenks A (2010) Osteopathy and the Treatment of Horses. Wiley-Blackwell. Figure 2.13, page 17. ©Anthony Pusey, Julia Brooks and Annabel Jenks.

can be palpated. From the upper cervical region to the withers, the dorsal outline of the neck is formed by the ligamentum nuchae. The caudal cervical vertebrae occupy a much more ventral position and the transverse processes are palpable above the jugular groove which runs between the brachiocephalic and sternocephalic muscles.

Anatomical components. The first two vertebrae are specialized, having a large vertebral canal to avoid damaging the spinal cord during movement of this highly mobile area.

The atlas is in the form of a ring and plays an important part in the positional requirements of the head. It has large transverse processes for muscle attachments supporting and participating in head movement. These muscles also provide proprioceptive information to the brain. The cranial surface of the atlas has deep cups to receive the large occipital condyles. They allow a considerable degree of flexion and extension, some lateral flexion, and a small degree of rotation (Fig. 5.4).

The axis has a strong odontoid peg which extends into the ring of the atlas, where it is held by strong ligaments. This articulation allows most of the rotational capability of the cervical spine. The axis also has a large dorsal process for the attachment of muscles and the ligamentum nuchae (Fig. 5.5).

The remaining five cervical vertebrae have low dorsal processes and plate-like transverse processes, giving attachment to the powerful cervical muscles.

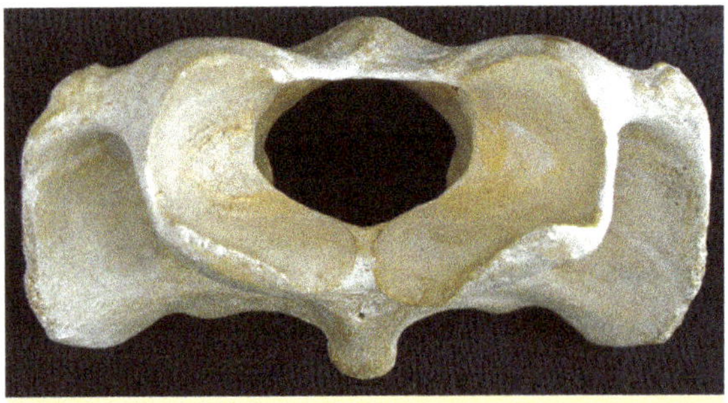

Figure 5.4
A view of the cranial aspect of the atlas showing the deep articular "cups" in which the occipital condyles sit.

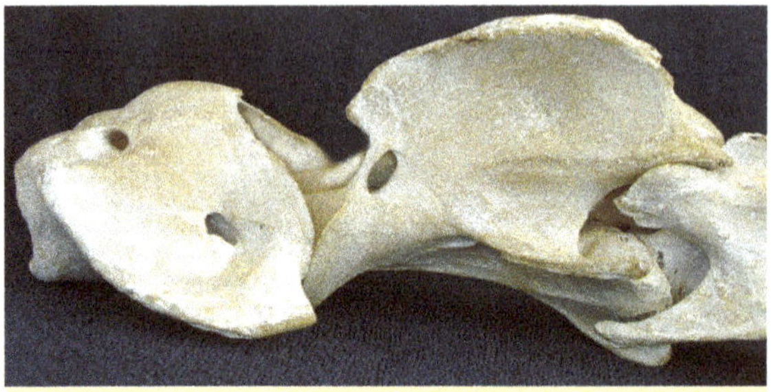

Figure 5.5
A lateral view of the upper neck showing the atlantoaxial articulation. Note the large dorsal process on the axis for the attachment of the ligamentum nuchae and neck musculature.

The transverse processes can be palpated in the muscle bulk above the jugular groove. The bodies have a rounded cranial surface and a concave caudal surface. The vertebral arches bear facets which facilitate flexion and extension movements.

The neck is supported and movement is aided by the huge elastic structure of the ligamentum nuchae. The strong funicular part gives the dorsal outline of the neck. It runs from the dorsal processes of the withers, across the spinous process of the axis, and attaches to the nuchal crest. From its under surface, there is an elastic lamellar part, which fans out to attach to the dorsal surfaces of the middle five cervical vertebrae.

Neck extension is initiated by contraction of the erector spinae and dorsal cervical muscles. Flexion is produced by the sternocephalicus muscles, which form the ventral border of the jugular groove. These also assist in lateral flexion, together with the scalenus, splenius, and brachiocephalicus muscles.

Thoracic spine

The thoracic spine is composed of 18 vertebrae positioned in a fairly straight line, with limited movement. There are paired ribs attached to the vertebrae.

Surface anatomy. The first few thoracic vertebrae lie deep between the scapulae and thorax, but the increasing height of the dorsal spinous processes means that the process of the 5th thoracic vertebra usually forms the highest point of the withers. The scapulae overlie the first seven thoracic vertebrae and the heads of the 3rd to 7th ribs. The varying inclination of the spinous processes makes determining the position of individual thoracic vertebrae difficult, but the last rib can be followed dorsally to locate the position of T18. The saddle usually sits with its front edge in the region of T12–T13.

Anatomical components. The typical thoracic vertebra has a short body bearing facets for the rib heads, short transverse processes with facets for the tubercle of the rib, and articular processes for intervertebral movement. The height of the dorsal spinous processes increase from the first thoracic (T1) spinous process, reaching a maximum height of around 10 to 15 cm at the 4th and 5th thoracic vertebrae (T4 and T5) at which point they begin to reduce in size (Fig. 5.6). They slope caudally until approximately T16 which is vertically orientated and termed the anticlinal vertebra, beyond which they slope cranially. The interspinous spaces are narrowest in the low thoracic region, where the proximity of the tops of the spinous processes can be involved in overriding or kissing spines.

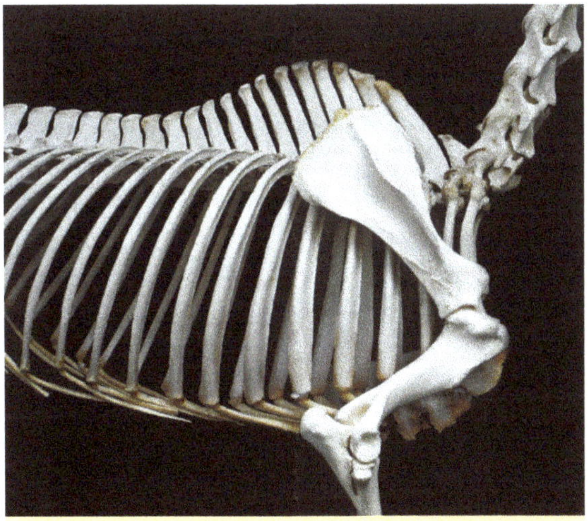

Figure 5.6
Lateral view of the skeleton of the horse (lower neck and thorax) showing the position of the cervical vertebrae and the variation in height of the dorsal spinous processes of the thoracic vertebrae.

Part of the limitation in thoracic movement is due to the ribs, the first eight pairs of which articulate with the sternum through their costal cartilages. The remainder are asternal ribs and their cartilages connect to form the costal arch. The 18th rib is "floating," and projects into the abdominal wall. The first rib, although the smallest, bears the imprint of the brachial plexus. If it is damaged, the nerves supplying the forelimb may also be involved. Radial nerve paralysis affects the extensors of the forelimb, with a characteristic presentation of a dropped elbow, carpal flexion, and inability to bring the distal limb forward. Occasionally the 1st rib is missing, and this may also be associated with lameness.

Lumbar spine

There are usually six lumbar vertebrae, although some animals may have an extra thoracic vertebra and five lumbar vertebrae. The vertebral bodies are longer than in the thorax, and the dorsal spinous processes slope forward, reducing in height till they are negligible at the sacrum. The transverse processes, projecting laterally, may be 7–10 cm in length and 2 cm wide. The transverse processes of the 5th lumbar vertebrae articulate with the 4th lumbar processes cranially and the wing of the sacrum caudally. These joints, together with the radially orientated facet joints, limit movement in all ranges. At the lumbosacral joint, the orientation of the facet joints and the widely spaced spinous processes allow a considerable degree of flexion and extension, although lateral flexion is limited.

Sacrum

The sacrum is a roughly triangular mass of bones, formed from five fused vertebrae. Occasionally the 1st coccygeal vertebra is also involved. The sacroiliac joint is a diarthrodial joint, but it is surrounded by fibrous ligaments which severely limit any movement.

Tail

There are approximately 18 coccygeal vertebrae forming the tail. They start to lose articular processes and central canals after the first three vertebrae, becoming short rods with cartilage connections toward the tail end.

Back muscles

The muscles of the thoracolumbar region can be divided into the epaxial muscles, dorsal to the transverse processes, and the hypaxial muscles, ventral to the transverse processes (Fig. 5.7).

There are two types of epaxial muscles:

- The cybernetic epaxial muscles: interspinales, intertransversales, and multifidus. These run between vertebral segments, are tonically active, and have an important role in proprioception.
- The hypaxial muscles: psoas and quadratus lumborum, and the abdominal muscles.

The psoas major (originating from the lumbar vertebrae) and iliacus (originating from the ilium) combine to form a common insertion onto the lesser trochanter of the femur. They act to flex and externally rotate the hind limb and together with the quadratus lumborum (running from the last ribs and lumbar vertebrae to the sacrum) they assist in stabilization of the lumbar spine.

The abdominal muscles, consisting of rectus abdominis, internal and external abdominals and transversus, form the ventral surface of the trunk. They act to flex the thoracolumbar spine and if working unilaterally, slightly laterally flex and rotate the spine. They support the considerable weight of the viscera and, by compressing the abdominal contents, assist in expiration, parturition, urination, and defecation.

There is a complex interaction of the musculoskeletal components of the trunk, which can be explained by the "bow and string" theory. At walk there is a degree of spinal movement in all ranges, but at higher speeds, a stiff core is an advantage. The core or "bow" is formed by the thoracolumbar vertebrae compacted by the epaxial muscles. The ventral "string" of the hypaxial muscles acts to flex the bow, countered by the weight of the viscera (suspended from the spine) which tend to straighten the bow. This interaction combines to form a stiff column on which the limbs can act to propel the body forward.

The limbs

To the student of human anatomy the limbs may appear unfamiliar. Most of the individual components, however, are present in man (Fig. 5.8). They differ primarily in proportion and form a long lever which is an energy-efficient system for covering the ground at speed.

The proximal limbs, with their power-generating muscles, are short, thick, and compact. Distally, the bones are longer, and with the weight of the horse borne on the equivalent of the human third finger or toe a number of structures have been lost. The muscles here are replaced by tendons. There are also a number of support and locking mechanisms to help keep the limbs straight. This enables the horse to remain standing with low energy cost.

Another source of confusion is man-made. The structures generally have a commonly used name as well as an anatomical name. The commonly used name differs depending on the vintage and nationality of the textbook, veterinary surgeon, or horseman consulted.

Complete descriptions of the musculoskeletal structures are beyond the remit of this text, but there

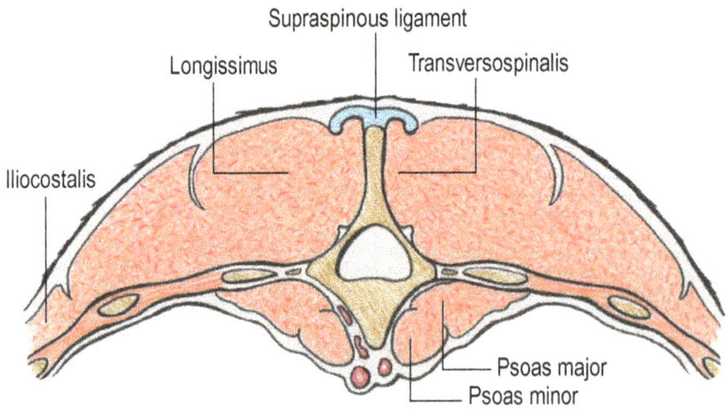

Figure 5.7
A transverse section of the thoracic spine showing the position of the spinal musculature. Redrawn with permission from Pusey A, Brooks, J, Jenks A (2010) Osteopathy and the Treatment of Horses. Wiley-Blackwell. Figure 2.15, page 19. ©Anthony Pusey, Julia Brooks and Annabel Jenks.

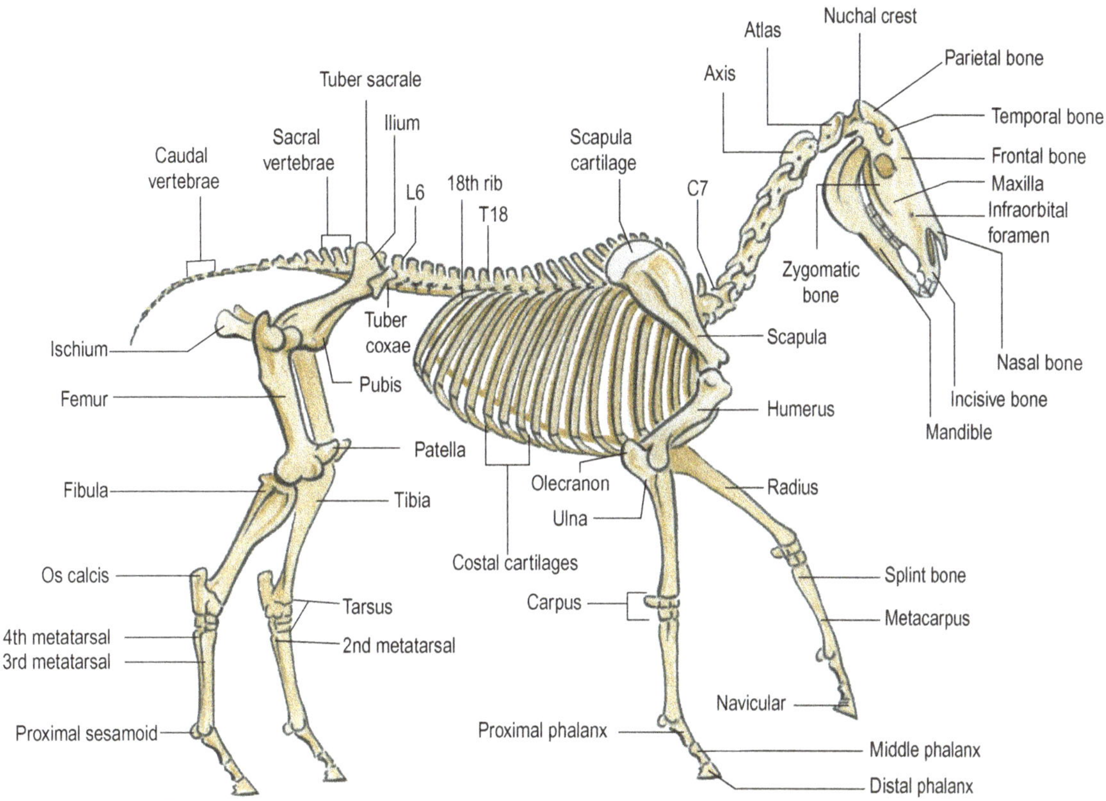

Figure 5.8
The equine skeleton.

are several anatomy textbooks devoted to the subject. An outline of the most salient features follows.

Thoracic girdle and proximal forelimb

The thoracic girdle and forelegs have no bony connection with the thorax. They form a musculoskeletal sling supporting the thorax and 60 percent of the body weight. The proximal forelimb is composed of the humerus articulating with scapula above and the radius and ulna below. The ulna is shortened and fuses with the top of the radius, excluding the possibility of limb rotation. The radius continues distally to the carpal joint (termed the knee).

Digital extensor muscles originate from the lateral epicondyle of the humerus and run down the cranial or dorsal surface of the limb, whereas the flexors lie on the caudal or palmar surface.

Thoracic girdle. The thoracic girdle is composed of the scapulae and their muscular attachments to the limbs and thorax. There are no clavicles, in common with many quadrupeds. The scapula is triangular, with a large cartilage attached proximally. Together they cover the first six or seven ribs, sloping caudally and dorsally from the shoulder joint to facilitate limb movement and shock absorption. The scapula forms a large expanse for the attachment of serratus ventralis, rhomboideus and trapezius muscles which hold it to the thorax (Fig. 5.9). This allows the body to rotate between the forelimbs during the flexion and extension range of limb movement. Contraction of the supporting muscles also lifts the thorax between the limbs, which moves the center of gravity caudally. The scapulae also rotate and slide over the thorax to aid limb movement. Their outer surface is divided by a scapular spine. This separates the infraspinatus and supraspinatus

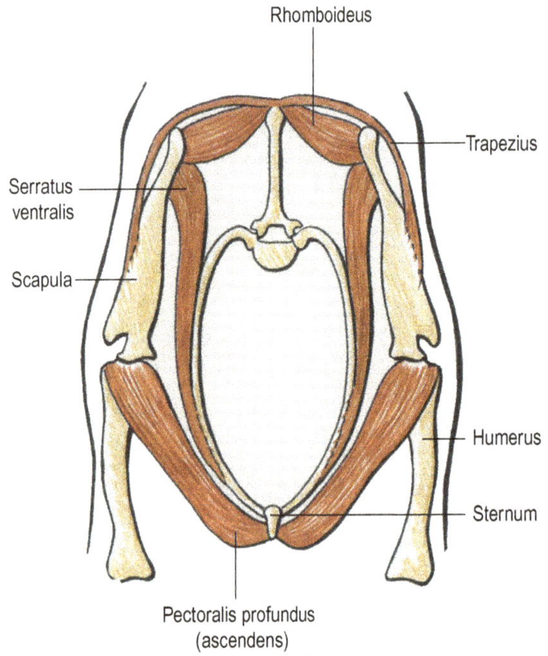

Figure 5.9
A transverse section through the thoracic region of the horse showing how the body of the horse is slung by muscles from the scapulae which allows it to rotate between the forelimbs during movement. Redrawn with permission from Pusey A, Brooks, J, Jenks A (2010) *Osteopathy and the Treatment of Horses* Wiley-Blackwell. Figure 2.23, page 24. ©Anthony Pusey, Julia Brooks and Annabel Jenks.

muscles which insert on the tubercles of the humerus. These muscles are supplied by the suprascapular nerve which runs anteriorly round the neck of the scapula, where it may be injured causing partial paralysis of the muscles - a condition referred to as "sweeny."

Surface anatomy. Viewed anteriorly, the trachea lies centrally and is covered by the sternothyroid muscle. On either side of the sternum bulge the pectoral muscles. The jugular grooves, under which lie the external jugular veins, appear on either side between the prominent bands of the brachiocephalic and sternocephalic muscles.

Viewed from the side, the scapula slopes at an angle of about 45-60 degrees to the horizontal and the scapular spine is marked by a shallow indentation between the masses of the supraspinatus and infraspinatus muscles.

Proximal forelimb. The humerus is a short, thick bone, with a number of tubercles for insertion of muscles (Fig. 5.10). The proximal head is hemispherical and suggests the possibility of a wide range of movement. In practice, however, movement is virtually limited to flexion and extension. The humerus lies at an angle of about 50 degrees to the horizontal, running down and back to the elbow which lies close to the thorax at the level of the 5th rib.

The triceps muscle is relatively bulky and acts to extend the elbow when flexing the shoulder. The cranial surface of the humerus is occupied by the main flexors of the elbow, the biceps, which also extends the shoulder, and the brachioradialis. The biceps may also participate in a stabilizing mechanism by virtue of a fibrous extension, known as the lacertus fibrosus, which blends with the extensor carpi radialis and helps to maintain carpal extension (part of the stay apparatus).

The humerus forms an angle of about 145 degrees with the ulna and radius to form the elbow joint. Unusually for joints in the limb, its resting position is midway between flexion and extension, held by its collateral ligaments and the antagonistic action of flexors and extensors. The radius drops vertically to the carpus. The carpal bones are arranged in two rows, the proximal row being composed of three weight-bearing bones: the radial carpal, intermediate carpal, and ulnar carpal. Projecting from the palmar surface is the equivalent of the human pisiform, termed the accessory carpal. The distal row consists of the 2nd, 3rd, and 4th carpal bones. Occasionally, residual 1st and 5th carpal bones may be present, but these have no weight-bearing function. Most flexion occurs at the radiocarpal joint and to a lesser extent the intercarpal joint, with very little occurring at

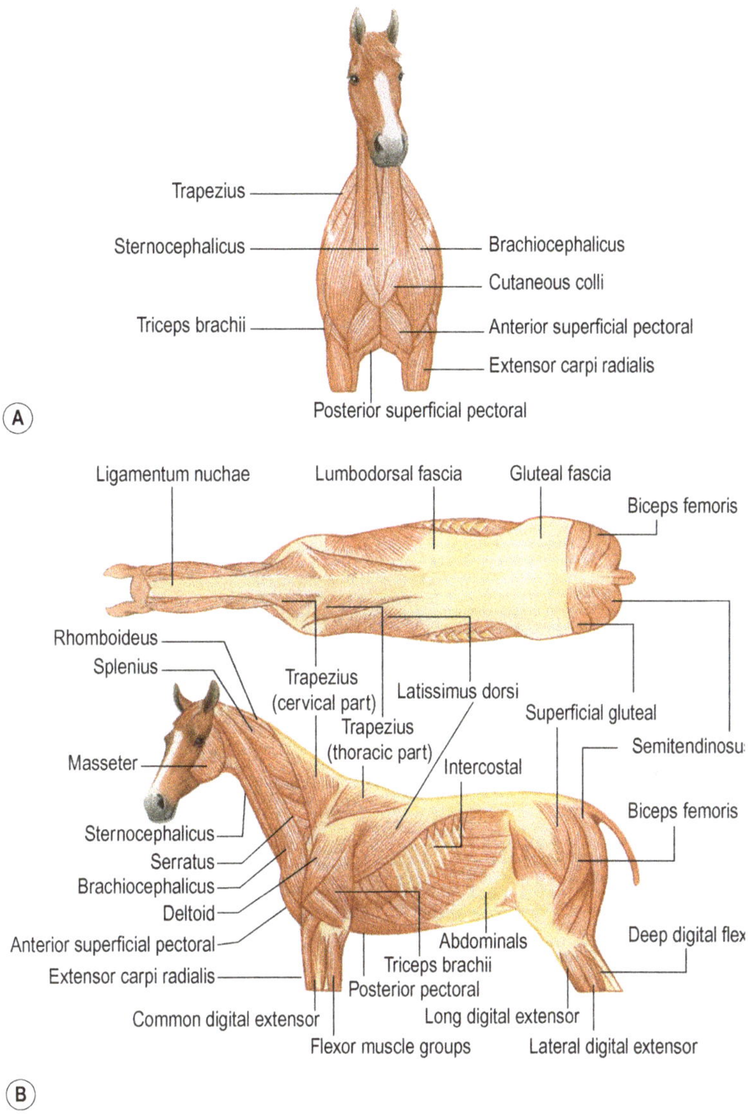

Figure 5.10
The principal muscles of the horse. (A) Anterior view. (B) Superficial layer of muscles. From Colles C, Ware R (2010) *The Principles of Farriery*. JA Allen. ISBN: 978 0 85131 973 5. Reproduced with kind permission from Crowood Press.

the carpometacarpal joint. Extension is limited by strong ligaments at the back of the joint. One of these, the volar carpal ligament, continues down to blend with the deep flexor tendon to form the subcarpal or inferior check ligament (part of the stay apparatus).

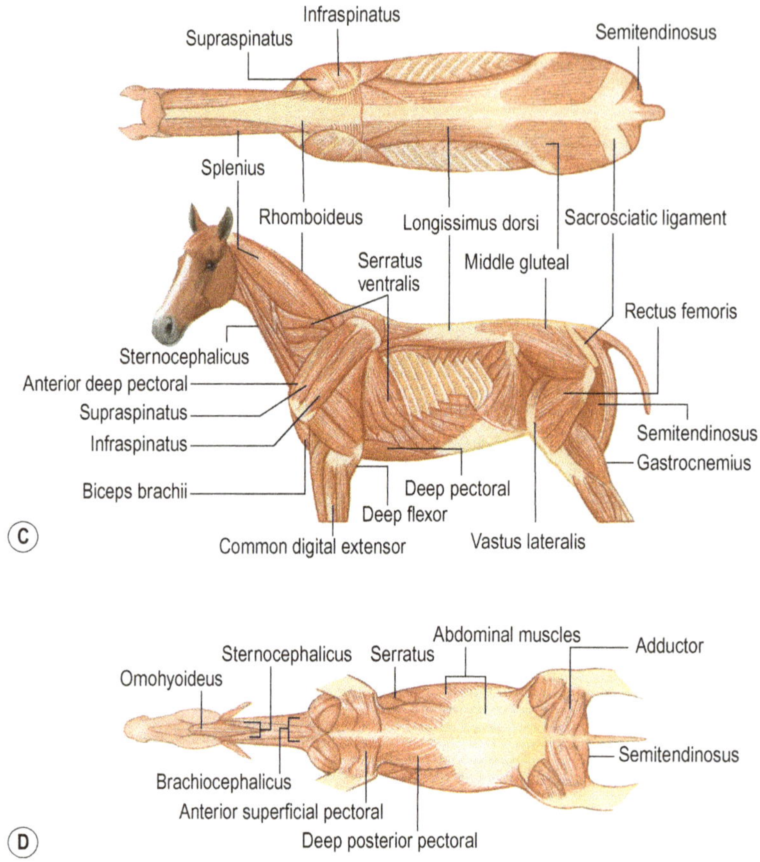

Figure 5.10—*Cont'd*
The principal muscles of the horse. (C) Deeper layer of muscles. (D) Ventral muscles. From Colles C, Ware R (2010) *The Principles of Farriery*. JA Allen. ISBN: 978 0 85131 973 5. Reproduced with kind permission from Crowood Press.

Surface anatomy. Palpable points on the humerus are the point of the shoulder (the cranial part of the greater tubercle) and the deltoid tuberosity on the lateral surface of the humerus (Fig. 5.11).

At the elbow, the olecranon process is obvious as the most posterior part of the elbow region.

Distally the medial and lateral styloid processes of the radius are palpable, and projecting caudally the accessory carpal bone can be identified.

Pelvis and proximal hind limb

The hind limbs are firmly attached to the vertebral column via the pelvic girdle. This allows the hind legs to generate most of the power for forward propulsion (85 percent). For this, flexion and extension of the hind limb joints are the principal requirement, and this is reflected in the structure of the joints.

The main components of the limb are similar to the human leg. The stifle joint, composed of the patella, femur, and tibia is the equivalent of the human knee, but there are three distal patella ligaments, and the fibula is reduced to a remnant fused to the proximal tibia. The area of leg below the stifle is often referred to as the gaskin, the tibia running as far as the hock joint, where the caudally protruding calcaneus, equivalent to the human heel, is an obvious visual landmark.

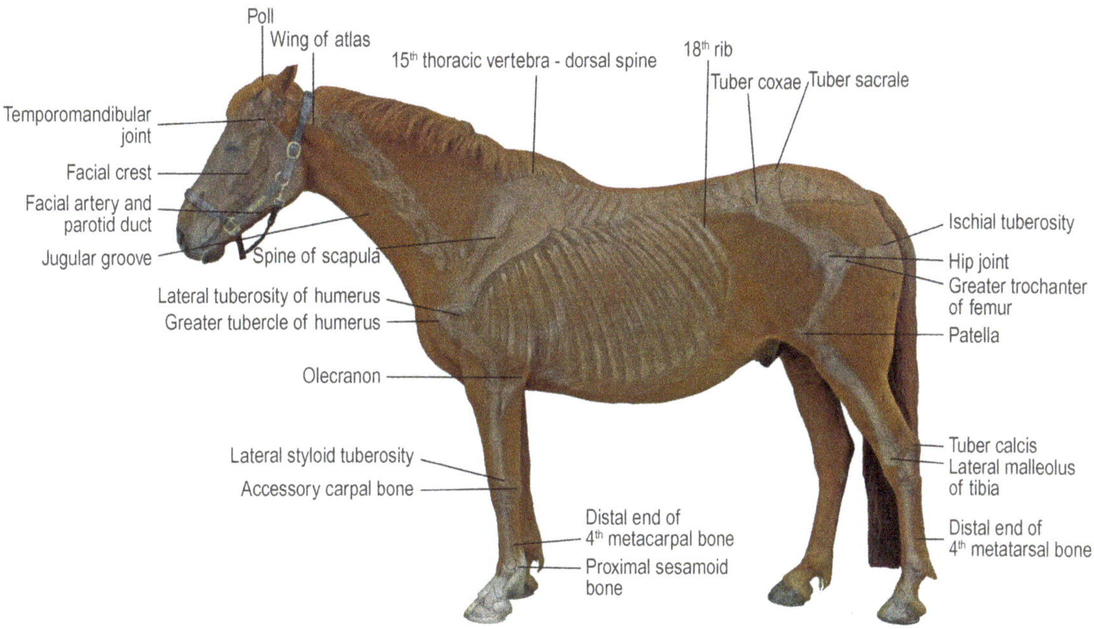

Figure 5.11
The surface anatomy of the horse pinpointing some of the significant anatomical landmarks.

The pelvis is formed from the fusion of the ilium, ischium, and pubic bones. They are joined to the sacrum by strong fibrous bands across the irregular articular surface of the sacroiliac joint. The three pelvic bones fuse to form the deep cup of the acetabulum. This receives the head of the short, thick femur to form the hip joint. Although this is a ball and socket joint, the accessory ligament attached to the head of the femur alongside the teres ligament limits abduction and rotation. Flexion is also limited by the position of the femur close to the body, and the hind feet rarely reach further forward than the umbilicus.

Much of the femoral shaft provides an area for muscle insertion (Fig. 5.10). Cranial, medial, and lateral surfaces are areas for insertions of the quadriceps muscle. The caudal surface has an attachment for the biceps femoris near the third trochanter, and the adductors extend distally. The iliopsoas inserts onto the lesser trochanter.

Distally the femur meets the tibia at the stifle joint at an angle of about 140 degrees. This articulation has femorotibial and femoropatellar components.

The femorotibial joint is formed by the condyles of the femur and the condylar surface of the tibia. The articular surfaces are made congruent by the crescentic fibrocartilage of the menisci. They are attached to the tibial plateau at each meniscal horn and also to the intercondylar fossa of the femur by a meniscal ligament. This articulation is stabilized by lateral and medial collateral ligaments and, within the joint, by the crossed cruciate ligaments which also prevent full extension of the joint.

The femoropatellar joint is formed from femur and patella. The patella rarely dislocates medially or laterally (except in miniature ponies), but can normally move proximally to fix the medial patella ligament over the medial trochlear ridge of the femur. This prevents the stifle flexing, forming an important part of the stay apparatus. This also affects the "reciprocal apparatus"; the opposing actions of the peroneus tertius and the superficial digital flexor muscle (which in the horse is largely fibrous) mean that the hock and stifle joints have to flex or extend together. By locking the stifle, effectively the hock is also fixed. The muscular control of the locking action of the patella is complex, and if disrupted upward fixation of the patella can occur, the hind limb being locked in extension. This condition, while most common in unfit young ponies, may occur at any age and in any breed.

The upper end of the tibia provides one site of origin for muscles of the hock and phalanges. From the lateral condylar area and the posterior surface of the tibia and fibula arises the deep digital flexor muscle. Laterally lie the lateral digital extensor and the anterior tibial muscles. The fibula may be totally vestigial or may be a thin bone tapering to a point at the lower third of the tibia. Distally, the tibia articulates with the talus (tibiotarsal bone) and, together with the calcaneus and other tarsal bones, forms the tarsus or hock which corresponds to the human ankle. The hock joint is held at the midpoint of its range with an angle of about 150 degrees in front. The largest bone is the calcaneus, the equivalent of the human heel, to which the hock extensors, including the gastrocnemius are inserted. The superficial flexor tendon runs over the point of the hock (the tuber calcis), to insert on the proximal and middle phalanges. The formation of a subcutaneous bursa here is referred to as a capped hock.

Below the talus and calcaneus lie the small tarsal bones, which contribute minimally to any movement.

Surface anatomy. Parts of the pelvis are readily palpable. The most dorsal of these prominences are the tubera sacrales which form the croup and are situated either side of the sacrum. Laterally the tubera coxae are very prominent. The tubera ischii project caudally to form the most caudal point of the buttocks and are palpable either side of the top of the tail. Approximately midway between the tuber coxae and tuber ischii, marking the position of the hip, the greater trochanter of the femur may be palpated deep within the musculature, and distal to it is the third trochanter. Both form points of insertion for the gluteal muscles which give the quarters their rounded outline (Fig. 5.11). Below the trochanters, the femur runs downward and slightly forward (about 70 degrees to horizontal) to end in the epicondyles of the stifle joint which lie in the musculocutaneous fold of tissue near the trunk.

The patella is easily palpated, as are the medial, middle, and lateral distal patella ligaments which attach to the prominent tibial crest. The muscle mass overlying the cranial surface of the tibia is the long digital extensor, and caudally lies the gastrocnemius which becomes tendinous distally, combining with the soleus to form the Achilles tendon. Together with the hock extensors and digital flexors, they form the prominent common calcaneal tendon descending to the point of the hock - the tuber calcis.

Distal limbs

Distal limb structures in both forelegs and hind legs are very similar, although the hooves are rounder and broader in the forefoot.

The basic structure consists of the 3rd metacarpal bone in the forelimb and 3rd metatarsal in the hind limb (known as the cannon bones), below which is a column of three phalanges. Residual 2nd and 4th metacarpal and metatarsal bones are situated medial and lateral to the cannon bones (known as splint bones). These are weight-bearing bones proximally, although they taper out at the lower third of the cannon bone. Held in place by interosseous ligaments at birth, these smaller bones frequently fuse to the cannon bones later in life. There are no muscle bodies below the carpus and tarsus.

Metacarpals and metatarsals. The cannon bones articulate distally with the first phalanx (long pastern) at the fetlock joint. This joint only has flexion and extension ranges of movement but is subjected to great stress. Overextension is prevented by the suspensory ligament (originating from the distal carpus or tarsus and the proximal cannon bone and inserting on the proximal sesamoid bones) and the distal sesamoidean ligaments, which insert on the proximal and middle phalanges.

In addition to their role of supporting the fetlock, the proximal sesamoid bones hold the superficial and deep flexor tendons away from the center of joint rotation, thus conferring a mechanical advantage during muscular activity. The fetlock and pastern joints are given further support by the superficial flexor tendons, the deep flexor supporting the coffin joint.

In the forelimb, extension of the deep digital flexor tendon is limited by a thick fibrous check ligament that runs from the palmar ligament behind the carpus to fuse with the tendon, level with the upper third of the cannon. A similar ligamentous structure restricts the extension of the superficial tendon, originating medially on the distal radius and fusing with the tendon above the carpal joint.

In the hind limb, a check ligament may be present on the deep flexor tendon, but is often absent (always absent in mules). There is no check ligament on the superficial flexor tendon, which attaches to the tuber calcis as it passes over its plantar surface.

Phalanges and interphalangeal joints. Below the fetlock, the phalanges slope down to the hoof. Together with the ligamentous and tendinous support structures, they absorb a considerable amount of stress during weight-bearing and movement (Fig. 5.12). The proximal phalanx (long pastern) articulates distally with the middle phalanx (short pastern) at the proximal interphalangeal or pastern joint. This is the least mobile of the phalangeal joints.

The middle phalanx is a short solid bone, approximately half of it being within the hoof. Together with the navicular bone on its distal plantar or palmar surface it forms the distal interphalangeal or coffin joint. Overextension of this joint is controlled by the deep digital flexor tendon. The navicular bone may be referred to as the distal sesamoid, and its palmar or plantar surface is separated from the overlying deep digital flexor tendon by a bursa.

The remnants of horny pads present in animals whose carpi and tarsi are in closer contact with the ground can be located as the chestnuts on the medial aspect of the carpal or tarsal area and the ergots located at the back of the fetlocks. These represent the metacarpal or metatarsal pads.

Surface anatomy. The distal limbs, with their tendinous structures and a well-developed ligamentous apparatus, are easy to palpate. At the knee, the lateral and medial styloid processes of the radius, and the small metacarpals below the carpals, can be identified. Behind the knee lies the accessory carpal bone (pisiform). In the hind limb, both the lateral and the medial malleolus of the tibia are palpable, as are the small metatarsals bones. Behind the hock the tuber calcis is visible. In both the forelimb and hind limb, the distal ends of the splint bones can be felt as rounded buttons about three-quarters of the way down the cannon bones on the palmar or plantar medial and lateral sides.

In front of the cannon runs the common digital extensor tendon, which inserts on the three phalanges. On the palmar and plantar surfaces of the limbs

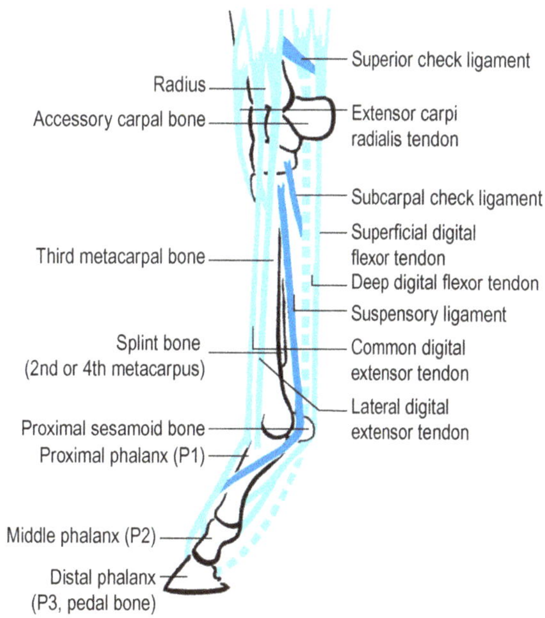

Figure 5.12
The distal forelimb of the horse showing the principal ligaments and tendons.

the deep and superficial flexor tendons are palpable, with the check ligament present level with top third of the cannon bone deep to the deep digital flexor tendon. Deep to these lies the suspensory ligament. This inserts onto the abaxial surface of the proximal sesamoids, which lie on the palmar and plantar surfaces of the metacarpophalangeal and metatarsophalangeal joints.

Feet

The anatomy and function of the foot are described below in the section on farriery.

Farriery

Anatomy of the hoof

Hoof wall

The hoof wall grows exclusively from the coronary band, growing down over the sensitive laminae, forming the major weight-bearing structure of the foot (Fig. 5.13). The wall is made up of horny tubules bound together by intertubular horn. This gives the hoof wall considerable strength against compressive forces acting down the length of the wall, but it is relatively weak if forces are orientated in a manner which bends or separates the tubules, or if shear forces are applied. At the heels of the foot, the wall is reflected forward to form the bars, which are also weight-bearing structures in the normal horse (Fig. 5.14). The bars also have a primary function in preventing the heels collapsing forward and inward. When standing the horse's weight is carried by the hoof wall, not through the sole of the foot. Increased loading of a section of the hoof wall will frequently result in a reduced rate of horn growth in that section. It will also in time cause the coronary band to be distorted proximally.

Sensitive and insensitive laminae

The parietal surface of the pedal bone (i.e., the "vertical" wall parallel to the hoof wall) is not covered by periosteum, but instead is covered by a layer of highly vascular dermal tissue. The outer edge of this layer is organized into leaves of dermal tissue formed at right angles to the surface of the pedal bone and running the entire height of the hoof wall. These are the sensitive or dermal laminae. The dermal laminae interleave with the insensitive or epidermal laminae formed in the horn of the hoof wall (Fig. 5.13). The laminae are thought to be responsible for attaching the pedal bone to the hoof wall and transferring the weight of the horse from the pedal bone to the hoof wall. Details of how this weight transfer occurs, and how the hoof wall can slide down over the laminae as it grows, are currently not fully understood. The laminae are present inside the entire hoof wall and bars. The posterior third of the foot is supported by the hoof cartilages rather than the pedal bone itself.

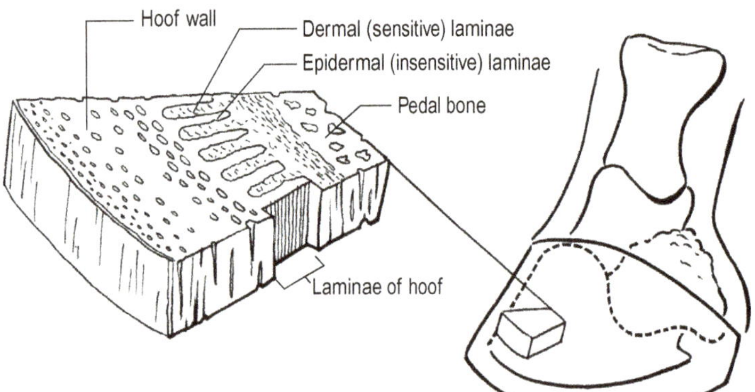

Figure 5.13
Diagram of the lower limb showing the sensitive laminae "suspending" the distal phalanx from the hoof wall.

Sole

The horny sole forms from a corium lying parallel to and just distal to the palmar surface of the pedal bone. The sole is also formed of tubular and intertubular horn, but has a softer consistency than the wall. The sole is slightly concave and in a normal foot the horn exfoliates as small flakes across the whole sole, when the sole flexes with movements of the hoof. At the outer margins of the sole the horn fuses with that of the wall forming the "white line" (or white zone). The sole of the foot is not normally a weight-bearing structure except on soft ground.

Frog

The frog is probably the most discussed and least understood part of the foot. It forms a rubbery wedge of tissue in the posterior part of the sole of the foot (Fig. 5.14). It is currently thought that its primary function is to allow expansion of the heels and allow flexion of the foot to occur during weight-bearing. In the past it has been suggested that it acts as a nonslip pad, a cushion against concussion, a pump to aid circulation, and a mechanism to expand the heels. All these functions are unproven.

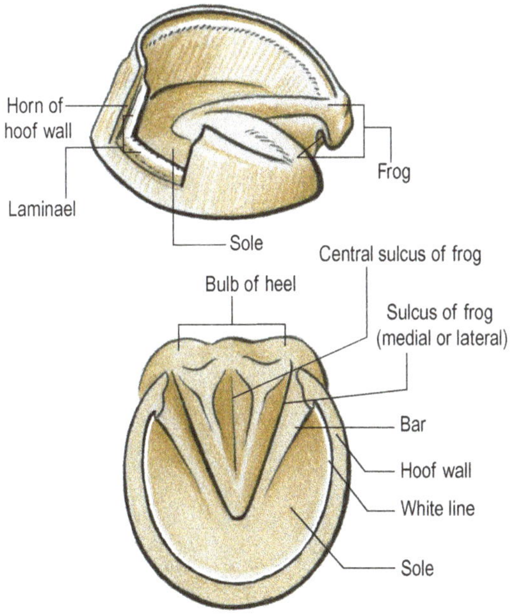

Figure 5.14
The hoof showing structures making up the horny wall, sole, and frog. From Colles C, Ware R (2010) *The Principles of Farriery*. JA Allen. ISBN: 978 0 85131 973 5. With kind permission from Crowood Press.

Movements of the hoof capsule

The weight of the horse is carried down the limb to the pedal bone, which is suspended inside the hoof wall by the laminae. Weight is not normally transmitted through the sole. During weight-bearing, the downward force on the pedal bone tends to cause the ground surface of the hoof wall to spread, because the hoof wall makes an angle with the ground (the hoof is not dissimilar in shape to a truncated cone) (Fig. 5.15). In the anterior two-thirds of the foot the spreading is restricted by the attachment of the hoof to the rigid pedal bone. In the posterior third of the foot, the wall has no such bone support, and the flexible hoof cartilages, bars, and bulbs of the heel allow the heels of the foot to spread further. As the heels spread more than the toe, the pedal bone rotates downward slightly at the heels, pulling the coronary band back at the dorsal aspect and allowing it to spread slightly at the quarters (sides) of the foot. As the horse travels forward, it passes over the foot, and as the pastern becomes more upright it will pull the coronary band forward at the toe of the foot. The hoof at the coronary band will become narrower at the quarters, and as the horse's weight moves forward the center of the load on the foot moves forward toward the toe. The heels of the pedal bone will start to lift, and the hoof wall at the heel starts to contract, even before the foot lifts from the ground.

As the foot takes weight, the pedal bone moves down inside the hoof capsule (a matter of 1-1.5 mm at the walk). This movement coupled with the movement of the elastic hoof wall helps to absorb concussion. The movements also put pressure on the underlying blood vessels, forcing the blood through the veins. This assists absorption of concussion, acting as a hydraulic damping system and also helps to pump blood away from the foot. In cases where the walls cease to flex normally, there is often significant interference with absorption

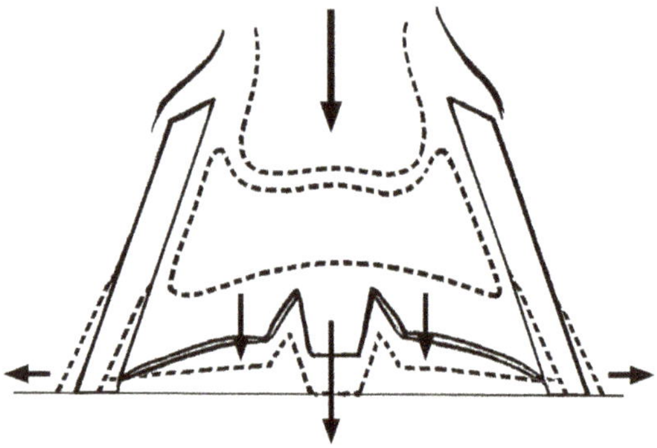

Figure 5.15
A transverse section through the horse's foot showing how weight-bearing pushes down on the hoof wall causing the wall to expand distally. This aids shock absorption and also plays a part in pumping blood through the foot.

of concussive forces and blood flow. This can affect stride length and possibly also cause lameness.

There is experimental evidence to show that horn strength is the same around the hoof wall and that this is not affected by color. Pigmented horn, however, is rather more resistant to abrasion than white horn (Leach 1980).

Horn hardness and flexibility is related to moisture content. In cool, humid climates, such as the UK and Ireland, feet tend to wear more readily and collapse more easily than in continental Europe. Normally the hoof wall has a moisture content of approximately 28 percent. This is higher in the sole and higher still in the frog.

Moisture content is highest in the deeper layers of horn, and the foot constantly loses moisture through the hoof wall.

Foot shape

The left foot and right foot of a pair should normally be the same size and shape. The front feet are rather more circular than the hind feet, the shape being dictated by the shape of the pedal bones (Fig. 5.16).

Three factors may result in uneven feet:

1. The horse may be born with odd feet. If so, attempts to correct this discrepancy (using corrective farriery) should be made while the animal is still a foal. The pedal bone ossifies from a single center. It is fully ossified at 18 months of age, and no further alterations to the bone can be made after this time.
2. Injury or disease may result in uneven weight-bearing and wear, or uneven growth, and cause changes in the size and shape of the hoof wall.
3. Careless or incorrect trimming or shoeing will give an uneven appearance. The normal hoof shape is shown in Figure 5.17. All corrective shoeing should attempt to bring feet back to this shape.

Shoeing

It is not necessary for all horses and ponies to be shod. Shoeing is carried out for three reasons:

1. *To prevent excessive wear.* Because many horses are ridden on hard or abrasive surfaces, the hoof wall will often wear quicker than it can grow. The resultant shortening of the hoof can result in pressure on sensitive tissues and can cause lameness. The fashion for barefoot trimming, i.e., working

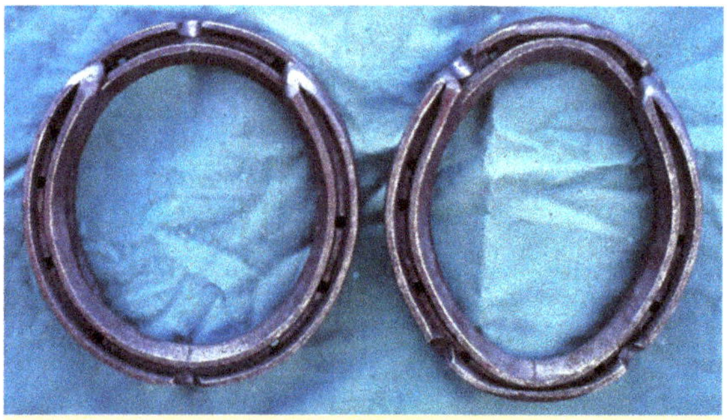

Figure 5.16
Left and right shoes superimposed on their contralateral pair to show the correct foot shape. This shape results from the shape of the pedal bones which control the direction the downward growth of the hoof wall.

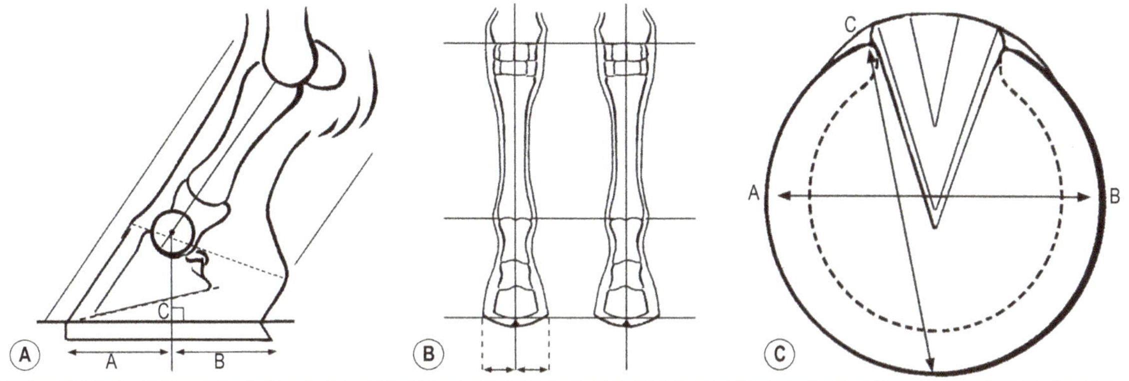

Figure 5.17
The guidelines for foot balance with the horse standing with all cannon bones vertical. (A) When viewed from the side the hoof pastern axis should be straight, and the horn of the heel should be approximately the same angle as that at the toe. The palmar aspect of the pedal bone should slope down by about 5 degrees to the toe, and the center of the distal interphalangeal joint should be over the center of the shoe. (B) When viewed from in front a line dropped vertically down from the shoulder should bisect the cannon, pastern, and hoof. The center of the coffin joint should be over the middle of the shoe. (C) The foot should inscribe a smooth elliptical shape. In the front foot, the widest point should be the same distance as from the middle of the toe to the back of the bearing surface of the heel. The hind foot, and front foot in some breeds of horse, is narrower across the widest point.

horses unshod, is acceptable if the foot can grow faster than it wears. It does, however, limit the use of most horses in moist climates where the feet become rather soft due to higher moisture content of the horn. In dry climates shoeing may not be so important. In the case of many ponies it is not necessary for them to be shod, or shoes may only be needed on the front feet.

2. *To spread the load and protect the foot on hard, uneven ground.* The shoe does give physical protection against uneven loading of the hoof wall, with the rigid shoe spreading a point load to include the adjacent areas of wall (as will arise if the foot is placed on a protruding stone). In some very uneven stony areas of desert, horses are sometimes shod with a complete plate of steel across the foot to protect the sole from damage by protruding stones.

3. *To correct hoof shape or limb angulation and support distorted feet.* The shoe effectively becomes an extension of the hoof wall. By placing it wide of the wall in certain areas, it can be used to help correct the hoof shape where it has become distorted. In young horses corrective shoeing can also aid in straightening limbs before the growth plates of the distal ends of the metacarpus and metatarsus or radius and tibia have closed. In older animals the shoe can be used to give support if needed to areas of distorted or injured hoof.

Hoof trimming (foot balance)

This is arguably the most important aspect of shoeing. The application of the shoe prevents normal wear of the hoof wall, and it is essential that the farrier trims the foot correctly to mimic normal wear. Failure in correct trimming and badly fitted shoes can result in changes in foot shape and function and alterations in limb flight and foot placement.

When assessing movement of a horse, it is important to differentiate between alterations in limb flight caused by musculoskeletal abnormalities and changes caused by poor farriery. Of course, in many cases they may be interrelated as abnormal limb placement from somatic dysfunction over a period of time frequently causes abnormal hoof shape. This may then interfere with attempts to correct the dysfunction by preventing normal limb movement returning.

The shoe

Types of shoe used vary around the world, based partly on the use to which a horse is put, but also to a large degree on local fashion. Certain basic principles, however, should always be present:

a. The width of the branch of the shoe should normally be twice the width of the wall and white line of the foot at the widest point in order to carry the weight of the horse. In heavy- or weak-footed horses this width may need to be increased, seating out the shoe to prevent excessive pressure on the sole. (Seating out means beveling the upper surface of the inner side of the shoe in order to reduce pressure applied to the sole of the foot.)

b. It is convention in many types of horse to place one clip at the toe of the front foot and one either side of the toe in the hind foot. Clips reduce the stress on nails as the shoe strikes forward into the ground. In hunter shoeing the horn at the toe of the hind foot marginally overlaps the front of the shoe to reduce the severity of injury if the horse over-reaches. Clips are not essential, and their positioning may be varied in certain conditions.

c. The shoes should be placed centrally under the bony column of the limb. In a normal limb and foot the shoe will fit exactly around the peripheral edge of the hoof. In an abnormal limb the shoe may be placed wide or tight on the foot in order that the ground surface is symmetrically under the cannon bone. This placement will encourage horn growth to alter direction, growing to fit the shoe that is nailed to it. If the shoe is correctly fitted, it will encourage the foot to break over at the center of the shoe and the limb to swing forward straight. If the shoe is placed to one side or other of the load-bearing line, then it will tend to cause the foot to break over to the opposite side of the midline, and the limb will swing medially or laterally after lifting from the ground.

d. The branches of the shoe should extend back under the heels until at least level with the posterior aspect of the lateral and medial sulci of the frog. In horses with collapsed or slopping heels, the shoe may be extended further back, to the point where the heels should be.

e. The shoe should inscribe a smooth curved outline with no sharp corners. The radius of curvature is smaller at the toe than at the branches but if two shoes are superimposed facing in reversed directions, the branches of the shoes should overlap exactly, to form a smooth ellipse (Fig. 5.16).

f. In young horses, extending a shoe laterally or medially will help support the limb and correct a limb deviation. The distal limb will grow toward the extension (but the medial-lateral balance must be correct).

The types of shoe and materials used in their manufacture are beyond the remit of this book. The reader may come across cases where horses are shod using pads (a layer of material across the sole between the sole and shoe) and/or wedges (a wedge-shaped insert between the wall and shoe intended to raise the heels of the foot). Other than advising that the reason for their use should be determined, further discussion of this cannot be entered into here, but the reader should be aware both systems are usually associated with attempts to cure sore feet and may indicate reasons for changes in gait.

Assessment of foot balance

Assessment of foot balance is an essential part of any lameness examination. Poor balance can cause lameness in extreme cases. It may predispose to joint effusions and can affect limb flight and foot placement.

Dorsopalmar or dorsoplantar balance

Ensure the horse is stood square, i.e., taking weight evenly on all four feet with the front and hind feet placed side by side and the metacarpal and metatarsal bones vertical. If the feet are then viewed from the side, there should be a straight hoof pastern axis (i.e., the slope of the pastern should be the same angle as the slope of the dorsal hoof wall (Fig. 5.17). The horn of the heels should make virtually the same angle with the ground as the horn of the dorsal hoof wall. If the foot is X-rayed, then the palmar surface of the distal phalanx should slope down toward the ground at the toe making an angle of about 5 degrees, and the center of curvature of the distal interphalangeal joint should be vertically above the middle of the ground surface of the foot (or shoe) (see Fig. 5.17).

Mediolateral balance

Forefeet. Mediolateral balance of the forefeet cannot be assessed with the horse weight-bearing on the limb, as collateral ligaments will stretch to accommodate imbalances. Stand beside the horse's shoulder facing the horse's tail and, with the hand closest to the horse, lift the foreleg, place your arm medial to the horse's radius, and support the limb under the metacarpus, holding the metacarpus roughly parallel with the ground and letting the phalanges hang free. It is then possible to look down on the back of the metacarpus and assess if the ground surface of the foot is at right angles to the long axis of the limb. The use of a simple T square may aid this assessment (Fig. 5.18A and B). Be aware that the coronary band may be distorted and cannot be used to assess balance. Also, the eye may be

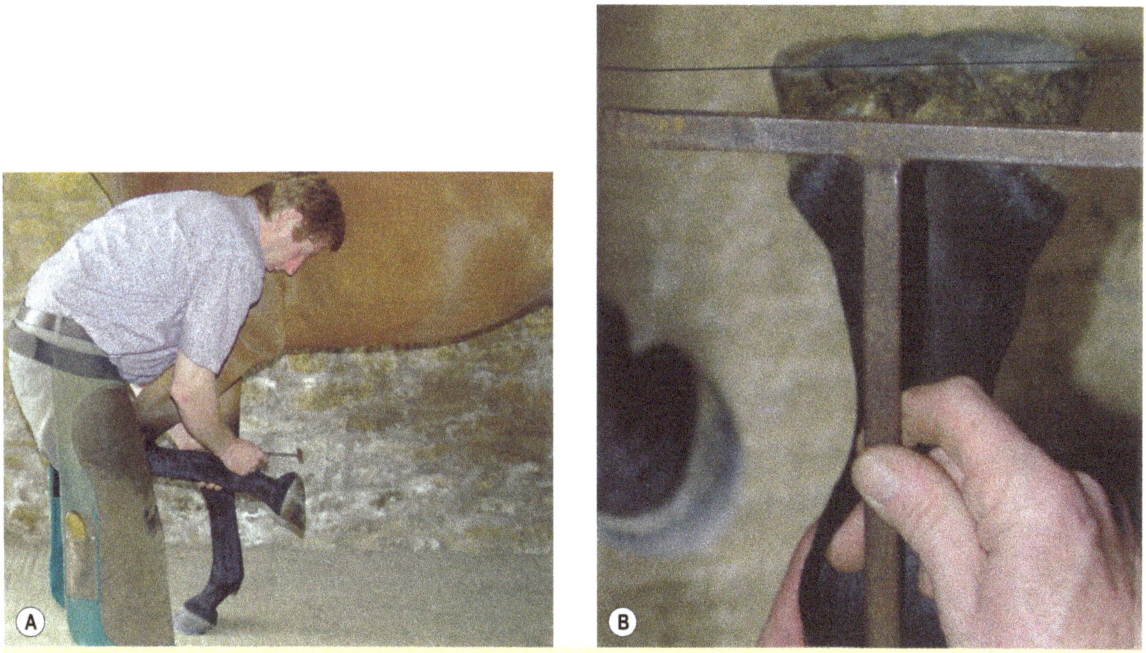

Figure 5.18

(A) A farrier assessing lateromedial balance of the foot. The cannon bone is supported with the farrier's arm medial to the bone, and the phalanges are allowed to hang naturally. (B) The long arm of a T square is positioned lying over the midline of the cannon bone, and the bone's distal end is over the central frog cleft. The ground surface of the foot should be in line with the top of the square if balanced correctly. From Colles C, Ware R (2010) *The Principles of Farriery*. JA Allen. Reproduced with kind permission from Crowood Press.

deceived by the differences in angles of the medial and lateral hoof walls.

Hind feet. The hind feet can only be assessed with the horse weight-bearing, as when the limb is flexed there is rotation of the limb at the stifle and hock joints and often also in the fetlock and/or pastern joints.

With the horse stood square as described above, stand behind the limb being assessed. Hind limbs will normally be slightly rotated with the toe outward, so stand behind the limb rather than the horse. Assess the metatarsus. Ensure it is vertical and that a line bisecting it will run down and also bisect the ground surface of the foot. If there is more ground surface to one side of this line than the other then the balance is incorrect. It is important also to assess the hind limbs from in front of the limb as sometimes imbalances are more obvious from this angle.

Palmar balance

When looking at the ground surface of the foot, it should be symmetrical around the frog. The wall of the foot, or shoe, should inscribe a smooth curved outline, with no sharp corners (Figs 5.16 and 5.17). The radius of curvature is smaller at the toe than at the branches. If two shoes are superimposed facing in reversed directions, the branches of the shoes should overlap exactly (Fig. 5.16) to form a smooth ellipse.

In the front foot, in the majority of horses the widest distance across the sole of the foot should be approximately the same distance as from the middle of the toe to either heel at the ground surface. There are some horses that have a slightly longer and narrower foot, but in no cases should the foot be wider than long. The hind foot of course is longer and narrower than the front, but again should be symmetrical around the frog and should have smoothly formed curves to the wall, with no flares or marked bends in at the heels.

Gait abnormalities ascribed to shoeing

Commonly used terms

- *Interference.* A nonspecific term to indicate any limb is striking any other limb between the coronary band and the knee during locomotion. There are a number of surgical shoes designed for use on horses which interfere. Most of the shoes are designed to minimize the resultant trauma rather than improve the gait to prevent interference. Correct foot balance and fitting of the shoe is more important than fancy ironwork and can usually prevent interference occurring.
- *Brushing.* An injury caused by striking one limb with the contralateral limb, usually about the fetlock level (or below). Although there may be other causes, the commonest is the medial side of the foot being overshortened. In this situation, at the beginning of the weight-bearing phase of the stride, the foot is placed wide of a vertical line dropped from the shoulder joint. At the end of the weight-bearing phase of the stride, the limb will swing inward (like a pendulum suspended from the shoulder joint), and may strike (brush) the other limb as it passes, before being swung out again so that the foot is again placed wide of the vertical. Treatment is preferably by correcting foot balance.
- *Speedy cutting.* This term is commonly used to denote an injury to the knee region, but definitions vary. In the UK it is used to denote an injury by the contralateral forelimb. Speedy cutting occurs at speed and is often assumed to be a conformational defect. There are surgical shoes available for horses that speedy cut. Once again check foot balance before employing fancy shoes!
- In the USA this term is also used to describe an injury to the knee region, principally in trotters, but in this case it may be caused by the outside of a hind foot cutting the inside of the front leg on the same side. Check foot balance in the front and hind legs.
- *Forging or clacking.* A gait anomaly occurring at the trot. The toe of the hind foot hits the sole of the front foot on the same side. It may strike the inside of the toe of the shoe or may hit the outside branch of the shoe. It is irritating to the listener, and may pull off shoes. It is corrected by shoeing to hasten breakover of the front foot and delay breakover behind. (Breakover is speeded up by shortening the toe and lengthening the heels.) Again surgical shoes have

been devised, but are of less value than correct fitting of the shoes.

- *Over-reaching.* The toe of the hind foot catches the heel of the forefoot on the same side, usually on the bulb of the heel. This is most common in short-backed or long-limbed horses and also in horses that are not well ridden. It can be corrected as above by changing breakover of the forefeet and hind feet.
- *Winging.* This is used to describe the action of the foot as it breaks over at the end of the weight-bearing phase of the stride. The sole of the foot is turned backward and outward. This may be due to conformational defects (e.g., the metacarpophalangeal joint slopes down to its medial aspect, the cannon bone rotates inward, or there is a lateral deviation of the distal limb). Most commonly, winging results from poor fitting of the shoes. Check the medial-lateral balance (medial side too short). Then check that the shoe is placed under the end of the cannon bone. Usually it will be found that the foot is breaking over the medial aspect of the toe. By placing the shoe wider at this point, breakover can be centralized and will stop the winging. Finally, if the limb is rotated place the shoe straight with the line of the horse rather than the foot, i.e., if the toe turns in, leave the branch of the shoe longer on the lateral heel and shorter on the medial heel. This repositioning of the shoe can be used to mask abnormal gait in horses with poor conformation and to correct poor shoeing.

Terms specific to the USA

- *Cross-firing.* This is usually confined to pacers. It consists of contact between the insides of the diagonally opposite front foot and hind foot.
- *Elbow hitting.* This is hitting the elbow with the shoe of same limb and is normally limited to gaited horses with weighted shoes.
- *Knee hitting.* This is generally seen in Standardbreds with a high knee action. The knee is hit by the contralateral foot.
- *Scalping.* The toe of the forefoot hits the coronary band of the hind foot on the same side, usually in trotters.

Saddle fitting

A major influence on the horse's movement is the comfort and fitting of the saddle and the ability of the rider. The saddle acts as a "junction" between horse and rider and should help spread the weight of the rider across the back muscles as comfortably as possible, allowing the horse to move as normally as possible.

Saddle fitting is a crucial part of any horse, rider, or performance assessment. It is a complex area and one where you would be well advised to seek the help of a professional saddle fitter if you have any doubts about the suitability of a saddle for a particular horse. Remember that a horse with somatic dysfunction of the back (which means it is using the back muscles asymmetrically) will show asymmetric muscle mass, and so the saddle will need to be reassessed and refitted as the horse begins to recover during and after treatment. Regular assessment of the saddle every few months immediately after treatment is essential.

Saddle structure

At the core of the conventional saddle is the "tree" (Fig. 5.19). This is traditionally a laminated wooden frame, onto which the padding of the saddle is fixed. In some more recent saddles the tree is made of plastic-type materials (some of which have the disadvantage of having little flexibility, which in itself may cause injury to the back). In some saddles the tree is completely omitted (treeless saddles). The tree is the core of the

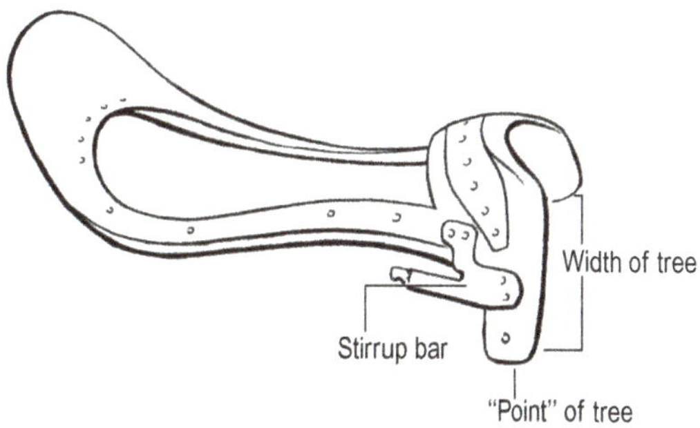

Figure 5.19
The saddle tree, traditionally made of laminated wood, is at the core of the saddle. The symmetry of the saddle and its fittings depend on this structure.

saddle, rather like the chassis in a car, and they come in a variety of widths, lengths, and shapes to fit different shapes of back. It is important that they are not curved dorsoventrally as this can also lead to abnormal pressure on the horse's back. The shape also varies to allow for the different uses to which the saddle may be put (e.g., show jumping or dressage).

Under the tree are the panels (Fig. 5.20) - large areas of padding that sit either side of the backbone and spread the rider's weight across the muscles. They should cover as large an area as possible, without impinging on the shoulder blades, lumbar or thoracic spine. The thickness and shape of the panels will also vary depending on the shape of the back (e.g., native ponies have a much higher rib cage than a thoroughbred). In the midline between the panels is the gullet. This is an unpadded channel that bridges over the dorsal spinous processes and ensures no weight

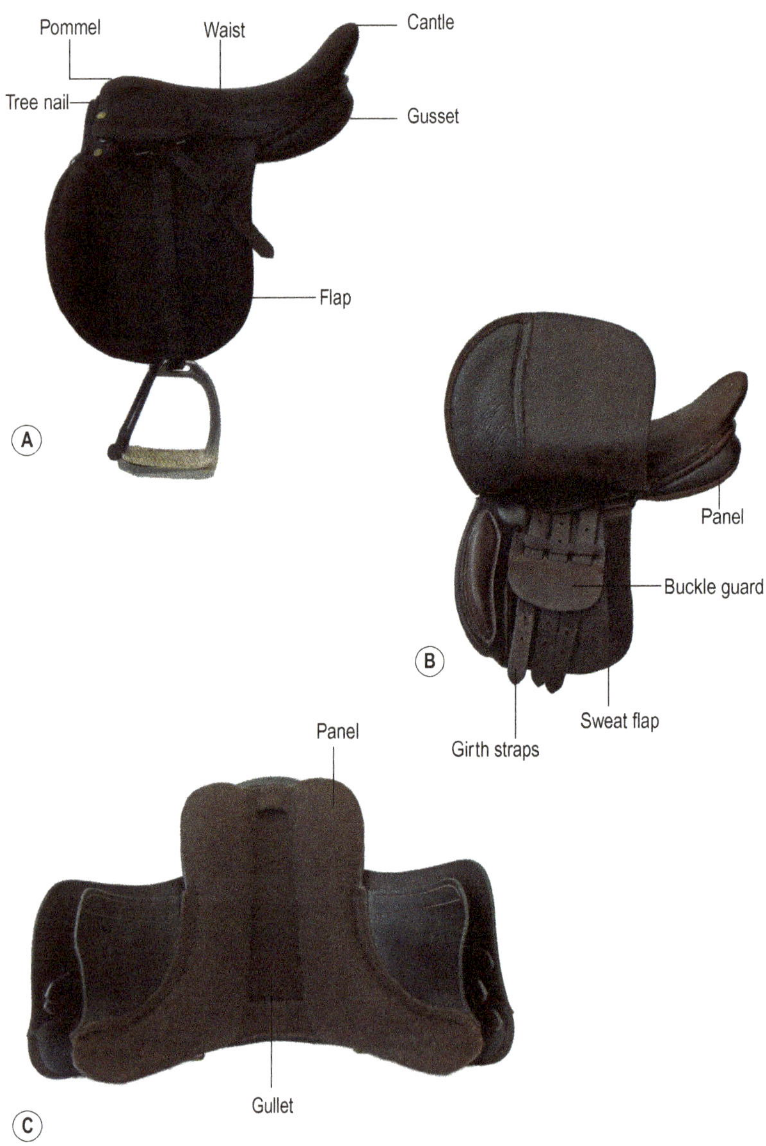

Figure 5.20
The parts of the saddle.

presses in on the spine. The width of the gullet is important.

Above the tree is the seat where the rider is supported. The front of the saddle is the pommel, and the back of the seat area is known as the cantle (Fig. 5.20).

Also attached to the tree are the saddle straps that attach to the girth and hold the whole assembly in place. These need to be placed so that the girth runs straight around the horse and does not pull the saddle forward into the shoulders or allow it to slip back along the spine when ridden. Check also that the girth and particularly the buckles do not impinge on the elbow of the horse at the back of the stride.

The stirrup bars are also attached to the front of the tree under the saddle skirts. These should be placed symmetrically either side of the saddle.

It is important that the saddle should be symmetrical about the midline (including the stirrup bars and saddle straps). The whole should be straight from front to back, and it must sit comfortably and evenly on the horse, with no tendency to move when being ridden.

Checking saddle fit

As stated above, saddle fitting is a specialist occupation, but you should have some idea of whether a saddle fits or not if you are to benefit the horse and advise the owner. You can make a reasonable assessment as follows:

1. Stand the horse squarely on level ground with its head and neck relaxed and looking straight in front. Place the saddle slightly forward on the horse's withers, do not use any saddle cloths or pads under the saddle. Push downward on the pommel and allow the saddle to slide back until it comes to a natural stopping point. You may need to repeat this several times to be sure you have the correct position. It should come to rest naturally behind the scapula, and the back of the saddle should be at least 12.5 cm in front of the whorls that lie over the loins.
2. Imagine a line running from the top of the pommel to the cantle. This should show the cantle to be approximately 2.5 to 7.5 cm higher than the pommel, depending on the depth of the seat of the saddle. A jumping saddle will normally have a shallower seat with a lower cantle. If the cantle is level with or lower than the pommel the saddle probably does not fit correctly. The center of the seat, which will support the rider's core, should be parallel with the ground. (With bespoke saddles, the cantle may be made lower to avoid catching back protectors, so be cautious when making this assessment.)
3. Check the panel pressure is even under the whole saddle. To do this, press down on the center of the saddle and run the other hand between the saddle and the horse, feeling for consistent pressure throughout. The panels should not "bridge" (i.e., have limited contact under the center of the saddle) nor should there be a tendency to rock because of too little support at the front or back. The back point of the panels and tree should not exceed the last rib, and in a croup high horse they may need to be slightly shorter in order not to interfere with the hind limb movement. The panels should feel smooth throughout, with no clumping or unevenness of the flocking (padding under the panel). With a brand-new saddle there may be some bridging until it has been used for 20 minutes, by which time the warmth of the horse and weight of the rider should mould the saddle to the shape of the horse's back.
4. Standing near the front of the saddle, run your hand between the front of the saddle and the withers, feeling in particular for any pressure areas especially under the front of the tree. (Known as the points, these can be found either side of the saddle in a small leather pocket under the saddle flap, just below the stirrup bars.) The panels at this point should run at an angle parallel with the horse's musculature. The shoulder blades must be able to move without impinging on the panels when the horse is ridden.
5. The depth of the front of the panel is vital to ensure it takes the bearing on the rib cage, holding the tree away from the scapula. The tree and therefore

the gullet must be wide enough not to impact on the spine. Normally there should be between two and three fingers' width of clearance between the top of the withers and the pommel when the rider is on the saddle. Check that the gullet is clear of the spine throughout its length.

6. The support given to the rider and the rider's position will also affect the horse. In the past saddles were made to fit the rider as well as the horse, addressing any specific issues such as limb-length discrepancy or past injury to the rider's pelvis, neck, etc. Cost implications, however, mean that in most saddles today, the tree and seat shape and knee and thigh blocks are the only aids the saddle fitter has to work with to help the rider.

Remember saddles should be checked regularly to ensure that the horse's musculature has not changed, and that the packing in the panels has not become too compressed. The Saddle Research Trust suggests a routine check every three months in a working horse. The days when one saddle fitted all the horses in a yard are no longer acceptable if the rider wants to get the best performance from the horse. A well-fitting saddle should allow the muscles to move freely, and the horse to develop a good top line.

Common orthopedic conditions and differential diagnosis

Forelimb lameness

Sixty percent of all lameness in horses is said to be in the front foot or fetlock. Space does not permit a full coverage of all causes of lameness in the horse, which is a vast subject. For further information refer to *Adam's Lameness in Horses* by Stashak (1987) or *Diagnosis and Management of Lameness in the Horse* edited by Ross and Dyson (2011). The present text aims to give some background information on the commoner back and hind-limb problems, but cannot cover all the common problems of the forefeet simply due to shortage of space.

When assessing horses prior to treatment, the reader should first consider if there is an obvious weight-bearing forelimb lameness. This is most easily seen if the horse is trotted in hand. The head and neck will drop when the sound leg takes weight. If there is obvious forelimb lameness, then the horse should first be assessed by an equine veterinary surgeon to ensure there is no pathological cause of lameness. Marked lameness in one forelimb is occasionally caused by somatic dysfunction in the lower neck or shoulder regions, but is more often caused by skeletal or soft tissue pathology.

Differential diagnosis of lameness in the horse is a lifelong study, but from the osteopath's point of view an obviously increased pulse in the digital arteries may be a useful pointer. An increased pulse in one foot, or one side of one foot, tends to suggest an inflammatory process distal to the increased pulse (e.g., bruising or infection). An increased pulse in both front feet or in all four feet may be indicative of laminitis. Distension, heat, or swelling in the limb or joints is also indicative of trauma or pathology and should be investigated before considering osteopathic treatments. Although osteopathy in these cases may be beneficial as an adjunct to medical treatments, it is unwise to proceed without the advice and cooperation of a veterinary surgeon.

Laminitis

Laminitis is a systemic disease that usually shows marked secondary problems affecting both front feet or all four feet. Signs, however, may occur in just one foot or in any combination and number of feet. Laminitis, despite having been recognized as a specific disease for over 200 years, remains something of an enigma. Current thinking is that typical cases are associated with chronically raised levels of insulin, resulting in spasm of arterioles, a rise in systemic blood pressure, and an acute vascular crisis in the feet. As a result, there may be rotation or total displacement of the distal phalanx within the hoof resulting in very serious secondary pathology (this may occur within four hours in acute cases or may takes weeks in more chronic cases). The condition is generally associated with overweight and overfed ponies, and rapid growth of grass. It can, however, occur in any type of equine, some of which may be in poor condition or have no access to grass. There are undoubtedly other causes of which we remain unaware, which may include mineral imbalance in the feed, toxic illnesses in the patient, and in some cases excessive concussion to the feet.

Laminitis requires a combined treatment between veterinary surgeon and farrier. In some cases there may be secondary somatic dysfunction, which may be treated osteopathically, but this should not be used instead of conventional treatments. All veterinary surgeons experienced in treating this condition agree that it remains one of the most challenging conditions in the horse. It is one condition where forming a prognosis remains a serious challenge, with apparently mild cases proving resistant to treatment and some acute cases responding better than anticipated. It has been quoted as the commonest cause of chronic lameness in the horse and in some cases may prove fatal despite intensive treatment.

Tendon injuries

Tendon injuries in horses are relatively common, usually in the front legs. Damage can range from a minor strain (tendinitis), which shows clinically only as some slight heat and pain to palpation of the affected tendon, through more significant strains resulting in some edema in the tendon tissues to complete rupture of the tendon tissue. Most tendon strains will fall between the two extremes. The superficial digital flexor tendon is the most commonly affected, in the mid cannon region, but almost any combination of flexor tendons and/or check ligaments and/or suspensory ligament may be involved.

The first signs seen are of increased heat in the affected tissue(s), which may occur some days prior to lameness occurring. The next signs will be of sensitivity to palpation of the tendon. Many horses resent tendons being squeezed, and so comparison with the contralateral limb and memory of previous reactions of the horse are essential. Swelling of the tendons will follow shortly after heat and pain, initially detected as slight loss of definition of the edges of the tendons which become rounded. Later there will be obvious swelling and possibly bowing of the tendon.

Lameness may occur at any stage of the onset, depending on the tendon involved, the pain threshold of the horse, and the ability of the rider or groom to detect lameness.

The prognosis is obviously very variable depending on the structures involved and severity of damage. Check ligaments will usually heal satisfactorily with rest. The digital flexor tendons may take six to 12 months to heal in severe injuries or may fail to heal adequately. The suspensory ligament generally takes longer to heal than the flexor tendons.

A condition known as proximal suspensory desmitis (mild strain of the proximal part of the suspensory ligament close to its origin) can occur in front or hind limbs. In forelimbs it will generally resolve. In hind limbs it often accompanies back dysfunction, and in chronic cases it may not resolve, or it may not resolve unless the back condition is also addressed.

Fractures

Fractures of the bones in the foot and fetlock are not uncommon, and many can be treated successfully, although internal fixation is commonly required. Fractures of the more proximal parts of the limb, however, become progressively more difficult to treat as they become more proximal. This is due in part to the nature of the patient, which, for example, cannot be put on bed rest and traction as might a human patient. Also the nature of the damage that occurs is often very extensive. Many equine fractures occur at high speed, damaging bone, but also causing catastrophic soft tissue injuries. The bones are also very dense compared with humans, so that rather than having a simple fracture to contend with, the bones tend to be shattered, rather more like breaking a piece of china. Because the horse is generally kept as a performance animal, lameness after treatment of fractures is not generally acceptable, and so with many fractures where the prognosis is poor treatment will not be attempted.

Arthritis

Arthritis and degenerative joint diseases are a common occurrence in horse joints as in many animals.

Commonly it will affect the distal limb joints, but various forms also occur in the carpus, tarsus, and stifle. In almost any joint this is a serious problem, as once again the standard for successful treatment is 100 percent recovery; no degree of lameness is acceptable in competing horses. In the early stages it may be managed with the use of good farriery, NSAIDs, and medication into the affected joints. In all cases, however, treatment can only be palliative to attempt to slow the progression of the condition. Obviously the significance will also depend on the use to which the horse is put.

Hind-limb lameness

Almost all the conditions seen in the lower forelimbs can occur in the lower hind limb, but do so less frequently. It is important to be aware that many bilateral hind-limb conditions may mimic back pain or be associated with it. Whether hind-limb lameness concurrent with back pain is caused by or results from such pain remains open to discussion, the evidence for which comes first currently being nonexistent. Veterinary treatment tends to center on hind-limb lameness as the primary problem, possibly because of the difficulty in diagnosing back pain in many horses.

Causes of lameness in the hind limb are briefly covered below, concentrating on conditions that may cause or be confused with back dysfunctions.

Sacroiliac strain

Strain of the sacroiliac ligament generally occurs after severe trauma, e.g., a fall. It usually results in tilting of the pelvis, which can be assessed by looking at the tubera coxae from behind. There is rapid and marked wastage of the gluteal muscles of the affected side. At least in the acute stage there is a marked pain response to pressure applied to the tuber coxae, especially directed dorsally while the spine is fixed.

Treatment of acute sacroiliac ligament strain requires rest (like any other ligament strain), probably for at least six months. Secondary somatic dysfunction is a likely sequel, and so gentle osteopathic treatment during the recovery phase may be helpful. Avoid more aggressive treatments in the acute and recovery stages of the condition.

Chronic strain with a history of gradual onset, but with no obvious trauma, is sometimes diagnosed, based on pelvic rotation and muscle wastage. These cases often respond readily and immediately to manipulation, suggesting that they may be associated with rotation of the lumbar spine and somatic dysfunction, rather than damage to the sacroiliac ligament or joints. (This is a speculative suggestion of the author (CC), not a generally accepted conclusion of the veterinary profession.) A proper differential diagnosis is important prior to treatment.

Hip and pelvis

Arthritic disease may be seen in the hips of older animals, and fractures may result from a fall at any age. These conditions, however, are unusual, and should be confirmed by X-ray, ultrasound, or scintigraphy. Arthritis and fractures involving the hip joint itself carry a very poor prognosis.

Hip dysplasia is rare, but does occur in the miniature breeds.

Fractures of the pelvis are not uncommon after major falls or accidents. If the fracture enters the hip joint the prognosis is hopeless. If the hip joint is intact then many horses will return to work after a period of rest. At the time of fracture there is usually severe pain with the horse being reluctant to move and frequently standing sweating and shaking when the fracture first occurs. There is initially marked muscle spasm in the pelvic area, and rapid muscle wastage (primarily of the gluteal muscles) occurs in days. If the standing horse is gently rocked side to side, crepitus may well be felt.

“Spontaneous” fracture of the pelvis is seen in two- and three-year-old horses in training, often associated with “jumping off” at the start of a training gallop. The prognosis depends on the position of fractures and the intended use of the horse, but with box rest and painkillers many cases will return to work. Osteopathic treatment later in the recovery phase may help control somatic dysfunction, which will be an inevitable secondary problem.

Stifle

In young animals, osteochondrosis dissecans and subchondral bone cysts in the distal femur are not uncommon causes of lameness. The degree of lameness and prognosis are very variable, and each case will need careful veterinary assessment before considering treatment.

Strain of the collateral ligaments (especially medial femorotibial) is very painful, but relatively uncommon. It may be diagnosed by palpation and ultrasound examination.

Rupture of the cruciate ligament causes very marked lameness, with secondary degenerative joint disease usually becoming present within three to four months.

Arthritis is rare except secondary to the above conditions. It requires diagnosis by X-ray and carries a hopeless prognosis.

Locking stifle. The horse can "lock" the stifle, by rotation of the tibia relative to the femur, causing the medial patellar ligament to drop into a notch formed above the distal end of the medial trochlear ridge of the femur. This prevents the stifle joint flexing (and because of the superficial flexor muscle and tendon also fixes the hock joint). This system allows the horse to stand while using minimal muscular energy. In some cases the medial patellar ligament fails to release from the femoral trochlear ridge, resulting in hind limb fixation. This is most common in ponies, but is becoming more frequent in larger horses.

This condition may present clinically as:

- Complete fixation of the limb, which cannot be flexed. The horse is generally found with one hind leg fixed straight, tending to drag it behind, with the fetlock partially flexed. It may release spontaneously, and fixation may be intermittent. The condition is not painful and does not normally result in any secondary joint problems. The horse (and owner) frequently panic, although ponies generally show little concern.
- Delayed or slow release of the patella. This causes a jerking action of the limb. The hind limb jerks upward on flexion when walking. There may be an audible clunk. If the stifle is palpated as the horse is walked slowly forward, the patella may be felt to jump in and out as the horse walks, but be aware this can occur in normal horses.

Treatment. If the leg is locked straight, turn the horse short (on the spot) with the affected leg on the inside of the circle. This may affect release. Alternatively try backing the horse. This causes the leg to straighten, thus taking the load off the medial patella ligament, and allowing it to release. Backing the horse, however, can also result in the stifle locking in some cases.

A third technique involves putting pressure upward and laterally on the patella while straightening the limb. This generally means standing behind the horse, and may result in the operative getting injured as the joint releases and the leg suddenly flexes.

Any of the above techniques may require sedation to be effective; this will relax the horse to allow release.

If the above techniques are not successful, then it may be necessary to carry out surgical section of the ligament under local anesthetic to release the limb.

Chronic cases. Chronic locking stifles are most often seen in ponies, and in immature animals the condition may resolve spontaneously as the pony matures. Unfit horses and ponies may also improve if worked. If the problem persists, they may require surgical section of the medial patella ligament. This has a very good prognosis in ponies, but larger horses may develop chronic problems subsequent to surgery, due to slight rotation of the patella relative to the trochlear groove. In larger horses therefore fenestration of the ligament may prove a useful alternative treatment.

Clinical observation suggests that in some previously normal horses this condition may occur after a fall. It is always worth assessing the back in such cases, and locking of the patella in some cases may resolve subsequent to treatment of back pain (author's opinion).

Note: intermittent locking or late release of the patella can be confused with stringhalt and shivering.

Hock

Spavin is the lay term meaning something that has gone wrong with a hock joint. There are two forms: bog spavin and bone spavin.

Bog spavin. This refers to a soft tissue swelling of the tibiotarsal joint. Distension will be seen dorsomedially and can easily be palpated. It indicates an inflammation of the tibiotarsal joint and should be investigated fully, even if the horse shows no lameness.

In acute onset cases the condition may be caused by trauma, with resultant synovitis, in which case a reasonable prognosis may be given assuming there is no ligament damage. In some cases, however, there may be a fracture of the distal lateral ridge of the tibia, which usually requires surgical intervention. After surgery a reasonable prognosis can usually be given.

In some young horses, particularly warmbloods and some heavy horses, bog spavin may be associated with osteochondritis. The prognosis in these cases will depend on the severity of the underlying condition.

Bone spavin. This term refers to a degenerative condition of the small tarsal bones. The etiology is unknown, but there is a progressive degeneration of the bones, frequently accompanied by formation of new bone. If this new bone formation results in fusion of the joint spaces, then lameness may resolve spontaneously. Any of the bones may be involved, but it is most commonly the central and 3rd tarsal bones that show change, involving the dorsomedial aspect of the distal intertarsal joint. The prognosis is worse if there is involvement of the proximal intertarsal or tarsometatarsal joints.

The horse may show lameness on the affected hind leg. If bilateral, this tends to be more severe on one leg than the other. Flexion of the leg will exacerbate lameness when trotted subsequently (not specific to spavin). The degree of lameness can vary between horses from showing virtually no clinical signs through to acute severe lameness. Usually if one limb is affected the other will follow suit in six to 18 months. Typically the gait changes, the affected limb being swung medially at the end of the swing phase, with some lateral movement immediately before placement of the foot. Typically when weight-bearing the foot is placed medial to the hock joint. Final diagnosis depends on X-ray (and possibly nerve block).

A number of treatments are recognized (which suggests none is very effective). Initially the foot placement should be altered, so that it is placed below or lateral to the hock. This is best achieved with some lateral extension to the hind shoe, with a 2.5 to 5 cm trailer at 45 degrees on the lateral branch of the shoe. It is essential to ensure there is adequate length of shoe, and that the mediolateral balance is correct. If the horse can then be worked on painkillers, this may encourage fusion of the affected joints, and resolution of lameness. If this is not successful steroid injection in the joint, surgical fusion, or chemical fusion may be tried. The prognosis must be guarded, as even with successful fusion of the joint and resolution of pain, the gait may be changed, and the horse subsequently be considered unlevel or irregular in gait.

Note: spavin may be hereditary (not acceptable for a stallion license). Spavin is often associated with back dysfunction. Which condition comes first is open to discussion but treatment of the back is likely to be beneficial.

Tendon injuries

The tendon injuries seen in the front limb also occur in the hind limb, but are less common. There are three conditions that do not occur in the front limb:

1. *Chronic degeneration of the suspensory ligament.* This may occur in older animals, often associated with straight hock joints. There is marked dropping of the fetlock joints, with subsequent changes in degenerative joint disease (DJD). Treatment is very unrewarding. Shoeing with long heel extensions

to the hind shoes will help slow progression, but eventually the suspensory ligament will rupture, or the fetlock joint will become too arthritic for the horse to continue.

2. *Dislocation of the hind superficial digital flexor tendon from the point of the hock (slipped tendon).* This usually occurs when a tired horse turns sharply. The tendon normally dislocates to the lateral aspect of the hock. Clinically the horse is initially very distressed, but is more upset by loss of control over the limb than by pain. The hock region becomes edematous very rapidly. If total dislocation occurs, then usually the horse will accommodate, and can jump and hunt, etc. afterward (requiring about six months to adjust). It is unusual for such a horse to carry out dressage without being marked as unlevel. In a small number of cases the tendon will flick on and off the hock intermittently. These cases carry a poor prognosis, as the horse can never adjust its gait to the inconsistent problem. Surgery on such cases is probably the best answer, either fixing it properly or resulting in permanent dislocation. Surgery should be undertaken within 24 hours of onset of dislocation if it is to have any real chance of success.
3. *Rupture of the peroneus tertius.* This is an uncommon condition. It will occur after relatively minor accidents, where the distal hind limb is caught, or extended passively, when the proximal part of the limb is flexed. Rupture does not necessarily cause lameness, but initially the horse will have difficulty in extending the limb forward at the front of the stride, and may catch the hind toe midstride. There is generally no obvious heat, pain or swelling, but pain may be detected by palpation at the proximal dorsal aspect of the hind cannon bone. Rest will not restore the ligament, but the horse will learn to accommodate. It may be left with inability to flex the distal limb fully, which can be significant especially in show jumpers. Diagnosis is simple. The hind limb is flexed, and it will then be found that the hock can be straightened, the gastrocnemius tendon appearing "wrinkled."

Conditions of the horse's back

There are a number of pathological and physiological causes of back pain in the horse, and these need to be considered before assessing a horse for manipulative therapy.

Equine rhabdomyolysis

Equine rhabdomyolysis is the term used to describe nontraumatic myopathies. It covers such terms as: azoturia, paralytic myoglobinuria, exertional myopathy, exertional rhabdomyolysis, tying-up, set-fast, and Monday morning disease.

The pathophysiology is open to much discussion, and there are undoubtedly several different conditions involved. This should perhaps be referred to as a syndrome (a collection of conditions or diseases giving similar symptoms).

Clinical signs. The incidence of the condition is higher in young fillies than in older animals, colts, and geldings, but it can occur at any age and in any breed or sex. It is more common in winter than summer, but any stress can precipitate attacks in susceptible animals. Cold and wet conditions also predispose to attacks.

Clinical signs most commonly start during work (65 percent). Fifteen percent may occur before real work is commenced, and about 20 percent show signs when resting after exercise. The clinical signs are:

- Stiffness (which may be so severe as to prevent walking completely).
- Muscle spasm (usually of the back, loins and hind limbs, but potentially of any muscle mass).
- Muscle boarding, trembling, or fasciculation.
- Severe pain, and sweating in more severe cases.
- In very severe cases, there may be temporary paralysis of gut movement, colic, recumbence, and death.

The differential diagnosis is not usually too difficult, but the most commonly confused conditions are colic, iliac thrombosis, laminitis, acute muscle strain, and tetanus. Confirmation of the condition can be made by measuring muscle enzyme levels in the serum (AST and CPK). These levels will rise within minutes of the attack, and may rise to more than 100 times their normal resting levels 24 hours after an attack. In animals suspected of being prone to the condition, measuring the enzyme levels before, immediately after, and 24 hours after a known amount of exercise may be helpful in confirming the diagnosis.

Management plays a large part in the occurrence of the disease, and 90 percent of cases have been subjected to overfeeding and irregular work. There are a small number of cases, however, which show recurrent attacks despite apparently carefully controlled nutrition and exercise, and these may require extensive investigation to resolve. The pathophysiology and treatment of this condition are under current research, and beyond the scope of this text.

Idiopathic rhabdomyolysis

Acute rhabdomyolysis has been seen in horses at grass, with no history of work, and often no supplementary feeding. A large percentage of these cases prove fatal, despite very extensive support and treatment. At the present time, the cause of this condition is thought to relate to ingestion of sycamore (*Acer pseudoplatanus*) and material from closely related plants.

Malignant hyperthermia

The pathophysiology of this condition is still not understood. It appears to be a hereditary condition that results in behavioral problems, chronically raised muscle enzymes, and exercise intolerance, with rhabdomyolysis attacks when worked. Research to date has shown no cure, although it may be possible to help control symptoms in some cases by reducing the carbohydrate in the feed and compensating with an increase in oil. The condition is rare and poorly understood.

Back disorders

Back disorders in the horse are frequently diagnosed by riders, but often doubted by veterinary surgeons. This is at least in part because of the difficulty of assessing backs in an objective manner. Horses do disguise pain very readily (something often seen in prey species), and so back disorders may be more a matter of loss of movement rather than acute pain. Clinical signs are largely the same whatever the cause of the problem and are listed below.

1. Clinical history

a. Stiffness in the back or generalized stiffness.

b. Failure to perform or drop in performance.

c. Inability, reluctance, or slow to form an outline. May demonstrate pain when worked on the bit.

d. Hanging on one rein, and/or reluctance to work one way, or inability to carry out lateral work.

e. Change in temperament.

f. Persistent rearing.

g. Occasional cases may collapse when the girth is tightened.

h. Lameness of one or more limbs.

i. Acute heat pain or swelling palpable over the back.

2. Clinical examination at rest

a. Limbs should normally be positioned under the horse with the cannon bones vertical. Look for a tendency to rest the same leg persistently, shift weight continually from one hind limb to the other, or reluctance to stand with the hind legs adjacent to each other (square).

b. The back should be straight, and symmetrical along the midline, showing a smooth regular curving dip from the base of the withers to the tubera sacrale.

c. The neck should be held freely in front of the horse, but when looking round to either side, the neck should flex smoothly from top to bottom.

d. The head should be held vertical and in line with the neck.

e. Muscle bulk should be symmetrical and appropriate for the work being carried out. Poorly developed muscles in the neck or along the top line of the back may be significant. The three thirds of the horse should match (neck, forequarters, and hindquarters).

f. Muscle tone should be symmetrical and normal in the neck and back. Flexion in the back should be readily carried out in all four directions.

g. With the horse stood square and weight-bearing, the tubera coxae and gluteal muscles should be level and symmetrical.

h. The dorsal midline of the back should show no thickening, heat, pain, swelling, or asymmetry in the dorsal spinous processes, dorsal spinous ligament, or back muscles.

3. Clinical examination of the horse moving. At walk and trot on a level, hard surface, preferably in a head collar, look for:

a. Symmetry of forelimb and hind limb stride length and failure to track up evenly.

b. Uneven strides and inconsistency of stride or limb placement.

c. Excessive movement of the head (swaying from side to side) or quarters.

d. Changes in movement of head, neck, back, and quarters between walk and trot.

e. Raising the head and neck in the upward transitions.

f. Failure to bring the hind legs forward under the body with resultant lack of drive from the hind limbs.

g. Turned short, the inside hind limb should be crossed over and placed in front of the outside limb during turning, and the neck and back should flex in the direction of the turn.

Causes of pain

Bone origin. < 10 percent of cases:

- Overriding dorsal spinous processes (ORDSP, also known as kissing spines)
- Arthritis of the facet joints
- Ossifying spondylitis
- Fractures.

Other causes are rare and include: TB, tumors, and infectious osteomyelitis.

Note: in horses, as in man, the relationship of radiological change to back pain is very inconsistent.

Soft tissue origin. > 90 percent of cases:

- Muscle strain
- Ligament strain
- Reduced joint mobility
- Somatic dysfunction (pathophysiological dysfunction of muscle-nerve complexes).

Differential diagnosis

- Requires an experienced clinician.
- Requires radiography by a fixed machine (i.e., not a portable), which is currently outside the range of most practitioners.
- May require ultrasound, scintigraphy, or infrared thermography.

Treatment

Bone origin

- *Overriding dorsal spinous processes (ORDSP).* This is frequently insignificant and overdiagnosed. It is likely to be secondary to another condition causing dorsiflexion (dipping) of the back. Treatment involves four months' rest and physical therapies, and steroid injections if necessary. Surgery should only be used as last resort.
- *Arthritis of facet joints.* There is no cure. The patient may be injected with steroids, may be able to perform on anti-inflammatory drugs, or at a lower level.
- *Ossifying spondylitis.* Fifty percent of cases were reported to be of no clinical significance (Jeffcott 1980). This opinion may now be superseded, with stiffness of the back being seen rather than frank pain. If significant, there is no cure. The patient may

be able to perform on anti-inflammatory drugs or at a lower level.

All the above conditions are likely to be concurrent with somatic dysfunction, so osteopathic treatment may be of value.

- *Fractures.* Treatment and prognosis depend on the site involved.

Soft tissue origin. Possibly more than 90 percent of cases of back pain are of soft tissue origin.

- *Muscle strain.* Muscles are hot, swollen, and painful. Strain can be confirmed with an ultrasound scan. Muscle strain will probably resolve with rest; however, most cases benefit from osteopathy.
- *Ligament strain.* Symptoms are heat, pain, and swelling of the involved ligament. Again, strain can be visualized with ultrasound in most cases. It may well resolve with rest and osteopathic treatment (but see the section on sacroiliac strain above).
- *Reduced joint mobility or sympathetic dystonia.* This requires manipulation. It will respond to varying degrees, depending on the position, the nature of the patient, and the duration of the problem (see Somatic dysfunction below).
- *Nerve irritation or pressure?* It is likely that such cases may exist in the horse, but they are very difficult to prove. They may respond to varying degrees to manipulation.

Somatic dysfunction

The concept of somatic dysfunction is fundamental to manipulative therapies. It is based on the assumption that somewhere in the process of collating information from the environment and body, processing the information in the central nervous system, and then generating a motor response, something has gone wrong. Clinically, this presents as a horse with symptoms such as stiffness, loss of performance, poor coordination or gait abnormality, where no pathological process can be identified. Manipulative therapies change the signals to the neural network, modify the way sensory information is processed, and thus correct the motor response generated in the central nervous system.

Incoordination

In horses the causes of incoordination can be very difficult to differentiate. Conditions such as bruising of the spinal cord are not generally diagnosed, although it seems likely they do occur. A diagnosis of incoordination is often assumed to be due to cervical stenosis, and so the manipulative treatment of such cases must be approached with great care for clinical and political reasons.

Cervical stenosis (wobbler disease)

Incidence. Cervical stenosis is more common in colts than fillies and is usually seen in Thoroughbreds in the UK. It may be seen in any rapidly growing horse especially of the larger breeds.

The onset is usually sudden, associated with increased activity or possibly trauma, for example, when being broken in. Cases may progress, but usually if work ceases signs stabilize or regress until work is resumed.

Pathology. Narrowing of the cervical spinal canal causes compression of spinal nerves, usually at the level of C2–C4 or C6–C7. The patient may have soft tissue swellings impinging on the spinal cord (usually C6–C7). This interferes with motor and sensory nerves to all four limbs.

Clinical signs. Cervical stenosis is not associated with pain. There is a rather straight-legged hind limb gait. This may be similar in front (hypermetric gait), but forelimb gait may appear normal.

When walked in hand, if the tail is pulled to one side the quarters will sway with the pull, and the horse will not resist or try to correct the movement.

There is a tendency for the hindquarters to drift to either side when trotting, and if the horse is stopped suddenly in a severe case the hind end may carry on, the horse falling over as the hindquarters overbalance. The horse generally appears relatively unconcerned about such a fall.

If lunged in a circle, the hind limbs are often used together if cantering (bunny hops), but this is also seen in other conditions.

When turned short (i.e., turned with one foreleg as the center of the turn), the horse pivots on the inner hind leg, throwing the outer hind leg wide. It may fail to cross the hind legs when turning or this may be inconsistent.

Note: all the above signs may have other causes, and are not specific to a diagnosis of cervical stenosis.

Confirmation of diagnosis

- The diagnosis is confirmed with X-ray, myelogram or CT scan. The significance of changes seen is often open to discussion (Butler et al. 2016).
- Slap test: when the horse is patted over the saddle area, the contralateral arytenoid cartilage and vocal cord will twitch in a normal horse. This reflex is arguably missing if there is interference of nervous transition in the cervical area.
- Cases are seldom clear-cut and are usually open to discussion and argument.

Treatment

- Steroids and NSAIDs are not much good.
- Surgery, to fuse the vertebrae causing the problem, may improve signs by one to two grades. This is still a controversial treatment as the horses are improved but seldom rendered 100 percent normal after surgery.
- This is usually a congenital malformation, and so no treatment will be 100 percent effective.

Cauda equina (polyneuritis equi)

Incidence. Cauda equina occurs equally in both sexes and tends to be seen in mature or older horses.

Pathology. There is chronic inflammation of the nerve roots of the cauda equina (the last part of the spinal cord).

The cause is unknown, but it may be associated with trauma. In some cases other nerves may be affected, principally cranial nerves.

Clinical signs. It is slowly progressive over several weeks, but may initially present as an acute onset. (This may be real or simply be because early signs were not detected.)

There is initially loss of sensation in the tail, progressing forward, with complete loss of muscle tone in the tail. Note that:

- With progression, paralysis of nerves further forward develops.
- Lameness or unevenness of stride may occur.
- Tail rubbing occurs initially, but not usually in the later stages.
- As the condition progresses the horse may develop fecal retention, and then urine dribbling.
- The horse may have hypersensitivity over the quarters (gluteal muscles).

Partial confirmation of the diagnosis may be possible by checking serum samples for myelin degradation products. This may give false negative results, and is not specific if positive.

Treatment

- Large doses of steroids, decreasing gradually if any response is seen.
- DMSO (dimethyl sulfoxide) has also been used intravenously.
- The prognosis is poor, but occasional cases do recover.

Protozoal myelitis

Incidence. Protozoal myelitis is not endemic in the UK or Europe, but is seen occasionally in horses imported from the USA and Canada where it is endemic. In the UK it is principally seen in Thoroughbreds, most common in horses that are one to four years old, although it can be seen at any age.

Pathology. The CNS is the site of protozoal infection. The organism is believed to be sarcocystis, but is still not definitely identified. It may affect any part of the spinal cord and may spread with time. It is not thought to be directly infectious between horses and requires an intermediate host, probably the opossum.

Clinical signs. It usually begins as an obscure lameness, progressing to ataxia. There may be slight muscle wastage, and this and nervous signs need not be symmetrical. The condition is slowly progressive, and may cause recumbency in days or months.

Treatment. The condition has been treated with sulphonamides and NSAIDs, steroids, and DMSO. Response to treatment is very variable. Some cases do recover. Others show no change, progress, or respond and relapse.

Fractured vertebrae

Incidence. Fractured vertebrae may occur in any age, sex or type of horse.

Pathology. Fracture of a vertebra or dislocation of an intervertebral joint usually results in paralysis or death. Hairline fractures without displacement or partial fractures may be compatible with life.

Clinical signs. Fracture of a vertebra is usually associated with a fall or other trauma. It occurs most commonly in the neck. There is usually acute pain and stiffness in the neck. There may be associated ataxia, which may be progressive to recumbency and/or death.

The exact signs depend on the site and severity of the fracture. Confirmation may be possible by X-ray.

Fractures of the thoracic spine and lumbar spine can be difficult to identify on X-ray and may require scintigraphy.

Note: the degree of pain shown can be very deceptive. Hairline fractures with no movement or separation may show minimal pain. Acute muscle spasm may be far more painful.

Treatment. The type of treatment depends entirely on the position of the fracture. Many have a hopeless prognosis. Some may respond to conservative treatment coupled with the use of painkillers and anti-inflammatories to reduce edema and swelling within the spinal canal.

Occasional cases may respond to surgical fixation (currently this would be unusual).

Movement should be restricted. The feed should be above floor level.

Do not manipulate.

EHV-1 virus (Rhinopneumonitis)

Incidence. It may occur in any age, sex, and type of horse. There is a vaccine which is becoming more widely used.

Pathology. It is the result of a viral infection. It normally causes a respiratory tract infection, but certain strains may cause neurological signs in a small percentage of animals.

Clinical signs. The signs are an infectious respiratory disease with an incubation period of seven days. Two to three days prior to the onset of respiratory signs the horse may run a temperature of 39 or 40 degrees centigrade.

Neurological signs occur sporadically, and may be associated with respiratory signs, but often occur one to three weeks after respiratory signs have passed. Neurological signs may be associated with stress. Note that:

- Symptoms vary from mild ataxia to recumbency.
- The patient may have urine retention and incontinence.
- The patient may lose sensation in the perineum.
- Lab tests may show changes in white cell count (but are not specific if positive).
- The complement fixation test may detect rising antibody titer.

Note: some strains may also be associated with late gestation abortion.

Treatment

- Supportive therapy may be administered.
- Respiratory cases recover over three to four weeks.

- Mild ataxia cases may recover in weeks to several months, but recumbent cases frequently do not survive.

Current vaccines (2018) for EHV-1 and EHV-4 do not claim to prevent paralytic signs. They do, however, reduce shedding of virus by infected horses, and so might help to reduce the incidence of disease in this manner. Vaccination should not be used on in-contact animals in the face of infection. (The paralytic signs may be associated with an antibody-antigen complex within the CNS.)

Motor neurone disease

Incidence. This is a very rare condition in the horse, but has been diagnosed at postmortem. It may occur at any age (two to 20 years), and in any sex and type, but it occurs most commonly in older horses with a peak incidence thought to be at 16 years. Usually at onset the horses have no access to grass or are on very poor grassing.

Pathology

- Neurological degeneration with ceroid lipofuscin inclusions.
- Lesions primarily in the ventral gray matter and brain stem nuclei.
- May be associated with low levels of α-tocopherol.

Clinical signs

- Neurological signs usually have a gradual onset, accompanied from early on by muscle tremors.
- Often increased periods of recumbency are seen, but these are easily confused with colic or grass sickness. There is gradual weight loss.
- The disease consistently involves the forelimbs (medial head of triceps) and hind limbs (medial and lateral vastus intermedius muscle and head of tail).
- Ataxia may be mild, but tends to be progressive leading to recumbency.
- Pigmentation of the retina tends to occur.

Lab tests

- Muscle biopsy may show atrophy of type 2 muscle fibers.
- Tests may show vitamin E levels of less than 1.0 μg/ml (normal = 1.5–4.0).

Treatment

- Supportive therapy may be administered.
- This is a rare condition, difficult to diagnose specifically other than at postmortem. Cases frequently do not survive, and if they do, do not return to normal work, 30 percent or more of the gray matter neurons being absent.
- It is not infectious.

Migrating worm larvae and lymphosarcoma. Both the above can cause any number of clinical signs and can occur in any age of horse.

Osteopathic evaluation of acute cases

This section provides an approach to evaluating and administering treatment to an unsedated equine patient. There is no one correct way to assess and treat a horse. The practitioner's technique will evolve as their knowledge increases and clinical skills develop. The approach detailed here provides some structure for a challenging but incredibly rewarding field of osteopathic work. A consistent and structured approach to assessment is important if evidence is not to be missed.

Evaluation

Evaluation of the equine patient should follow the taking of the case history. Together these two elements of the consultation provide the basis and rationale for treatment. If these first two elements are accurate and sufficiently detailed, the treatment protocol can be effective and will provide the horse with the desired relief. It may well be necessary during the initial consultation to spend extra time performing a thorough evaluation to detect all the minor changes in the animal's movement. This is time well spent, as once a clear diagnosis has been made treatment techniques can be more precisely directed. It also helps the practitioner to formulate a clear prognosis for the owner and provide treatment that is the least invasive with the maximum benefit for the horse.

There are many ways to make an osteopathic evaluation of the equine patient, and the practitioner should choose a sequence of examinations best suited to him- or herself, that covers all aspects. The following protocol is the one the author (BA) uses and is offered as a guide, which others may use as a basis from which to develop their own model:

- Observation of the whole horse, including its emotional state, conformation, gait patterning, muscle tone, symmetry of limbs, and overall structure.
- A passive palpatory examination to identify areas of dysfunction, providing some clarification of the presenting complaint.
- Dynamic assessment is then performed to reinforce palpatory findings, to check for overt clinical lameness, and to reveal any restrictions that were not detected during palpatory examination.
- A further passive palpatory evaluation can then be made if the dynamic assessment did not appear to match the initial findings, otherwise a diagnosis should have been reached and treatment can commence.

The individual components of this sequence are discussed in more detail below.

Observation

This aspect of the evaluation is crucial, with the process beginning from when the horse first steps out of the trailer, or is first seen standing in its paddock or stable, or is led toward the clinic for the consultation. The horse should be assessed first for clinical lameness and suitability for treatment, with an immediate veterinary referral if necessary. This initial visual impression can provide significant information about the horse's biomechanics and its emotional state.

Although most horses are used to being handled, it is always wise to observe and approach with the respect that they deserve. It can be useful to have the horse present during the initial history taking process in order to allow it to read the dynamic between client and practitioner. A horse that has adjusted to the consultation process, and is calm in this environment, will save the practitioner and handler significant time later in the consultation. A component of trust can develop during the taking of the case history, with the horse observing this trust built between the handler and the practitioner. This tends to have a roll-on effect to a trust between the practitioner and the horse. Achieving this before physically "introducing yourself" to the horse pays dividends when contact is eventually made.

Careful observation should be made of the horse's conformation and its suitability for the type of work required. There is a certain predictability of movement, depending on breed and physical conformation. When assessing the conformation of a horse, a useful guide is to use the rule of thirds. An imaginary box should be made to section the horse into three equal parts, with the head and neck in one section, the forelimb and thoracic cage in another section, and the hindquarters in the final third. This technique can be used to determine if a horse is using itself evenly and developing muscle accordingly. Often when a horse is avoiding a chronic injury in its hindquarters, the forelimb girdles, cervical musculature and pectoral muscles will appear overdeveloped when using this method of assessment. This uneven development is a result of the horse attempting to pull itself forward using its forelimbs, rather than driving from behind.

A full conformational analysis is beyond the scope of this text; however, many equine conformational texts are available to research this topic further (e.g., Hedge and Wagoner 2004).

Once general conformation has been assessed, more specific observation should be performed from either side, from behind and from in front, looking for evidence of asymmetry of muscling. This can be present for many reasons, including but not limited to:

- An underlying injury resulting in an avoidance and disuse atrophy.
- Significant tension in the muscle, reducing the appearance or actual bulk of muscle.

- A biomechanical compensation (for example a pelvic tilt or rotation leads to the pelvis appearing dropped on one side when compared to the other). This can result from an issue in the limb on the affected side, a compensation from the opposite forelimb, or any other fascial, ligamentous, visceral, or muscular connection to the affected side.

The same appreciation should be made for symmetry of bony landmarks, especially that of the structures readily identifiable on visual appraisal, for example, the tubera coxae, tubera sacrales shoulder joints, thoracic cage, and atlas. Should there be a bony asymmetry present, it may be indicative of a tissue strain (of any origin) and indicates a more detailed assessment is required.

The inspection continues with a visual scan of the horse for any contusions, cuts, abrasions, or swellings. Check also for splint formation in the limbs, evidence of tendon strain, or evidence of trauma of any kind. Findings such as these should be investigated by feeling for a raised temperature when palpating later in the assessment. If these injuries are acute or active, they usually generate a significant amount of heat. Skin or coat changes may indicate changes in the autonomic nervous system, sometimes resulting in significant sweating in a particular region. This should be noted and verified during the passive assessment. A coat or skin change may also be due to an allergy or infection, in which case the horse should be referred for veterinary examination for treatment of this condition.

During observation, particular attention should be paid as to whether the horse is resting a leg or is altering its stance, as this may provide an insight into where discomfort lies. Usually a horse will try to offload the affected limb, resting this leg in preference to any other. Occasionally the limbs being rested are continually altering. In the experience of the author this may be indicative of discomfort centrally, such as within the pelvic mechanics, but do not overlook veterinary problems such as laminitis, navicular disease, and other bilateral orthopedic diseases.

Once the observation has been completed, the practitioner should have a preliminary understanding of the horse's biomechanics, its mental and emotional state, its potential for movement, and an insight into the presenting complaint.

Passive examination

Following the initial observation, a focused clinical assessment can begin. The most important aspect of the clinical examination is to develop a routine system and be methodical with each horse, to ensure that nothing is missed. Commonly equine osteopaths begin by assessing the limbs. This author has found it to be least intimidating and safest for everyone involved to start with the nearside forelimb as this is familiar territory for horses that have had any level of training or basic handling.

Limbs

The limbs in the horse vary significantly between breeds (compare a draught horse with a young thoroughbred); however, the assessment remains similar for all breeds. Begin with palpation; feel for the contour of the cannon bones and follow the limb down into the foot. Palpate the texture of the overlying skin and connective tissue; warmth can be a sign of injury or active inflammation, as seen in splint formation or simple contusion. Feel for any swelling present and perform a check of the hoof wall and feet. Of particular interest is the area of the coronary band, where inflammation of the hoof can be detected relatively easily. From this position, the practitioner is able to place two fingers over the abaxial surface of the sesamoid bones to assess the digital pulses; if strong and bounding in more than one limb this may suggest laminitis, which should immediately be referred to a veterinary surgeon. Increased strength of pulse is associated with any inflammation distal to the point at which the pulse is felt, such as bruising and infection.

A hoof pick is an essential tool for investigating subclinical lameness. It is not uncommon to be requested to assess a lame horse and find it to be footsore. This is often from a stone or other foreign object compressing sensitive structures in the foot and leading to discomfort.

Running a hand down the back of the limb from the shoulder should stimulate the horse to pick the leg up and redistribute its weight. Once the feet have been cleared, continue to palpate up the limb for heat and also look for any bruising present. Following palpation, passive range of motion testing is indicated. Start to articulate the forelimb with the fetlock joint resting in your hand. Test for range and equally importantly the quality of motion present in the fetlock, knee, elbow, and shoulder joints.

A combination of ligaments in the limbs forms a system known as the stay apparatus. This provides a support or "locking" mechanism which allows the horse to stand for extended periods while expending minimal energy. Utilizing this mechanism in the forelimb, the practitioner is able to facilitate passive extension and flexion of the fetlock, knee, elbow, and shoulder, all yielding together when guiding the fetlock and knee. This provides the practitioner with an insight into the functioning of the entire limb and its relationship with the whole horse. This gives more information than a simple test of flexion or extension, as the practitioner can observe the horse's compensatory mechanisms within the thoracic cage, the cervical unit, and across the remainder of its body. Further motion testing can be performed with accessory motions. Medial and lateral movements at each articulation of the limb provide more information about its function. Careful palpating during motion testing is vital, feeling for signs of crepitus and reduced quality of motion, which may be suggestive of joint pathology. This same method of evaluation can be used for the hind limb; however, more care should be taken as this places the practitioner in a more vulnerable and potentially dangerous position, especially in an unsettled or easily spooked horse. As with the forelimb, motion testing here can give the practitioner an impression of the functioning not only of the hock, stifle, and hip, but also the smooth rocking of the pelvis, abdominal contents, and pelvic floor tone. Should an impression of heaviness or congestion be palpated through the movement of the limb, this can be assessed more closely later in the evaluation.

Body

Assessment of the body of the horse is methodical and measured and as a preference, the author finds it most useful to palpate and articulate the regions as one moves around the horse as this allows you to perform a closer inspection should there be an indication to do so.

Beginning with palpation, an open-handed broad contact may be used to palpate from the limbs, caudally across the expanse of the rib cage, and caudally from the withers, across the back, loin, flank, and to the croup, feeling for the normal motion of the thoracic cage during respiration, feeling for any bony or connective tissue abnormalities, areas of swelling, or perception of tenderness. Areas of swelling or tenderness may be a sign of trauma or inflammation beneath the area palpated, which can be from a joint sprain, muscle strain, ill-fitting saddle (especially if located beneath the points of contact for the saddle), or an internal pathology that requires veterinary referral. Following palpation of the flank, specific diagnosis can be made of the spinal facet joints and their rib attachments with a refined palpation at the dorsal articulations. The practitioner should then continue to the lumbar spine using the method described above. During this palpation, watch for the horse shifting away from the practitioner, watch for any involuntary muscular spasm, and palpate for changes in tone or heat within the tissues. This may be suggestive of a problem in that particular segment or in a structure that the segment supplies. Be mindful of the normal cutaneous spinal reflexes present in the horse, where light palpation causes the horse to move away and laterally flex (side-bend) its trunk around the stimulus (de Lahunta et al. 2014).

To determine whether true hyperalgesia is present, and to eliminate false positives, perform the deep palpation along the spinal and costal joints several times. Attention should be paid to the health, mobility, and inherent motility of the thoracic and abdominal organs, as the potential always remains for somatovisceral or viscerosomatic reflexes as the primary etiology.

Passive motion testing of this area can commence with translation of the spinal joints, springing over the ribs to assess tissue yield. To assess the thoracic inlet and thorax, place one hand over the wither and the other hand under the horse's sternum, and gently compress the two; a normal response is to feel some tissue slack between the hands, with an elastic end feel. Should this feel overly hard, the practitioner needs to direct treatment to this area, which is discussed later in this chapter.

From the horse's flank, continuing caudally, palpate over the lines of the sacroiliac joints from cranial to caudal. This can be useful to diagnose any pelvic dysfunction. A horse with an acute injury here will normally show marked discomfort upon palpation, with some horses seen almost to buckle at the stifle with light palpation. This should not be confused with the normal cutaneous reflex present in every horse, where the patient will immediately move away from the stimulus. Once again, repeat palpation will help to reveal a true sacroiliac issue. Once a true discomfort is detected, it is usually seen on active gait assessment as a dropping of the pelvis on the same side as the lesion (which is discussed more fully later in point 3 of the section on Dynamic assessment).

Palpation of the abdomen and evaluation of the abdominal viscera is vital. Alongside a thorough palpatory exploration for masses, tenderness, edema, or any other abnormality, the osteopath should also perform a fine-tuned palpation of the healthy functioning of each organ, also taking into account its arterial supply, venous return, innervation, and lymphatic drainage.

Neck

Systematic assessment of the cervical spine includes palpation, passive motion testing, and specific active motion testing to form a working diagnosis.

Palpation of the horse's neck begins immediately cranial to the shoulder, and the practitioner should palpate for the markers of inflammation (heat, swelling, and tenderness), as well as for the overlying tissue elasticity and texture. The neck contains extensive fascial structures and dysfunction can quickly involve this fascial network, turning acute issues into more chronic somatic dysfunction. Identifying tension in the cervical region can be achieved by standing in line with the horse and assessing and comparing both sides of the neck simultaneously. Osteopaths usually describe a segment as dysfunctional on palpation if it feels hard. The author often has the impression that one segment doesn't belong to the horse when compared with the remainder of the cervical spine. Passive motion testing may follow the palpatory assessment. The author finds accessory movements to be particularly helpful in forming a specific diagnosis. This can be performed from the same position as palpation, with a translatory force applied laterally between the practitioner's hands. There should be a sense of give and fluidity in the tissues. A hard end feel or a boggy or restricted motion may be a sign that treatment is required. Careful attention should be paid to the ventral structures of the neck at this point of the assessment (in particular, the vascular supply and drainage and the freedom and balance between each side, the areas of dense lymphatic accumulations, the cartilaginous structures of the thyroid cartilage, trachea, and larynx, and the investing tissues surrounding the hyoid bone and its sling of connective tissue from the mandible and cranial base).

Generalized active motion is observed when the horse demonstrates a walk and trot (as discussed later); however, active assessment of the cervical spine can be checked at this point of the consultation by using a carrot or similar treat and asking the horse to flex laterally (side-bend) toward the point of each hip. A restriction here can be either a frank joint restriction (i.e., the horse is physically unable to yield and appears to have a "block" in the neck) or a reduction in the quality of the movement, which may be suggestive of a muscular or ligamentous issue. Horses will often evade this maneuver by tilting the head sideways before laterally flexing the neck. This is just as strong an indication for treatment as a frank restriction. Despite this being quite a crude test, it provides an insight into the function of the region and can be repeated following treatment to demonstrate to both the practitioner and the owner whether or not treatment was successful.

Head

Palpation of the horse's head needs to be performed with care and precision. Begin by palpating for abnormalities in the bony structures. By running a flat hand over the cranial bones, the practitioner is able to detect heat (a sign of inflammation), and irregular margins of bone (suggestive of trauma). It is important to watch for the horse's reaction during this assessment. The author finds that keeping a close watch of the horse's eye provides a good measure of comfort and helps to predict if the horse may react adversely. This assists with safety, as an indicator of pain, and a more comfortable horse will be more relaxed, making the tissues easier to assess. Assessment of the musculature over the frontal and temporal bone, and the mandible, can be useful to determine tensions that may be affecting the mechanics of the jaw. Alignment of the bite should be assessed by looking into the front of the cooperative horse's mouth, where the suture line of the maxillae and the mental suture (middle of the incisors) should form a vertical line. If a malalignment is detected, it is appropriate to involve an equine dental technician in the integrative management of the horse. The importance of the function and equilibrium between the poll, occiput-atlas-axis (OAA) joints, and temporomandibular joint (TMJ) and their influence on the equine bite cannot be underestimated as this region forms a functional junction for much of a horse's activities, including support and influence from the bridle. As such the area has an enormous impact on performance. The ligamentous connections between the TMJ and the cranial cervical region result in an interdependence of these two areas for optimal function. They also impact on the muscular sling between the hyoid bone and the sternum.

An osteopathic cranial assessment (OCF) is also performed at this point, palpating for the involuntary motion and quality of the primary respiratory mechanism of the horse, taking into account the fluid, vascular, membranous, and bony relationships, should the practitioner be familiar with this approach.

At this point the practitioner should have a thorough picture of the presenting complaint, and also have formulated a working diagnosis.

Dynamic assessment

It is this author's preference to perform the dynamic assessment after the palpatory evaluation. It provides an instant confirmation of the passive assessment, or if the gait analysis does not match the palpatory findings a reassessment can be made immediately prior to treatment commencing. This sequence of examination also ensures that the feet have been checked for heat, swelling, and inflammation. The sequence of evaluation, however, is flexible and can be performed in any order. In some circumstances it may be preferable to perform the active motion assessment prior to any hands-on evaluation; if the practitioner is concerned the horse should be referred for veterinary examination, as with cases of overt clinical lameness.

The dynamic assessment consists of many elements. In all movements, fluidity and symmetry of motion should be observed, together with limb flight and deviation.

It can be helpful to tailor the active assessment to highlight the symptoms that the handler reports, and so occasionally a ridden assessment or lunged evaluation may be helpful. On most occasions, however, the following assessment is sufficient:

1. Ask the handler to lead the horse in a straight line, at a walk, with a loose lead rope, on an even surface, so that the horse takes approximately 20 paces away and toward the practitioner. Further information on the horse's movement can be observed from the side, including the footfall and the head and neck posture. Note if the horse tracks up (i.e., the hind foot is placed where the forefoot was), overtracks, or is short-striding in any limb. This is most easily seen on a soft surface. Any abnormalities seen should reflect a dynamic representation of the restrictions palpated. The practitioner should watch for the head-bob of the horse during motion, most easily viewed from in front of the horse. The head-bob should be fluid in its motion and should normally

be symmetrical. Increased lifting of the head during weight-bearing is an indication of soreness in that forelimb. The author finds two of the most useful measures of a horse's soundness and overall function are the symmetry of its limb flight (best viewed from in front or behind) and symmetry of ground clearance of the feet (best viewed laterally) (Atkin 2013).

2. The same sequence should be performed at a trot. Many deviations from symmetry are more obvious in this gait. Some restrictions, however, can only be seen in one type of gait, and may be hidden during other movements of the horse. For this reason, it is important to assess both the walk and trot, and should a canter be required, assessment during lunging is normally more appropriate than seeing the horse ridden (when other factors caused by tack and rider may complicate the assessment).
3. Following a straight-line evaluation, the handler should turn the horse short around themselves, allowing assessment of the lateral flexibility of the musculoskeletal system. The horse should lead by flexing through the head and neck, and follow with the thorax and lumbar region, crossing the hind limbs under itself with each pace (the limb on the inside of the turn being placed in front of the outer limb). The whole movement should be smooth and comfortable. In many horses, this test will prove difficult, with a shuffling of the limbs or complete avoidance of this action, which can be strongly indicative of a restriction that requires attention. A horse with a cervical restriction will turn with the neck and whole body stiff or straight, with the head often failing to look in the direction of the turn. Also check for the ability of the forelimbs and hind limbs to perform a smooth movement, coordinated with each other. A dysfunction in the hind limb, pelvis or caudal lumbar spine is often seen in the horse as an inability to step fully underneath itself during the turn. The avoidance of this maneuver is usually a shuffling "side-stepping" motion. This and excessive tail swishing during the movement (which may indicate lumbar pain), may mean a closer examination of the lumbar spine is required.
4. The final aspect of the dynamic evaluation is asking the horse to back up a few paces. This is useful in assessing the flexibility of each hind limb and the lumbosacral region. This area needs to flex and extend through its range during this part of the test. Significant discomfort within the cervical spine can also produce a resistance to backing, as the movement requires a counterbalancing movement of the cervical region. A young horse, or one that has not been well schooled, may be confused by this test and appear to be resistant to it. This needs to be taken into consideration before assuming a dysfunction.

If the passive evaluation has been performed with a high degree of accuracy, the active evaluation will normally reflect the palpatory findings, and a working diagnosis can be reached. Once a working diagnosis has been formulated, a treatment plan can be devised.

Osteopathic treatment of acute cases

Treatment is a dynamic process, undergoing modifications within each consultation. It is a dialogue with the horse's tissues, the treatment plan remaining flexible so it can be adapted to the response seen and felt in the horse as the treatment progresses. An important aspect of this is the recognition that the practitioner has invaded the horse's "personal space" and therefore the approach and the palpatory interaction must respect the horse's response. A practitioner aware of this will move around the horse with ease, will recognize a safety issue before it becomes a problem, and ultimately will bring about a greater therapeutic change in the patient. This approach can be likened to the "old horsemen" interaction where the communication is constant between horse and horseman. From a health and safety point of view, it is the responsibility of the treating osteopath to ensure the safety of the horse, the handler, and themselves when performing all of the techniques described. At a minimum, this means always having the handler on the same side of the horse as the practitioner, and ensuring there is always an exit available that is closer to the people involved than to the horse.

Techniques available to equine osteopaths

There are many treatment techniques available for osteopaths to create change in a horse's tissues, including but not limited to:

- soft tissue massage and stretching techniques
- articulatory approaches
- high velocity manipulation
- indirect approaches, such as balanced ligamentous, membranous, or fascial tension techniques
- visceral approaches
- osteopathy in the cranial field (OCF) or biodynamic approaches (Pusey and Brooks 2010).

There are no devices used as an adjunct to treatment, and the osteopath's hands are the only facilitators for creating change and the subsequent tissue response. This sole reliance on palpation becomes an advantage, as feedback from the patient's tissues can be obtained continuously (DiGiovanna et al. 2005; Hartman 1996).

Techniques by region

The following section will provide examples of techniques used by the author (BA), that are designed for trained and experienced practitioners in this field, but it is by no means exhaustive. These techniques are intended to provide an introduction for the practitioner, who should then expand upon the techniques, applying basic principles to the region to be treated.

Cervical region

In the cervical region there is often muscle guarding of a soft tissue or joint injury. This will affect the control and communication of the horse through the reins. The ever-changing tensions through this area mean the horse must accommodate this, potentially predisposing to soft tissue strain. The rider may comment that the horse finds it difficult to perform lateral movement, also the responsiveness is reduced when asking for bending, or the horse may be tossing its head. A counterstrain technique is very useful for this presentation.

The practitioner stands to the affected side of the horse's neck and locates a tender point by palpating the cervical musculature for an area of localized tissue tension, hypertonic muscle (this feels like a gathering of tissue). Usually the horse will provide a subtle indication that this location is correct (by a change in its eye, flickering of the ears, or another body signal). The practitioner then places a steady, firm contact over the tender point within the hypertonic tissue. With the other hand, cradle the contralateral side of the muzzle, and laterally bend the cervical spine toward the practitioner (Fig. 5.21). This serves to crowd and shorten the tissue underneath the palpatory hand, which should become more comfortable for the horse. This position

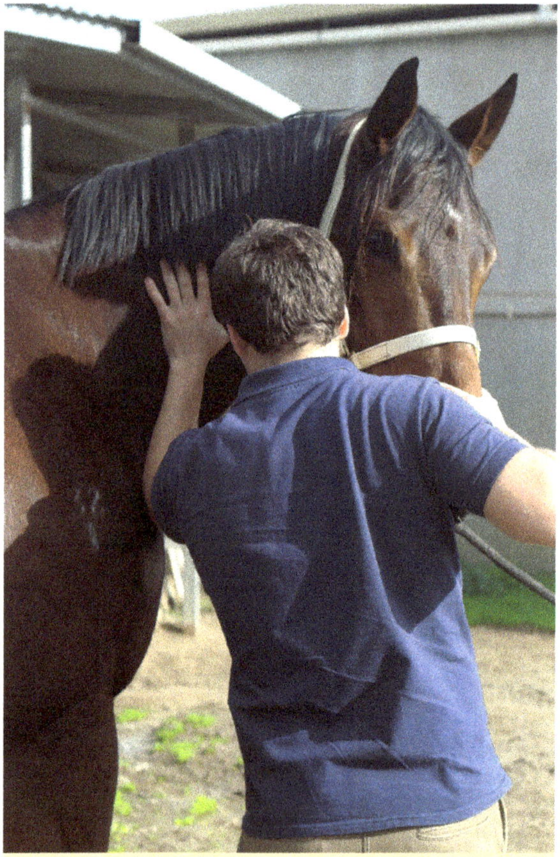

Figure 5.21
A counterstrain technique applied to the horse to release tension in the neck.

of ease can then be fine-tuned, and taken to a finer point of ease. Begin stacking other vectors such as slight flexion or extension of the cervical spine, using rotation or lateral translation, compression or distraction, or a combination of any of these vectors (Chila 2010a). Monitor the point of ease through palpation, the horse's body language, and observation of the horse's eye. The eye of the horse can provide information for many techniques, indicating the comfort level at that moment in time (Fig. 5.22). When applying the counterstrain effectively, the horse's eye should soften and look less stimulated. Occasionally the horse will appear to fall asleep. The pressure applied should remain unchanged until the tissue begins to yield and soften. Warmth is a feature that many osteopaths observe, as is a feeling of melting under the hand. It is always wise to retest the area following the treatment to ensure enough change has taken place.

Base of neck: anterior thorax

Working further caudally, in the author's experience, the thoracic inlet is an area that is essential for forelimb function, thoracic cage mobility, lung function, and therefore overall health. The rider may report a lack of extension in the forelimbs, resulting in a choppy action. Occasionally a description of girthiness also accompanies a dysfunction in this region. If a dysfunction is found in the fascial structures surrounding the thoracic inlet, the following technique may be useful.

The osteopath stands alongside the base of the neck. The best contact for treatment is one hand on the cranial portion of the sternum, and the other contact over the wither (Fig. 5.23). Applying slight compression between the hands can create engagement with the fascial structures, and tune into the compression that is often palpable resulting from past trauma, forelimb or cervical dysfunction, or some other mechanism. The practitioner can then use a fascial unwinding

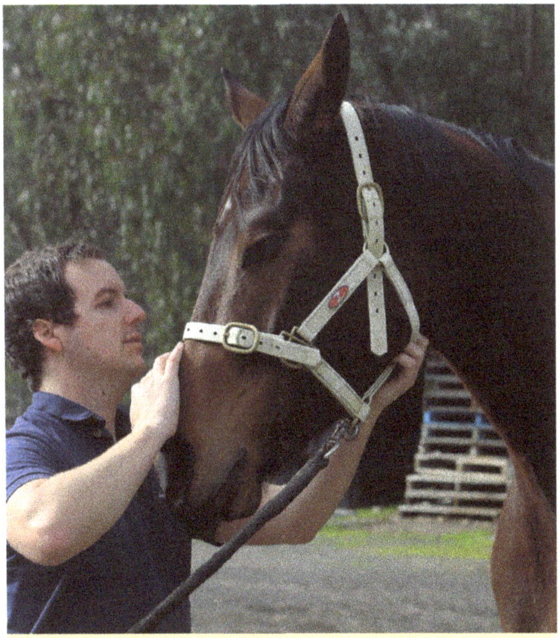

Figure 5.22
Monitoring the horse's eye helps to indicate the horse's comfort level. Here the eye is relaxed.

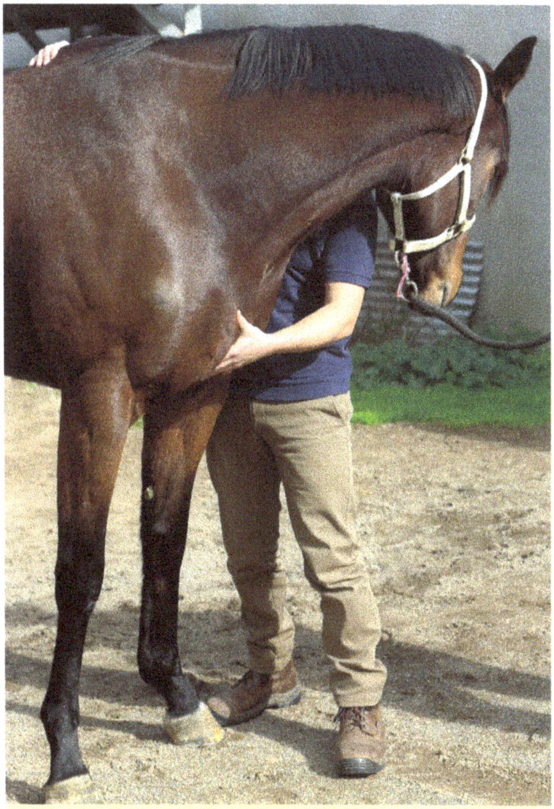

Figure 5.23
Treatment of the thoracic inlet. The osteopath applies gentle pressure between the front of the sternum and the withers.

approach or a balanced fascial tension approach, to address the strain pattern. Fascial unwinding follows the fascial tissues in the direction of ease. That means engaging the tissues and constantly correcting the position according to the tissue change that is continually evolving under the practitioner's hands. Ultimately a position of ease is detected, having facilitated an "unwind" of the fascial structures. Balancing fascial tension involves a balancing technique where the practitioner takes the tissues of the thoracic inlet to the relative position of balance, creating a fulcrum for the horse's tissues to initiate the reorganization process around this fulcrum (Chila 2010b). The practitioner waits and holds this fulcrum until the process has completed and a new neutrality is restored for the region.

Should these methods have limited success, or if the practitioner is having trouble engaging with the tissues, the least intrusive and most effective way of achieving effective change in an unresponsive thoracic inlet is to attempt to meet the compression within the tissues with the assistance of body weight. The practitioner stands in front of the horse and leans with a shoulder against the horse's sternum, palpating with the shoulder. The horse will push forward, and the practitioner can gently meet this compression leaning into the patient and perceiving the change through to the withers. This often feels as though the tissue slack needs to be gathered up and the compression met. Respiration will take over the process once this has occurred. This technique should not be limited by considering only fascial structures. Acknowledging and respecting the palpatory sense of function of the heart and lung, and their charge dynamic from this contact, will allow space for observation and deeper integration of changes throughout the horse. This technique is particularly effective if significant trauma has occurred, such as a fall cross-country or falling over a fence in showjumping. It is also hypothesized that this technique may be effective at releasing the shock in the tissues that often accompanies trauma, especially considering the proximity of the middle cervical sympathetic ganglia of the nervous system, located dorsally at the thoracic inlet (Furr & Reed 2015).

Forelimb: thorax

A method of treatment that can be applied to any region of the horse is a harmonic or articulatory technique. Articulation techniques are direct, where a short gentle pressure is directed toward a restrictive barrier. A repetitive motion is applied to the region to increase the range in all planes (DiGiovanna et al. 2005). Harmonic technique is defined as a rhythmic and cyclical motion of an object between two spatial positions, which brings on a state of resonance within the body (Lederman 2000). The author finds this approach particularly effective in the limbs, to increase the range and quality of motion. The same applies to the thoracic spine. The thoracic spine is an area that is under immense pressure due to the saddle and weight of the rider. Lying immediately beneath the spine are sensitive structures such as the thoracic paravertebral sympathetic ganglia and the continuation of the sympathetic chain (Furr and Reed 2015), and given horses remain instinctively and physiologically prey animals, this region is highly sensitive to changes in function of the corresponding vertebral segments. The respiratory and circulatory system and the cranial end of the gastrointestinal system also relate to the thoracic region, and the interplay between function at the spinal level and the visceral structure ventrally is significant.

In order to perform articulation techniques, the practitioner should be standing comfortably with access to the thoracic spine. It is often easier to treat this region with your hands at a comfortable height, which may necessitate standing on a box, as with many other areas of the body (Fig. 5.24). The technique is applied to the thoracic segments either broadly or very specifically between two segments. The applicators will change from a portion of the hand to a forearm depending on the target area (Fig. 5.25). Articulation should be performed toward the restrictive barrier, and a harmonic-type rhythmic impulse can serve to spring the ligamentous components surrounding the joint (Chila 2010c). The aim is to improve the range and quality of the motion while increasing the blood supply and fluid exchange within the joint capsule.

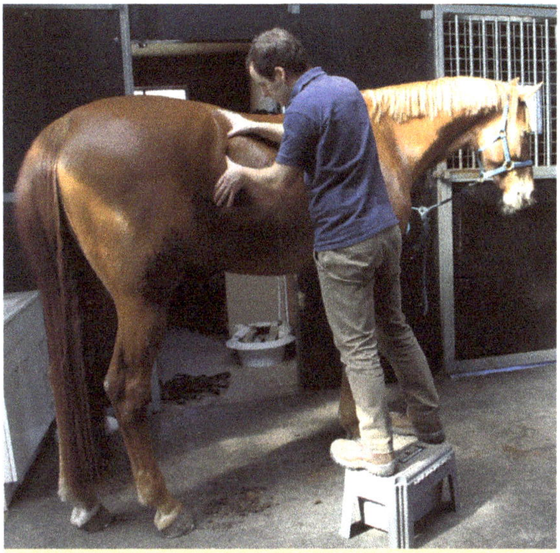

Figure 5.24
Treatments are most easily carried out with the hands at a comfortable level. The use of a box to bring the osteopath up to the height of the horse is an invaluable aid.

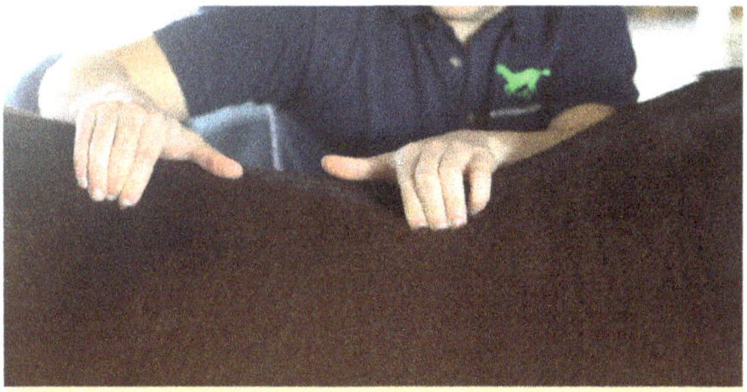

Figure 5.25
Performing articulation techniques on the thoracic spine.

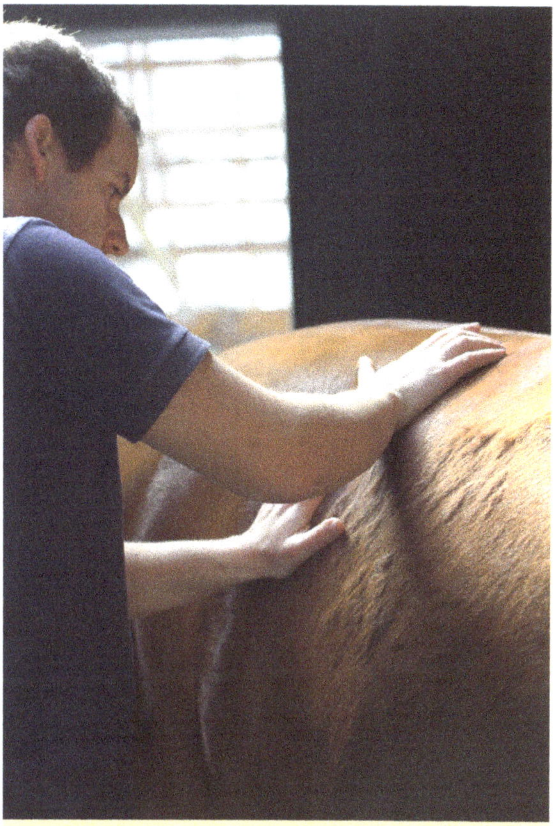

Figure 5.26
Balancing the ligamentous tension at the 18th rib.

Thoracolumbar area

Balanced ligamentous tension techniques can be extremely effective in the equine patient, with many applications. One such application is at the 18th rib, where one hand is placed over the angle of the rib, and the other is placed midshaft on the same rib (Fig. 5.26). Susan Turner (a preeminent teacher in this field of work) describes the technique on humans, where the practitioner synchronizes with each breath and gently encourages the 12th ribs laterally, only doing as much as the tissues will naturally yield on each outbreath, without creating any resistance or recoil in the tissues (Turner 2008). Although this description is for humans, the principle remains the same for equine patients, but with a change of focus to the 18th rib. This method facilitates disengagement and allows the rib to complete its therapeutic process. It may be necessary to support the rib in a variety of small vectors, to achieve an ultimate position of ease. Some clinicians describe the "dance" of the tissues immediately prior to a balance point being reached.

A variation on this technique is a change of intention to a balanced fascial tension technique applied to the thoracic diaphragm. The diaphragmatic fibers attach directly onto the caudal ribs, before blending with the cranial lumbar vertebral segments. This treatment can be performed using a change in depth of intention, or a slight variation on the previous contact, moving one hand to the opposite rib (Fig. 5.27). The completion of the technique can usually be recognized by a change in respiration rate or depth in the horse. This accompanies the fluid-like swelling change that infiltrates the tissues being treated. This method can be adapted to virtually any articulation in the horse, with extensive interconnections with tendon, fascia, muscle, nerve, blood, and lymphatic tissues in the limb. This is particularly useful considering the anatomy of the stay apparatus in the equine limb (Fig. 5.28).

Lumbosacral joint

A more direct method for releasing a joint is the high velocity, low amplitude thrust (HVLAT) technique. When applied with precision and speed this can be incredibly effective at releasing spinal facet joints and creating a reflex muscular relaxation via the corresponding spinal neurological loop. The HVLAT technique is described as a short rapid thrust, once the restrictive barrier is engaged. Care should be taken in a horse with articular hypermobility or significant pain, and HVLAT is contraindicated in cases of osseous or ligamentous disruption (Chila 2010d).

An example where HVLAT may be useful is treatment of the lumbosacral joint. This can be manipulated by asking the horse to lift a hind limb, and, while supporting the hind limb by the cannon bone, the practitioner can palpate through the limb into the lumbar region. It will often be found that the vector of force needs to be fine-tuned prior to delivering the manipulative thrust. A monitoring contact can be placed on the lumbar spine while the other hand provides the stacking for the vectors of motion to reach the point of barrier (Fig. 5.29). The thrust itself is administered after gently lifting the hind limb until a point of tension is palpated then a short, controlled impulse is applied dorsally, using both hands on the cannon bone, creating a local rotatory force at the level of the lumbosacral articulation. Often there is an audible cavitation accompanying improved mobility and increase in local blood supply. The joint that is targeted during this manipulation is the facet joint, and restriction in this

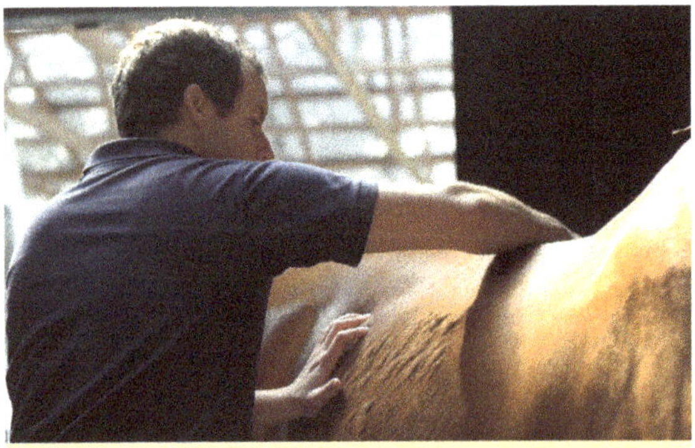

Figure 5.27
Progression from Figure 5.26 to involve the diaphragm.

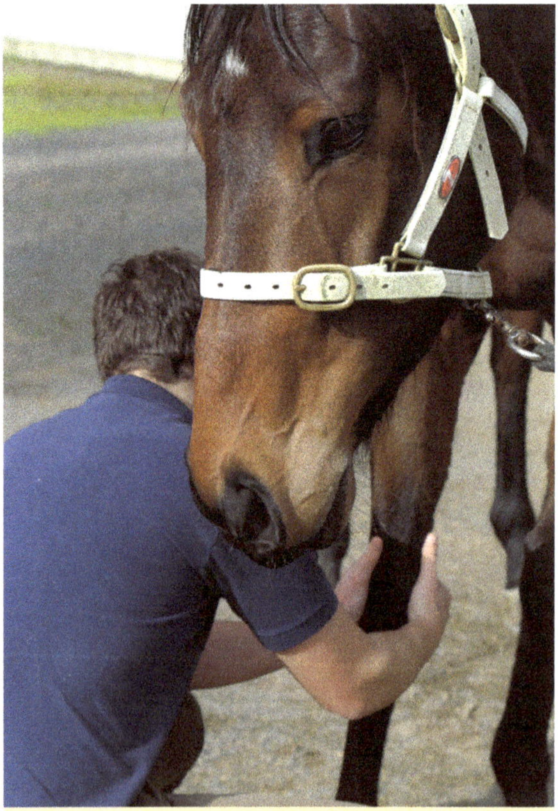

Figure 5.28
Balancing the tensions of the stay apparatus.

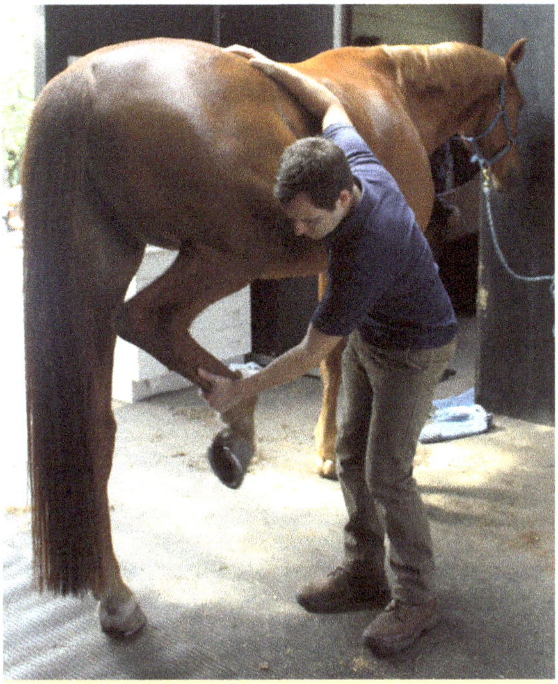

Figure 5.29
Applying a high velocity, low amplitude thrust to the lumbosacral region.

region can produce symptoms such as a lack of power in propulsion during jumping or a reluctance to move forward or track up in the hind legs. An astute rider may comment on the horse "bracing" underneath the rider, and dropping through a shoulder, becoming heavier on the forehand. This is a pain-avoidance mechanism for the horse, reducing local extension through the lumbar spine, so that the pain-sensitive joint is not aggravated. Pain in this area can also cause the horse to avoid stretching this articulation, losing the ability to collect in its gait, shortening the hind-limb stride, and resulting in an asynchronous action and lack of connection between the forelimb and hind limb.

Craniocervical junction

Another treatment approach available to the practitioner is osteopathy in the cranial field (OCF). This approach recognizes the subtle mechanics and fluids of the body, and utilizes the inherent forces for optimizing health, in order to create changes that will support normal function of the horse. The hallmark of the OCF approach is that it is respectful to the body, and administered gently, with a focus on a particular layer of tissue and fluid in order to facilitate interchange of fluids that will provide nutrition to every cell (Chila 2010e). Using osteopathy in the cranial field at the craniocervical junction can be particularly useful because of its close relationship with dural membranous attachments, the central nervous system, and blood supply and drainage from the skull.

The equine TMJ is utilized for most of the day for mastication as horses are natural grazers. The mandible also houses the bit when ridden. There is a strong link between the TMJ and the occipitoatlantal joint. During extension of the poll, the mandible glides caudally approximately 3–10 mm, with the opposite occurring during poll flexion (Liyou 2005). This rostrocaudal biomechanical interplay requires both of these structures to be functioning optimally. Embryologically, the mandibular portion of the first branchial arch and the cranial cervical spine vertebral segments develop together in very close proximity (Hartwig 2008). This intimate relationship appears to persist throughout life. For this reason, these structures can be treated as a unit using osteopathy in the cranial field.

In the case of the mandible-atlas relationship, the practitioner places a hand on each of these structures (Fig. 5.30) and draws attention to the space between both contacts, with the intention of bringing about the uninterrupted fluid loop through the mandible and the atlas. It is thought that finding a balance of the joints and tissues involved in preparation for this fluid technique, with balanced membranous and balanced ligamentous tension, can help to increase the potency of the fluid. The change in palpatory perception is often the only trigger required for the change to take place. During this technique the patient frequently responds on quite a deep level, with the horse significantly lowering its head toward the ground while the changes are taking place. Completion of the technique is noted when the loop appears to "connect up" and an expansion and occasionally warmth is palpated.

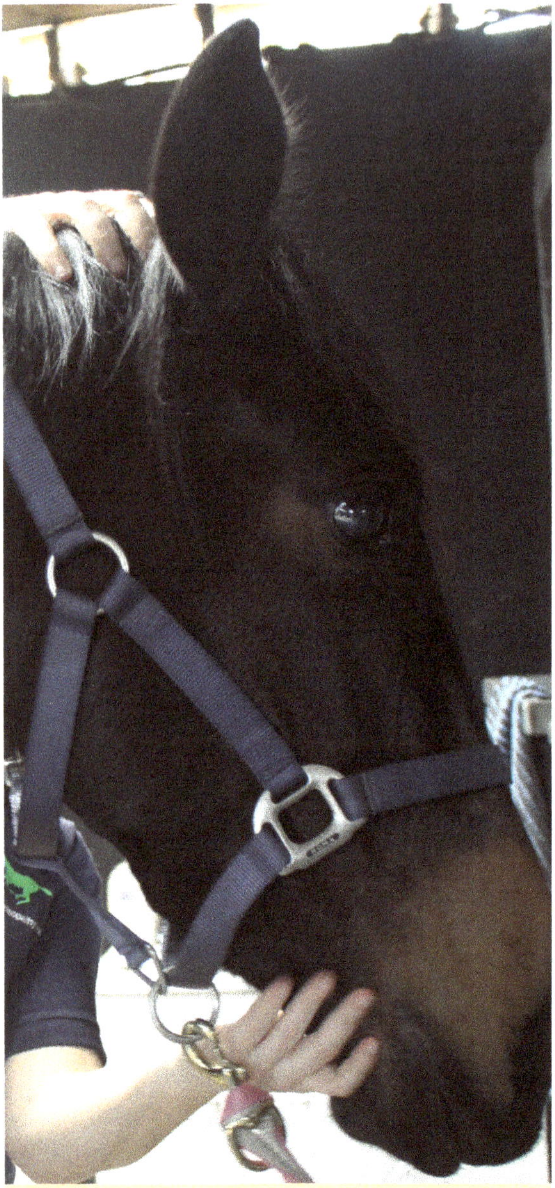

Figure 5.30
Cranial osteopathy applied across the mandible and atlas.

Although this is a description of a specific technique using OCF principles, the primary respiratory mechanism described in OCF and biodynamic osteopathy is engaged and utilized throughout the consultation regardless of the osteopathic approach applied.

When considering any of the above techniques, it is important always to engage osteopathic thinking and judgment for each horse treated. It is most effective not to be prescriptive when choosing techniques, but rather select a treatment technique or approach that will best suit the particular horse's tissue at that moment in time. Remain open to a flexible treatment plan as the horse responds to each technique.

An osteopathic approach to treating the chronic horse

Every aspect of equine work is fascinating and comes with its own challenges. Many horses present with chronic, long-standing problems, but the osteopath is often being asked to treat an acute episode on top of an underlying chronically compromised musculoskeletal system. Owners, riders, and trainers are often so focused on getting the horse back to work that they are unaware that these underlying issues are probably why the horse is struggling with the level of work it is being asked to carry out.

This section covers the assessment, treatment, and rehabilitation needed to return these patients to normal work. It is the single most challenging area of equine osteopathy, but also the most rewarding.

Due to the longevity of the presenting problems, taking an accurate case history is often not possible. In many cases the horse has changed hands several times or may have spent protracted periods away from the owner while in training. This means getting accurate details is very difficult, especially if the horse has injured itself in any way. Trainers are often reluctant to admit anything has happened to a horse while it has been in their care.

Obtaining the horse's veterinary history may help, although it is not always fully comprehensive. Often owners will also have sought nonveterinary treatments for musculoskeletal issues, being unaware of the need to contact their own vet first.

Observation and palpation of the chronically injured horse are therefore critical, along with the need to work alongside a veterinary surgeon in order to treat these cases, as most will require intravenous sedation in order to relax enough to work with the osteopath. Many of these cases may require a treatment under a general anesthetic in order to unravel the complex soft tissue tension patterns held within the myofascial structures before the horse can be successfully rehabilitated back into work.

These cases will be referred from primary care veterinary clinics and also from secondary referral practices. They will often have carried out extensive examinations and lameness workups as well as radiography and nuclear scintigraphy. Colles et al. (2014) found the results of these different procedures rarely match closely with the symptom patterns and clinical signs of the patients.

The use of infrared thermal imaging, when used under strict clinical conditions, has been shown to highlight irritation through the sympathetic nervous system via subcutaneous blood flow (Holst 2000; Vollmer and Möllmann 2010), and this has been used successfully in the horse (Colles and Brooks 2011) (Fig. 5.31A and B).

The whole process of applying osteopathic principles to treat the chronic horse requires a different mind-set to that for the acute patient. The vast majority of these cases will have to be withdrawn from any form of work. They will need to be allowed freedom to move, yet not enough space that they can get up to any serious mischief. The exact amount of space is not easy to determine. For some they can happily graze and behave in a paddock comprising of several acres. For others a few square metres are all they need in order to fall over or get caught up in something.

Owners will often have their own impression of what constitutes a small space. There was one memorable occasion when the vet and author (TN) explained the need for the horse to be turned out to grass in a small area. The owner said that they had a small paddock that would suit. This turned out to be 10 acres and the horse in question got up to plenty of mischief before the problem was addressed.

Osteopathic evaluation of chronic cases

Static observation

When viewing the stationary horse, it is a useful tip to divide it mentally into three distinct sections when looked at from the side:

1. the head, neck, and forelimb
2. the thorax
3. the lumbar region, pelvis, and hind limb.

Decide whether the three areas all look in proportion to each other. Are one or more areas overdeveloped or underdeveloped? This, more than anything else, will give you a good idea as to how the horse moves, and its general condition, along with the longevity of its movement problems (assuming that this is why you are being asked to look at it).

Next, perform a cursory overview of the horse before focusing on the finer details. Look at the way the horse stands, the general musculoskeletal development, and the condition of the coat. Note the eyes and any telling signs from the body language as to the state of the individual. Note the breathing, and whether you can hear anything that might suggest difficulty or congestion.

The first third (head, neck, and thorax)

The head. View the head from the front and then each side. Assess the position of the head in relation to the neck.

1. Is the nose stuck out, with the occiput-atlas (OA) joint held in extension, or is the chin tucked in, creating a flexed resting state for the OA joint?
2. Is the head rotated or laterally flexed?
3. Is the mandible relaxed or held tense?
4. Are there any marks or scars to the head, ears, or face, including around the mouth where biting issues can arise?
5. Are the nostrils level or asymmetric in size and position?

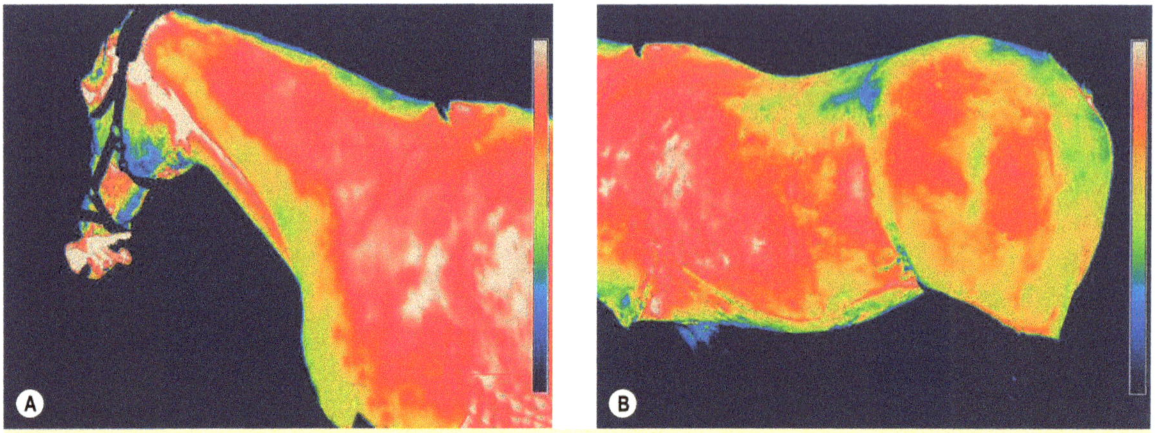

Figure 5.31
(A) An infrared thermogram of the front of a horse showing a normal image. The jugular groove is slightly cooler (yellow) than the upper neck. There is a band of increased temperature at the back of the mandible (white). (B) An infrared thermogram of the hind end of a horse showing significant cooling over the spine in the posterior thoracic and lumbar regions and over the middle gluteal and semitendinosus muscles.

6. Look at the frontals for symmetry and size of muscling and check for any fascial tethering to the skin and hair.
7. What facial expression does the horse have? Is it relaxed, nervous, tense, or angry? Look at and around the eyes for signs.

The neck

1. From in front look for any scoliosis. From each side look at the muscling and the shape of the neck, and compare the top line with the throat structures.
2. Is the neck evenly muscled?
3. Is the neck heavily muscled with a smooth top line running from the occiput down through the withers and into the thoracic top line, or is there underdeveloped muscling dorsally with much more bulk ventrally, giving a camel-like appearance? Do the throat structures appear tense?
4. Are there any scars, lumps, or bumps visible?
5. What is the condition of the coat, and are there any signs of patchy sweating?

Shoulders and forelimb. When viewing this region it is essential not only to assess each of the limbs, but also to compare left with right. The observer should view from the side, in front, and from behind the horse, as some conformation anomalies will be easier to see from different perspectives.

Standing back, and to the side of the horse, view the lateral conformation of the shoulder and forelimb. Are the limbs straight, or is the stance one where the limbs are camped out (anterior to the vertical line), or camped under (posterior to the vertical line)? Once you have assessed this then you can break your observation down into component parts as follows:

1. Look for the outline contours of the scapula. Are they clearly defined? What muscling is evident? Can you see the spine of the scapula itself and if so is there any visual evidence of past trauma, such as a break or deviation in the line of the spine?
2. Is there evidence of fascial tethering over the scapula and periscapula soft tissues? What is the skin tone and condition like?

3. Immediately cranial to the dorsal aspect of the scapula does the neck meet at the withers in a smooth line, or is there a dip followed by a sharp rise with the muscles attaching to the spinous processes of the most cranially palpable dorsal vertebrae?
4. Following the line of the scapula downward assess the outline of the shoulder joint and the associated muscles. Triceps can appear overdeveloped or underdeveloped in relation to the other muscles. Very often there will be a greater difference in one limb, therefore it is essential to compare the two.
5. As you look further down the distal limb assess the elbows for size, conformation, scars, and discoloration before looking further down the length of the radius and ulna. Look for any changes to the contours of the soft tissues and skin, paying particular attention to the tendons and any evidence of soft tissue swellings and edema.
6. View the limbs from in front and above, and look down for any splints, which can be seen as small raised areas of skin and hair on the lateral or medial aspects of the cannon bone.
7. Moving more distally note the shape and size of the coronary band and fetlock, and assess the pastern angle. At the same time, check for any signs of hair loss, swellings, or lumps and bumps which can signify foreign bodies, mud fever, or trauma.
8. Looking at the foot itself, note the size, shape, and wear patterns. Is the foot trimmed or shod? Look at the length of the toe and also any indications of altered hoof growth patterns when looking at the growth rings. Just like growth rings on a tree these can be indicative of altered health states over time.

When viewing from in front, look at the relationship of each section of the limb and note if there is any rotation, valgus, or varus conformation. Bear in mind that a young horse or foal may well show signs of these. Development of the chest at four and seven years old can cause some medial rotation of the forelimbs (more marked in the heavier breeds). Look at the loading through the foot. Then compare what you see with the other forelimb.

The middle third (thorax)

View the thorax from both sides as well as from in front and from behind the horse. Look at the overall shape and ask yourself if it is representative of the breed or mix of breeds. A narrow-chested thoroughbred or a barrel-chested cob would not be considered as being a problem as long as the overall condition, weight, conformation, and muscling are within healthy ranges.

1. View the top line from the withers caudally. Ideally there should be a smooth line with even muscling. Hollowed-out areas over the caudal portion of the trapezius should be noted, as this indicates a horse with movement issues. If this is present, ask the owner if you can see the saddle fitted, but also note that a horse with an altered gait will often cause a saddle to impinge on this part of the trapezius muscle. Note any dipping along the top line as you view it caudally. Also look for any hair loss or whitening of the hair. This occurs if there has been repeated or excessive pressure directly over these spots.
2. Look for any lumps or bumps and cast your eye over the ribs, paying attention to the rib angles and the quality and size of the muscling longitudinally, before assessing the rest of the rib cage. Note whether or not you can actually see the rib outlines, and if these are clean and free of any signs of previous trauma. Look at the symmetry of the rib cage itself, and whether it is held in any degree of rotation or lateral flexion around its longitudinal axis. Note any hair loss or discoloration.
3. Look at the ventral part of the chest. Assess the size and position of the pectoral musculature and the weight-bearing position through the thoracic sling. Note whether the outline of the sternum is visible, and if it appears to run in a straight line craniocaudally.

4. From a lateral aspect view the ventral surface of the thorax and look for any sagging of the chest or visible tension. Do the structures look sucked in where the thoracic diaphragm attaches? Note any swelling or apparent edema at this level.

The hind third

When viewing this area one needs to assess whether it merges seamlessly with the middle third of the horse or not. Looking caudally along the top-line musculature, note the tone, size, and evenness of the longissimus dorsi. Are the loins sucked in or rotund, creating the impression of a barrel on legs? Becoming more specific, work your way visually through each area that you can see.

1. From a lateral view examine the top line of the lumbar spine. Note any roaching (arching) or dipping of the back in this region, any lumps or bumps, or any signs of trauma.
2. Assess the size and development of the quadratus lumborum muscles bilaterally. If these appear unusually large they may well indicate an altered gait.
3. Are the tubera sacrale the highest points? If so this usually indicates poor gluteal muscling. Note their symmetry. This is best done from behind the horse.
4. Viewing the rest of the pelvis from various angles look for symmetry and check the positions of the tuber coxae and hip joints. Note any scars or obvious muscle wastage.
5. Looking at the hind limbs note their position in relation to the rest of the horse. Are they very straight, camped under, or back? Stand back and compare with the forelimb positions, and whether the horse stands square or keeps shifting its weight between each limb. Look for any valgus or varus within the horse's conformation. (Hind limbs usually rotate laterally slightly in the normal horse.)
6. Look at the muscle development of the proximal part of each hind limb. This is best viewed from several angles. Note from a posterior view point whether the lateral aspect of the limbs appear well muscled or hollowed out. From a lateral view note any fascial tension, and also whether the TFL appears tight.
7. View the hamstrings and note whether their origin is clearly defined. Look at their size and development and compare them with the quadriceps mechanism on the anterior aspect of each limb.
8. View from an anterolateral angle, assess the stifle and patella position. In particular look for any signs of previous trauma or surgical intervention. Note the size of the joint and compare bilaterally.
9. From a posterior view note the size, symmetry, and resting state of the adductor muscles. From this position also note the orientation of the hind limbs through their vertical axis and note if one limb is held in more rotation than the other. Also note their positions relative to the midline of the horse.
10. Assessing the distal part of the limb note the contours of the tendons and bony structures. Note any marks, scars, and swellings, along with any hair loss. Compare joint sizes between each hind limb.
11. Note the pastern angles before viewing the foot. Move around so that you can trace the hoof wall outline, assess the size and shape of the feet, and see if the horse is standing squarely on each foot. Note the load bearing, if the toes are long or short, and what state the heels are in. If the feet are shod also note nail marks and shoe positioning along with any differences in toe clip positions and heel development.
12. Note the position and carriage of the tail. Does it hang straight down or away from the horse, and is it held lateral to the midline? Is the tail held still during your observation?
13. If you can see underneath the tail look for tension to the perineum, and whether there appears to be good integrity to the anal sphincter and genitalia

(female). If the horse's stance is wide enough look along the ventral line of the linea alba to see if it deviates at all. For geldings and stallions look for any abnormality around the genitalia.

Observation of controlled movement

For the purposes of assessing how the horse can move it is essential to perform a series of controlled procedures that make it virtually impossible for the horse to disguise any difficulty with moving in a normal, unimpeded way.

Observe the horse in walk and trot in straight lines on an even, flat surface and then turning in a tight circle around a handler before being asked to rein back. If we are undecided after seeing these maneuvers we can have the horse lunged. When observing the chronic horse, remember that some of these animals have been adapting their movements to cope with various mechanical impairments for several years, and often do not show any signs of pain or discomfort. They are very rarely "lame" in the normal sense of the word.

Be aware that the environment in which you observe the horse moving can affect what you see. Weather conditions, the proximity of other horses or animals, and even traffic can alter the way the horse behaves and make it very difficult to assess properly.

The handler must be able to follow simple instructions. It will amaze you how few can actually do this without guidance.

Although osteopaths talk about wanting to see symmetry, this can lead to all sorts of problems if we aim for this above wanting to see freedom of movement throughout the entire patient's body. No patient will ever be totally symmetrical, and if we were to find one it would probably struggle to perform! Therefore, when viewing the chronic horse please bear this in mind and realize that what we want to achieve is smooth, fluid movement, with all soft tissues and bony structures contributing and working as they should.

Examination of walk

Position yourself so that you can watch the horse walking away from and then back toward you. Once you have assessed it from this angle, then move so that you watch it from a lateral perspective. In each case you will be looking at how the horse moves as well as watching its body language as it moves and how it behaves toward the handler when asked to perform each test.

Posterior viewing. Watch the pelvis and gluteal muscles and limb flight as the horse walks away from you. Note if the pelvis rotates to allow the hind limb to protract in its suspension phase, or whether it laterally flexes via the lumbar spine causing the hind limb to travel in a horizontal arc in protraction before swinging medially in retraction. Look at what the tail is doing, and whether the root is held to one side or even alternates from left to right rather than hanging centrally. Note also if the horse swishes the tail or raises it (be aware that in some breeds it is considered a good trait to raise the tail in work).

If the ground surface is dry and loose, note any dust kicked up, and listen to each footfall (Fig. 5.32).

Note whether you can see the head, neck, and ears from behind, and if so whether they deviate laterally and/or show rotation. Note the state of the perineum and whether it moves cranially and caudally as the horse moves.

Anterior viewing. Watch the head carefully. What are the ears, eyes, and nostrils doing? Check if the mandible is held tight or if there is freedom of movement, or even excessive movement. Check for any scoliosis in the neck. Look at the thoracic sling and whether this moves with freedom and symmetry. Note whether the forelimb flight is straight or whether the limbs dish.

Look for symmetry of body roll and excessive body roll.

Lateral viewing. From the side it is much easier to assess stride length, symmetry and length of limb movement, and any areas of increased soft tissue

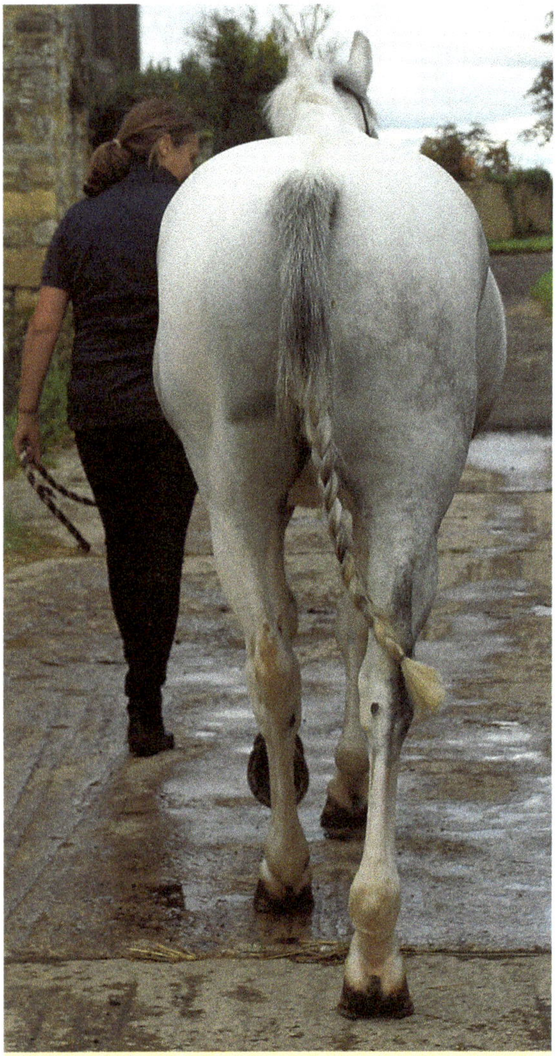

Figure 5.32
Watching the horse being walked away. Try to stand directly behind the horse, which should be walked in a straight line.

tension. In really chronic, fibrotic cases it is possible to see fascial binding around the periscapular structures, in the quadriceps and gluteal muscles, and along the top line in the longissimus dorsi muscles.

It is also possible to see which limbs are providing forward propulsion (Fig. 5.33).

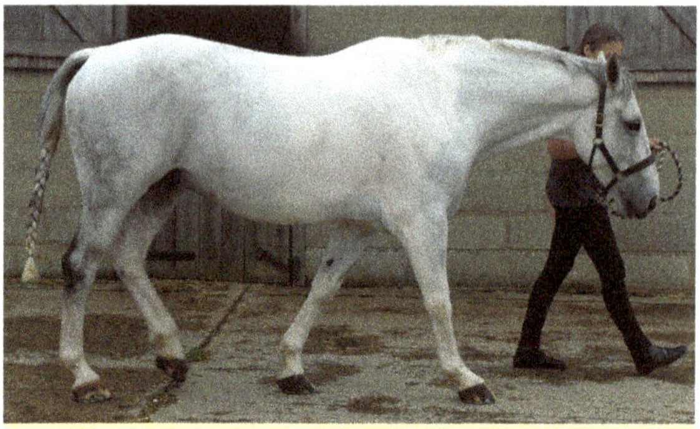

Figure 5.33
Watching the walk from the side of the horse allows assessment of stride length and gives better indication of which limbs are providing forward propulsion.

Examination of trot

- Look from posterior, anterior, and lateral viewing points.
- Watch how the horse transitions from walk into trot. Does it hop or jump with one forelimb? What do the head and neck do? Some horses will hop and raise their head in order to throw a forelimb forward in its cranial phase. Look for any anxiety in the facial features. Note any swishing of the tail and whether it is held high or to one side.
- Watch the flight of each limb and assess overall movement. Note where movement appears to originate from, and also where areas of stiffness arise.
- Watch what the main trunk of the body does, and whether you can see more of the rib cage swinging laterally to either side when viewing the horse from the front or from behind (Fig. 5.34).

Note: try not to be drawn to one joint or muscle. This is easily done, and can render the osteopath blind to the causative reason for the horse not moving correctly.

Turning short

In this maneuver, ask the handler to turn the horse in a tight circle around themselves, with the handler

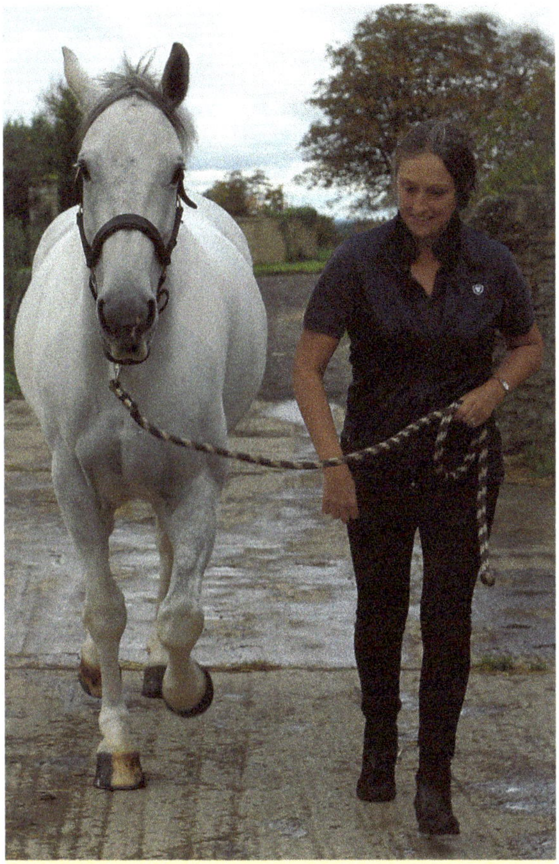

Figure 5.34
Watching the horse being trotted. Again the horse should be trotted in a straight line, and is best observed from directly in front.

standing at the center of the circle facing the horse's shoulder. The horse is encouraged to step forward and laterally flex around the handler or even to turn with the inner front leg on the same spot as the center of the turn. If it can achieve this comfortably it will be able to rotate the head and neck around the axis (C2), rotate and laterally flex the rest of the cervical spine, laterally flex the trunk, and cross the inside hind limb over in front of the outside hind. Watch both facial expression and what the tail does during these turns to the left and to the right as well as any flicking of the head and snorting (Fig. 5.35).

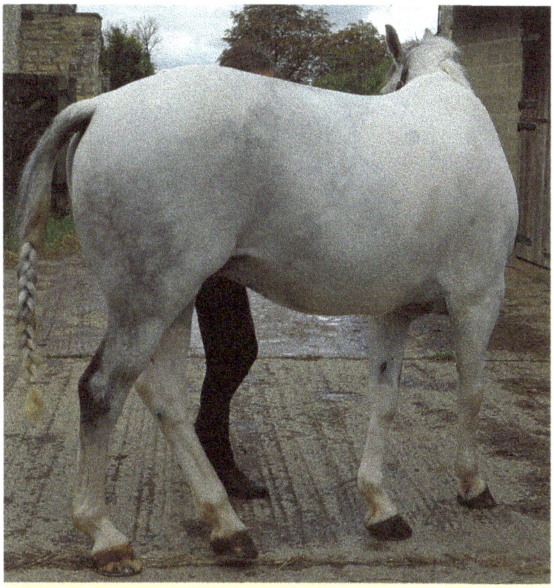

Figure 5.35
The horse should be "turned short" to the left and right.

Rein back

With the horse standing square get the handler to ask the horse to walk backward slowly. Watch for ease and symmetry of movement, along with the ability to move each limb evenly. Watch the individual foot placement. Note what the back does - does it dip or roach? Again, note the facial expression and any tail movement or snorting (Fig. 5.36).

Palpation

With the majority of chronic cases palpation is best performed once the horse has received intravenous sedation. The true chronic cases will resent palpation while fully conscious, and at best will guard against it, rendering the osteopath's ability to feel tissue quality very difficult. Sedation is fast acting and allows the osteopath to assess tissue quality and joint motility quietly, and to a much finer degree than with the fully alert horse.

As with all palpation it is best to have a routine that you stick to. As with all other animals, try not to

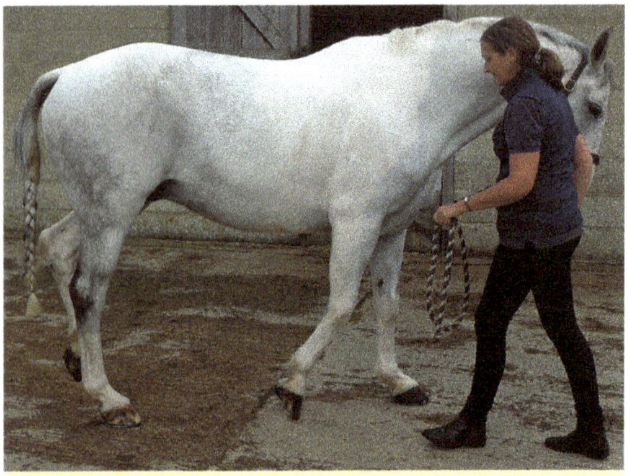

Figure 5.36
Moving the horse backward. This is a movement seldom performed by many horses, but it can provide a lot of evidence of movement problems.

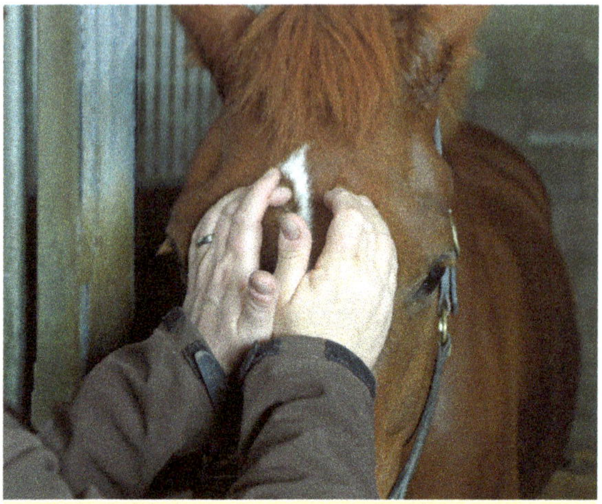

Figure 5.37
Palpating the temporal and frontal (interscutularis) muscles.

jump from one part of their body to another, which may surprise or alarm them. Be particularly aware that a sedated horse can react to this without giving the normal warning signs that a conscious horse will give.

The sedated patient should be examined and treated in a stall or box that has adequate rubber matting or thick bedding placed upon an even dry floor. This ensures that if the patient drops onto a knee it doesn't cause any damage. Before beginning the examination the author would suggest placing a hand on the horse's shoulder as a way of introducing yourself.

Head

The sedated horse can still be sensitive, so it is important that you position yourself safely to avoid getting injured. If the horse is sleepy it may well lower its head. Ensure that you are not standing over it when you begin your examination.

Begin with feeling the temporalis muscles - their size and resting tension (Fig. 5.37). Trace the outline and note any signs of trauma. Due to the position of the head on a long neck, as well as the activities they are expected to carry out, it is not uncommon to find signs suggesting past trauma which can give clues to the horse's present condition.

Next check the temporomandibular joint. This synovial joint allows for opening, closing, and lateral movement of the mandible when masticating food. There is also protraction when the head is flexed ventrally and retraction when the head is flexed dorsally while the horse is moving, due to the various muscle attachments and mechanics of this region.

Feel for symmetry around the cranium, the ears, and then rostrally along the nasal bones. Note any deviation and the size and shape of the nostrils. It is worth noting that horses can fracture their maxillae, and careful palpation should allow the osteopath to feel for any such previous trauma.

Feel along both sides of the mandible and the attachments and size of the masseter muscles.

Palpate the floor of the mouth and the ventral aspect of the mandible. Compare both sides as it is not uncommon to discover healed fractures or dental anomalies, and not just in the younger horse.

The neck

As your hands trace up the caudal aspect of the vertical ramus of the mandible, they will approach the gap created by the occiput and the wings of the atlas. Check for both symmetry and depth of this gap. Note whether cranial neck muscles appear enlarged and at what angle the OA joint sits, i.e., is the head held in extension or flexion?

Then allow your hands to trace caudally over the axis and again note both the position and orientation in relation to the OA joint and C3. This region of the horse is critical to how it can function from a biomechanical point of view.

Trace the outline and orientation from C3 to about C6. How far caudally you can palpate depends on the breed and condition of the patient. In most cases you can palpate the cranial part of C6.

The natural orientation of the equine cervical spine is such that the C1 and C2 present in dorsal flexion, whereas the main body of the cervical spine is in ventral flexion with the vertebral bodies much more ventrally placed within the neck itself.

Note the shape and tension within the nuchal ligament as well as muscle development. Apparent overdevelopment of the brachiocephalicus and sternocephalicus, amongst other muscles, can indicate an altered or adapted gait.

Ventrally trace from the floor of the mouth in a caudal direction. Note the position and orientation of the hyoid. Due to its muscle attachments and function this is a particularly important piece of the jigsaw, just as it is in human osteopathy (Fig. 5.38).

Moving in a caudal direction feel and note the soft tissues and the resting orientation of the entire neck. Although the sedated horse may hold the head and neck lower than when fully awake, this will not alter the overall orientation, and any lateral flexion, rotation, or general dorsal or ventral flexion will still be apparent.

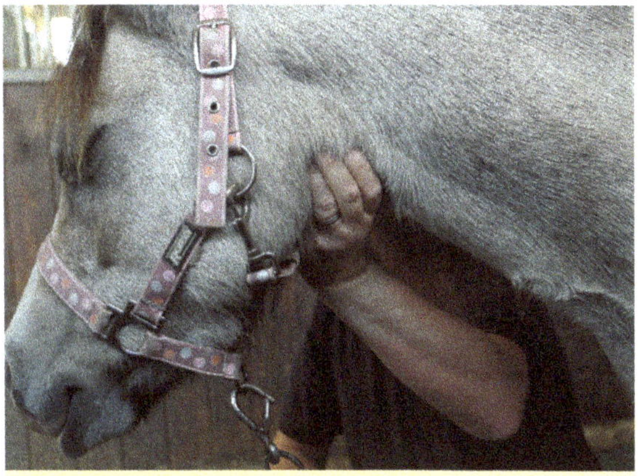

Figure 5.38
Palpating the hyoid apparatus.

Cervicothoracic spine

The cervicothoracic (C/T) junction lies deep within the thoracic sling. It is not possible to palpate it directly; however, the osteopath can get an idea of its orientation and mobility by taking contact with one hand over the spinous processes at the apex of the withers and placing their other hand ventrally on the cranial part of the sternum. Try to compress this area between both hands, and you should be able to feel "give" through this mass, indicating a cervicothoracic junction that is mobile. If it feels as if you are squeezing concrete, this would suggest a C/T junction that is not moving freely (Fig. 5.39).

You can also assess weight-bearing through the thoracic sling apparatus by standing at an oblique angle cranial to the shoulder and gently rocking the horse slightly in a lateral direction left and right.

The C/T junction is another critical point where normal function is required for the horse to move freely throughout. In the "chronic" horse, movement here is often restricted. Mechanically any restriction will affect forelimb action, as well as head and neck movement, when the horse moves. It can also have a bearing on grazing bias if there is a rotational element as well. From a neurological viewpoint this area is the autonomic gateway to the head, neck, and forelimbs.

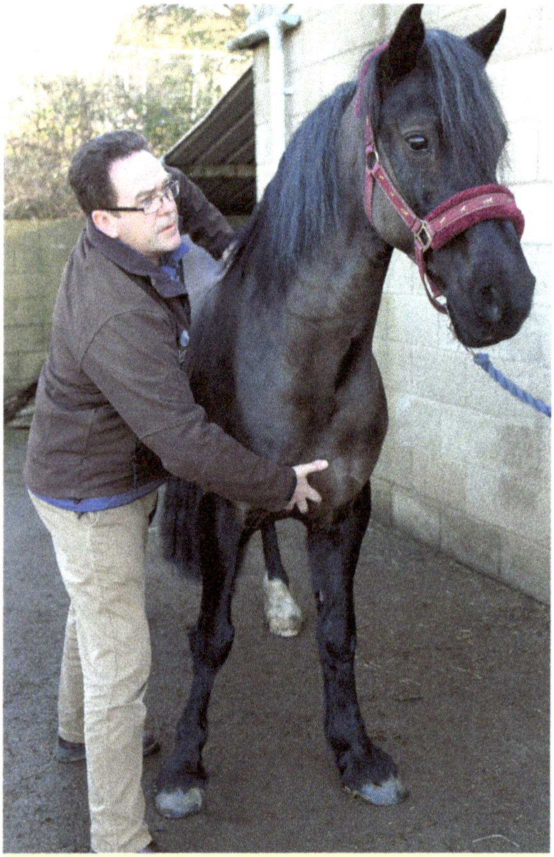

Figure 5.39
Palpation of the cervicothoracic junction. There should be a feeling of give between the two hands.

Impaired movement through this area does show up well on thermography when performed under strict clinical conditions.

The shoulders and forelimbs

Trace around the outline of the scapulae. Note the size and distribution of muscling, especially with regard to the supraspinatus and infraspinatus muscles. Note whether you can easily feel the spine of each scapula and check the overall orientation and height (Fig. 5.40). If one scapula is higher than the other this could denote the limb is taking more weight, or that the muscle attachments have less tone than those on the other side.

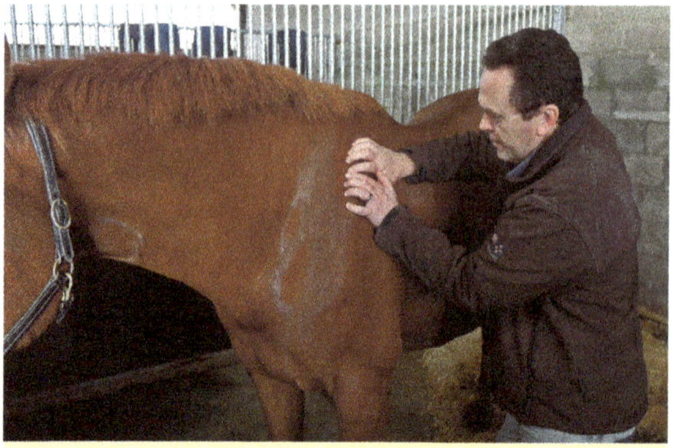

Figure 5.40
Palpation of the scapula should include assessment of the size and tension in the supraspinatus and infraspinatus muscles.

From your visual observations you will have noted limb orientation. Now feel each muscle and trace tendons and bony landmarks to assess for signs of previous injuries or present conditions. Heat and swellings in the limbs of the equine patient are common and can indicate compromised movement elsewhere in the horse.

Please note that when palpating the sedated horse it is unwise to try raising any of the limbs. Not only can they be unsteady, but if they don't want you performing such a task they can kick out at lightning speed with no warning.

Thoracic and lumbar spine

The cranial part of the thoracic spine is buried deep between the scapulae. Depending on the state of the nuchal ligamentous attachments you will be able to feel either the T3 or T4 spinous process cranially. Remember that from T1 through to T16 the dorsal spinous processes point caudally, whereas caudal to this through to the lumbosacral junction they point cranially. The thoracic vertebrae from T2 to T16 have facet joints allowing for some rotation and limited lateral flexion between approximately T9 to T14. Around T16 the facet joints alter their orientation to face relatively medially. Generally ventral and dorsal flexion is limited due to the attachment of the ribs and the shape and orientation of these facet joints.

When palpating this region note muscle development and symmetry caudal to the withers. Poor muscling here will denote impaired movement. Feel either side of the dorsal spinous processes, as the supraspinous ligament is wide throughout its length. Note any changes along its course and any signs of sensitivity in the patient to light pressure.

Trace the ribs and compare muscling dorsal to their angles. Remember that horses have 18 pairs of ribs. Also note that your patient may be sensitive around its girth, along the ribs themselves, and the intercostal muscles. Tracing the 18th rib in a dorsal direction will help you to locate T18.

Palpate the ventral surface of the chest and note the size, tension, and symmetry of the pectoral muscles. Be aware that some horses can be ticklish around this area, even when sedated. Trace along the sternum, and note any scarring or edema.

The lumbar spine should be well covered in muscle; however, if the quadratus lumborum is overdeveloped this can indicate an altered gait. In the lumbar spine each of the six vertebrae has an interlocking facet joint that creates a very sturdy structure capable of transmitting forces longitudinally when the horse moves.

The lumbosacral junction is where most ventrodorsal flexion occurs and there should be a relatively larger space between the dorsal spinous processes of L6 and first sacral segment than either side of this junction.

The pelvis and hind limbs

From the lumbosacral junction, move your hands over the cranial part of the ilia to the tubera sacrales. Note their levels and orientation cranial and caudal to each other. In a healthy horse in work there should be large enough gluteal muscles either side to make this point a slight depression. In the compromised horse this is very often the highest palpable point of the hindquarters.

As you trace the outline of the pelvis note any lumps and bumps and the degree of muscling on each side. If you stand directly behind the sedated horse you should be able to reach around each side of the pelvis to compare symmetry and orientation, but note that this is another area that can elicit a defensive response from the patient. By placing your extended index fingers on the outer edges of the tuber coxae you will get a good impression as to whether one half of the pelvis is more cranial than the other (Fig. 5.41).

Note the feel around each of the hip joints before moving caudally and locating each of the tuber ischii. Dorsal to these you can palpate the segments making up the tail. Usually there are 18 tail vertebrae.

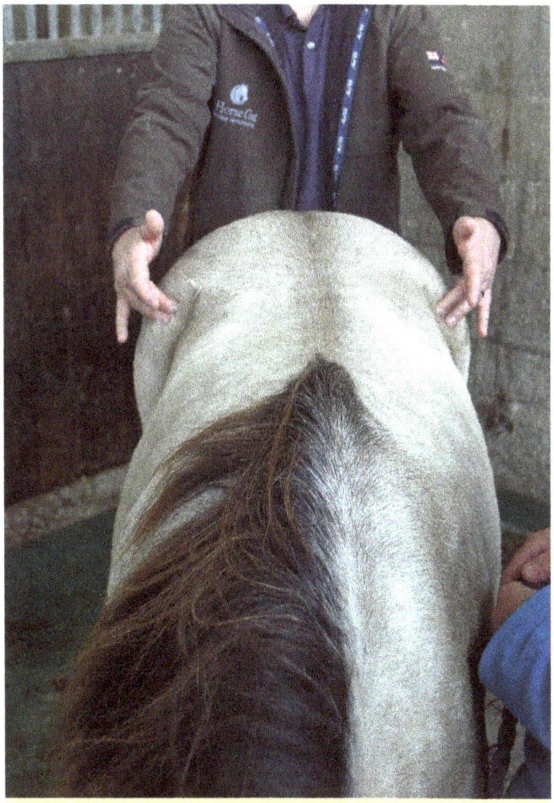

Figure 5.41
By palpating the dorsal aspects of the tubera coxae it is possible to assess how the pelvis is positioned.

Moving down the hind limb, check for all of the usual signs of previous trauma or present conditions. Note any edema around joints or along tendons and any abnormal heat. Be sure to place yourself safely so that you can avoid getting hurt if the horse kicks out suddenly. Be particularly careful when palpating around the stifle and patella. When placing a hand to palpate the medial structures of the limb, be aware that many horses resent palpation in this area, especially when you are assessing the adductor muscles.

Moving distally, the hamstrings are often overdeveloped in many of the chronic horses, and the texture of the muscles is often rather fibrous and unyielding when compared to the normal horse.

Check around the hip joint, then moving in a distal direction feel for the tension and quality of the iliotibial band (ITB). Moving further down the limb, assess the condition of each of the hocks and compare them. Note any heat, lumps or bumps, and scarring.

The distal part of the limb from this point comprises tendons, ligaments, joint capsules, bone, and finally the hoof structure, which is almost identical to that of the forelimbs.

Palpate carefully down the hind limb, but with the sedated horse it is best to avoid trying to lift any of the limbs to examine the palmar aspect of the foot. Do this while the horse is still fully conscious.

Osteopathic treatment of chronic cases

The chosen method of treatment for these cases is to use intravenous sedation with the horse standing. Care needs to be exercised with this procedure as a sedated horse does not give much warning if they are going to react to any aspect of your work.

A suitable sedative cocktail is made up of an α_2-adrenoceptor agonist such as romifidine (20 µg/kg), and an opioid such as butorphanol (0.1 mg/kg). The former affects the synthesis and release of noradrenaline, which reduces the alertness of the horse, whereas the latter helps to reduce sensitivity, thus reducing the chance of getting kicked, bitten, or otherwise injured.

When sedating for other purposes vets will usually use less of the opioid drug. When working with your vet please ensure that they understand that you will require enough opioid to avoid eliciting a reaction when you palpate. Remember most vets are trained to elicit a pain response when they are trying to locate the site of a problem. They may not be aware of the palpatory skills of the osteopath or the fact that we want to avoid raising sensitivity via unnecessary stimulation, especially if we are going to have to stand behind said patient during the treatment.

The drugs only take a few minutes to reach full effect and are relatively short acting, allowing a treatment window of about 20 minutes before the patient starts to regain normal consciousness. They then need about another 20 minutes to fully wake up before they can travel (this is if the osteopath is based in a veterinary clinic or hospital). No food should be offered until the patient is fully alert, and the vet working with you can guide the owner as to how long this period should be. If sedation needs “topping up” then the time required to fully wake up increases substantially when compared to the same quantity injected as a single dose. Dosage levels do vary depending on the breed, size, and excitability of each patient. Some native ponies require several times more than an Irish Draught. This is where the skill of the veterinary surgeon is required to gauge the amounts required. They can always give more if needed, but you can’t take it out once it’s been put in!

Once palpation has been performed it is best to have an able-bodied colleague stand in front, and slightly to the side of one forelimb, with their knee placed just above that of the patient’s, thus acting as a brace to dissuade the horse from letting its knee flex. A further colleague is also required to be available to act as an anchor on the tail should the horse wish to stretch through its spine. This is a frequent occurrence when the osteopath is performing direct input to stimulate the horse to release patterns of tension associated with an altered gait.

There are many myths surrounding the treatment of animals while they are sedated. Most originate from sources that have no actual knowledge or practical experience of working this way. When you palpate a sedated horse you will discover that it is actually easier and more accurate to assess the patient than if it was fully alert. With the horse relaxed, feedback from the soft tissues is clear and uncluttered. It is the one time when you actually have more time to assess the overall patterns throughout the horse, and collate these with your visual findings and case history.

A sedated horse undergoing treatment can be easily startled by sudden noise or sudden movements from those working around it.

A very interesting observation is with those patients where the OAA joints are most reluctant to move, even with passive input from the osteopath. When sedated, these cases will very often fight the sedative, and will often twitch and brace themselves. They usually need a small additional dose administered by the vet, before they are able to relax enough to allow any meaningful treatment to commence. These cases occasionally release the OAA muscle tension suddenly. This can startle them and you, causing them to jump, and a very small number to kick out before again standing very still. This is why it is paramount that everyone involved understands the importance of being focused and works as a coherent member of the treatment team.

The colleague holding the tail needs to be aware that this is one of the most important contributions to the entire treatment process. From here they can deftly feel their way cranially up the spine segment by segment. By matching any pull that the horse exerts, and maintaining a constant counterforce, this colleague can allow the horse to release entire myofascial strain patterns (Schultz and Feitis 1996) while the osteopath, who is more hands-on, can encourage release to begin from specific areas or regions. This often involves the hands-on osteopath acting more like a fulcrum with the horse dictating what and how much is achieved during each session.

How you structure each treatment will depend on the individual case, and how the patient responds. As mentioned in Chapter 1, there are no "prescription" treatments as no two cases are ever exactly the same. However, you will want to have a framework to begin with, and for the purposes of this book we will begin at the head, working caudally, and describe methods for assisting the chronic patient to unravel complex compensatory patterns as they manifest throughout the musculoskeletal system as a whole.

The head

The head can be injured during falls where there can be compression associated with the occiput and an altered resting state for the junctions with the atlas and axis, along with ventral or dorsal compression of the frontal and nasal bones and associated joints where the horse has either tipped over backward or landed at speed on its front end.

The mandible, temporomandibular joints, and their supporting soft tissue structures are another area of importance to the osteopath in helping to restore normal biomechanical function.

Through some of the reciprocal nerve supply from the associated cranial nerves it appears possible to initiate considerable changes by either stimulating, via trigger points, or inhibiting some of the facial muscles and muscles of mastication (Fig. 5.42).

By combining pure osteopathic techniques such as functional with craniosacral modalities the osteopath can achieve multitissue release especially around the

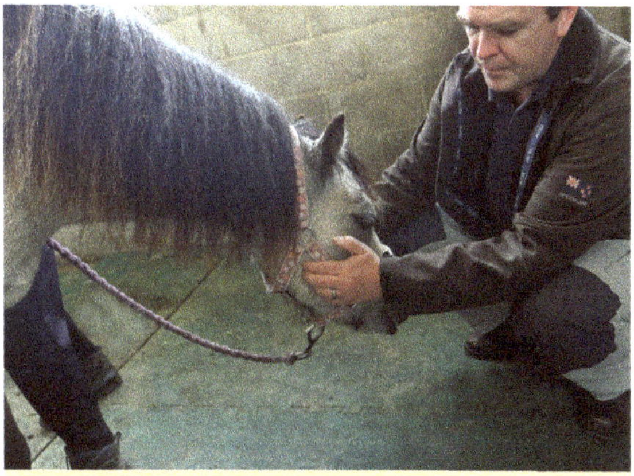

Figure 5.42
Treatment will often begin with the facial muscles and muscles of mastication.

ears and the underlying joints between the frontals, parietals, sphenoid, and temporal bones. These synarthroses are often the key to achieving a lasting return to normal function throughout the entire musculoskeletal system. They can be adversely affected when a horse takes a heavy fall or has been subjected to harsh riding conditions along with poorly fitting tack (TN's own clinical experience).

Working on the structures that make up the head is very often the key to initiating a cascade sequence of tissue release throughout the entire body. If you consider the biotensegrity of an individual body (Scarr 2014) then this starts to make sense. The chronic patient really shows us how we, as osteopaths, have to embrace the practical aspects of this concept in order to successfully treat a longstanding biomechanical problem.

The fascial connections around the cranium, mandible, and face continue, and exert their presence throughout the rest of the body. The dura mater at a deeper level and its involvement with the involuntary mechanism (IVM) contribute to this pattern as well.

For the above reasons, the chronic horse always receives a lot of attention around the head once sedated – many of them do not want you anywhere near it without sedation.

Fascial techniques for gaining release can involve gentle holds on the ears, nostrils, mandible, and cranial vault. The amount of compression that the cranial vault can receive from a traumatic fall should not be underestimated.

With the horse we generally attempt to release around the occiput and frontals first, followed by applying a lift to the parietals, and then temporal bones. These procedures may be accompanied by simultaneous release to the mandible by offering both traction and distraction or compression, depending upon what is required.

Unhindered movement of the mandible in all planes is essential for overall freedom of movement through the horse. Special attention should be given to this prior to moving on to the cervical spine.

The cervical spine and neck

In the chronic horse, the author (TN) believes that the cervical spine and its associated structures are always compromised (author's own clinical experience). Only if these structures are functioning normally, and with total freedom in both range and quality, can the horse move normally. This is only true for these long-standing cases. As described earlier in Chapter 5, the acute horse can present in a very different way. Every horse that you see with chronic movement problems will have an altered state of soft tissue function in the neck and cervical spine as part of its overall pattern. This is a dogmatic statement borne out by decades of observation and treating this type of patient. If you remember only one thing from this section, the author would suggest it is this.

Due to the way horses move, and looking at the intrinsic myofascial web, if a horse is moving freely then the mandible must be free floating (relative term). It follows that the occipitoatlantoaxial (OAA) joints must also have a full, free range of movement continuing caudally through each and every joint, ending in the final tail vertebral segment. It will also include all of the joints of each of the four limbs. Anything less is not free movement.

In reality we will never see this, but we do need to aim at it. By falling short near to perfection, we should be able to return a chronically compromised horse close enough to pure, normal movement, so that it no longer exhibits any symptoms or signs of compromised movement.

Mechanically the most mobile part of the neck is around the first three joints. Beyond the C2–C3 articulation the facet joints interlock much more to give the neck the structural integrity required for the muscles attached and the functions it is required to perform.

When treating the sedated horse the best techniques appear to be functional, sustained positional release, oscillation, and craniosacral. These can be performed with the head and neck in either compression or decompression depending on what the tissues require (Fig. 5.43A and B). It is not uncommon for both compression and decompression to be needed with the osteopath alternating from one to the other during the course of a treatment session.

Checking for symmetry in the resting state of the atlas and axis are good indicators as to how the horse is coping biomechanically. This has been covered under palpation, but is worth repeating. If the soft tissues are maintaining any rotation, lateral flexion, flexion, or extension, then this is going to affect how the horse moves and its balance and coordination. Remember that the head and neck are needed for good locomotion, utilizing energy recovery via the pendulum action when the horse moves forward.

Due to the soft tissue attachments to the cervical vertebrae, treating the rest of the cervical spine involves releasing through the entire column using the various osteopathic modalities and sometimes combinations of them. The author finds visualizing the three dimensional aspect of the structures while unraveling the resting imbalances in tissue tension essential. At the same time allowing the horse to guide in what order it is able to allow changes to take place is essential to gaining a positive treatment outcome. The author often blends final palpation with a "functional" walk through of the cervical spine to help initiate a continuation of the treatment process, having moved caudally from the head. The skill is in encouraging the horse to work with you and resisting the urge to focus on what you want to release during any given part of the treatment.

With the chronic patient there is usually less reaction to any stimulus the osteopath provides when compared to an acute condition. However, there is usually more resistance felt, in the form of stiffness when the osteopath initiates movement. This is where the techniques mentioned earlier come into their own. By placing the mandible onto the osteopath's shoulder this frees up both hands to guide a controlled pattern of soft tissue release through from the OAA joints caudally to the thoracic sling, and link up with a second operator providing traction via the tail (Figs 5.44 and 5.45).

Thoracic sling

With the chronic patient the thoracic sling is the other key area to consider when trying to restore normal equine movement. Many musculoskeletal problems that do not resolve over time

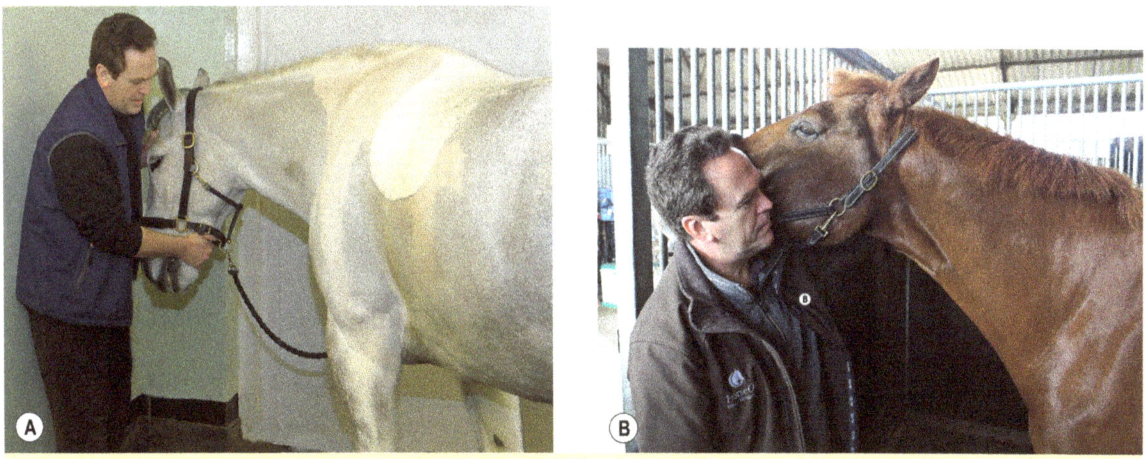

Figure 5.43
Sustained positional release of the head and neck. (A) Compression (flexion). (B) Decompression (extension).

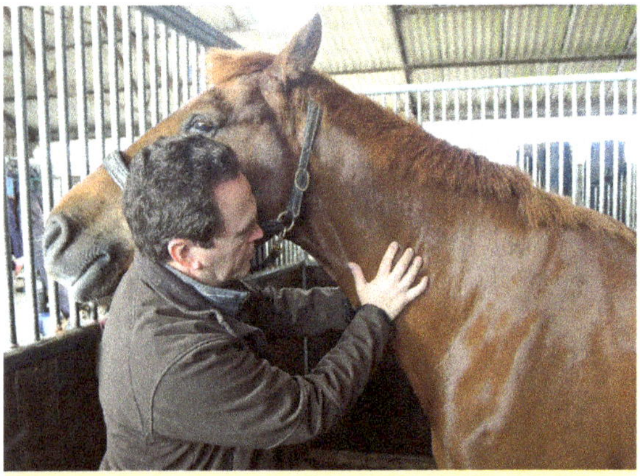

Figure 5.44
Supporting the mandible on the operator's shoulder (maintaining extension of the upper neck) frees up the operator's hands to control the soft tissue release through the OAA joints caudally to the thoracic sling.

will result in the horse adapting its way of moving so that it no longer engages properly from behind and adapts to pulling itself along through the forelimb structures to allow it to remain mobile. This creates the classic front-heavy horse with overdeveloped ventral neck and pectoral muscles (Fig. 5.46). The osteopath is therefore going to be particularly interested in this area and the way it is affecting any overall pattern in the horse.

We described above (under palpation) the best way of ascertaining whether the thoracic sling as a "unit" has any "give" or correct motility; from this you will be able to build a picture of any traumatic falls or recurrent rider patterns (author's clinical experience). Many of the chronic horses we see appear desperate to release the thoracic sling and will plant their weight through the sternum and onto the osteopath, who often feels reduced to nothing more than an organic fulcrum while delivering a sustained positional release (Fig. 5.47). Sometimes these patients are so keen to release through the entire range of tissues that they will let their front legs flex and relax. It is wise to have a third assistant who can keep at least one forelimb propped in extension (Fig. 5.48) to ensure the safety of the "fulcrum."

When treated using this procedure, the horse will often alter its position while maintaining a constant downward pressure through the "fulcrum," thus creating its own functional unwind at the same time. The "fulcrum osteopath" may need to adjust the vector of the upward pressure in order to facilitate a better pattern of release for the patient, but again emphasis needs to be placed on the osteopath being guided by the horse. If the vector is not precisely correct the horse will stop leaning on the osteopath and will attempt to reposition itself. This technique may only take a minute, or may last for up to 20 minutes, and is best not carried out on a full stomach!

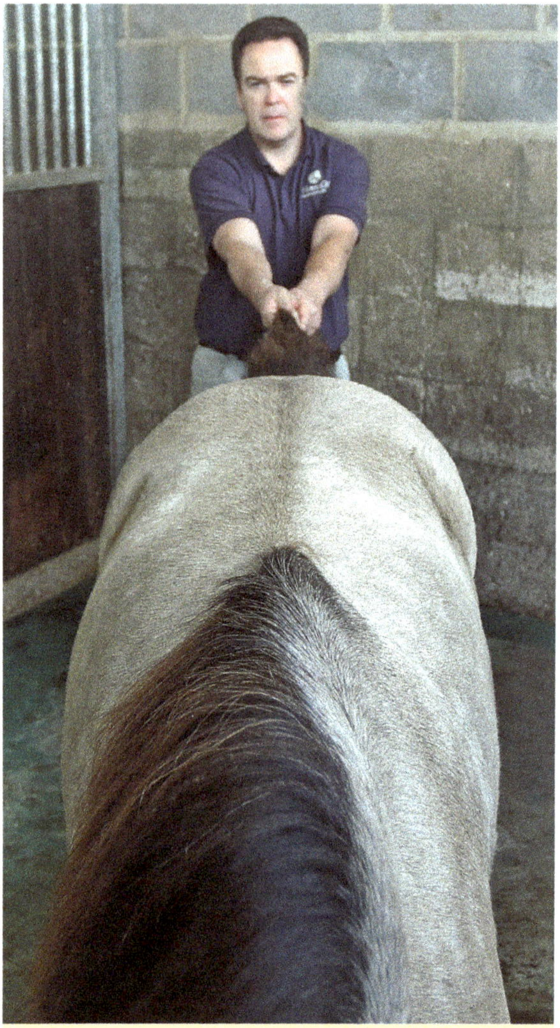

Figure 5.45
A second operator applying traction on the patient's tail will often aid in the release of chains of muscles along the spine.

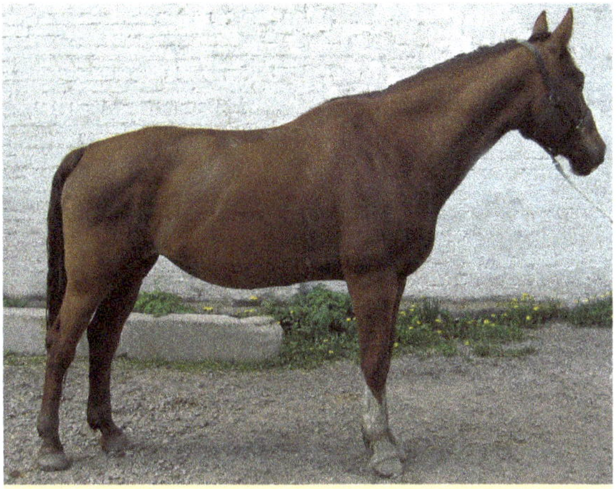

Figure 5.46
In this chronic case the horse has been overusing the forelimbs for forward progression and has the appearance of a classic "front-heavy" horse. There is increased development of the ventral cervical and pectoral muscles with atrophy of the back and hind quarters.

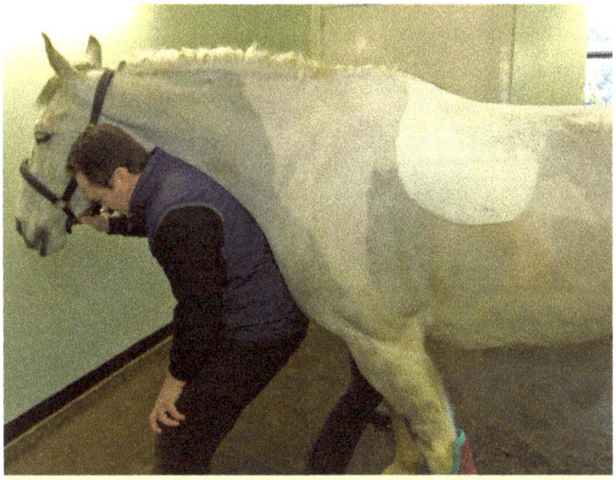

Figure 5.47
The operator acts as a fulcrum, to allow the patient to push down through the sternum, and delivers a sustained positional release to the muscles around the thoracic sling.

Releasing fascial tension overlying the scapulae can be achieved when using the preceding technique, or when the patient is pulling through its tail, by applying strong inhibition through the supraspinatus and infraspinatus muscles. The best result may be achieved

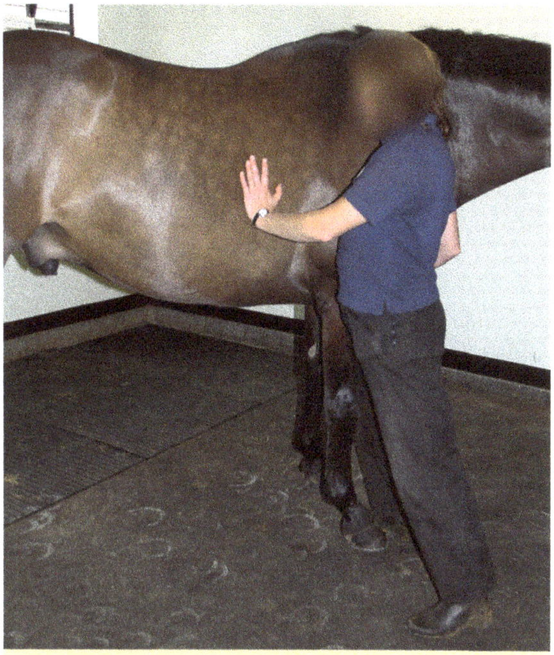

Figure 5.48
When treating chronic cases, it is advisable to have an assistant support a front limb to prevent sudden collapse of the front end of the horse.

using inhibition combined with cervical release and tail traction simultaneously.

Many cases also benefit from careful inhibition through the caudal cervical spine where the osteopath guides their flattened hand between the scapula and rib cage, again while the horse is stretching longitudinally against an operator maintaining a constant pull from the tail (Fig. 5.49).

Thoracic spine and rib cage

As a region the thoracic spine and rib cage is relatively rigid with limited movement, but it is an area in which some breeds seem to be particularly susceptible to problems. Probably the most common condition that owners will be concerned about is that of overriding dorsal spinous processes (ORDSP) or kissing spines. There are, however, many other problems that can affect this region, many of which may actually result in dipping of the thoracic spine and may actually precipitate ORDSP.

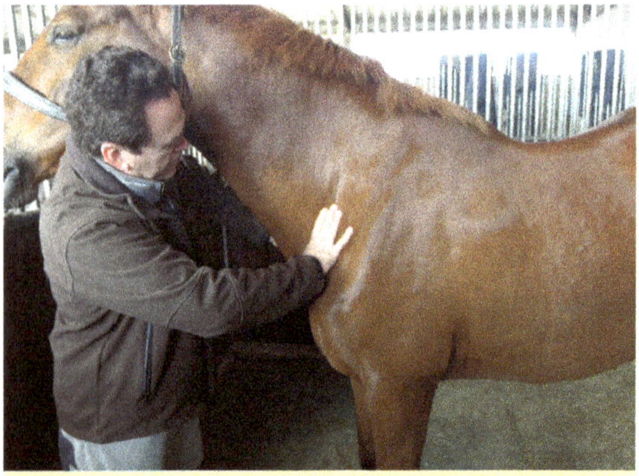

Figure 5.49
Inhibition of the caudal cervical spine.

The spinous processes at the withers can fracture if a horse takes a very bad fall. An ill-fitting saddle, or pressure caused by bad riding, can cause pinching behind the withers. This can result in pressure constricting the blood and peripheral nerve supplies to the caudal part of the trapezius muscle. Overtight girths can cause increased sensitivity to the ribs and intercostal muscles as well as affecting the action of the serratus ventralis and its role in supporting the thoracic sling. Too tight a fit of the saddle can also create irritation to the sympathetic nervous system, which has reciprocal innervation to some of the paravertebral muscles. Direct saddle pressure can also cause the development of hard skin nodules under the saddle, which can make the area more sensitive to pressure.

The weight of the horse is also important. Overweight can cause an altered gait, especially if fat deposits have been laid down caudal to the scapulae. Certain breeds (e.g., cobs) are predisposed to this.

Inhibition of the diaphragm can be performed from either side of the horse with one hand on the spinous process of T18 and the other covering the attachments of the costal cartilages to the sternum along the ventral aspect of the horse (Fig. 5.50). Where stronger inhibition is required this can be applied with two operators using an opened towel or blanket which is carefully lifted so as to create a sling for the caudal part of the chest and abdomen, creating suitable conditions for release of resting tension within the diaphragm itself.

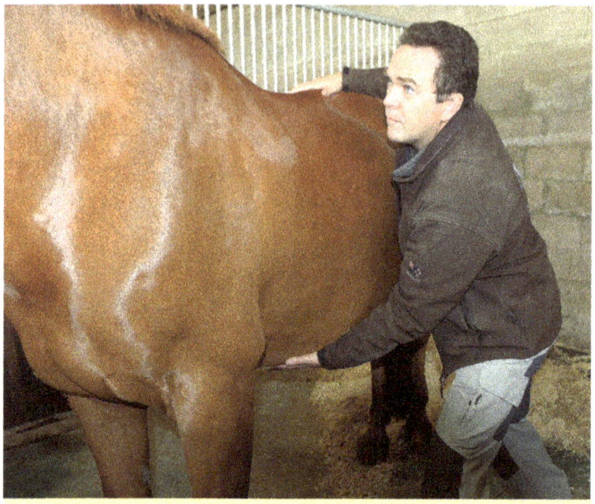

Figure 5.50
Inhibition of the diaphragm.

Lumbar spine, pelvis, and hind limbs

This is an area which is commonly injured, and where somatic changes are very often first noticed. The lumbar spine provides a very flexible connection between the thoracic spine and rib cage and the pelvis, so it can be subjected to incredible forces when accelerating the horse forward, changing direction suddenly, or attempting to slow down and come to a standstill. The bridging nature of the lumbar spine means that the various bony and soft tissue structures can incur vectors and combinations of force that put excessive stress through these joints. These injuries are described in more detail above in the section on osteopathic evaluation of acute cases.

Where this region is important in the chronic patient is in the strong compensatory patterns that transect this part of the body. Using the biotensegrity model (Scarr 2014) the dynamic forces involved in an initial trauma, such as a rotational fall, will involve entire myofascial chains. Once these injuries have become chronic the patient is already adapting its movements to compensate for the original trauma.

Continue palpation caudally from the thoracic spine over the paravertebral musculature until you reach the tuber sacrale and tuber coxae. Long-standing problems respond well to a mixture of functional, cranial, and stretching techniques. Many cases exhibit sensitivity between T11 and T13. The author believes this is where tissue change is greatest after adapting to a rotational fall, which often results in an altered gait through one or other diagonal pair of limbs. Where this sensitivity is found the patient will very often respond to a functional release using contacts over the withers and tuber sacrale rather than any direct input over the sensitive segments themselves (Fig. 5.51). Sometimes this can be followed by a careful lift through the abdomen, which appears to assist in gaining relaxation of the iliopsoas musculature. It may subsequently be possible to offer direct muscle inhibition along the paravertebral muscles working in a caudal direction along the lumbar spine.

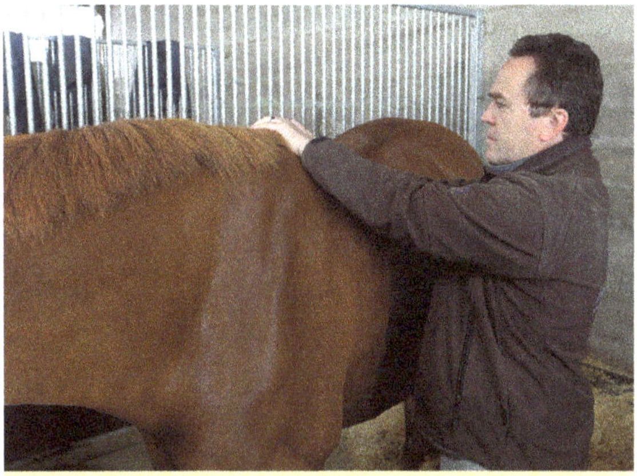

Figure 5.51
Functional release in the spine using a double hand contact over the withers.

If the lumbosacral junction is restricted on observed movement and palpation then this will usually benefit from offering squeeze resistance and release through the coccygeal segments of the tail while simultaneously finding the best angle at which to create a soft tissue release through the lumbosacral junction itself (Fig. 5.52). In many cases the horse will respond by leaning forward to make use of the osteopath as a point from which they can perform the desired release themselves. It may require two operators to perform this procedure with one holding onto the tail.

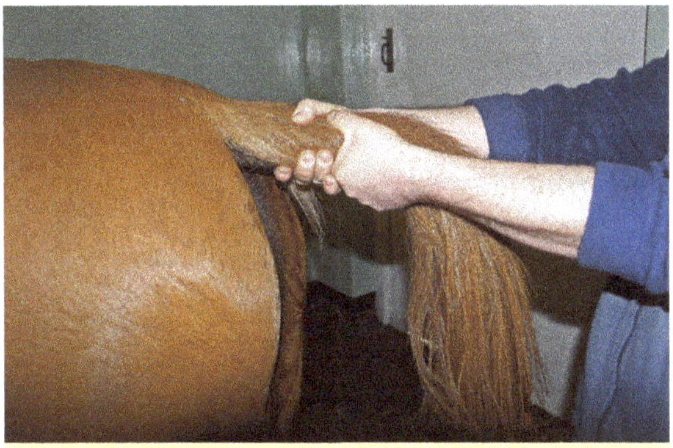

Figure 5.52
Soft tissue release through the lumbosacral junction via traction of the tail.

In cases where one or other of the sacroiliac joints are involved in maintaining an altered movement pattern, or if there is undue tension within the pelvic floor, it may be necessary to offer a sustained pelvic lift via a contact on either of the tuber ischii. This will be apparent if the horse does not wish to take a stretch through the tail, but has restricted movement behind. When performing this treatment take care to avoid sudden movements, and remember that you are working very near to a sensitive region (Fig. 5.53). With any mare in season this technique is best avoided even with a sedated patient.

When performing this technique successfully, it is not uncommon for the horse to clamp their gluteal

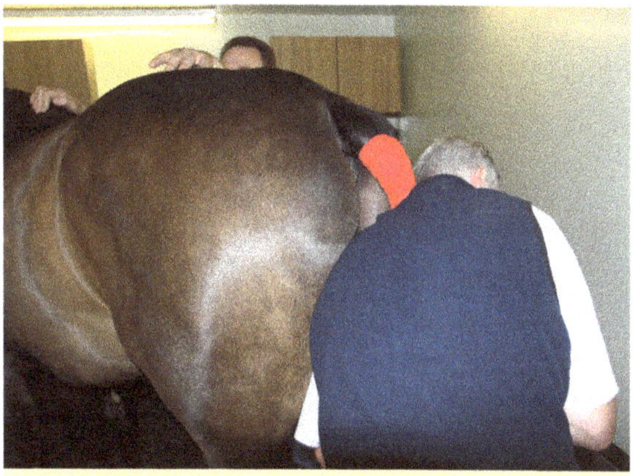

Figure 5.53
A sustained pelvic lift is a very effective technique that must be performed with great care.

and hamstring musculature so that it fixes the osteopath in position. The osteopath offers an oblique upward vector of resistance while bracing against the considerable posteroventral pressure from the horse. In some cases it is necessary to involve more than one operator, and in more than one case the author has had to resort to using the worktop in the treatment room to take the weight of the patient while it has literally sat down in order to relieve tension through the sacroiliac joints!

If there is undue tension within the gluteal, quadriceps, and hamstring muscles these will often benefit from direct inhibition, functional fascial release, and sustained positional release methods. These are often combined with stretching from the tail or with a sustained pelvic lift.

Where there is a need to work on the hamstring muscles, these respond well to cross-fiber stretching and strong inhibition (Fig. 5.54) and allow the horse to achieve positional release by using either tail stretch or pelvic lift procedures.

The tail itself can be used as a short lever (by holding around the coccygeal segments) to create functional and positional release of the sacrum within the sacroiliac joints (Fig. 5.55).

The tail is also a useful tool for assessing the effects of osteopathic treatment once a session has come to an end. By holding the tail and maintaining a degree of traction longitudinally, the osteopath can gently rock the horse backward then reduce the tension and allow it to rock forward again. This can be repeated gently and slowly to assess segmental mobility and the overall level of "give" or "resistance" within the soma. With this technique always be aware of the body language of the patient. If a horse has performed a particularly strong treatment it may not appreciate this last act, and experience will need to be developed to ensure your safety.

When finally releasing your hold on the tail, ensure that tension is reduced very slowly, in much the same way as when performing inhibition. This should ensure that there is no reflex contracture through the lumbar multifidus and sacrocaudalis dorsalis muscles. If this contracture should occur it is important not to let go of the tail suddenly; instead try to maintain a small amount of contact resistance and very slowly release this before stepping away from the patient.

Following any sedated treatment it is important to allow the patient to become fully conscious before traveling (if seen at a veterinary clinic), and also to ensure that no food is ingested until the veterinary surgeon is happy that the patient is fully awake.

Treatment programs will usually require several sedated sessions and depending on each case they may well benefit from being taken out of any ridden work during this phase of their recovery. In certain cases,

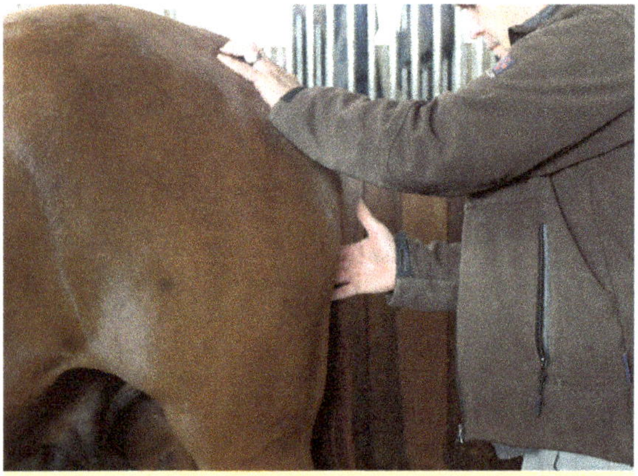

Figure 5.54
Stretching and inhibition of the hamstring muscles.

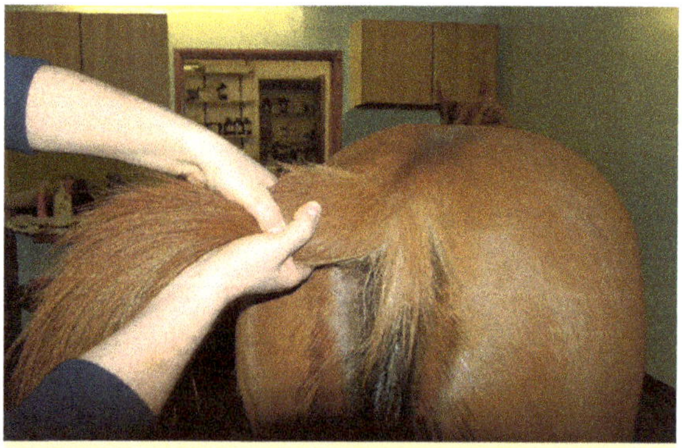

Figure 5.55
The tail can be used to create functional and positional release of the sacroiliac joints.

where the primary somatic pattern will not release fully and allow normal locomotor function, it has been found that a treatment with the horse under general anesthetic is required to facilitate this.

Treatment under general anesthetic

This is never undertaken lightly and does require a slightly different mind-set. As with most exotic large animal work, however, it is often the only way to successfully resolve a somatic dysfunction issue. In equine osteopathic practice, it has often been the only way to relieve a patient fully of the presenting signs and symptoms. It is only undertaken if a series of sedated treatment sessions have failed to fully release the underlying tension patterns of the patient at rest. With a much better understanding of myofascial strain patterns emerging, we are able to explain more of what is going on at a nonpathological level. For the best results the author has found that a team is needed, all of whom can work closely and take direction from each other. Ultimately the anesthetist will call the shots with the patient's welfare being paramount.

Once the patient has been anesthetized it is positioned on its back and propped up with airbags. The ideal place to examine and treat is on a heavily padded floor in an operating theatre. Once the anesthetist is happy, the osteopath can palpate all of the structures and carry out mobility tests from nose to tail, as much for quality as for range of movement. Before touching the patient it is important to note the way the horse lies in this supine position. All of the chronic patients that the author has examined in this way have exhibited scoliotic postures, and they all revert to this even when placed as centrally and as straight as possible. Photographs obtained under anesthesia, before and after treatment, are useful indicators to show how well each procedure has gone (Fig. 5.56A and B).

Palpation and mobility testing are similar to that for the standing horse. The only difficulty most osteopaths encounter is in remembering the horse's right from left when the horse is positioned in a supine manner.

Once the patient has been physically assessed the osteopath will need to initiate release of tension within the myofascial system, and along with at least two other manual assistants they will functionally unwind the patient using any or all four limbs, the head and neck, and tail as levers. Rhythmic cervical traction can be employed using a rope looped through the head collar (Fig. 5.57).

Due to the unique soft tissue patterns of each patient, there is no single way to prescribe treatment under GA. The palpation and mobility testing phase will give an idea as to how the body will accept or deflect osteopathic intervention, but the sequence in which it will accept this varies considerably. The vast majority of these cases have suffered a severe fall at some stage in the past. Many of these are documented, but in others one must rely on circumstantial evidence such as skid marks in their turnout area, along with marks on the face and body of the animal.

In every case that the author has treated under GA the focus and driving element of a full body unwind has shifted from one operator to another. Very often this focus will shift several times before the tension patterns within the soft tissue framework release. It is essential that each member of the GA team can feel what is happening when one or other operator guides the patient through this process. From an observer's point of view it is often difficult to appreciate the multitude of factors that have to happen simultaneously in order for the procedure to lead to a successful conclusion (Fig. 5.58).

The act of several practitioners combining to offer full body soft tissue unwinding requires that force through any of the structures be avoided without allowing the patient to evade treatment. If certain patterns of release cannot be initiated then a different approach is tried until sequences of release can be reached with the compliance of the structures involved. It is this aspect that makes each and every GA treatment session unique. As the treatment session unfolds, the horse will be carefully maneuvered into different positions in order to enable full body functional unwinding to be carried out.

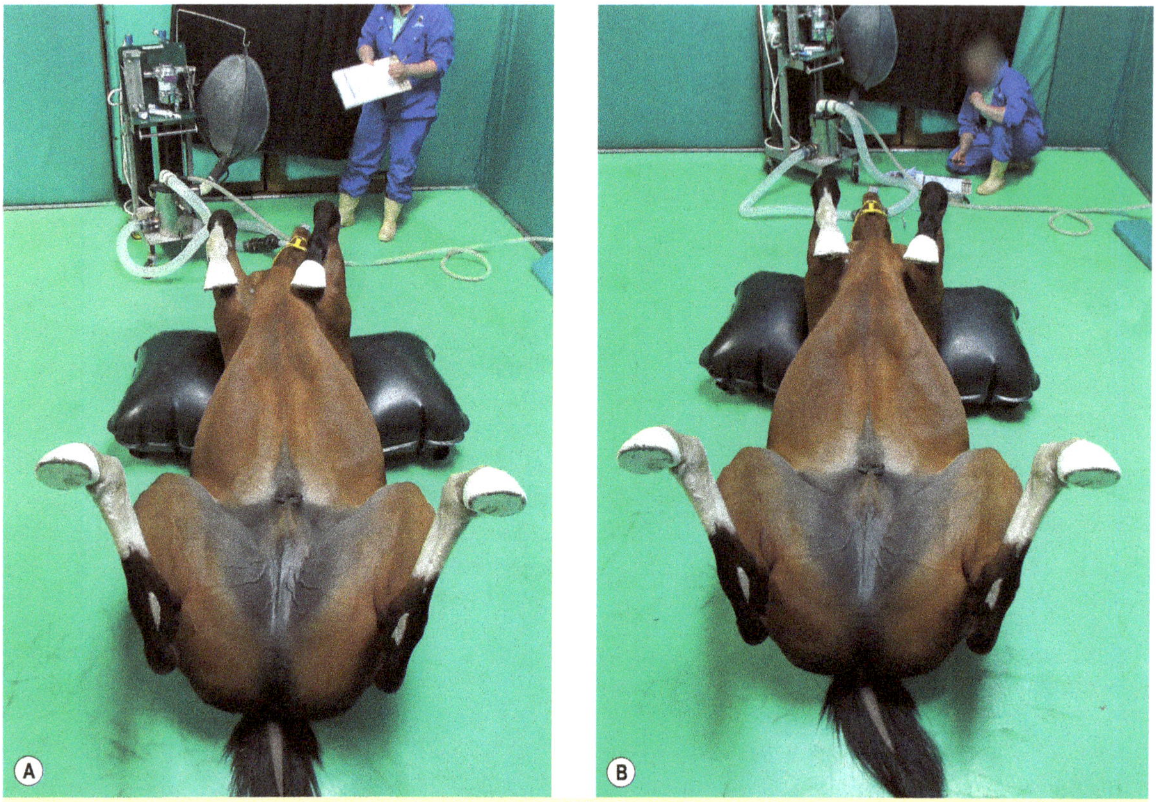

Figure 5.56
(A) A patient under general anesthesia prior to treatment. Note the rotation along the spine between front and hind legs, the asymmetry of the thoracic sling, and the deviation of the head. (B) The same patient as in image (A) after treatment.

It is important to note that normal ranges of movement and combinations of movement must be kept within normal parameters for the patient, and at no stage should excessive force be applied to any region of the body (Chaitow 2007). Once the team are happy that they have achieved all that is possible at this point, the patient is repositioned onto its back and visually assessed for symmetry in the supine position before the osteopath manually assesses individual joints and then groups of joints for their mobility and, importantly, motility (Fig. 5.56B).

In most cases the author has found that the patient's soft tissue injuries will indicate when a GA session has achieved as much as it can. In most cases there will be some residual somatic tension, but most will resolve with further standing sedated treatment. In a very small number of cases more than one treatment under GA may be required to achieve sufficient release to allow a return to normal movement throughout the entire soma (Colles et al. 2014).

As soon as treatment is finished the osteopath instructs the anesthetist that the treatment session has concluded, and the horse is placed in a secure padded recovery box. It is allowed to regain consciousness and stand in its own time, closely monitored by one of the nursing staff to ensure that all remains quiet.

Returning a horse to work

Following any lengthy withdrawal from ridden work as a result of undergoing a course of osteopathic treatment, it is essential to introduce a graduated return to work. This needs to be tailored to the individual;

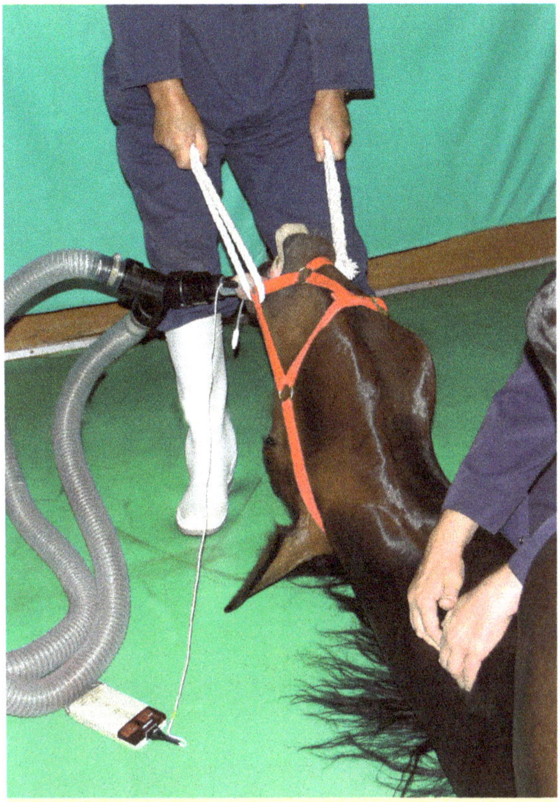

Figure 5.57
Application of rhythmic traction to the neck of a horse under general anesthesia.

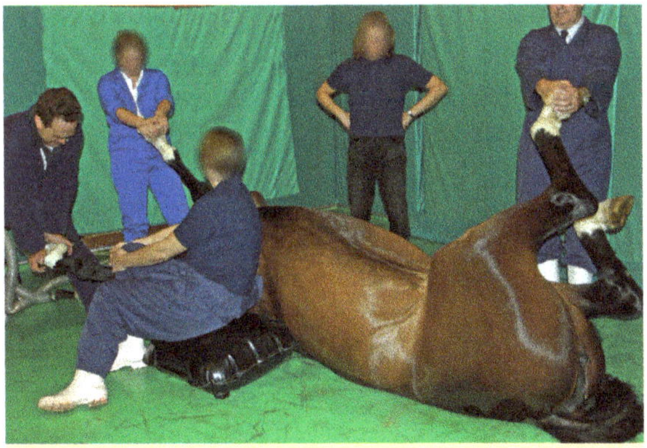

Figure 5.58
A team of operators give osteopathic treatment to a patient under general anesthesia.

however, certain protocols need to be considered. The author would suggest using the following as a basis to work from, adjusting aspects to better suit the patient where needed.

Walking in hand

Start walking in hand for about 20 minutes each day. The emphasis should be on allowing the horse to walk in a straight line without applying force through the lead rope. An alternative to this would be long reining, depending on the patient and handler competence.

The time spent walking can be increased over a two to four week period until each walk lasts for around one hour. Hill work where the horse has to walk both up and down an incline can be introduced where possible (not for the entire walk though). Leading from another horse should be avoided as it tends to stretch the neck in one direction.

Active stretching exercises

Active controlled stretches can be introduced to activate key core stability muscle activity at the same time as the walking in hand. These are critical to the longer term recovery of the patient and should not be underestimated or forgotten about. It is beyond the remit of this book to cover all of these. For a comprehensive guide to stretching please refer to *Activate your Horse's Core: Unmounted Exercises for Dynamic Mobility, Strength and Balance* by Stubbs and Clayton (2008).

Introducing ridden work

Walk in hand for 10 minutes with the horse tacked up, then ride in walk for 10 minutes, and then finish with 10 minutes of walking in hand still tacked up. Gradually increase the time ridden to about 40 minutes per session, but maintain the in hand work before and after the ridden work.

Introducing trotting

Maintain all of the above work, but once the horse is being ridden for 40 minutes at a time begin introducing two minutes' trotting for each 10-minute section of walk, ensuring that you always walk first, trot, walk, trot, and so on for the session.

Assuming all is going well you can introduce pole work in the school, where the horse is walked over poles on the ground spaced such that there is room for one stride length between poles. Once the horse has got the hang of this you can raise alternate ends of these poles by as much as 30 cm to encourage better axial rotation through the lumbar spine, along with better hind limb engagement and overall action. Hill work can be included at this stage as well (if not before).

The above is a general guideline, and should be modified to suit the patient (and not the owner's or trainer's desire to speed up the process). The majority of cases that fail to return to work at a decent level fail at the rehabilitation phase (Colles et al. 2014).

Case study *5.1*

An 18-year-old cob

Signalment

The patient was an 18-year-old cob x 15.3hh hack. He had been owned for 13 years

History

There was no previous history of back or neck-related problems. The horse was out of work for approximately one year when the owner was pregnant. On returning to work, there was a very gradual onset of the horse "not feeling right" when ridden. There were no specific overt symptoms initially, but the rider was sufficiently concerned to keep asking if there were any signs of lameness.

The horse was checked by a vet who could not find any specific problem. As the owner was going abroad, the horse was turned out for a week. At the end of the week the horse was found to be extremely lame on his left forelimb and had great difficulty walking. No signs of any trauma were evident.

The vet was recalled and a diagnosis of left forelimb lameness was confirmed, but no obvious cause was found. No specific workup was performed at the time, and the horse was put on box rest. The foot was checked by a farrier during routine shoeing, and there was no evidence found of laminitis or foot abscess.

Box rest resulted in slight improvement. The horse was symptom free in the morning following rest, but within an hour of being ridden the lameness recurred. The horse now began to stumble on his left foreleg when ridden, and he was seen to fall several times when loose in the field. The horse appeared depressed, and became increasingly head shy and apprehensive toward other horses.

A second veterinary opinion was sought and a likely diagnosis of arthritis was made, but with an offer to perform a full neurological and orthopedic workup. Prior to the workup osteopathic assistance was sought.

Osteopathic examination: static

- The horse stood with a low head carriage paying scant attention to its surroundings.
- There was tenderness in the suboccipital and upper cervical areas especially on the left.
- Extension of the occiput on the atlas was limited.
- Passive rotation and side bending of the cervical spine was limited to the left.
- The left deltoid and upper trapezius muscles were slightly wasted.
- Tenderness over the lower lumbar region was present bilaterally.
- There was slight wasting in the left gluteal muscles.
- Pulling through the tail revealed tension through to the thoracolumbar junction.
- No swelling or heat was present in the left leg or hoof capsule. There was no palpable tenderness in the tendons or ligaments in any leg.

Osteopathic examination: movement

Movement tests were carried out resulting in the following observations.

Walk away: Slightly high left pelvis. Short behind. Lack of drive through hindquarters.

Walk toward: Low head carriage. Slight lameness left foreleg. Tightness through thoracic sling. Drags himself along on forelegs.

Trot away: Head rises on transition from walk to trot. Poor drive from behind. High in left pelvis but tendency to balance out as horse loosens.

Pivot left: Neck fixed. Very stiff. Tendency for head to poke rather than flex into direction of bend.

Pivot right: Better mobility throughout upper cervicals, but showing some resistance.

Backing up: Tight through lumbars and pivoting at thoracolumbar junction.

Osteopathic diagnosis

Primary OA and AA restriction with secondary caudal cervical and cranial thoracic dysfunction was diagnosed with compensatory lumbar and pelvic dysfunction.

Treatment

Osteopathic treatment of this horse was performed with the permission of and under sedation by a veterinary surgeon.

Initial treatment was directed at the cervical spine which was considered the primary cause, specifically occipitoatlantal fixation. Traction was applied to the poll area to release the OA articulation before introducing side bending, rotational to the right to release the mid to lower cervical spine. Good mobility was achieved to the right, but some restriction was present in the lower cervical spine on side bending rotation to the left.

Attention was next directed to the lumbar spine and pelvis. Initially tail traction was performed until a good release was obtained through to the thoracolumbar (TL) junction. This was followed by a bilateral pelvic lift up though the ischial tuberosities, noticeably worse on the left side from the left sacroiliac (SI) joint through to the TL junction.

On returning to the neck, good free movement was achieved to the left. To obtain more relaxation in the lower cervicals gentle pressure was applied through the area by pushing ventrally up through the anterior lower neck, then through the cervicothoracic junction and up into the upper thoracic spine and withers, releasing any areas of tension found. There was increased tension present on the right side of the thoracic sling up to the T6–T7 area.

The cervical, lumbar, and pelvic areas were rechecked using further tail traction and pelvic lifts to ensure all tensions had been adequately treated. Nothing of any consequence was found and the treatment was concluded.

The owner was advised the horse should be box rested for the rest of the day but could be turned out the following day. The horse was not to be ridden or exercised for a fortnight although cervical mobility should be maintained by gentle carrot stretching twice daily.

An appointment was made to reassess the horse after two weeks.

Follow-up

The owner reported that after a couple of days stiffness post-treatment, the horse had shown tremendous improvement both physically and in his temperament.

He was back to his old 'naughty' self and was much more alert. There were no signs of any lameness present and the horse was moving much more freely.

On examination, occipitoatlantal and cervical mobility was good with no sensitivity behind the poll or through the lumbar spine. The pelvic mobility was well balanced and he was engaging his hindquarters. A further two weeks off work was prescribed before a gradual return to work. On returning to work no further problems were found and good progress has been made since.

Summary

Although this horse had not had a full veterinary workup, the owner had requested an opinion and possible treatment prior to further investigation.

Although there was no history of any specific trauma, it is quite possible that the horse had suffered trauma in the five years prior to the present owner's purchase. If so, the animal had compensated extremely well, and one can only postulate that a second trauma occurred while the horse was turned out, or something occurred leading to the breakdown of any compensatory mechanism that was present.

In this case after freeing the occipitoatlantal problem successfully there were some issues in the lower cervical and upper thoracic spine which, although improved, did not fully resolve until the thoracolumbar area had been treated.

It is unusual in a case like this for a horse to respond so quickly and so effectively with just the one treatment. Most chronic conditions will take three to four treatments, spread out over a number of months, to achieve a similar result.

Editor's comment: it is surprising how horses left to their own devices in a field can injure themselves. It seems possible that in this case this was a relatively recent self-inflicted injury. This would fit with the rapid response to treatment – but we will never know!

Case study 5.2

A 10-year-old Irish Sport Horse

Signalment

A 10-year-old gelded Irish Sport Horse, bought as a backed four-year-old from Ireland, with the intention of building him up to compete at eventing, and more latterly focusing on dressage where he has progressed to Advanced-Medium level.

History

The owner reported that there had never been any incidence of trauma noted; however, she had been aware that he always seemed to try to pull himself along with his right shoulder and with some propulsion through his left hind-limb apparatus. When ridden she noted that he would push his trunk laterally to the right (convex right axially) and also tilt his head to the right.

His saddler had noted that the right shoulder (periscapular) musculature was better developed than that on the left side.

As with many young horses he was noted to be nervous of doing anything new for the first time.

His vet could find no pathological explanation for his movement pattern and so was happy to refer to the author (DG) for an osteopathic evaluation.

Presenting signs

On visual examination he appeared calm and inquisitive. When standing he appeared to have a slight dominance in muscle development through the right lateral and ventral throat structures, right shoulder, and through his right periscapular musculature. This then continued caudally crossing to the left of the midline around the T16–T18 region, through to the left gluteal and hamstring muscles. The root of the tail was held slightly to the left of the midline.

Watching him move in walk and trot, turning short to left and right, and reined back in walk confirmed this pattern while in locomotion.

Osteopathic treatment

Having assessed this biomechanical problem the author and veterinary surgeon concluded that the best way to proceed would be to administer a short course of functional release treatment sessions, carried out under sedation.

The author also decided to blend in some engagement with the involuntary mechanism (IVM), and also sustained positional release (SPR) work in response to the patient's feedback during treatment.

The patient responded well to these early sessions, and feedback from the owner stated that he appeared happier and more confident when faced with new challenges.

The original movement pattern still persisted, and so it was deemed prudent to offer follow-up sessions between his training and entering low level competitions.

The owner's circumstances changed and she decided to focus on dressage, which he seemed to really enjoy, and soon he was climbing the ranks.

Frustratingly he still has a bias toward pulling through the right shoulder; however, he will soften and yield when warmed up carefully and encouraged to engage from behind.

When observed standing he presented as almost symmetrical, with good muscling in the hindquarters.

Outcome

This horse was bought as an inexperienced four-year-old with an inherent movement asymmetry. There were no signs of any pathology, and he has remained sound throughout his ownership. Osteopathic treatment has improved his movement, and integrated treatment with his saddler, dental technician, and farrier has helped produce a well-rounded dressage horse. His confidence has grown, and he appears to thoroughly enjoy competition work.

Summary

This horse did not present with a specific injury. As with so many horses, he presented with a pattern of movement at odds with normal, free locomotion. Left unaddressed this would have increased the odds of creating real pathology in one or more limbs and a myriad of other issues related to areas innervated from the same spinal cord segments. Osteopathy works very effectively in the preventative role, and when an owner is as observant as this one was, serious lameness issues can be avoided. Human athletes do not wait for an injury to occur. They have a team of experts working at preventing injuries from happening in the first place. Osteopathy can be a major part of this process with the equine athlete as well.

References

Atkin B (2013) The effect of osteopathic treatment on the symmetry of gait in sport horses. (Masters dissertation). University of Wales, UK.

Butler JS, Colles CM, Dyson J, Kold SE, Poulos P (2016) Clinical Radiology of the Horse. 4th edn. Wiley Blackwell, pp. 531–568; pp. 733–743.

Chaitow L (2007) Positional Release Techniques. Churchill Livingstone Elsevier, pp. 259–263.

Chila A (2010a) Foundations of Osteopathic Medicine. 3rd edn. Philadelphia: Lippincott Williams and Wilkins. Philadelphia, p. 752.

Chila A (2010b) Ibid. p. 831.

Chila A (2010c) Ibid. p. 766.

Chila A (2010d). Ibid. p. 45.

Chila A (2010e) Ibid. p. 743.

Colles CM, Brooks J (2011) Osteopathic treatment of the axial skeleton of the horse. In: Ross MW, Dyson SL (eds.) Diagnosis and Management of Lameness in the Horse. 2nd edn. Saunders Elsevier, pp. 907–914.

Colles CM, Ware R (2010) The Principles of Farriery. London: JA Allen.

Colles CM, Nevin A, Brooks J (2014) The osteopathic treatment of somatic dysfunction causing gait abnormality in 51 horses. Equine Veterinary Education. January; 26 (3) 148–155.

de Lahunta A, Glass E, Kent M (2014) Veterinary Neuroanatomy and Clinical Neurology. 4th edn. St. Louis, MO: Saunders Elsevier.

DiGiovanna E, Schiowitz S, Dowling D (2005) An Osteopathic Approach to Diagnosis and Treatment. Lippincott Williams and Wilkins, pp. 577; 602–606.

Furr M, Reed S (2015) Equine Neurology. 2nd edn. Iowa: John Riley and Sons, p. 18.

Hartman L (1996) Handbook of Osteopathic Technique. Nelson Thornes.

Hartwig W (2008) Fundamental Anatomy. Philadelphia: Lippincott Williams & Wilkins, p. 188.

Hedge J, Wagoner D, Equine Research Inc. (2004) Horse conformation: Structure, Soundness and Performance. Equine Research Inc. Guilford, Connecticut: Lyons Press.

Holst GC (2000) Common Sense Approach to Thermal Imaging. SPIE Press and JCD Publishing.

Jeffcott LB (1980) Disorders of the thoracolumbar spine of the horse – a survey of 443 cases. Equine Veterinary Journal. October; 12 (4) 197.

Leach DH (1980) The structure and function of the equine hoof wall. PhD thesis, University of Saskatchewan.

Lederman E (2000) Harmonic Technique. London: Churchill Livingstone.

Liyou O (2005) Wolf teeth in horses-equine dentistry. Australian stock horse journal, Artarmon. 1(1) 76–77.

Pusey A, Brooks J (2010) Osteopathic treatment – overarching principles. In: Pusey A, Brooks J, Jenks A. Osteopathy and the Treatment of Horses. Wiley-Blackwell, pp. 100–105.

Ross MW, Dyson SJ (2011) Diagnosis and Management of Lameness in the Horse. 2nd edn. St. Louis, Missouri: Elsevier Saunders.

Scarr G (2014) Biotensegrity: The Structural Basis of Life. Pencaitland, East Lothian: Handspring Publishing.

Schultz RL, Feitis R (1996) The Endless Web: Fascial Anatomy and Physical Reality. Berkeley, California: North Atlantic Books.

Stashak TS (1987) Adam's Lameness in Horses. 4th edn. Philadelphia: Lea & Febiger.

Stubbs NC, Clayton HM (2008) Activate your Horse's Core: Unmounted Exercises for Dynamic Mobility, Strength & Balance. Sport Horse Publications.

Turner S (2008) Principles of osteopathic treatment. In: Moeckel E, Mitha N (eds.) Textbook of Pediatric Osteopathy. Churchill Livingstone Elsevier, p. 193.

Vollmer M. Möllmann K-P (2013) Infrared Thermal Imaging: Fundamentals, Research and Applications. Wiley – VCH Verlag GmbH and Co. Chapter 10.

Further reading

Audigié F, Pourcelot P, Degueurce C, Geigert D, Denoix JM (2001) Kinematic analysis of the symmetry of limb movements in lame trotting horses. Equine Veterinary Journal. April; 33: 128–134.

Buchner HH, Savelberg HH, Schamhard HC, Barneveld A (1996) Limb movement adaptations in horses with experimentally induced fore- or hindlimb lameness. Equine Veterinary Journal. January; 28(1) 63–70.

Chaitow L (2007) Positional Release Techniques. Churchill Livingstone Elsevier.

Clayton HM, Almeida PE, Prades M, Brown J, Tessier C, Lanovaz JL (2002) Double-blind study of the effects of an oral supplement intended to support joint health in horses with tarsal degenerative joint disease. Proceedings of the Annual Convention of the AAEP 2002, Vol. 48.

Colles CM, Ware R (2010) The Principles of Farriery. London: JA Allen.

Dyce K, Sack W, Wensing C (2009) Textbook of Veterinary Anatomy. 4th edn. Saunders Elsevier.

Muñoz A, Cuesta I, Riber C, Gata J, Trigo P, Castejón F (2006) Trot asymmetry in relation to physical performance and metabolism in equine endurance rides. Equine Special Issue: Proceedings of the 7th International Conference of Exercise Physiology. Equine Veterinary Journal. Supplement. June; 38 (S36) 50–54.

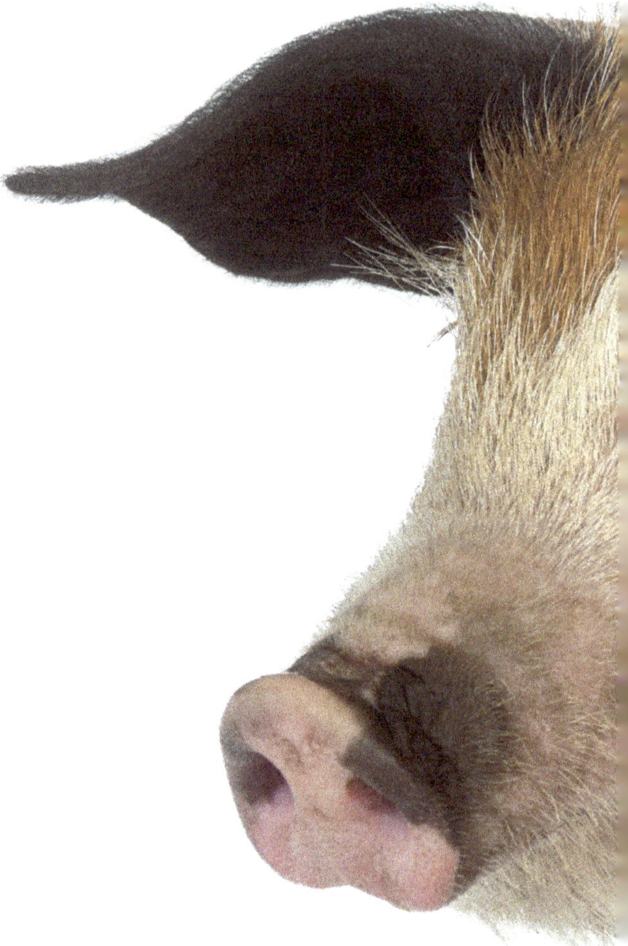

Chapter 6
LIVESTOCK

Chris Colles, Julia Brooks, Tony Nevin, Brendan Atkin

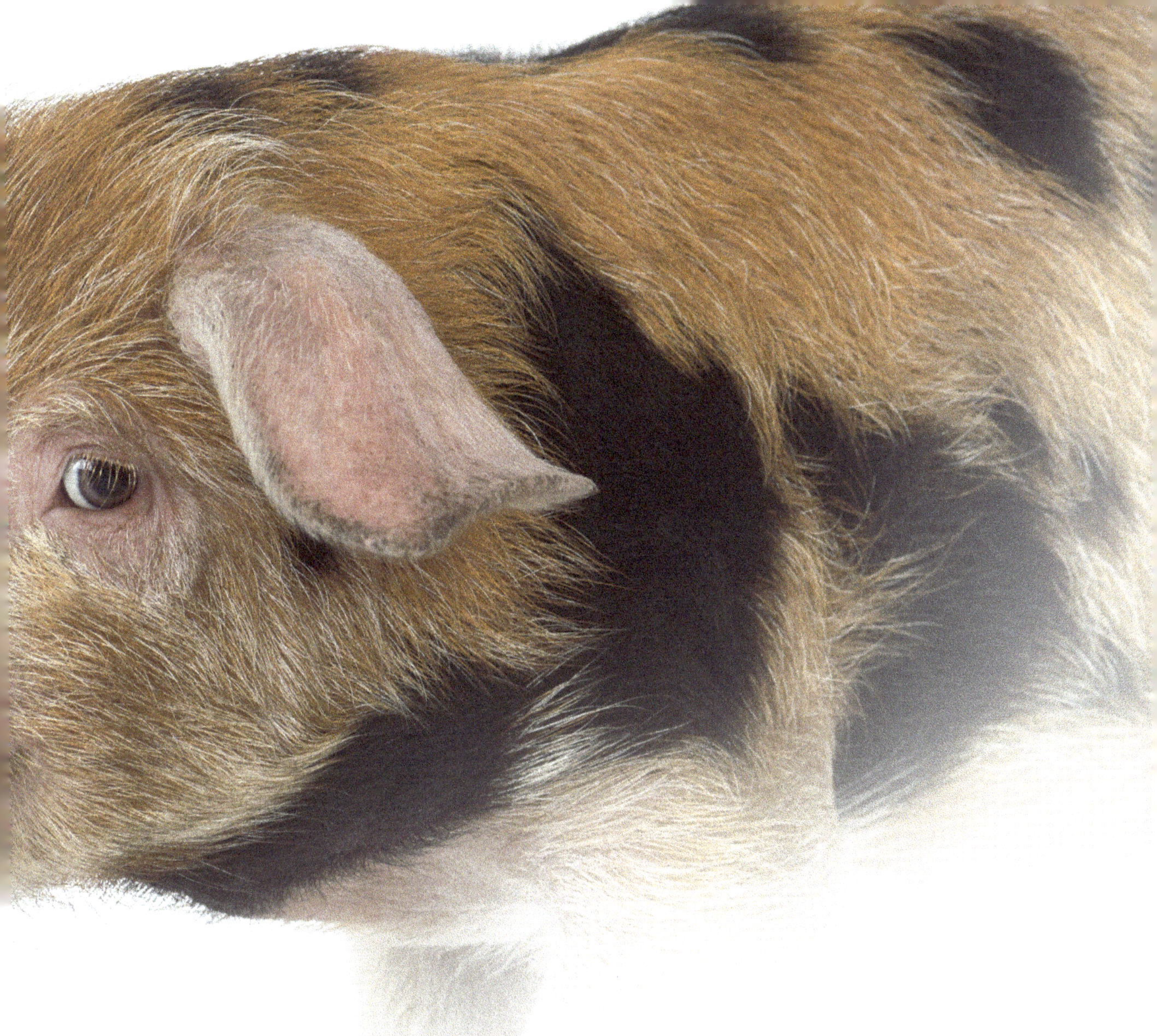

Introduction

Osteopathic treatment is greatly improved when the practitioner has accurate anatomical knowledge of the animal undergoing treatment. If the reader has studied the anatomy of the dog and horse in Chapters 2 and 5, the basic structures of farm livestock will be familiar. However, there are variations between species, and breed characteristics, which are outlined later in the chapter.

Animals are farmed for meat, milk, or fiber. The product needs to be produced quickly and economically, with some stock held back to breed the next generation. A painful musculoskeletal problem may affect an animal's ability to forage which, combined with the stress of pain, will cause loss of condition, affecting weight gain, production of milk, or the quality of wool or fiber. It may interfere with a male's libido and ability to serve females of the flock or herd. Good physical condition can prolong the number of breeding seasons possible for an animal, which is particularly advantageous where a valuable bloodline has been established. On a practical basis, most farm animals are unlikely candidates for extensive musculoskeletal treatment for financial reasons; however, valuable or rare breeding stock and some pet animals may be candidates.

Cattle, sheep, goats, and pigs are the main large animals to be found on farms. Goats and ewes may be kept for milk production as well as meat. Red deer and some fallow deer are farmed for meat, with some body parts used in Oriental medicine. They remain semiwild, however, and are unlikely candidates for treatment. In recent years, alpacas and llamas have become a feature of the countryside, producing lanolin-free fiber for clothing. Fowl are covered in Chapter 8.

Animals bred for meat have a relatively short life span. The slaughtering of cattle for beef occurs at 18 to 36 months, and in calves for veal it occurs at 18 to 20 weeks. Lambs are slaughtered at between eight and 12 months, and pigs are slaughtered at around six months. Goats may live for 10 to 12 years, but their productive life is around seven years.

Deer aged between 15 and 18 months produce a good-quality, low-fat carcass.

Bulls may be kept for four or five breeding seasons, starting as yearlings with peak fertility from two to four years but exhibiting a rapid decline after seven years. Heifers begin breeding from 15 months and may be culled for meat at around five years old.

There are considerable variations in the local names given to all types of domestic animals and to their management. The terms given below apply principally to farming in the United Kingdom.

With cattle, calf refers to either gender with no specific end age. Heifers are females that have not yet bred, becoming cows after their first calving. Bullock in the UK refers to a castrated male of any age, whereas in the USA it usually means a young entire male, and in Australasia it tends to refer to an animal kept for draft purposes which is usually but not always castrated.

Sheep are referred to as lambs in their first year of life. Shearing is carried out annually, either to harvest wool or for welfare reasons, so that sheep do not carry a heavy fleece through the heat of the summer. A year-old sheep may be referred to as a shearling. A ram, or tup, is an uncastrated male. Breeding in sheep may be carried out to preserve a line, or they may be crossbred with other breeds to select for characteristics which maximize the health and productivity of the flock. The peak productivity of sheep is three to six years of age, declining after seven years. Most are culled before their natural life span of 11 to 12 years.

Boars are uncastrated male pigs more than six months of age. They begin serving females at 28 to 30 weeks and are usually culled at two to four years. The term gilt generally refers to a female that has not yet produced her first litter. Sows (female pigs that have been bred) may produce two litters of 10 to 15 piglets a year and are pregnant or lactating for most of the year. Breeding sows are generally replaced every three to five years. Weaners are piglets of either sex that have been separated from the sow and are usually around five to 10 weeks of age.

Llamas and the smaller alpacas may be kept for fiber production. They also make exotic pets and good guards against predators. Llamas have characteristic long, banana-shaped ears compared to those of the alpaca which are short and spear-like. Alpacas produce a finer fiber at annual shearing. Both llamas and alpacas start to breed at about 18 months and have a gestation of 350 days, which usually produces a single offspring known as a cria. The female can produce 10 to 12 cria over a 20-year lifetime.

By far the most common conditions that will be brought before an osteopath will be of an MSK nature. Depending on the breed involved this could involve compression, such as with cattle and sheep, following butting; or strains and sprains, which are more commonly seen in pigs and camelids.

Sometimes a farmer will call and ask an osteopath to have a look at one or more of their animals in the belief that it will be cheaper than calling the vet out. In many territories, the UK included, this can put an osteopath on the wrong side of the law. Livestock can be similar to wildlife, masking pain and giving poor feedback when examined. In the case of pigs their sheer bulk and shape can render a purely physical examination almost null and void with observed posture and gait giving the best clues as to what is going on (Fig. 6.1). It is essential to obtain a veterinary surgeon's diagnosis, as well as permission, before attempting to help these patients.

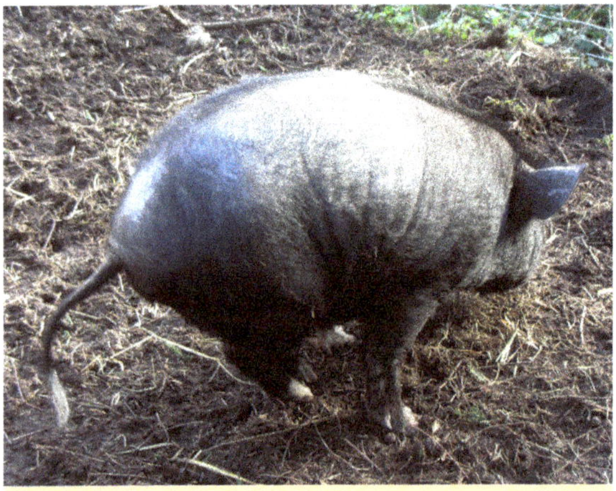

Figure 6.1
A Kunekune pig with severe pain avoiding load-bearing through the hind limbs.

Health and safety

Although livestock are domesticated, this must not be confused with them being tame. Most farm animals are seldom handled. The osteopath will usually need assistance in restraining and handling these patients, and will need to be aware of the defence mechanisms they may employ. Working around livestock requires a sharp mental attitude. Always ensure that you have exit routes worked out before commencing any hands-on work. Ensure that everyone involved has a good idea of what you intend to do during a treatment or consultation session. Be prepared to take advice and heed any warnings given. When treating any animal you are responsible for everyone's safety, not just your own. Cattle have killed stockmen, and pigs can be extremely dangerous. Many breeds of sheep and especially rams can be vicious if they catch you off guard, so the osteopath needs to be constantly alert. Never turn your back on farm livestock when in the same pen as the patient!

Osteopaths are generally looking at the physical biomechanical health of patients. When visiting farms, however, it is important to realize that we must ensure that we do not act as vectors for any infectious diseases. Suitable barrier defence as well as regular changes of clothing and disinfecting of footwear are essential. The sanitizing of hands between each patient treatment also reduces the risk of any contact infection being spread.

Female osteopaths should also remember that if they are or suspect they may be pregnant they should not work with, or handle, sheep due to the risk of listeriosis to their own unborn.

Anatomy

The following is a brief anatomical description with an emphasis on the variations in the musculoskeletal system specific to farm animals (see Figs 6.2–6.5). Some attention will be given to the specialized digestive system and the reproductive system in view of the emphasis on growth and breeding in these animals. Much farm animal anatomy is similar to that of other animals, but there are some features that diverge from the basic pattern.

Overview

A number of anatomical inferences can be made initially by looking at the toes! Most farm animals are ungulates, meaning that they have hooves. They are Artiodactyla - even-toed ungulates. They have evolved to weight-bear on the 3rd and 4th toes which have become encased in horn. Camelids are the exception, where the 2nd and 3rd phalanges lie flat on the ground, with a large "pad" (rather like that of a dog) under the back of the foot, and the hooves are rather claw-like on the front of the feet.

Typically, farm animals are herbivorous, and have developed specialized dentition and a digestive process involving a three- or four-compartment stomach to digest cellulose. The odd-toed ungulates (horses and rhinoceros) weight-bear through the 3rd toe and digest cellulose in the hindgut.

Pigs differ from other farm animals as, like humans, they are omnivores and obtain nutrition from both plant and animal matter. They have simple stomachs, but to accommodate their largely plant-based diet they have developed the ability to degrade carbohydrates in the upper part of the digestive tract. In addition, the large intestine has a well-established ecosystem for partial fermentation in order to utilize fibrous material.

Ruminants and camelids

Cattle, goats, sheep, and deer are ruminants (from the Latin *ruminare* meaning "to chew over again"). In order to digest an herbivorous diet, these animals ferment plant-based food utilizing microbial action. This takes place in a specialized stomach which has four chambers. Camelids, such as llamas and alpacas, are often referred to as modified ruminants, as they have three rather than four stomach chambers.

Skull

The skull in cattle is angular and pyramidal with the addition of horns in many breeds. Horns arise from bony cornual processes of the frontal bones, set at the lateral angles of the forehead. They have a bone core. The horn sheath grows from the epithelium covering these bony processes. The growth is continuous and pushes old horn out to the apex which is virtually solid horn. Growth is slow and can be affected by stressful events such as calving as well as changes in nutrition. In times of stress, thinner, softer horn is produced, and ridges are formed on the surface of the horn.

The horns are innervated by the maxillary branch of the trigeminal nerve. Horn development may be prevented by cauterizing the germinal epithelium in calves, but there are a number of naturally polled (or hornless) cattle.

The cranium of sheep and goats is more domed than that of cattle. The horns develop close together in a central position behind the orbits, overlying the parietal bones. The frontal sinus is not involved with the base of these centrally positioned horns, whereas in cattle the sinus extends up into the horn. Polled breeds in sheep are common, but where horns do occur they are generally seen in both sexes. In cross-section, goats' horns are oval whereas sheep's horns are triangular.

Horns are a permanent feature, with a central core of live bone covered with keratin. Antlers of deer are not permanent. Antlers are a bony growth, formed annually from the skull, with the size and shape depending on age, sex, and species. They begin to grow in spring and may grow several inches in a week. Initially they are covered by highly sensitive skin known as velvet. Around July, the antlers stop growing, and the velvet dies and is rubbed off to reveal the antlers in time for the breeding season or "rut" in October. The bone of mature antlers is dead. A fall in testosterone levels at the end of the winter causes the antlers to drop off.

The heads of ruminants may bear a number of glands associated with territorial marking. Sheep have an infraorbital cutaneous pouch in front of the eye whose secretions often stain the face. Goats have groups of musk glands at the base of the horns which, stimulated by testosterone in the male, can be seriously pungent.

The skull is covered with mimetic muscles, for facial movements, supplied by the 7th cranial nerve. The auriculopalpebral branch supplies the external ear and eyelids, and if damaged results in a drooping ear and sagging eyelid. The dorsal buccal branch supplies the muscles of the nose and upper lip. Its relatively exposed position on the side of the face leaves it prone to injury, causing facial asymmetry with the face drawn toward the unaffected side. The facial artery crosses under the mandible, in front of the masseter muscle, where it may be used to palpate the pulse.

A large part of the skull is formed by the nasal passages, although these are smaller than outside appearances might suggest as much space is devoted to sinuses and conchae.

The salivary glands are very productive in ruminants. Saliva serves to lubricate fodder during mastication, but also buffers acids produced from the fermentation processes in the stomach chambers. The parotid gland lies between the ear and the angle of the jaw. The more productive mandibular gland forms an arc around the inner surface of the mandible and is active during mastication. The sublingual gland lies lateral to the tongue.

Teeth. Ruminant teeth consist of a lower arcade of eight incisors, arranged in a crescent, which act against the dental pad of the upper jaw (there are no upper **incisors**). The outer incisors are actually modified canine teeth. A large gap or diastema occurs between the canine and the six cheek teeth. This gives a dental formula of 0033 (upper)/3133 (lower). The grinding surface of the cheek teeth wears unevenly to give a rough shredding surface. The permanent teeth are complete by three and a half to four years and will erupt continuously to compensate for wear. The incisors are rather spatulate in shape and do not erupt continually with increasing age. By six to nine years the gums retract, and the incisors become level and badly worn before gradually being lost.

The upper arcades of cheek teeth are broader than the lower, and so chewing is unilateral, with each side being used alternately. The main muscle involved is the masseter, which has horizontally orientated superficial fibers and deep vertical fibers. This is complemented by the medial and lateral pterygoids. The temporalis is relatively weak as there is no requirement for powerful mouth closure to crush food because chewing is the main activity. Cattle and sheep are primarily grazers (eating grass), whereas goats also tend to browse on leaves, soft stems, and woody shrubs.

Llamas and alpacas are grazers and browsers, and have developed a slightly different dentition. The deciduous dental formula is 1123 (upper)/3112 (lower) and the permanent formula is 1123/3123. The upper incisor count is unusual. As in ruminants there is a toothless upper dental pad. One incisor persists, however, and has migrated caudally. Together with a modified canine, they form the "fighting teeth" or fangs - two in the upper arcade and one in the lower. They erupt at two to three years of age in males and may erupt at four to five years in females. They may be removed in males to avoid injuries to other males.

In cattle, the temporomandibular joint allows considerable movement in the horizontal plane. The postglenoid process is small, and the condylar process of the mandible is concave transversely and articulates with the convex mandibular fossa of the squamous temporal bone. The joint is divided by a fibrocartilaginous disc, to smooth incongruity of the joint surfaces.

Pharynx. The pharynx is divided into nasopharynx, oropharynx, and laryngopharynx. The pharynx receives regurgitated cud in the form of a bolus and transmits it to the mouth. It also receives the large amounts of gas produced by fermentation in the stomach which leave through the mouth (eructation or belching) which occurs around once a minute

Eyes. The eyes, set at each side of the skull, give a good range of monocular peripheral vision with a small degree of binocular vision in front. In addition to the upper and lower eyelids there is also a third eyelid or nictitating membrane which protects and moistens the eye. Only a small part is visible in the medial corner of the eye, but it becomes more visible when the eyeball is retracted or pushed in.

Compared with the vertical slits of predatory animals, the bovine pupil, in common with most herbivores, is widened from side to side to give a broader field of vision. The ciliary muscle is weak and so visual accommodation is poor.

The vertebral column

The vertebral column provides a stiff body axis, which aids locomotion and protects the spinal cord. It is divided into cervical, thoracic, lumbar, sacral, and caudal segments with the number of vertebrae in each varying between species and to some extent between individuals.

As in all mammals, with very rare exceptions, ruminants have seven cervical vertebrae. There is some distinction between large and small ruminants in terms of thoracolumbar, sacral, and coccygeal components: cattle have 13 thoracic, six lumbar, and five fused sacral segments, and 18 to 20 caudal vertebrae.

Smaller ruminants, such as sheep and goats, have 13 to 14 thoracic vertebrae, six or seven lumbar vertebrae, and four fused sacral vertebrae. Sheep have 16 to 18 caudal vertebrae forming the downward hanging tail, which is often docked within the first week for health reasons. Goats have four to eight caudal vertebrae, which project in an upward direction.

Llamas have 12 thoracic, seven lumbar, four fused sacral, and 15 to 20 caudal vertebrae.

The neck is very mobile. Thoracic spinal movement is limited by the rib cage. The lumbar spine is quite stiff, with the short intervertebral discs forming 10 percent of column length. It is subject to degeneration especially at the lumbosacral joint. Osteophytes form around the vertebral bodies and degenerative synovial articulations. This may have significance in bulls where degenerative changes may affect their ability to serve the female.

Thoracic girdle and proximal thoracic limb

Proximally, this follows more or less the same format as equine anatomy. The obvious difference is the distal limb where, instead of a leg being composed of a single supporting structure, the ruminant limb has two weight-bearing digits.

Pelvis and proximal hind limb

Pelvic conformation, with its effect on the ease of parturition, is of significance in breeding stock. Together with the hind limb, the pelvis also influences the power generated during locomotion.

Surface anatomy

In bovines (Fig. 6.2) the contour of the spine is slightly raised over the withers but is otherwise generally straight down to the sacrum, with the line of the neck varying with the carriage of the head. In sheep and goats (Fig. 6.3) the thoracolumbar spine tends to be slightly arched with a raised neck. Camelids (Fig. 6.4) have a relatively flat thoracolumbar spine with a long, upright cervical spine.

In bovines, the dorsal line of the neck, from the upper cervical region to the withers is relative to the length of the ligamentum nuchae. The first to third vertebrae are near the dorsal surface of the neck, the large wing of the atlas being easily identified caudal to the temporomandibular region. Between the angle of the jaw and the transverse process of the atlas, the largest of the salivary glands, the parotid, can be palpated. The caudal cervical vertebrae occupy a much more ventral position but, although the spinous processes cannot be felt, the transverse processes are palpable above the jugular groove, between the brachiocephalicus dorsally and the sternocephalicus ventrally

A series of lymphatic structures run in the neck including a palpable superficial cervical node in front of the scapula which may be used as part of a screening process for the health of the animal. The trachea is palpable toward the upper end of the neck. The esophagus cannot usually be palpated, but can be seen during swallowing and eructation. In the smaller ruminants and camelids palpation of these areas is easier.

Thoracolumbar spinous processes can be palpated except in the interscapula area where they are enclosed by the scapular cartilage. Dorsally, the paraspinal muscles run along either side of the spinous processes and lateral to this the flank sinks down into a concave surface. The ends of the transverse processes of the 2nd to 5th lumbar vertebrae can usually be palpated. The 6th is tucked under the tuber coxae and is covered with muscle. The 1st may be difficult to palpate because of

Chapter 6

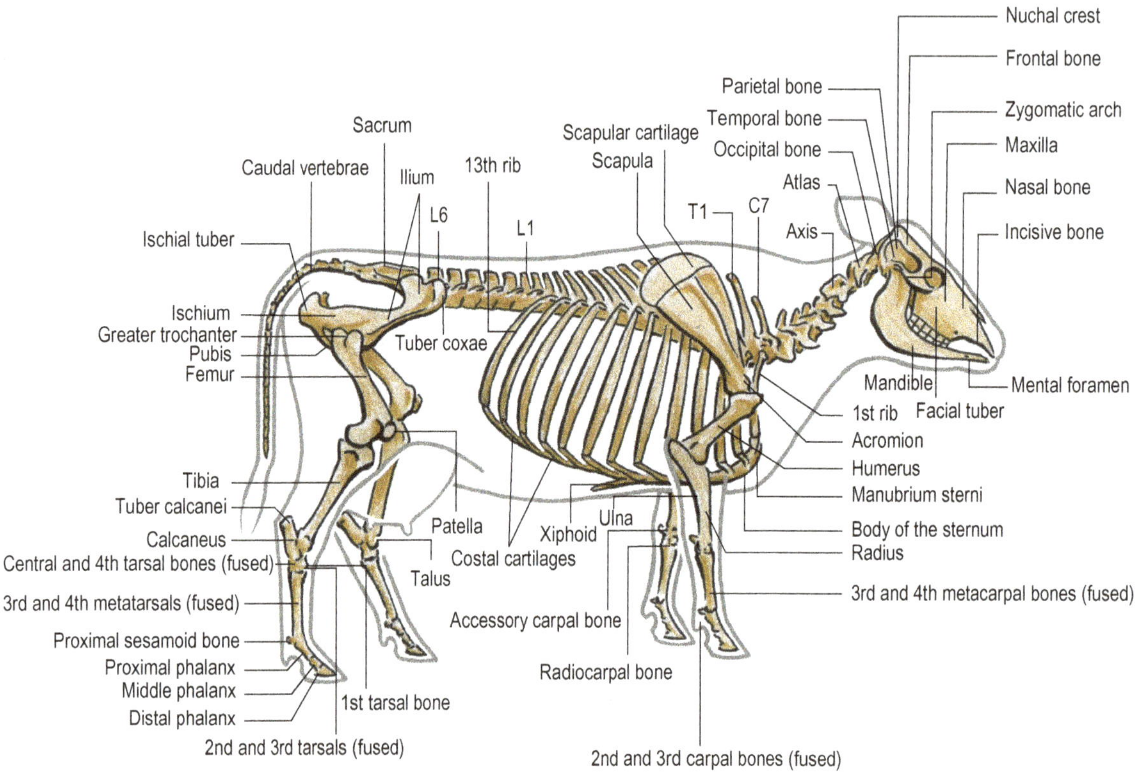

Figure 6.2
Ox skeleton.

the costal margin. In the smaller ruminants and camelids (Figs 6.3 and 6.4) palpation of these areas is easier.

Identification of individual vertebrae is most reliable if the vertebrae are counted forward from the large lumbosacral space which lies between the tuber coxae of the pelvis and is created by the upright 5th lumbar spinous process and the caudally sloping sacral crest.

In the bovine the sacrum maintains a level with the thoracic vertebrae. In smaller ruminants and camelids, the sacrum slopes down caudally to its articulation with the first caudal vertebrae.

The shoulder girdle is composed of parts of the thoracic spine, the scapula, and the humerus which lie level with the trunk. The cranial and caudal angles of the scapula can be palpated. Between these angles extends a semicircular plate of cartilage lying parallel with the spinous processes of the 2nd to the 6th thoracic vertebrae. The spine of the scapula divides the lateral surface into two fossae for the infraspinatus and supraspinatus muscles. It ends ventrally as the prominent acromion. The shoulder articulation overlies the middle of the first two ribs, and movement is primarily restricted to flexion and extension. The greater tubercle of the humerus forms the palpable point of the shoulder. Some way below this the deltoid tuberosity can be palpated.

The elbow joint is approximately level with the ventral extremities of the 4th and 5th ribs. The olecranon of the ulna projects backward and is readily palpable.

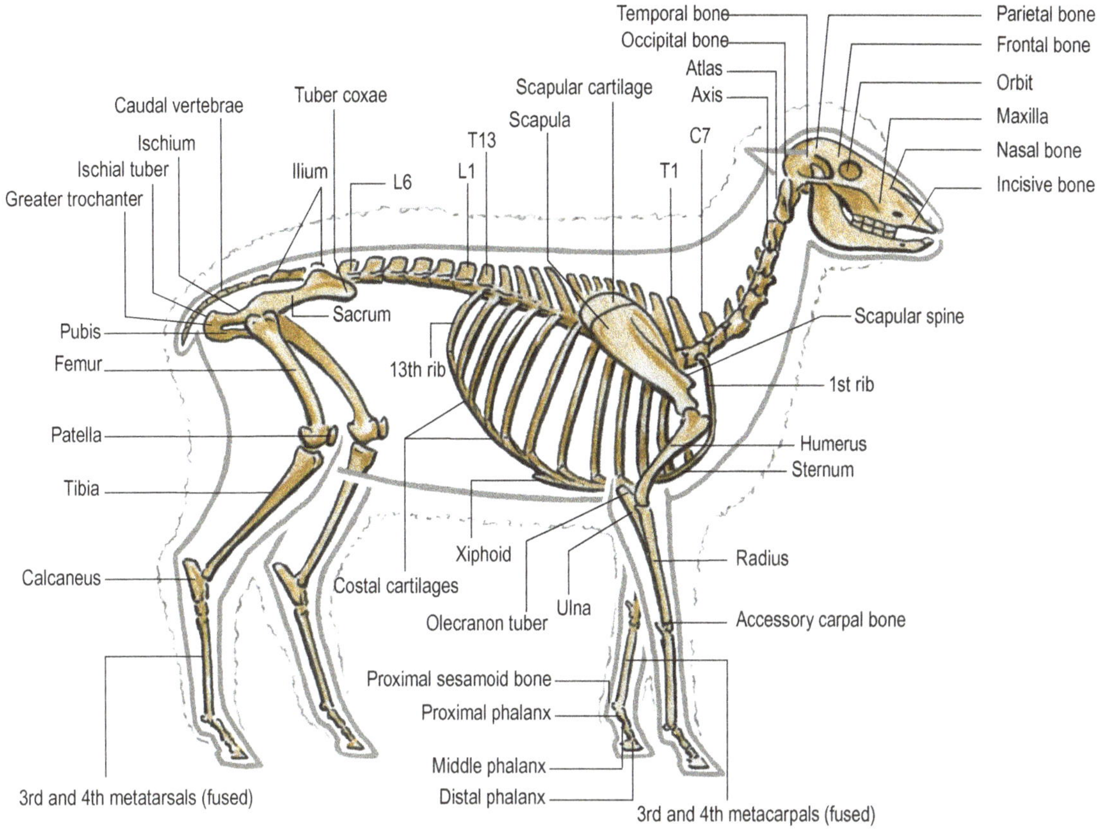

Figure 6.3
Sheep skeleton.

The medial border of the radius is palpable along its length, marking the division between extensor and flexor muscles. The shaft of the ulna and radius are fused, but at the carpus the styloid process of the ulna is palpable laterally, as is the accessory carpal bone on the caudal surface.

The carpus consists of six bones. The proximal row has the radial, intermediate, and ulnar carpal, with the accessory carpal bone palpable posteriorly. The two bones of the distal row are the 4th carpal and the fused 2nd and 3rd carpal bones. This arrangement allows flexion and extension, with most movement occurring at the radiocarpal joint. There is very little movement at the carpometacarpal joint.

A number of bony landmarks are easily identified, particularly in dairy cattle. The human equivalent to the posterior superior iliac spine is the sacral tuber, which gives the position of the lumbosacral joint lying below. If this projects above the level of the convex sacral crest, dislocation of the sacroiliac joint should be suspected. The iliac crest, thinly covered by the gluteus medius, runs forward to the prominent tuber coxae or "hook bone," which equates to the human anterior superior iliac spine. Projecting backward is the ischial tuber or "pin bone."

These landmarks may be used to determine the orientation of the pelvis. The angle between the horizontal and a line drawn between the coxal and ischial tubers

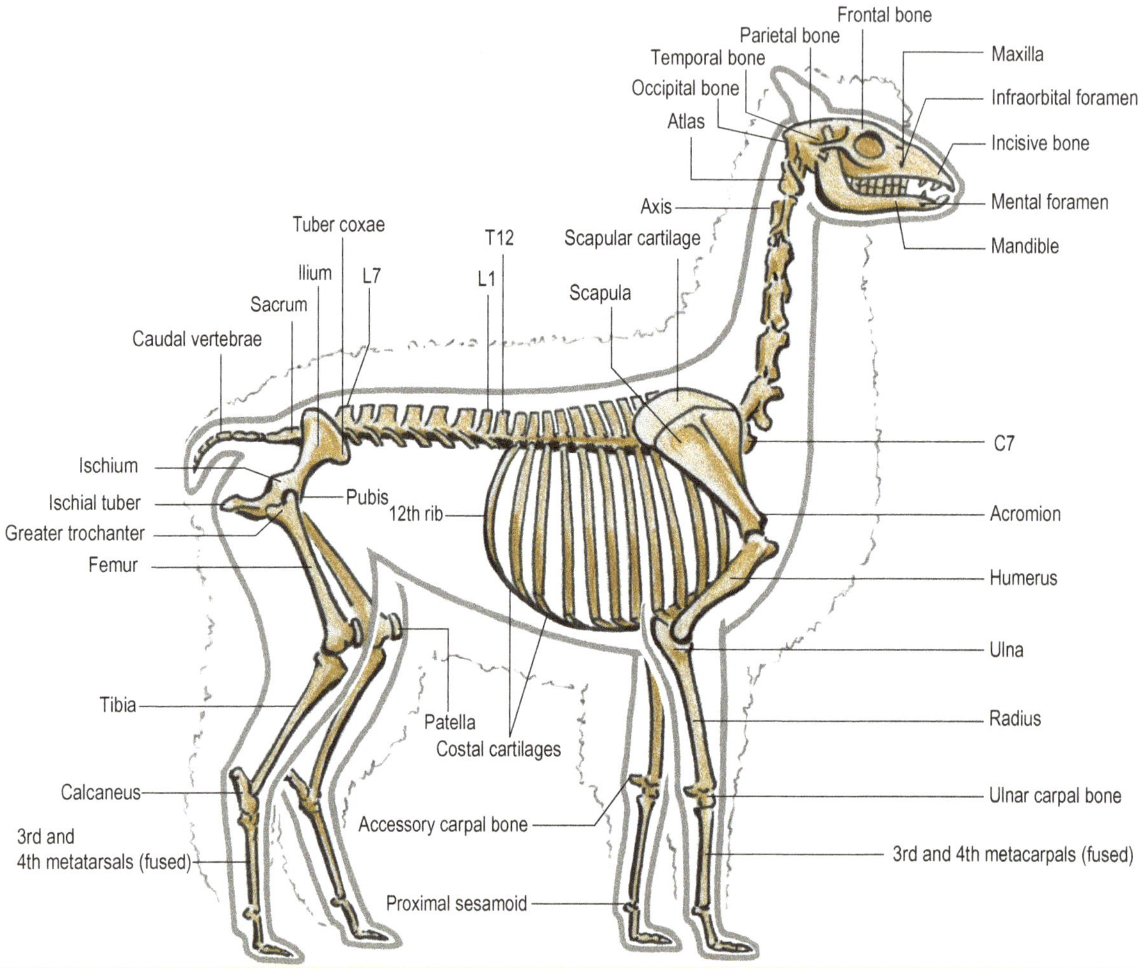

Figure 6.4
Llama skeleton.

indicates the slope of the pelvis. A small angle indicates a flattened rump, so that the femur is relatively straight under the animal, which may predispose to increased concussive forces through the hip joint. The distance between the backward projecting ischial tuberosities is significant, and wide spacing will facilitate parturition. Cattle lack an internal obturator muscle and, without this protection, the obturator nerve which supplies the adductors, external obturator, and gracilis is vulnerable to injury, especially during parturition.

The hip joint lies medial and slightly cranial to the greater trochanter, which may be palpated through the biceps femoris. The trochanter lies slightly below a line joining the coxal and ischial tubers, but projects above this line in dorsal dislocation of the hip or fracture of the neck of femur.

The stifle is situated just caudal to the skin fold formed where the leg meets the body. Cattle have three distal patellar ligaments, of which the middle and medial, together with the patella, create an energy-conserving locking mechanism for the stifle employed during standing. While the stifle is similar to that found in the horse it is less efficient. Smaller ruminants have only one patellar ligament.

The patella, the patellar ligaments, and the tibial tuberosity are all palpable. In cattle two gaps between the three patellar ligaments can be identified.

The tibia has a tibial crest on the upper third of the cranial border of the tibia. Its medial surface, ending in the prominent medial malleolus, is palpable, as is the lateral malleolus of the fibula. Caudal to this, the tuber calcanei forms the point of the hock. The hock may be used to establish conformation of the limbs. From behind, if the points of the hocks are too close, the animal is said to be cow-hocked and if too far apart bow-legged. From the side, the hock forms an angle of around 145 degrees. Smaller angles result in a sickle-hocked animal. Conversely, a greater angle is described as straight-hocked. These conformation defects may predispose to joint injury and tendon strains.

The fibula is residual. Its shaft is totally absent, and the proximal head is fused to the tibia. The distal part remains as the malleolar bone, a palpable quadrilateral bone which articulates with the tibia and contributes to the hock joint.

The hock joint is a composite of a number of different joints, arranged in three rows. The first row is made up of the calcaneus and the talus. The talus, in common with other artiodactyls but unlike that of a horse, has a grooved structure, the trochlea, at both ends. Proximally, it articulates with the tibial and malleolar bones to form the talocrural joint. The distal trochlea articulates with the calcaneus caudally, and distally, with the fused central and 4th bones of the second row. These joints allow flexion and extension.

The distal row articulates with the metatarsal, and is formed from part of the 4th tarsal which lies lateral to the fused 2nd and 3rd tarsal bone, and a small 1st tarsal lying on the plantar surface of the joint. The intertarsal and tarsometatarsal articular surfaces are relatively flat and movement is limited.

The hock allows flexion and extension. Extension is achieved by five muscles inserting on the calcaneal tuberosity by way of a calcaneal tendon (the tendon is made up of the gastrocnemius and the superficial digital flexor, as well as the biceps femoris, gracilis, and semitendinosus).

Distal limbs

The distal limb is composed of metacarpals or, in the hind limb, metatarsals, and the three phalanges which make up each digit, in addition to a number of sesamoids. They form the articulations of the fetlock, pastern, and coffin joints.

Metacarpus and metatarsus. By early fetal life, four cartilaginous metacarpals are present - the 2nd, 3rd, 4th, and 5th metacarpals. The 3rd and 4th gradually unite in utero to form a cannon bone, or large metacarpal, although this union is incomplete and there is a discernible internal septum. The 2nd metacarpal disappears completely or may be present as a small rod, while the 5th persists as an approximately 4 cm rod lying alongside the lateral border of the upper end of the large metacarpal. The metatarsals of the hind limb follow the same pattern, although the large metatarsal is longer by about 3 cm and the small metatarsal is a quadrilateral disc of about 2 cm articulating with the proximal end of the large metatarsal.

The cannon bone is shorter, wider, and flatter than in the horse. It divides distally into two condyles for articulation with the two digits at the fetlock joint.

Phalanges of the digits. Of the four digits, digits 2 and 5 are vestigial dewclaws, and lie behind the fetlock. Only digits 3 and 4 are fully formed ending in two toes or "clays." Each digit consists of three phalanges, with two proximal sesamoids at the fetlock joint, and a distal sesamoid at the distal interphalangeal joint. The phalanges lie together within the skin, with only the hooves appearing as two distinctly separate structures. Sheep have an extended pouch of skin extending up between the two toes.

The proximal phalanges are three-sided in cross-section. The area between the two phalanges is flattened, and caudally there is a prominence for the attachment of the interdigital ligament and facets for articulation with the proximal sesamoid bones. The middle phalanges, also three-sided, are shorter than the proximal phalanges with which they articulate. Together they form the pastern joint, which allows a degree of flexion and extension.

The middle and distal phalanges articulate at the coffin joint, which lies entirely within the hoof. The structure of the two distal phalanges each resembles one half of that of a horse. Each distal phalanx has four surfaces. The sole surface is narrow and slightly concave. The wall in front slopes at a 25-degree angle, while behind the angle is steep and there is a facet for the distal sesamoids. There are no hoof cartilages as found in the horse.

The distal phalanges are encased in hooves which curve inward toward each other. The lateral hoof is usually larger and bears more weight. The weight-bearing surface is formed by the walls and sole. The horn of the walls grows at a rate of about 5 mm per month and may require trimming.

The extensor tendons are palpable on the front of the metacarpals or metatarsals. These tendons run down to either the lateral or the medial digit or, in the case of the common digital extensor, both digits, bifurcating at the fetlock. Similarly, the superficial flexor tendon splits at the fetlock. The tendons are enclosed in synovial sheaths and are held in place by annular ligaments.

Abdomen

In ruminants a significant proportion of the abdomen is occupied by the stomach which is modified to allow the digestion of fodder obtained by browsing and grazing.

Muscular layers of the abdominal wall, as in other species, include rectus muscles, the external and internal obliques, and the transversus abdominis. These muscles contribute to the inguinal canal through which herniation can occur. A deep fascial layer contributes to the support of the viscera.

The superficial fascia provides a pathway for cutaneous nerves and some palpable lymph nodes. One of these, the subiliac node can be found in the skin fold of the limb and trunk. The subcutaneous "milk" veins run forward from the udder over the lower abdominal wall.

In ruminants the stomach is composed of four compartments - the rumen, reticulum, omasum, and abomasum- through which the food passes successively. In adult cattle this accommodates around 60 liters of macerated fodder, most of which is held in the rumen.

The rumen and reticulum are involved with maceration and microbial breakdown of complex carbohydrates. This breakdown is assisted by regurgitation and masticating the fodder again, known as "chewing the cud." Ruminants may spend a third of their time chewing the cud. A byproduct of the microbial action is the production of carbon dioxide and methane, with cattle producing 30–50 liters of gas per hour, and goats and sheep 5 liters per hour, depending on the fodder being digested. This is dispersed by belching or eructation, and any interference with this activity is life-threatening as the expanding rumen interferes with breathing.

From the rumen and reticulum the macerated food passes to the omasum where fluid is removed. It then passes to the abomasum, which resembles the stomach of monogastric species and produces pepsin and mucosal secretions.

From the stomach the partially digested food is passed to the intestines, which lie mainly on the right of the midline.

Llamas and alpacas are camelids and are often referred to as modified ruminants. They are browsers (eating bark, stems, and leaves) as well as grazers. They have a high digestibility coefficient, 25 percent higher than sheep, enabling them to survive in harsh environments.

The camelid stomach has only three compartments. The first, representing 83 percent of total stomach volume, is analogous to the rumen. The second, contributing to 6 percent of stomach volume, is composed of absorptive cells and mucous glands and is the equivalent of the reticulum. The third is the counterpart of the abomasum and contains mucosal, gastric, and pyloric glands. The glands of the three compartments secrete significant amounts of bicarbonate to aid absorption and digestions of cellulose. Camelids are also able to secrete urea from the blood into the rumen for protein synthesis. This reutilization mechanism accounts for their survival on low-protein diets. Regurgitation, eructation, and remastication are also part of their digestive process.

Pelvic viscera

Much of farming relies on reproduction, so it may be helpful to know some aspects of the reproductive processes.

Cattle begin ovulation at around 8 to 10 months and the estrus cycle is repeated every 21 days throughout the year. Gestation is 280 days (40 weeks). Although twins do occur, single calves are more common.

Sheep estrus cycles occur every 16 to 17 days, in most breeds between August and October-November depending on weather conditions. Gestation is 147 days. Twinning is common, and many farmers will aim for twin conceptions. Triplets are not uncommon, but can be difficult to rear.

Goats' estrus cycles occur every 18 to 21 days, usually between September and February, and are again dependant on climate and seasonal changes in the length of light periods. Gestation is generally about 154 days. As in sheep, twins are not uncommon.

In llamas ovulation is induced by coitus and may occur at any time of year. Pregnancy lasts 11 months, and generally birth is aimed for the spring or early summer. Although twins do occur, singletons are generally preferred.

Pigs

The requirement for musculoskeletal treatment for most pigs is limited, as the life span, from birth to slaughter, is only about six months, and their generally uncooperative disposition can cause handling difficulties. Veterinary concerns are more those of infection and congenital abnormality. There is, however, a pool of breeding sows and boars where treatment may be of value. Some problems will have their origin in selective breeding for meat mass which has outstripped the ability of the structure to support it. A pig may achieve a weight of 100 kg in six months compared with 70 kg 150 years ago.

The skull

In modern breeds there is a height to the skull above the brain. The front of the skull has an extensive sinus structure so that the brain lies about 5 cm deep to the skin surface. The brain itself is elongated and the occipital lobes do not conceal the cerebellum. The frontal lobes do not cover the very large olfactory bulbs which contribute to the pig's keen sense of smell. The snout and mouth are important in its rooting behavior for feeding. The snout is the central part of the upper lip and takes the form of a movable disc incorporating a rostral cartilage and moved by the levator labii superioris. Putting a ring through the dorsal part of the snout discourages rooting behavior.

The shape of the mandible, which slopes sharply back from the point of the chin, also facilitates rooting. The mandible and maxilla bear teeth, and at one and half years, well after the usual six-month age for slaughter, full dentition is present. This dentition is the most complete of domestic species, having a formula 3143 (upper)/3143 (lower). The six upper incisors and six lower incisors come together in a grasping action. Behind these lie the curved canine teeth, or tusks. In the boar, they can grow at a rate of 2 cm every six months, and regular detusking to remove all or part of the tusk is often performed for dental health as well as safety reasons.

There are seven cheek teeth on each side. The first premolar is usually separated from the second by a small gap, although the latter may be absent. The cheek teeth increase in size from front to back, and the irregular occlusal surface is adapted for crushing.

Chapter 6

At birth, piglets have eight laterally projecting, deciduous "needle teeth," which are occasionally clipped shortly after birth to avoid damage to the sow's teats and their littermates.

The coronoid process of the mandible is small and thin, and the condylar process is low and convex in both directions. The temporomandibular joint is capable of considerable protraction and retraction of the lower jaw, while limiting lateral movement. The mandibular symphysis is fused as in humans. Mouth opening is limited.

The vertebral column

The cervical spine (Fig. 6.5) is composed of seven vertebrae, but numbers in other regions can vary considerably with the breed with most pigs having 14 or 15 thoracic and six or seven lumbar vertebrae. The sacrum usually consists of four partially fused segments. There are between 20 and 27 caudal vertebrae.

The dorsoventral dimensions of the neck are almost the same as the trunk and the thickset nature of the neck means that cervical movement is limited.

The thoracolumbar spine is made up of 19 to 23 vertebrae, with higher numbers being desirable in terms of producing more loin for meat.

Articulating with the thoracic vertebrae are a variable number of ribs, usually 14 or 15, with unequal numbers on each side being common. The first seven ribs are attached ventrally to the six segments of the sternum. The vertebrae and the strongly curved ribs give structure to the barrel-shaped thorax, which encloses the heart and the lungs. The heart is relatively small in view of the animal's bulk, comprising only 0.3 percent of total body weight compared with 1 percent in the horse.

There are six or seven lumbar vertebrae, which have long bodies and broad, forward-directed spinous processes, except that of the last lumbar vertebra,

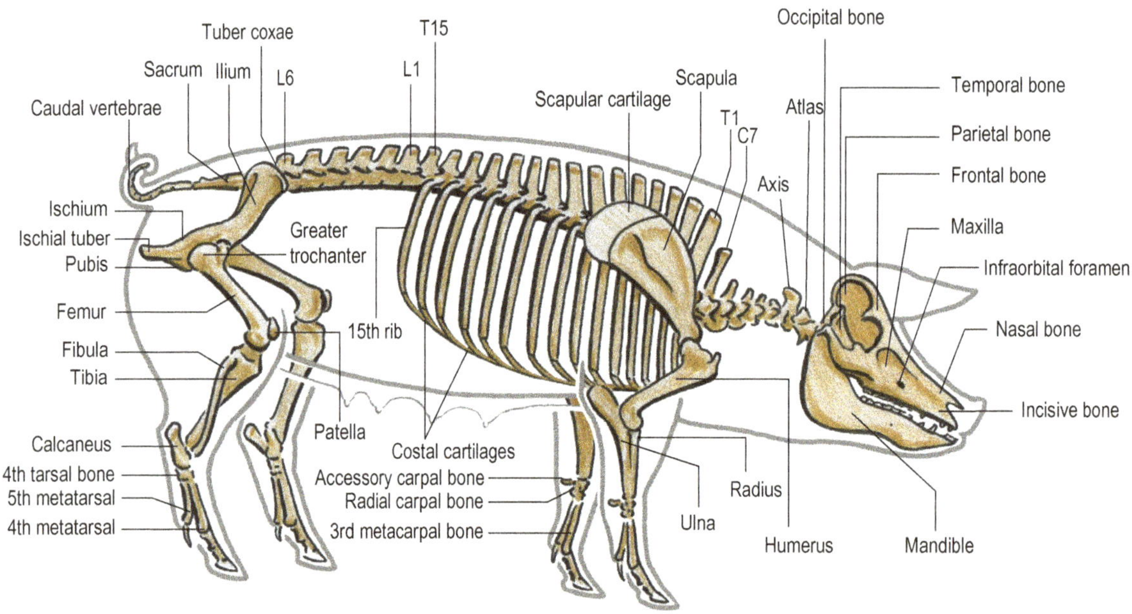

Figure 6.5
Pig skeleton.

which is narrow and vertically orientated. The transverse processes project ventrally and slightly forward, and do not articulate with each other or with the sacrum.

The muscles supporting the vertebral column dorsally follow the usual pattern, with the longissimus having the largest diameter. Ventrally, support is given by the psoas minor and psoas major. Lateral to the sixth lumbar vertebra are the iliac crests. In young pigs, the spinal cord ends within the sacrum. In older animals it ascends to terminate cranial to the sixth lumbar segment.

Caudal to the last lumbar vertebra, the back drops away as the four partially fused sacral elements have no spinous processes. The first caudal vertebrae resemble normal vertebrae, with articular processes. The last 15 are rod-like, with spiral arrangements for the insertions of the sacrococcygeus muscles, forming a curly tail.

The thoracic limb

The scapula is wide and has a less extensive scapular cartilage than cattle. Its external surface has a broad spine with a palpable tubercle midway along its length. The spine ends in a rudimentary acromium. The origin of the trapezius extends from the occiput to the 10th thoracic vertebra, inserting onto the scapular spine. The rhomboids, the latissimus dorsi, and the pectoral muscles all contribute to the attachment of the thoracic limb to the thorax.

The scapula articulates at the shoulder joint, with the curved head of the humerus. Laterally is the extensive external tuberosity onto which shoulder muscles such as the supraspinatus and infraspinatus insert and below which are attachments for the deltoid and teres minor. The shaft of the humerus is compressed from side to side, covered in front by the biceps and the more substantial brachialis, and covered behind by the triceps. The shaft ends distally in a condyle, which articulates with the radius and ulna.

The radius is short and thick, increasing in size distally where it articulates with the radial and intermediate carpal bones. Most of its posterior surface is firmly attached to the ulna by interosseous ligaments that allow only negligible movement between the two. The ulna is longer and heavier than the radius and extends from the olecranon process through a curved shaft to a relatively small distal end, which articulates with the ulnar and accessory carpal bones.

The carpus is composed of eight bones, four in each row. The distal row articulates with the four metacarpals, the first being absent. The third and fourth are the chief metacarpals either side of which are the much smaller second and fifth accessory metacarpals. The metacarpals all articulate with each other and with the distal carpals.

Each metacarpal articulates with a digit, made up of three phalanges, with two proximal sesamoid bones at the metacarpophalangeal joint, and a distal sesamoid at the distal interphalangeal joint. The phalanges end in hooves, with those of the 3rd and 4th phalanges supporting the animal's weight, whereas those of the 2nd and 5th phalanges are much smaller and do not usually touch the ground. The digits are moved by the digital extensors in front, which insert either on one digit or, by a series of bifurcations, on several of the digits.

The pelvic limb

The pelvic bone is elongated with the ilium and ischium in line with each other in a sagittal direction. The ilial wing is less outwardly orientated than in cattle. The palpable ischial tuber fuses late with the body of the ischium and may be displaced which causes considerable pain and dysfunction. The pubis is thick with the two sides coming together at the symphysis in an almost horizontal plane. The acetabular fossa is deep to receive the strongly curved head of the femur at the hip joint. Beyond the head is a distinct neck and the large trochanter and trochanteric ridge. There is no third trochanter.

The muscles around the pelvis with vertebral origins include the united psoas minor and major and the quadratus lumborum. Giving the rump its rounded form, and acting across the hip joint, are the gluteal muscles, biceps femoris, semitendinosus, and semimembranosus, with the broad expanse of the laterally positioned TFL reaching almost to the patella. These muscles cover the posterior and lateral surfaces of the four-sided femoral shaft. Medially and cranially lie the sartorius and the gracilis below which are the adductors and a well-developed pectineus. Acting both to flex the hip and extend the stifle are the large muscles of the quadriceps which lie over the cranial surface of the femur.

The stifle is composed of the femoropatellar and femorotibial joints principally allowing flexion and extension. The distal end of the femur has two equal, sagittal ridges on the trochlea for articulation with the patella. The patella only has one distal patellar ligament. Behind the trochlea, the femoral condyles articulate with the condyles of the tibia via semilunar cartilages.

The tibia is slightly curved with a tuberosity in front and a facet for articulation with the fibula behind. The fibula extends the whole length of the tibia, separated by a wide interosseous space. Forming the outline of the leg cranially are the peroneus tertius and tibialis anterior which insert into the metatarsals. Caudally the soleus and gastrocnemius insert onto the tuber calcis. Distally the tibia forms part of the hock joint, which, with the seven tarsal bones, is composed of the tibiotarsal, intertarsal, and tarsometatarsal joints.

The four metatarsals are similar but somewhat longer than the metacarpals in the forelimb. The two smaller metatarsals, the 2nd and 5th, lie more posterior to the principal digits.

Surface anatomy

The scope for palpation of the pig is somewhat limited by its compact nature and the quantity of subcutaneous fat. However, the following points do give some idea of the position and level of some structures (Fig. 6.5).

The skull has a high nuchal crest positioned well above the cranial cavity. From the base of the skull, the cervical spine runs in a straight line, as does the thoracolumbar spine of older pigs. In young piglets the thoracic spine is convex dorsally. There is little distinction between the neck and thorax, and the division is marked only as a depression in the muscle between the jowls and the shoulder joint.

In the thoracic limb, the tubercle on the spine of the scapula and the point of the shoulder are palpable, as is the manubrium sternum between the shoulder joints. The elbow lies lateral to the line of the 5th rib, and the medial and lateral epicondyles of the humerus and the olecranon of the ulna are palpable. Distally the accessory carpal bone protrudes backward to mark the position of the proximal carpal bone.

Despite the considerable layer of fat, the tubera coxae may be palpated, from which the position of the lumbosacral joint may be inferred. The ischial tuber may also be palpated. At the stifle, the patella, patellar ligaments, and tibial crest are palpable. At the hock, the medial and lateral malleoli of the tibia and fibula can be located and the calcaneal tendon is visible as it attaches to the calcaneus. Here, a bursitis or "capped hock" may result from lying on hard surfaces.

Abdominal and pelvic cavities

The abdominal cavity contains the organs of digestion, which includes a simple, monogastric stomach suited to an omnivorous diet where the digestion of complex carbohydrates is not essential. The abdominal walls are composed of muscular sheets of the external and internal oblique muscles and the transversus abdominus muscle. The inguinal canal, with its deep and superficial rings, gives a potential space between the internal and external oblique muscles. Inguinal and scrotal hernias are not uncommon in male weanlings, and may be repaired surgically.

Female pigs have two rows of about seven teats, providing an outlet for milk from the mammary glands.

The pelvis contains the reproductive organs. Estrus occurs for about 21 days all year round, but especially in spring and autumn. Gestation is 114 days, with sows giving birth to 10 to 16 piglets, although they seldom raise more than about 12. In most intensive systems sows will have two litters of piglets each year.

Common orthopedic conditions

Cattle

Neurological conditions

There are several conditions that can affect the nervous system of cattle. The most common ones are listed below.

Bovine spongiform encephalopathy (mad cow disease). This is a transmissible disease of cattle, notifiable in the UK, and hopefully becoming less common. Nonetheless it should be considered in any case of incoordination or instability seen in cattle. It is infectious, through eating infected meat, and the causal organism is probably a prion. It is infectious to humans, in which it is known as a variant of Creutzfeldt-Jakob disease.

In cattle the condition has a long incubation period, possibly two to three years. It is first evident as a slight change in gait, often associated with slight tremors and changes in behavior, such as hypersensitivity or aggression (but see Metabolic disease below). Once signs are present they tend to progress over a period of several weeks to months. Hind limb ataxia will become more obvious with time.

This condition should not be treated, and if suspected should be referred to a vet immediately or to the local authorities.

Metabolic disease. Modern farming puts increasingly high demands on farm animals. Milking and breeding cows are often under stress and severe metabolic demand, particularly around parturition.

Cattle are prone to several types of metabolic disease. Hypocalcemia, hypophosphatemia, and hypomagnesemia are all relatively common and are seen primarily in milking cattle usually around the time of calving, in spring, or when otherwise stressed. All three conditions may present initially as incoordination, progressing to recumbency. Hypomagnesemia is generally associated with excitability with the animals concerned often showing signs of convulsions and paddling when recumbent. The clinical signs alone are not adequate to diagnose which condition is present. They may all present as acute onset (often found dead) or slowly progressive conditions. Correct treatment by mineral supplementation is essential and must be instituted rapidly.

Spastic paresis of gastrocnemius muscle

Seen in calves generally six months old or less, this presents as tightening of the gastrocnemius initially, with progressive increasing tension as time progresses, with resultant hyperextension of the hind limb. It may be unilateral or bilateral. Attempts by the animal to move result in spasm of the extensors and flexors of the hind limb or limbs.

The condition is inherited, caused by a recessive gene, and no treatment is available.

Obturator paralysis

In cattle the obturator nerve is particularly vulnerable on the floor of the pelvis and is prone to damage during parturition. Affected cows will develop a base-wide stance of the hind legs (the obturator nerve innervating the adductor muscles). Damage to the ischiatic nerve may also result with knuckling of the fetlocks and possible recumbency. The wide-stance gait also leaves the animal prone to slipping and traumatic damage to the pelvis.

Treatment is basically allowing time for recovery with good management. The cow should be moved to a surface where the floor is not slippery and is reasonably soft. Sometimes the hind legs can be tied together below the hocks using a soft strap, restricting movement apart of the two limbs to about a meter. As with all nerve damage recovery tends to be slow and is not guaranteed.

Chapter 6

Lameness

Fractured pelvis. Fracture of the pelvis is not uncommon in cattle if they slip on hard floors. Particularly if affected by obturator paralysis, cows may do the splits, and this can result in separation of the pubic symphysis or fracture of the head of the femur. Treatment is problematic and generally not financially viable.

Foot-and-mouth disease. Foot-and-mouth disease is an acute infectious viral disease. It is accompanied by a raised temperature and the development of vesicles (blisters) chiefly in the mouth and on the feet. It is highly infectious and affects all cloven-hoofed animals such as cattle, buffalo, camels, sheep, goats, deer, and pigs. It is notifiable in the UK and many other countries. Lameness is generally seen in several animals in the herd and may be accompanied by salivation and drooling. Do not touch or engage with the animals and take serious biosecurity measures. Do not engage with any other animals without first seeking veterinary advice.

Foot lameness. Ninety percent of lameness in cattle is in the foot, mainly in the hind feet. Much lameness can be prevented by careful regular hoof trimming, and high standards of hygiene. Types of lameness are:

a. *Sole ulcers.* These occur at the back of the foot and are generally associated with poor foot care and hard surfaces. They can result in the corium of the foot being exposed. Treatment is by careful foot trimming.

b. *White line disease.* This is basically a traumatic condition involving separation of the hoof wall from the sole and secondary infection of the hoof wall. It is associated with hard or stony ground. Treatment is again by foot trimming and management considerations.

c. *Digital dermatitis.* This is an infectious condition and is generally associated with poor hygiene and cows standing in slurry. It tends to be infectious to other cattle. Treatment is by foot trimming, removing dead tissue, and application of topical antibiotics coupled with improvement of overall hygiene.

d. *Laminitis.* This is probably less common than in the equine, and is possibly underdiagnosed. It is associated with overfeeding and high-energy rations.

e. *Foul in the foot.* This is an infectious condition caused by *Fusobacterium necrophorum.* It infects the foot between the clays and is associated with a strong pungent "foul" smell. It may be associated with swelling of the foot, and possibly the pastern, and infection may progress to involve joints or bones in the foot if not treated promptly. Treatment generally requires systemic antibiotic treatment.

Arthritis. Arthritic changes can occur in any animal and in any joint. Generally associated with wear and tear and old age, it is not a common problem in cattle as they seldom attain old age in commercial situations. Arthritis of joints can occur as the result of infection, however, and occasionally changes related to old age may be seen in pets or animals belonging to smallholders. As with other species there is no long-term treatment, and anti-inflammatory treatments are not compatible with food production, although they can be helpful, along with osteopathy, in alleviating pain in pet animals.

Sheep

Neurological conditions

There are a large number of conditions that cause neurological signs in sheep. Differentiating between them is difficult as the principal symptom is a loss of the will to live. Differential diagnosis should be left to suitably experienced veterinary surgeons.

a. *Tetanus.* As in most species, this is seen as generalized stiffness and progresses to recumbency, often with prolapse of the third eyelid in early stages. Sheep generally die in three to four days.

b. *Copper deficiency (enzootic ataxia or sway back).* This generally only affects unweaned lambs It may be seen at birth, but is generally seen in one- to two-month-old lambs. Symptoms in older animals show less severe onset. Lambs affected in the first few months of birth may well die in two to three days. Older animals may survive, but always show some ataxia and atrophy of the hindquarters.

c. *Scrapie (spongiform encephalopathy).* This is an enzootic disease in the UK, Europe, and occasionally New Zealand, Canada and the USA. It is caused by a prion, and has a long incubation, generally being seen in animals of three to five years of age. Signs include pruritus, with rubbing and biting at the fleece. This is accompanied by a general loss of condition and gait abnormality which starts as incomplete flexion of the hock and leads on to weakness and loss of balance.

d. *Listeriosis.* In sheep the commonest form of listeriosis is encephalitis which causes inappetence, depression, and circling to one side. The condition is caused by infection with *Listeria monocytogenes* and is a zoonotic disease, which causes abortion, still birth, or severe illness in newborn children. Pregnant women should keep away from lambing ewes. The incidence of the disease tends to be seasonal and may be associated with feeding of silage. About 1 percent of a flock may be affected.

e. *Coenurosis (gid or sturdy).* This is a parasitic disease of the CNS caused by the cystic stage of the dog tapeworm *Taenia multiceps.* In acute cases young lambs of six to eight weeks may show signs of listlessness and occasionally the disease results in convulsions and death. In the more chronic form animals of about 18 months will show neurological signs, such as standing away from the flock, becoming depressed, and showing signs of circling, incoordination, and paralysis. In some cases there is evidence of slight softening of the skull overlying the cyst, and in these cases it may be possible to aspirate and remove the cyst using a large hypodermic needle and syringe. Cysts can infect humans and it is not uncommon for them to develop in the eye in children.

Metabolic disease

As with cattle, sheep suffer from metabolic diseases largely as the result of domestication and intensive livestock production. Once again symptoms tend to be depression and death, and differential diagnosis should be left to an experienced ovine veterinary surgeon. The commonest condition is pregnancy toxemia (twin lamb disease). This is seen in late gestation, where the diet is insufficient to provide for the needs of the ewe and developing fetus or fetuses. As usual in sheep, the signs are depression, anorexia, and death. Diseases due to mineral imbalance do occur but are less common than in cattle.

Lameness

Fractures. Lambs, and to some extent older animals, are prone to fracture of the lower limbs. In very young animals this may be treated by the use of a plaster cast, but economics may make this impractical.

Foot lameness. The commonest cause of lameness in sheep is "foot rot," which is infection of the feet with *Fusobacterium necrophorum* and *Dichelobacter nodosus.* It causes irritation, inflammation, and necrosis in the central cleft of the feet, which develops into underrunning of the sole and heel with necrosis of horn tissue. Although it is often treated by curettage of infected tissue, prevention with vaccination or routine footbaths is becoming more common.

Goats

Goats suffer many of the same problems as sheep and show similar symptoms, for example, depression, inappetence, and death:

a. They suffer from tetanus, copper deficiency, coenurosis, and metabolic and mineral diseases, the latter possibly manifesting as physitis or rickets.

b. Goats have their own specific retroviral disease – caprine arthritis encephalitis (CAE). Seen primarily in European dairy breeds in two- to four-month-old kids, it is usually evident as progressive paresis and incoordination. In adult animals it is seen as progressive arthritis involving one or more joints. There is no known treatment.

c. Goats do suffer from foot rot if kept in damp conditions.

d. Although generally agile, goats are prone to fracture of limbs, especially if frightened or poorly handled.

e. Newborn kids are subject to contracted tendons. There is possibly a hereditary predisposition, although this is still uncertain. This is particularly common in Angoras in Australasia and Anglo-Nubians in the USA, Canada, Australia, and New Zealand. Treatment by splinting may be possible in some cases with osteopathy to follow.

Camelids

Camelids are generally not under the stress of intensification and rapid growth rates seen in other farm animals. There is little known about the incidence and causes of lameness in camelids. The results of a survey carried out by Ohio State University suggested that lameness occurred as follows:

- Foot injuries 28.5 percent
- Muscle injuries 22 percent
- Neurological conditions 11 percent
- Bone disease 4.75 percent
- Back injuries 3.2 percent.

Camelids are generally resistant to "foot rot" as seen in sheep and goats, but it does occasionally occur in animals kept in very wet conditions. Generally, it responds well to basic hygiene and care.

Rickets has been reported as a problem in alpaca crias in Eastern Victoria in Australia. The symptoms are mild lameness, but few other signs are seen other than possible limb deviations.

Pigs

Although they are compact and muscular, pigs suffer many problems as outlined below, largely as the result of domestication and intensive rearing.

a. Damage and secondary infection to limbs and feet as the result of housing are not uncommon, as pigs are commonly housed on hard, slippery surfaces and grids to allow the clearance of slurry. This results in erosion of the soles of the feet and sores on the knees of suckling animals.

b. Biotin deficiency can result in the failure of hoof horn. Vitamin E deficiency may cause muscle damage, and deficiency of pantothenic acid may be associated with nerve damage.

c. Foot rot can occur in older animals.

d. Osteochondrosis is seen, especially in sows.

e. Damage to the pelvis and back resulting from injuries when mating is common.

f. Infectious arthritis is commonly seen in growing piglets and is often associated with injuries to the tail.

Osteopathic examination

Observation

This will depend very much on what type of patient you are observing, and what type of farm is involved. Some farms have mixed pasture and barn grazing, whereas others are solely indoors or outdoors. Observing a specific animal may prove difficult. Isolation of the patient by the farmer prior to your arrival is an option, although flock animals can become nervous when separated from their group. Another useful tool is if the farmer takes a video of the patient when it is moving and static in its normal environment. If the quality of filming is sufficiently good this can be more accurate than watching in person as the animal will behave naturally.

The usual criteria should be requested when having any filmed work done as outlined below:

1. Film the subject on a level area.
2. Avoid filming into the sun.
3. Keep the camera static, preferably fixed on a tripod.
4. Avoid zooming in and out while recording. Frame the subject first.
5. Ensure that the background does not distract the viewer from the subject.
6. Avoid giving a running commentary as it can be distracting.
7. Try to locate the camera so that the subject is viewed walking away and toward the camera, and then reposition so that the subject moves across the camera from left to right and from right to left.

Obviously, this will not always be as easy as it sounds, as animals have a habit of doing anything but what is asked of them. Adhering as closely as possible to these guidelines will help the osteopath and veterinary surgeons to acquire a much better understanding of any movement and postural problems.

Handling and restraint

Some livestock will be used to attending agricultural shows and will therefore behave well when walked in a head collar and lead rope, while others will behave in a feral manner.

Some breeds of bull cattle are renowned for being dangerous, with the Jersey probably top of the list of Western breeds, and it is usually best to examine and treat these animals from a protected contact position. Examining in a chute or crush prevents the patient from turning and using its head as a weapon. The osteopath will still need to ensure that they cannot be kicked from this position, or have their limbs caught between patient and crush.

Sheep can be difficult to manage and are best examined in a confined space, or with an expert stock person restraining them for the osteopath. There are many breeds worldwide, and they vary in behavior as well as build and temperament. Even a small ram can inflict serious injury if it can get you on the ground. Never turn your back on one!

Camelids are often best examined out in their pasture. One of the best ways the author (TN) has experienced of catching llamas is to place an outstretched arm across the path of the animal's neck as it goes past the handler. This slows the animal and then the handler can apply a gentle downward pressure behind the withers with the hand of their other arm to encourage the llama to lie down. This works very well unless the animal is moving at great speed.

Pig breeds are very easy to stress, especially if they are in any degree of pain. Take care to ensure that any contact is as noninvasive as possible or seek veterinary help with regard to sedating the patient. There can be issues regarding this if the patient is likely to enter the human food chain, and the veterinary surgeon will be able to advise.

Palpation

Where this is performed will be dictated by the species and sex of the patient. Camelids are easily restrained within a flock, whereas sheep, pigs, and cattle are best separated, and in many cases restrained using a chute or crush, for everyone's safety. Seek advice from the handler.

Most livestock are only handled for veterinary treatment, moving and separating individuals, weighing, and administering specific treatments. They are therefore often jumpy when palpated, especially around the head and face, and can be known to defend themselves!

If you are palpating through or over a crush or chute avoid putting arms, hands, and legs anywhere that they can be trapped. Although this sounds obvious, it is amazing how many injuries occur in this way - the author has witnessed several during his career. It is very easy to become so focused on the palpation that personal safety is ignored. Livestock can be very unpredictable, and are immensely strong. When their flight response is stimulated, you need to be well clear of them. All livestock may spook unexpectedly at things going on around them.

As a rule of thumb, the author would suggest the osteopath sticks to a standard routine for palpation and begins by making contact over the scapula, then examines the face and head using as flat a contact as possible, before working caudally, leaving the limbs until last, thus avoiding the chance of being kicked early in the process. Try to keep constant contact throughout by sliding the hands from one region to another.

As with other categories of animals, note any changes in posture, weight-bearing, breathing, and facial expressions as you perform the physical examination. It is often the subtle alterations that will indicate physiological changes to the underlying structures. Pigs in particular may well give vocal input, and in extreme cases of pain will grind their teeth (the author has personal experience of this where there is a serious underlying pathology, and it has helped veterinary surgeons isolate where to focus their examination).

Cattle

The osteopath will notice a difference between dairy and beef cattle, and between cows and bulls. Muscling and conformation will differ, with older dairy cows often developing a drooping top line, large udders, and increased abduction of the hind limbs with more pressure on the medial portion of the hoof.

Beef cattle are usually more muscled with a flat top line and usually have a leg set wide at each corner.

Due to their digestive system, be aware of any abdominal sensitivity to touch, generally on the left-hand side, as well as any obvious asymmetry, which might indicate a buildup of trapped gases or other forms of gut irritation (Fig. 6.6).

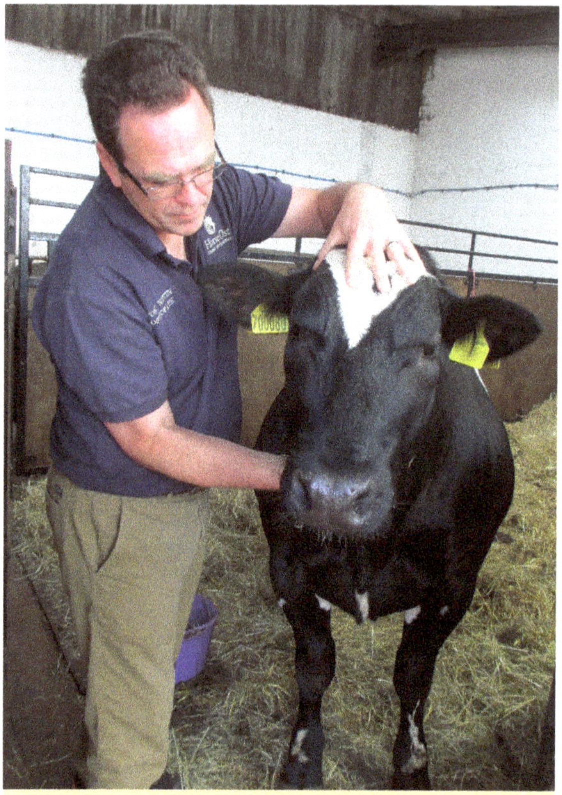

Figure 6.6
Assessing the involuntary mechanism (IVM) in a milking cow.

Sheep

In most cases the osteopath is only going to be asked to look at rams or high-value ewes, such as rare breeds (Fig. 6.7).

Young rams are good at testing themselves out on anything and anyone. A common sight for the osteopath is forelimb lameness. A dislike of the head and ears being touched is also common. The author has noted that most patients present with guarding to soft tissue compression in their cervical musculature and periscapular structures.

Due to the length of the fleece at certain times of year sheep can be rather difficult to palpate accurately, with what at first might appear to be a large patient actually having quite a small frame.

Some farmers now keep milking flocks and, as with dairy cows, their hind limb conformation will differ slightly, with more pressure being put through the medial half of the hoof structure which usually results in slightly externally rotated hind limbs.

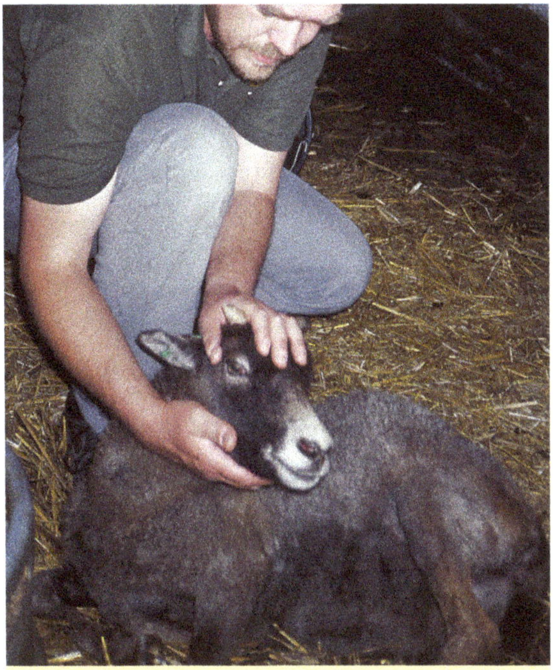

Figure 6.7
Assessing the IVM in a rare breed (Hill Radnor) ewe.

Camelids

Depending on the size of the flock, camelids can be examined in their pasture or separated into a confined space. Be aware that when stressed they will vocalize, flatten their ears, and can spit regurgitated food matter. In most cases , however, they will be fine. Like sheep, they can grow a long fleece, which can make observation of any anomalies difficult, making palpation more important. By remaining quiet and calm it is easy to examine them methodically. All camelids have seven cervical vertebrae, the bodies of which are deeper than those of humans thus giving height to the neck.

As most camelids are kept for their fleece, they will usually have a lighter frame and MSK system when compared to other farm stock. They are easier to examine when they are lying down, although to assess limbs it is probably better to have them standing.

Pigs

Pigs are extremely strong and unless very tame it is best to examine them in a chute or crush. Remember that they stress easily, and it is important to remain quiet and to move slowly when palpating. The nature of their surface anatomy is such that for the most part you will be feeling for any anomaly rather than being able to pick out specific landmarks and anatomical features.

When examining around the face, head, and cervical regions please be aware that pigs can give a very nasty bite, and some breeds possess tusks that can easily cause severe trauma to the unwary. The author would recommend that you keep things simple, use a methodical approach to palpation, and keep the examination time short. This will reduce the likelihood of the animal being stressed and minimize the potential for accidents to all parties.

Osteopathic treatment

In all but extreme cases treatment will be performed with the patient fully conscious. For stud, cost, and food chain reasons sedation can cause problems for a farmer. Therefore, techniques that can be successfully applied will depend on the species, breed, and temperament of the individual, as well as the circumstances the osteopath will be required to work in.

Cattle

Although they will often respond well to soft tissue massage the author (TN) has found that the majority react much quicker to functional release methods and myofascial unwinding (Fig. 6.8). These are often blended together, along with working through the involuntary mechanism (IVM). Treatments are usually short, and the patient rarely needs more than a couple of sessions to achieve lasting changes (Fig. 6.9). Avoid standing directly in front of the patient, and when working from the side be aware that cows can kick forward with the hind legs when defensive.

Unlike the equine patient, one must never use strong tail traction methods as bovine coccygeal joints are far less robust structures.

Sheep

Concussive injuries, which rams will often inflict and receive, benefit from soft tissue and articulatory

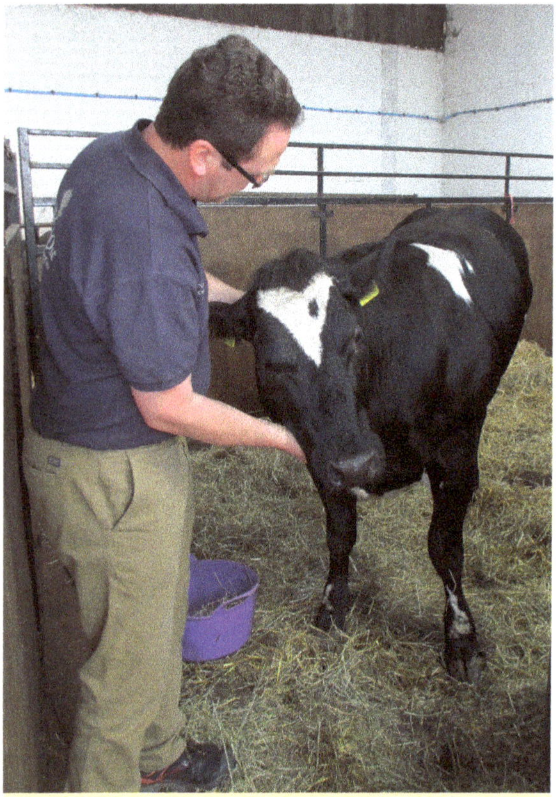

Figure 6.8
Myofascial unwinding through the cervical spine in a milking cow while supporting under the mandible.

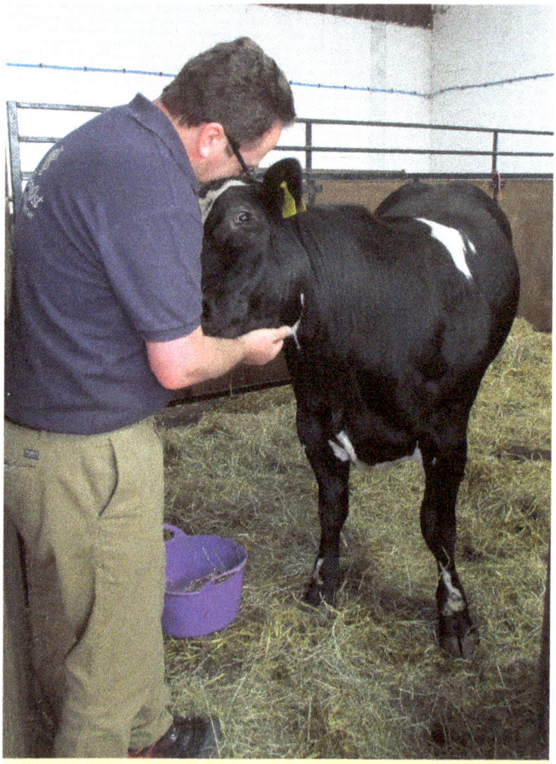

Figure 6.9
Sustained positional release (SPR) applied from the occiput–atlas junction through to the cervicothoracic junction of a milking cow.

techniques, as well as traction methods, especially through the cervical and thoracic sling regions.

Lameness issues require a slow, calm approach to avoid further injury.

Many of the rare breeds, which are often quite nervous by nature, respond better to functional-fascial-IVM blends, and they may resent a soft tissue approach.

Camelids

The author has found that these will respond to all of the major osteopathic modalities. As a general rule, high velocity, low amplitude thrust (HVLAT) techniques should only be used where there are clear radiographs eliminating any possible pathologies and the patient has not responded positively to other less dramatic techniques.

Once a camelid is restrained it will accede to osteopathic treatment without fuss as long as the operator maintains hand contact throughout and moves in a methodical manner around the patient (Figs 6.10 and 6.11).

Pigs

As a group these are often the most sensitive to manual treatment. A slow approach appears the best way to begin, with functional-fascial-IVM blends often able to achieve the most, although some of the rare breeds (which are also kept as pets in some parts of the world) will often like soft tissue massage and gentle short lever articulatory treatments (author's own experience).

Where possible work from the side of the patient and keep constant contact through your hands and body (Fig. 6.12).

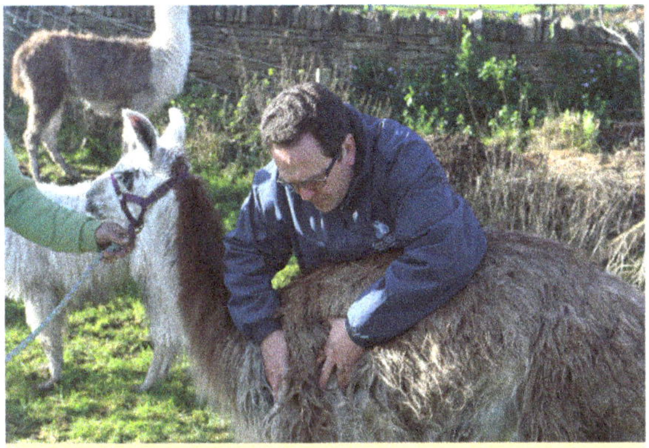

Figure 6.10
Periscapular release in a llama.

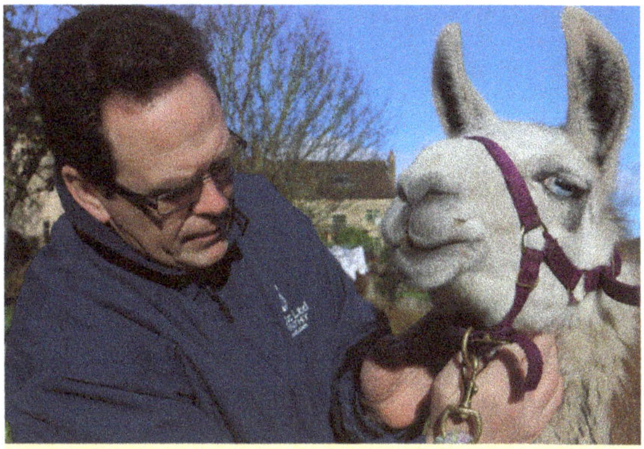

Figure 6.11
Functional release around the hyoid structures of a llama.

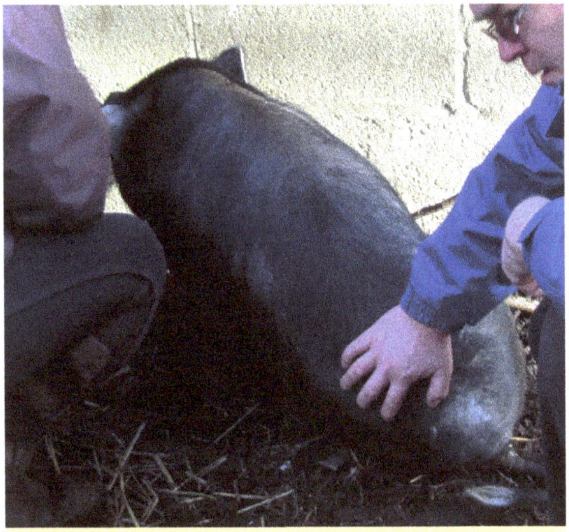

Figure 6.12
Functional release around the left hip and associated structures of a Kunekune.

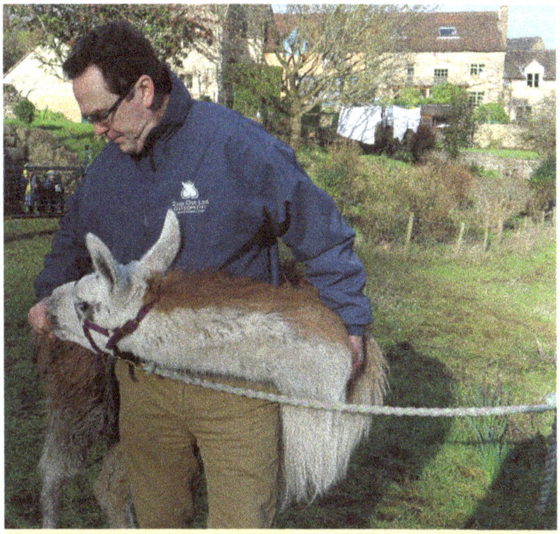

Figure 6.13
A baited stretch exercise with a llama. The practitioner can use their own body as a fulcrum.

Management

This is likely to be simpler than for other categories of patient. Generally, a conservative approach is going to work best. Avoidance of any noxious stimuli or adverse environment is essential. Husbandry issues such as providing extra warmth and lower humidity may be required to assist a patient's recovery, as well as adjustments to diet if they are being confined during this period.

The farmer should also be advised on any grazing or free-ranging issues, such as steep gradients, excessive mud, or overexposure to extreme weather conditions, which might have a bearing on the patient's condition. Where possible some rehabilitation work can be carried out (Fig. 6.13).

Chapter 6

Case study 6.1

Serving ram

Signalment

The patient was a serving ram with spinal pain.

History

The following case details the osteopathic assessment and treatment of a serving ram. A farmer from Eastern Victoria (Australia) requested an osteopathic consultation following advice from his veterinary surgeon. One of his prized rams was displaying signs of discomfort and increasing difficulty mounting ewes. The veterinary surgeon suggested the significant pain the ram was in might be having an effect on his testosterone levels. It is accepted in the livestock husbandry literature that pain is a stress on the body, leading to multisystem distress (Moberg and Mench 2000). Stress serves to activate the hypothalamic-pituitary-adrenocortical (HPA) and hypothalamic-pituitary-testis (HPT) pathways, increasing secretion of CRH from the hypothalamus (Stephens 1980). This stimulates the release of ACTH (Rivier and Vale 1987) and the release of endogenous opioid peptides (EOP) from the hypothalamus and pituitary (Gindoff and Ferin 1987), which serve to inhibit the testicular axis (Petraglia et al. 1986). Knol (1991) concludes that because of this inhibition, stress usually causes a rapid and dramatic decrease in plasma testosterone concentration. This rapid reduction in plasma testosterone has been shown in Ayrshire bulls to have a positive correlation with poor sperm motility and an overall decrease in fertility (Andersson 1992). The stress of pain and failure in serving would have an effect on the EOP release, increasing the response the longer the ram is exposed to the stress.

On this occasion, the treatment room was the back of the farmer's vehicle, as he brought the ram to be assessed from the farm (Fig. 6.14). It meant that a dynamic assessment was not viable, and a palpatory examination was the only form of assessment possible. If possible, it is preferable to see the animal moving in its own environment.

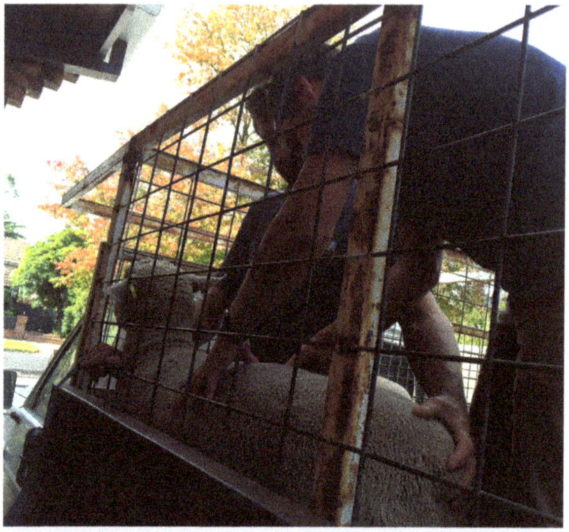

Figure 6.14
Examination of the ram while it was restrained in the trailer.

The ram displayed significant spinal pain on palpation of the thoracolumbar region, extending to the first two cranial lumbar vertebrae and bilateral in its distribution. The palpatory sense of this spinal region was one of dampened function and turbulence, lacking the expected vitality that is present in health. This area also felt dragged ventrally, giving the impression that the thorax was heavier than the ram was able to support on its feet. There was increased tone in the diaphragm and surrounding congestion, leading to a chronic "boggy" feel to the overlying tissue. The excursion of the caudal ribs was reduced and there was restriction in the articulations at the spinal attachments.

The working diagnosis was a chronic sprain and group dysfunction of several thoracic and lumbar segments. However, as there was no specific mechanism of injury (aside from the role of mounting a ewe), and because of the boggy tissue quality and the distribution of the palpatory findings, a viscerosomatic etiology was suspected. The decision was made to treat the ram symptomatically on the proviso that the farmer had the ram assessed and diagnosed by its veterinarian to rule out potential pathology.

Osteopathic treatment

The treatment applied included balanced ligamentous tension (BLT) techniques, rhythmic articulation, and harmonic technique to the caudal ribs, spinal joints, and supporting ligaments, leading to a fascial unwind of the thoracolumbar region. Acknowledging the irritable palpatory quality in the fluid body and appreciating the arterial, venous, and lymphatic circulation greatly increased the potency of the techniques. This was successful for the most part, and some meaningful positive changes were observed, with the ram's tissues relaxing significantly. We were able to observe the ram's breathing change and it settled during the process of treatment and stood square for most of the consultation.

Soon after this treatment, the ram was taken to the veterinarian and he was found to be suffering from urinary calculi, which eventually led to a rupture of his urethra. It is possible that the pain experienced by the ram may have been from both local and referred pain as a result of significant inflammation from this condition. The end product of visceral pain can be affected by osteopathic treatment, and it is always prudent to refer if unsure of a definitive etiology, as in this case. This highlighted the importance of having a sound working diagnosis and knowing one's limitations and when to refer to make sure that an underlying pathology is not mimicking a musculoskeletal presentation.

From this clinical encounter and further research, the author (BA) became more aware of where osteopathic treatment may be of assistance in optimizing musculoskeletal function in rams. As discussed, the negative correlation between pain and the hormonal cascade is significant, and this clinical reasoning can be transferred to any breeding animal. With this in mind, it can be postulated that a consultant osteopath working within a sheep or other animal stud may be a valuable part of the overall health and well-being of the animals and may result in higher fertility levels and quality across the stud.

Case study 6.2

Female alpaca

Signalment

Patient C. was a juvenile female alpaca who had been locally bred on a farm in the UK.

History

The farmer discovered one morning that Patient C. was reluctant to stand, and when encouraged to stand she was unsteady on her feet and appeared to sway as if she were intoxicated. The veterinary surgeon could find no pathology, and all blood tests appeared normal. He did find that her cervical musculature was asymmetrically tight, creating a slight scoliosis centered at the mid-cervical region.

Presenting signs

When the author (TN) first saw the patient, she presented with the unsteady gait of a newborn. There was no hypermetric aspect to her movement; however, he was concerned that there was some deficit to her proprioceptive function. There were no signs of any physical trauma, although the farmer did state that the paddock containing the juveniles did contain some rather high-spirited individuals, and he suspected that the patient had been involved in some rough play.

Upon examination there was a marked imbalance to the cranial cervical musculature resulting in a functional left rotational presentation to the occipitoatlantoaxial (OAA) joints. This tension then carried on caudally as a spiral through the rest of the cervical spine and into the thoracic sling, culminating in fascial tension as far as the sacroiliac joints.

Osteopathic treatment

Osteopathic treatment followed a functional release pattern through from the OAA articulations caudally to the sacrum. At certain stages this was combined with sustained positional release (SPR) at particular points of tension. The patient was in a recumbent position for the duration of treatment making it easy to administer treatment and keep the patient under control (Fig. 6.15A–D). Due to the young age of the patient HVLATs were not used, although the author did perform some cervical traction toward the end of the session.

After this first session Patient C. was kept isolated from the herd for a couple of hours to allow her body to settle and start integrating the changes effected before she was reintroduced to the group in their pasture.

A follow-on session took place seven days later whereupon it was noted that Patient C. was much more agile and had better coordination and proprioception. The rotational pattern through her neck and body was vastly reduced but could still be observed affecting her gait when she was moving. Treatment followed a similar pattern to before; however, she was returned to the group straight afterwards as she was much livelier and there was more risk of her trying to get to them once we had left.

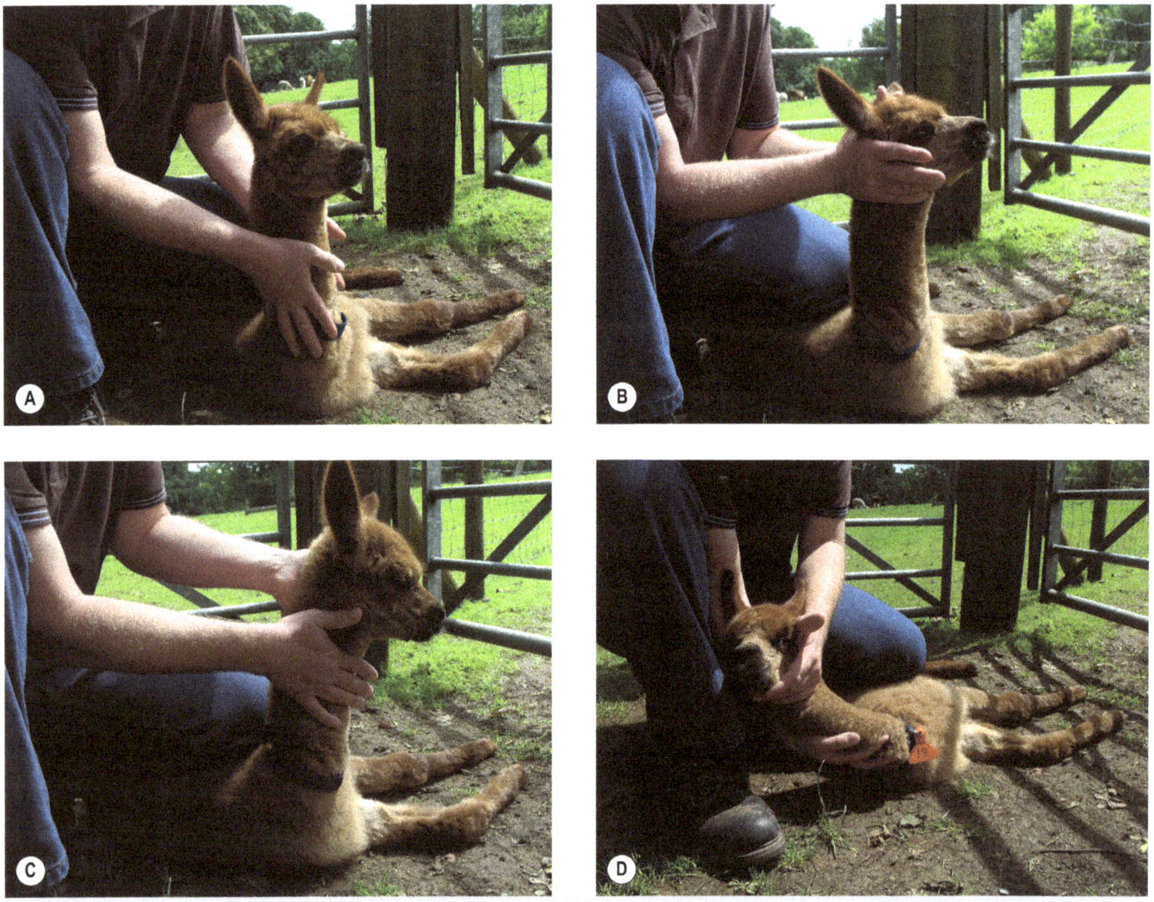

Figure 6.15
(A) Palpation through the caudal cervical spine. (B) Functional release through the cranial cervical spine. (C) Functional release through the midcervical spine. (D) Functional unwinding release through the entire cervical spine and into the cranial thoracic structures.

The author asked the farmer to phone a few days later with an update which he did, confirming that she appeared to be "back to normal." No further visits were planned unless the farmer noticed a deterioration in the patient.

Outcome

This juvenile alpaca presented with symptoms suggesting a biomechanical strain. No pathologies were detected by the veterinary surgeon, and nothing the author found contradicted this finding. The patient responded to straightforward osteopathic intervention and made a speedy recovery. These animals are known to be pretty rugged and so the prognosis for a long-term resolution of her condition was good. The author never had to treat her again.

Summary

This was a very straightforward MSK-related injury that responded well to osteopathic treatment. These are the most common livestock cases that an osteopath will be asked to treat. Due to the value and nature of this category of patient, only higher value species, breeds, or individuals will command this level of care. Treating livestock can be more dangerous than any other sector. The patients may be "domesticated" but that does not mean they will be easy to handle. A juvenile alpaca should be relatively easy to contain and treat. The main concern for the osteopath will be to administer safe treatment that is suitable and relevant to that individual.

Most livestock are not used to being physically handled on a day-to-day basis, so the osteopath must keep treatment to a minimum to avoid undue stress. Animals like alpacas are very observant and will recognize a stranger immediately. Making accurate observations is often difficult if a herd is playing up, therefore the author elected to use the farmer for more accurate feedback. Most will give an honest assessment and are more likely to notice when anything is out of the ordinary.

Livestock can and do respond as well to osteopathic medicine as any other group of animals and birds, and there is definitely a valid role for it in modern farming alongside an ethical approach to producing our food.

Summary

Farm livestock, like all other main groups of animals and birds, will respond well to osteopathic intervention. Due to their role in human society most cases an osteopath will see will be of particular value to the farmer; however, there will always be other cases where the osteopath may be asked to "have a look at out of interest."

The experience an osteopath can gain from this sector of the animal world can be invaluable if they are also interested in wildlife work. Farm livestock can be great patients to learn from, and in return they can benefit from the osteopathic work administered to them.

Public awareness is growing as to how our food is produced, and it is likely that osteopaths will play a greater role in farm animal husbandry in the future alongside our veterinary and allied professional colleagues.

References

Andersson M (1992) Relationships between GnRH-induced testosterone maxima, sperm motility and fertility in Ayrshire bulls. Animal Reproduction Science. April; 27 (2–3) 107–111.

Gindoff PR, Ferin M (1987) Endogenous opioid peptides modulate the effect of corticotropin releasing factor on gonadotropin release in the primate. Endocrinology. September; 121 (3) 837–842.

Knol BW (1991) Stress and the endocrine hypothalamus-pituitary-testis system: a review. Veterinary Quarterly. April; 13 (2) 104–114.

Moberg GP (1985) Influence of stress on reproduction: measure of well-being. In: Moberg GP (ed.) Animal Stress. Bethesda: American Physiological Society.

Moberg GP, Mench JA (2000) The Biology of Animal Stress: Basic Principles and Implications for Animal Welfare. CABI Publishing, pp. 172–173.

Petraglia F, Vale W, Rivier C (1986) Opioids act centrally to modulate stress-induced decrease in luteinizing hormone in the rat. Endocrinology. December; 119 (6) 245–250.

Rivier C, Vale W (1987) Diminished responsiveness of the HPA axis of the rat during exposure to prolonged stress: a pituitary-mediated mechanism. Endocrinology. October; 121 (4) 1320–1328.

Stephens DB (1980) Stress and its measurement in domestic animals: a review of behavioral and physiological studies under field and laboratory situations. Advances in Veterinary Science and Comparative Medicine. 24: 179–210.

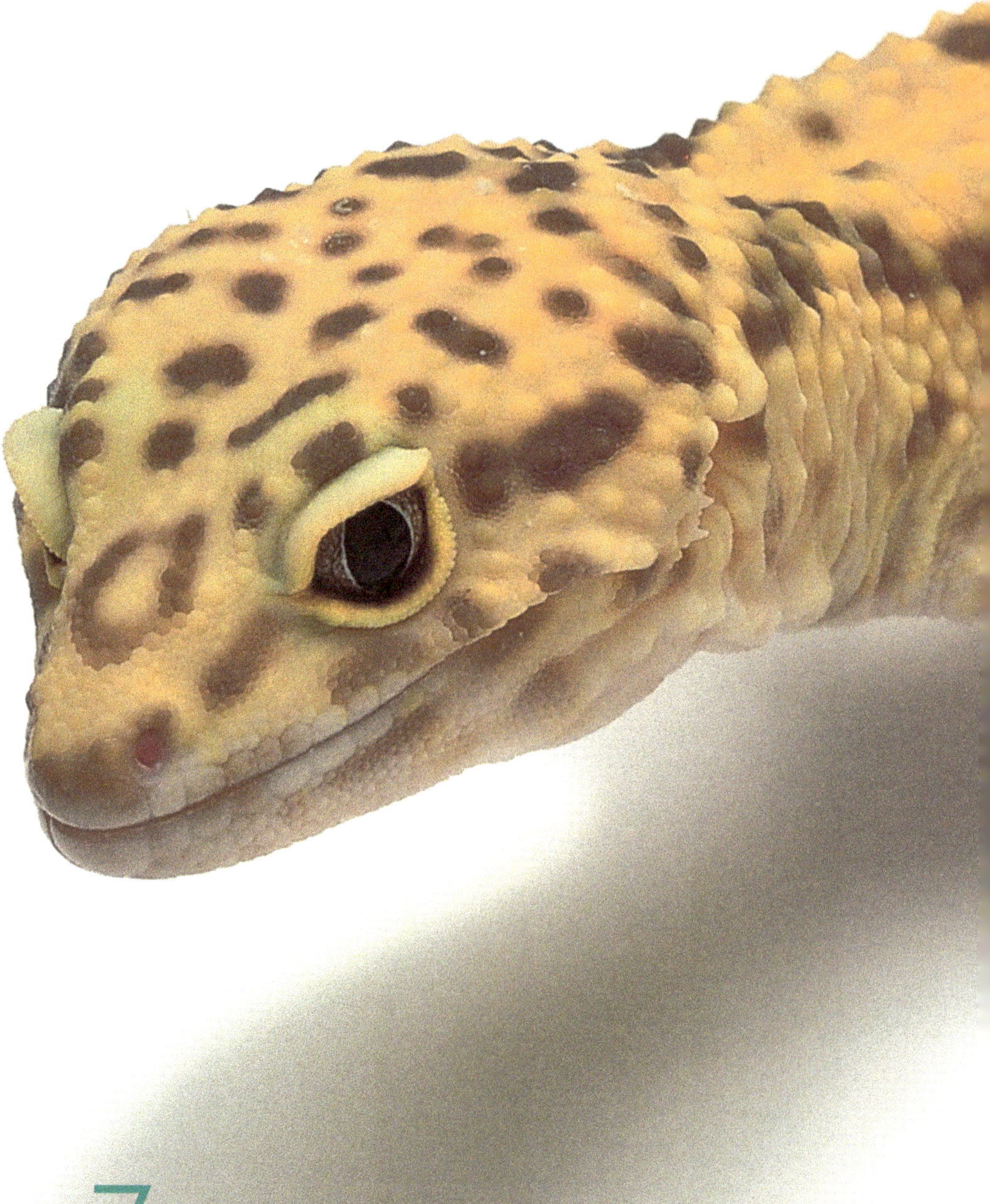

Chapter 7

REPTILES

Paolo Tozzi, John Hope-Ryan, Leonidas Christodoularis

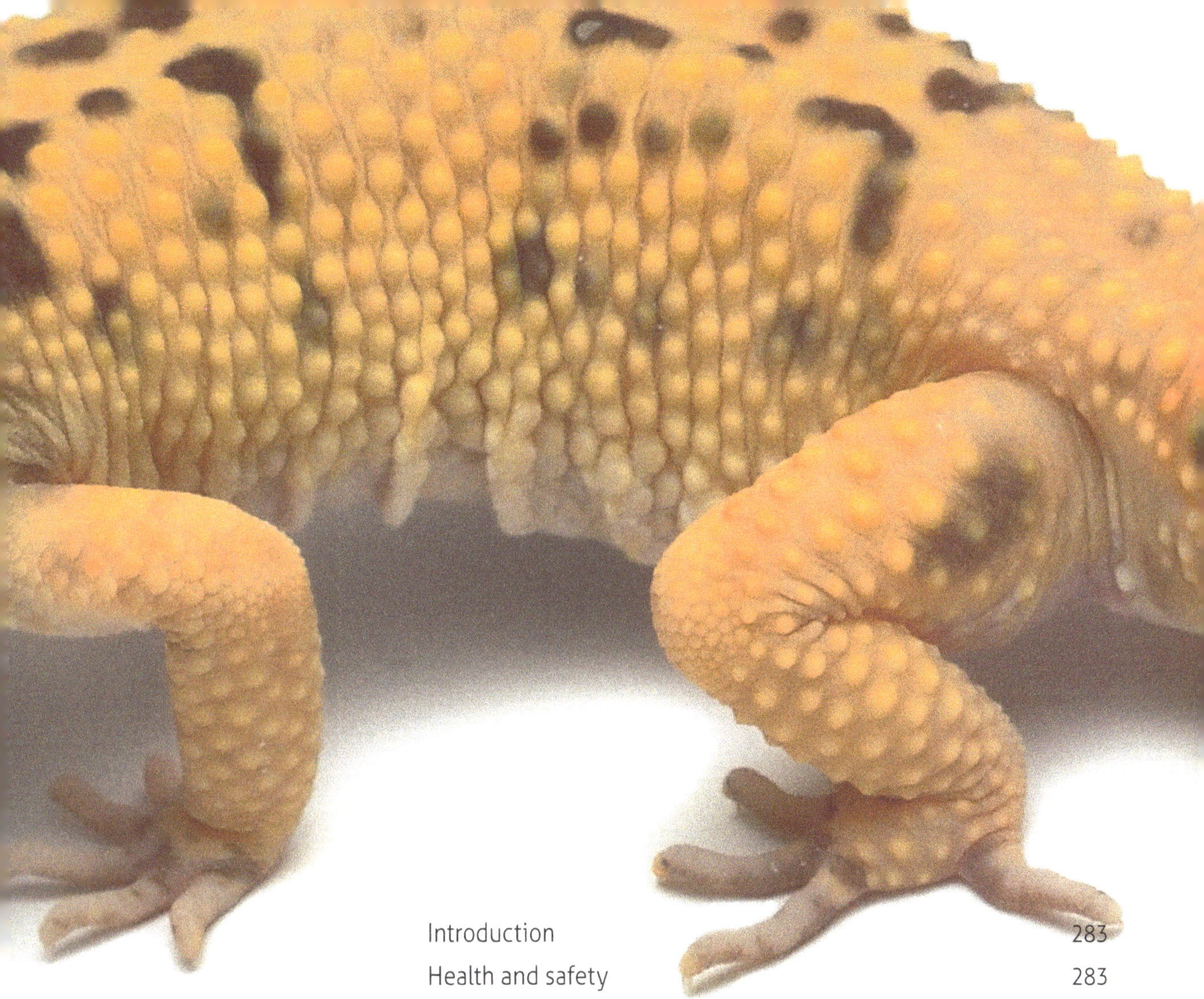

Reptiles

Chapter 7

Introduction

From an osteopathic perspective, reptiles are fascinating animals to work with. Although it may be uncommon to encounter these patients in everyday practice, there are estimated to be over 9,546 species of reptile in existence today (Pincheira-Donoso et al. 2013). Several of them have become popular in the pet trade and are now bred in captivity (Jacobson 1993). This chapter will mainly focus on shelled species, and snakes and lizards. Despite their appearance, the variation in anatomy, physiology, behavior, and clinical presentation makes reptiles a true challenge even for the most experienced and skillful practitioner. It requires careful observation and thorough examination of the animal's condition and husbandry, together with consideration of any issues concerning safe handling and management. Although osteopathic principles and objectives remain basically the same as those applied to humans, their application to reptiles requires specific adaptations for each species. This must encompass size, weight, age, sex, and defensive mechanisms as well as protective reactions and reflexes. This makes osteopathy of reptiles a unique art applied by a limited number of specialist clinical practices.

With most snakes and iguanas the practitioner must constantly and promptly adapt his evaluation and treatment as dictated by the animal's response to manipulation. Reptiles may not always be in the mood or in a condition to be touched and worked on, so caution is always necessary. Most reptiles have poor hearing, with sight as their primary sensory organ and skin sensors as the second (O'Malley 2005). This means touch may be one of the main entrances into the homeostatic potential of these animals, and osteopathic manipulation may be a possible activator of this self-regulatory system (Fig. 7.1). As far as the authors are aware there is no material in the osteopathic literature about treatment of reptiles. This chapter therefore represents the first attempt to offer basic knowledge and general guidelines for the osteopathic evaluation and treatment of these intriguing animals. The reader should not, however, regard this chapter as providing comprehensive information for the osteopath to be competent to work safely and efficiently on reptiles.

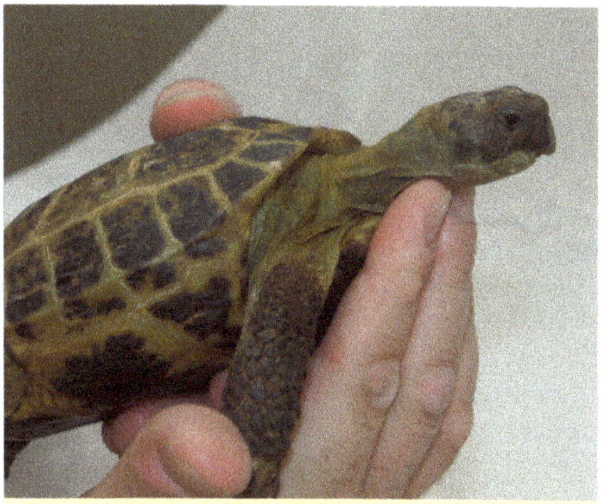

Figure 7.1
A gentle touch with therapeutic intent may produce a calming effect in reptiles, enhance their self-regulatory mechanisms, and thus promote health.

Finally, the collaboration of veterinary surgeons is paramount to achieving the best clinical outcomes, especially in complicated patients with underlying pathology and/or recurrent dysfunctional patterns.

Health and safety

There are particular protocols to ensure safe handling of reptiles. Some are general and others are specific to the anatomical make-up of the patient in question.

Before taking any reptile out of its transit carrier or vivarium you should assess the examination area for potential problems. These could be unsecured exits (doors and windows), narrow spaces between fixtures and fittings, and unprotected heat sources such as radiators.

Snakes

The way the patient is picked up can vary. Snakes need to be confidently held and lifted with support provided at roughly one-third and two-thirds of the way along their length. When picking up a snake try not to move quickly or grab at it. Make a smooth movement and take a secure yet gentle hold. Do not make movements head on, as some snakes will be spooked by this, triggering a flight or fight response. Once secured the osteopath should allow enough time for the snake to relax before trying to examine it.

The use of latex gloves may allow for a better grip and also protects the osteopath from basic allergens and micro-organisms (more of a problem when handling wild snakes).

It is not advisable to handle a snake if it has just eaten, or is due to slough its skin - signs of which are lethargy, opaque eyes, and dullness of the skin.

Lizards and legless lizards

Most species kept as pets are fairly easy to handle. The golden rule is to pick them up by taking hold of them around the shoulders and thorax. Depending on their size, they may also need another hand supporting under the pelvis and root of the tail. It is never a good idea to catch or lift a lizard by the tail as some species can spontaneously detach the caudal part, and heavier species can sustain injury if lifted this way. Holding around the shoulders prevents a nervous individual from escaping the osteopath or handler.

As with any reptile, lizards' expressions are often difficult to read, so care needs to be taken to avoid an inadvertent bite. As with snakes, it is best to avoid handling animals that have just eaten, or that are due to slough their skin - signs of which are discoloration and flaking of the skin, and general lethargy.

Tortoises

Tortoises are easy to handle, although the handler needs to maintain a secure hold of the carapace with a grip similar to holding a burger in a bun. They can give a strong peck but very rarely do. Some will panic when lifted up so take time to let them settle. Many like to be stroked under their chin, and this also encourages them to extend the neck forward of the carapace and allows for easier examination.

Terrapins

Freshwater terrapins are handled in a similar manner to tortoises; however, they do carry quite potent external bacteria and are best handled wearing latex gloves. Many are carnivorous so are slightly more likely to bite than tortoises. As with all exotics, please be aware of the potential risk of zoonotic disease.

Anatomy

Introduction

There are approximately 9,500 species of reptile, belonging to four orders: Chelonia (turtles), Crocodylia (crocodiles), Rhynchocephalia (tuatara), and Squamata (lizards and snakes) (Uetz 2000). The Chelonia and Squamata make up most of the species likely to be seen in practice and so this chapter applies mainly to these orders. Reptiles can be found in a wide variety of habitats from arid desert conditions to tropical rainforest. They can vary in size greatly from Giant Anacondas (5.2 m long) to leaf-toed gecko (*Phyllodactylus reissii*) (55 mm long). Most species are, however, smaller than mammals and birds.

Metabolism

All reptiles are ectothermic. They rely on behavior and habitat selection to provide them with the right conditions for their metabolism and life cycle. This means that they require between one-fifth and one-seventh of the caloric input of similar sized mammals, but it also means habitat plays a vital role in their survival. They are much more intolerant than many other species to environmental and habitat challenge. They do, however, have a great deal of behavioral and metabolic flexibility to cope with a given habitat. An example would be the Galapagos marine iguana using basking to assist with the digestion of algae and raising body temperatures to cope with cold water temperatures when grazing. This lack of thermogenesis leads species from more temperate regions to undergo hibernation during the colder months of the year, with the more tropical species being able to thermoregulate during the whole year. The day-night temperature variance in more temperate habitats makes species in these climates relatively tolerant of temperature fluctuations, unlike tropical species. The trigger for hibernation in reptiles is almost always temperature dependent, unlike mammals that may hibernate due to food scarcity. The close reliance on the environmental temperature of each individual species and their relative tolerance to changes in this temperature is a very important aspect of the management of these animals and in practice forms one of the cornerstones of treating any ailment.

Cardiovascular and respiratory system

Chelonia and Squamata have a three-chambered heart (one ventricle and two atria) the oxygenated blood from the lungs and the deoxygenated blood from the body are kept apart partially by a ridge in the ventricle. Blood can be shunted to either the lungs or body through changes in the resistance of the pulmonary arteries. The heart rate varies greatly with environmental temperature, body size, stress, and activities such as diving. Blood volumes are around 5–8 percent of the body mass. The arteries and veins follow a similar pattern to higher vertebrates except for the presence of a renal portal system that can channel blood from the caudal body through the kidneys before entering the rest of the circulation. This ability is under neurohormonal control and is poorly understood. Reptiles have a highly developed lymphatic system but no lymph nodes. The lymph is moved around by smooth muscle dilations that act as pumps. While only crocodiles have a diaphragm, breathing is achieved through a combination of smooth muscle contraction of the lungs, intercostal muscle contraction, and coelomic expansion. The limbs may assist especially during higher oxygen demand such as chasing or being chased. Breathing is triphasic with inspiration, expiration, and a rest period, which can often be misinterpreted as apnea in aquatic species. These rest periods can be very long and frustrating for an anesthetist. Reptiles are very tolerant of hypoxia especially if muscle requirements outstrip respiration of oxygen. The lactic acid produced by anaerobic respiration will be eliminated after the hypoxic episode has passed.

There is a great deal of variation in the anatomy of the upper and lower respiratory systems in all species (Fig. 7.2A–C). The need to swallow prey whole, which compresses glottis, trachea, and lungs has led to

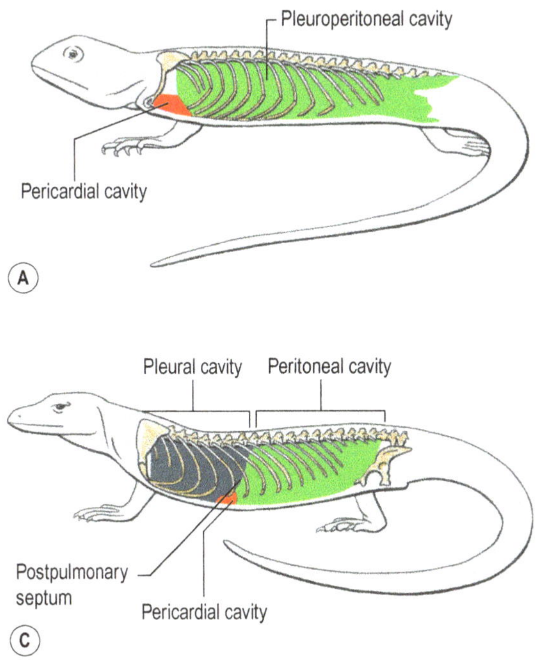

Figure 7.2
(A) Unicameral lizard. (B) Paucicameral lizard. (C) Multicameral lizard.

various adaptations such as the tracheal lung in vipers. In some species there are thin-walled air sacs after the lungs that may be used as buoyancy aids and air reservoirs in aquatic diving species.

Urinary system

Reptiles have metanephric kidneys derived from the posterior embryo. The primary excreted product is uric acid in the terrestrial species and a combination of ammonia, uric acid, and urea in aquatic species. The urine produced is isosthenuric (there is no loop of Henle) and it undergoes no water resorption in the kidneys. The urine passes from the kidneys through the ureters to the cloaca and then to a bladder (Chelonia and some lizards) or is kept in the distal colon where water resorption can take place. Urine is passed with or without feces through the cloaca.

Osmoregulation in reptiles is very different to mammals. Water is obtained from food and drinking, but also through the skin which is porous, and it can be absorbed from water condensing in the respiratory tract. Losses are from urine and feces and also respiration and cutaneous water loss. The thickness of the keratin layer of the skin determines this loss. Some reptiles can survive with very little water intake using reduced renal blood flow and salt glands to excrete excess salt. Prolonged dehydration leads to formation of uric acid deposits in the kidneys (renal gout) and other areas of the body such as joints.

Reproduction

Reproductive cycling is triggered by a combination of environmental stimuli acting on the pineal gland. These include temperature, food availability, rainfall, and increasing daylight - all of which have been shown to affect reproductive behavior.

Most species show sexual dimorphism. The male testes are located intra-abdominally. Lizards and snakes have paired hemipenes, which are located caudal to the cloaca, and Chelonia have a single phallus which is intracloacal. Females have paired oviducts which open into the cloaca (Fig. 7.3). The structure of the oviduct will depend on whether the female is viviparous. Viviparous species have a more muscular oviduct to hold the developing embryos.

Fertilization is internal, and sperm in some species can be stored for several seasons in the oviduct. Reptiles can be viviparous or oviparous. Viviparous females produce live young, whereas oviparous females lay eggs (with varying degrees of calcification of the shells) with gestation taking place in nests built by the female. There are also ovoviviparous females where the eggs are laid immediately prior to hatching.

Integument

Reptile skin is divided into the dermis and epidermis. The dermis is composed of connective tissue, blood, lymph, nerves, and pigment cells. Chromophores lie between the dermis and epidermis, and these produce changes in color such as those seen in the Chamaeleonidae. The epidermis is heavily keratinized to help maintain hydration and is divided into scales. In Chelonia the shell consists of epidermal bone plates and the epithelium.

Although the epidermis is essentially dry, there are various glands that may be found around the head and cloaca that produce pheromones. The degree of porosity can also depend on the species' contact with water, with a significant amount of water being able to be absorbed by immersion of the skin.

Ecdysis or shedding of skin takes place as one piece in snakes, with lizards shedding in parts over time and Chelonia shedding individual scales. The skin becomes vulnerable during this time and dehydration or damage by parasites can take place.

Skeletal system

Reptiles share common ancestry with mammals and thus direct comparisons with mammalian anatomy can be made.

Lizards have pentadactyl forefeet and hind feet. There are ribs present attached to all vertebrae except the tail (Fig. 7.4). In some species the tail will spontaneously detach (autotomy) as a means to distract a predator while the body makes an escape. Rough handling

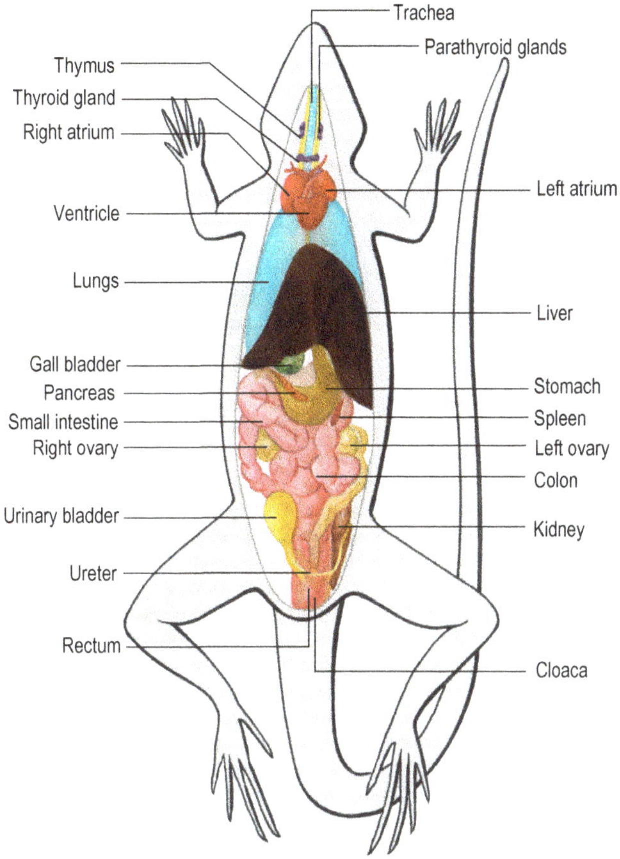

Figure 7.3
A ventral view of the internal anatomy of the female lizard.

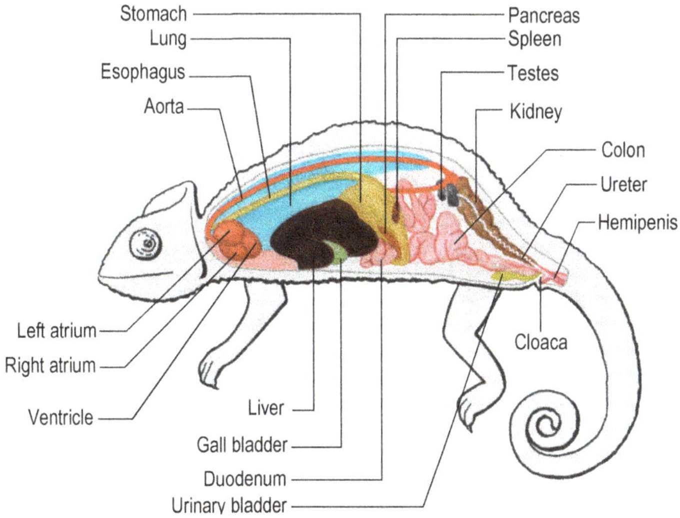

Figure 7.4
A lateral midsagittal view of a male chameleon.

when examining can result in this happening, and owners need to be warned of this prior to examination and treatment. In most species tails will regrow after autotomy but with darker skin, and the resultant tail is shorter and blunter.

Snakes do not have visible limbs (Fig. 7.5), although in boas and pythons there may be spurs present as vestigial remnants of pelvic limbs. Movement is achieved through a series of techniques that depends on the size of snake and the environment and substrate present. Locomotion relies on a large number of precloacal vertebrae that can number over 400. Most of these vertebrae have ribs with very small regional variations. There are several different techniques that allow the snake to move forward. Lateral undulation is the common serpentine locomotion seen in snakes. It is very energy-efficient and requires sequential unilateral contraction of the dorsal muscle groups. The body follows the winding path of the head and neck. Sidewinding is similar to lateral undulation but relies on the points of contact with the ground being static and the body lifting off from these static points to contact and gain purchase further forward. Concertina movement moves the body by pulling the body into a series of bends once the cranial part of the body has purchase on the ground. This is then followed by pushing forward once the caudal part of the body has gained purchase. Rectilinear locomotion is the classic caterpillar crawling with the alternate lifting and placing of the belly scales on the ground.

The skull of the snake has a solid brain case (Fig. 7.6), but in order to facilitate the ingestion of prey items that are larger than the head the mandible articulates with the quadrate bones, palate, and maxillary

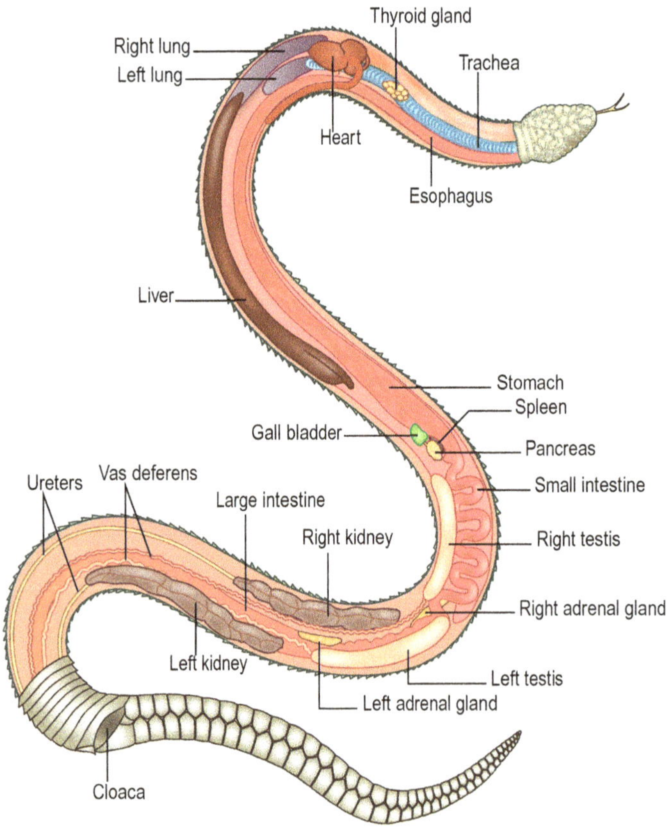

Figure 7.5
The internal anatomy of the male snake.

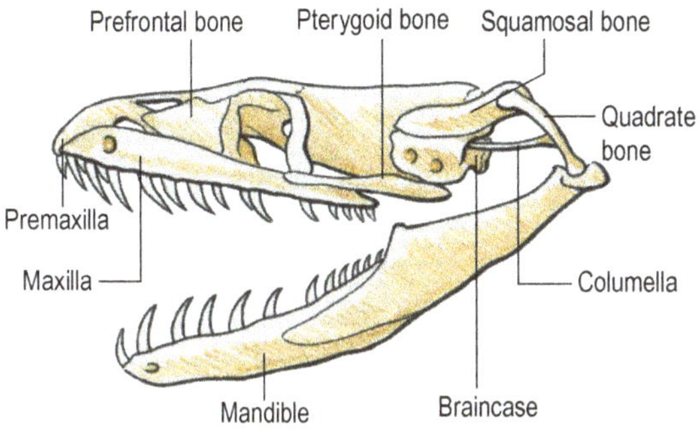

Figure 7.6
The skull of a simple snake.

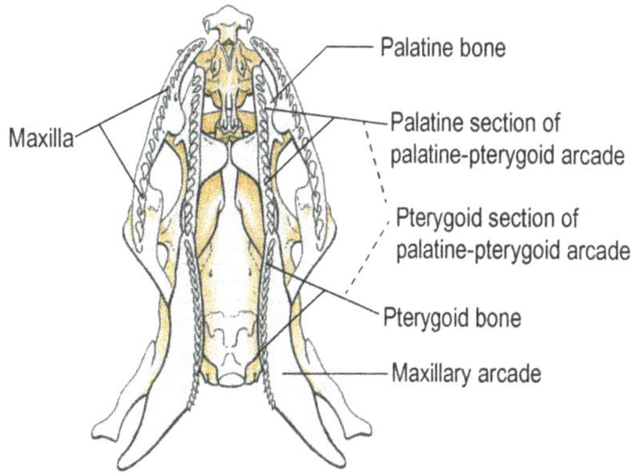

Figure 7.7
A ventral view of the maxilla of a simple snake.

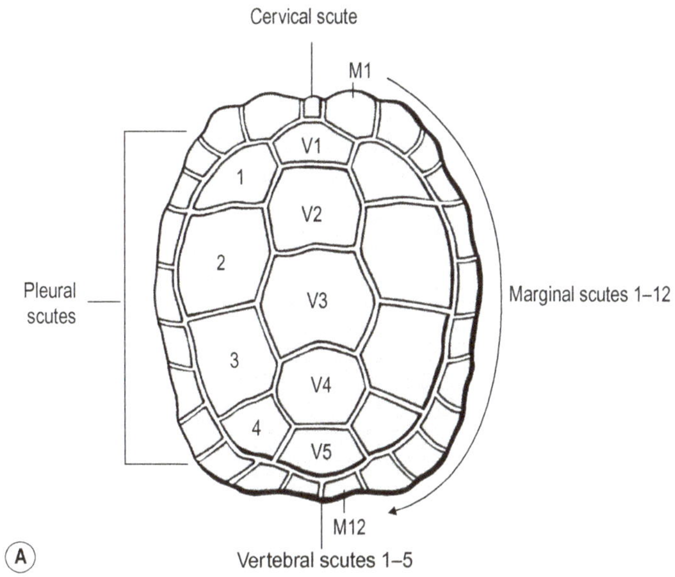

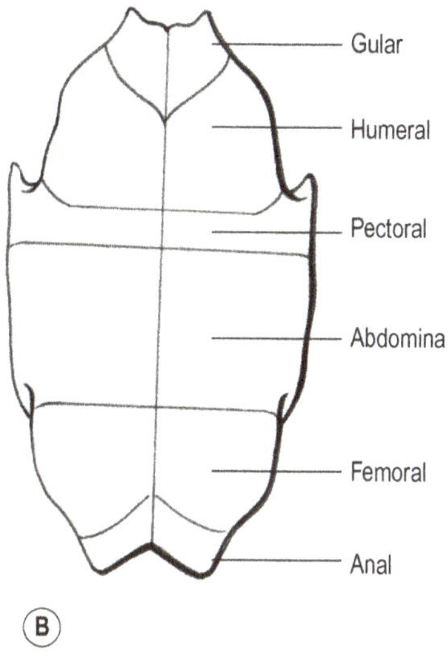

Figure 7.8
(A) The epidermal scutes of a tortoise carapace. (B) The epidermal scutes of a tortoise plastron.

arch (Fig. 7.7). There is also no mandibular symphysis. These anatomical arrangements allow large prey to pass into the body.

The Chelonia are distinguished by the presence of their shell. The upper carapace is connected to the lower plastron with bony bridges. The carapace is derived from the ribs, vertebrae, and epithelium. The plastron is derived from the abdominal ribs, clavicles, and interclavicles. The shell is covered by a keratinized layer called scutes (Fig. 7.8A and B). Scutes can be retained or shed depending on species and growth cycles. In most land-based tortoises they are retained. The pelvic and pectoral girdles are kept within the rib cage and are orientated to provide support for the shell and anchors for the limbs (Fig. 7.9). The appendicular bones are similar to all vertebrates and can be easily identified on radiographs. There are large groups of muscles associated with the head and neck to provide retraction of the head.

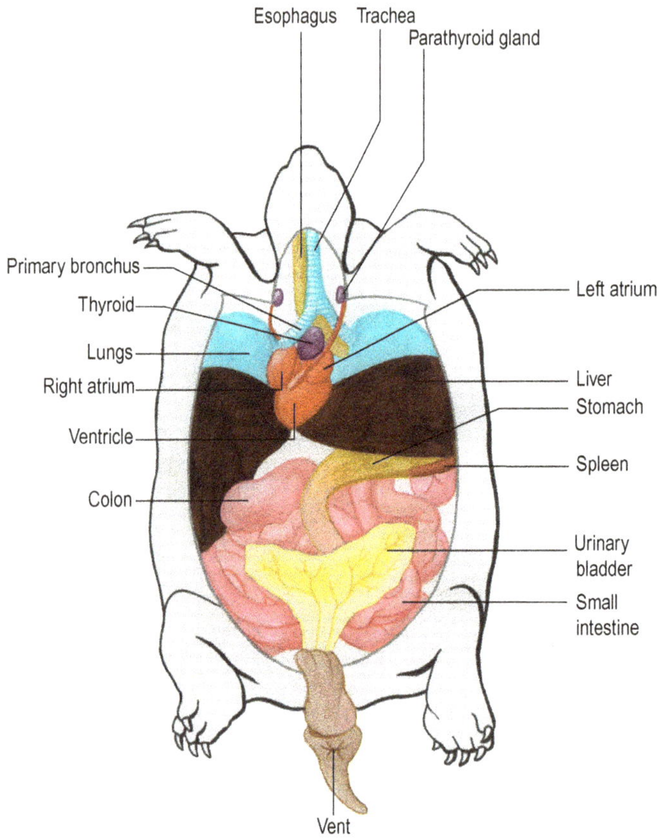

Figure 7.9
A ventral view of a chelonian.

Common orthopedic conditions

Introduction

Almost 90 percent of all reptile orthopedic injuries are related to trauma or structural changes associated with bone demineralization. The occurrence of metabolic bone disease and its relationship to the environment and nutrition of the reptile cannot be overestimated. History taking becomes extremely important in determining causes and treatment pathways for any orthopedic condition. A minimum historical database should include: provision of UVB (ultraviolet radiation band region B), thermal provision (and the gradient of this inside the vivarium), humidity, substrate and furnishings, nutrition including water, and in-contact animals. The practitioner needs to be able to identify whether the provisions are adequate for any given species, if they are contributing to the problem, or if the environment itself is the problem.

Metabolic bone disease (MBD)

Calcium is required by all reptiles for bone formation in addition to being needed for muscle contraction and nerve conduction. Calcium deficiency of whatever cause leads to bone demineralization and hence to weakening of the bones or softening of the shell. In order for a reptile to absorb and utilize sufficient amounts of calcium several factors need to be working optimally as outlined below (Mader 2006; Klaphake 2010):

- *UVB lighting* is required for the conversion of vitamin D_2 to D_3 in the skin, which is then required for absorption of calcium in the gut. This will be hampered by improper or exhausted UVB lighting provision in the enclosure. The efficiency of UVB fluorescent tubes has been the subject of much controversy, and manufacturers' claims for tube longevity are almost always inaccurate (Antwis and Browne 2010).

- *Healthy gut, liver, and kidneys.* The absorption of calcium, and the production of vitamin D that is required for this absorption, requires a healthy reptile. Deficiencies that lead to bone disease may not just be related to diet: they may stem from other issues such as renal disease or disease affecting the gut and liver.
- *Adequate calcium in the diet.* An improper ratio of phosphorous to calcium in the diet can lead to bioavailability issues of naturally occurring calcium in the diet. Supplemented calcium may be improperly applied in live feeding regimens.

Lack of available calcium in the bloodstream leads to the overproduction of parathyroid hormone which causes the release of calcium from the bones. If the overproduction is due to lack of dietary calcium, or lack of absorption due to inadequate vitamin D_3, then this is called nutritional secondary hyperparathyroidism or nutritional metabolic bone disease (NMBD). The end result of the overproduction of parathyroid hormone is the release of calcium from bone into the circulation to support the body and the gradual demineralization of the bones. Low bone calcium levels lead to lethargy, anorexia, lameness, jaw deformities, joint swelling, and ultimately fractures. The fractures can be found anywhere in the skeleton, and hence any presenting fracture should be evaluated in the light of possible bone calcium depletion (Fig. 7.10).

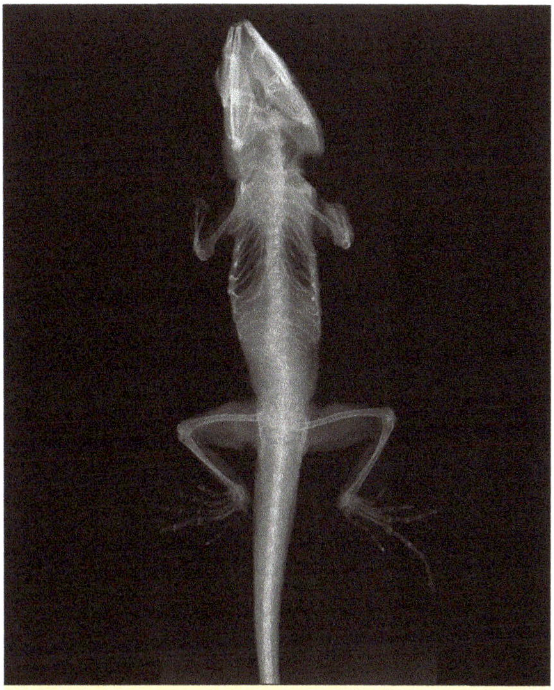

Figure 7.10
Severe spinal folding fractures associated with metabolic bone disease.

Diagnosis of NMBD is achieved through clinical history, examination of the patient, radiographs of the skeleton, and biochemical testing. Examination of the patient needs to involve careful manipulation of the joints and long bones and also the spine and jaw. The practitioner is looking for new fractures, swellings from previous healed fractures, angular limb deformities, jaw deformities and swellings, neurological deficits, and weakness of movements. In some affected reptiles the severe loss of calcium may lead to tremors, hyperreflexia, and spasms. The younger the affected animal the more severe the signs, as calcium is required for the growth that is trying to take place and for maintaining normal calcium homeostasis.

In chelonians the shell often has upturned and soft scales. Biochemical testing, if carried out, will often fail to provide insight into body calcium levels as these are often normal when tested. Biochemical tests should be performed to rule out concurrent renal or liver disease that may be contributing to the problem. Whole body radiographs are the most accurate way to evaluate a patient for MBD. All reptiles will show generalized decreased bone density. This is evaluated by the opacity of the bones gradually becoming similar to surrounding soft tissues on the radiograph. The long bones will show decreased cortical thickness and may have angular deformities. In lizards the best areas for evaluating this are the skull (Fig. 7.11) and the bones of the limbs. In chelonians it is best to evaluate the bones of the pelvic girdle and pectoral girdle.

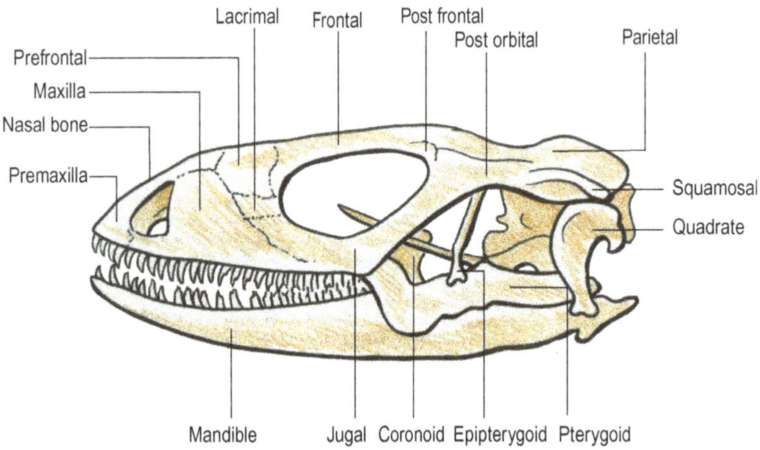

Figure 7.11
The skull of a lizard.

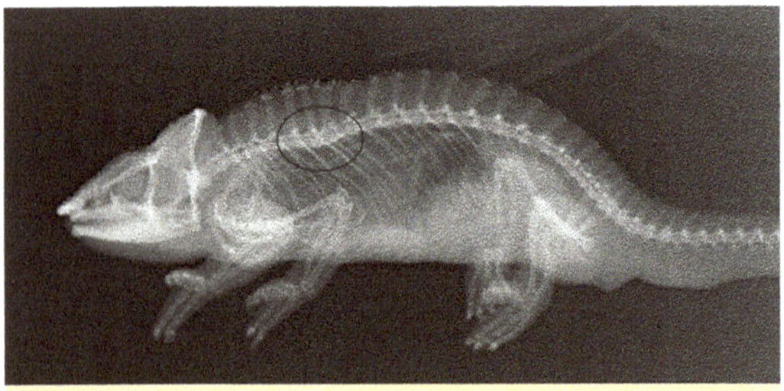

Figure 7.12
This chameleon presented with severe neurological deficiencies and was falling off branches in its vivarium. The bone density is normal but the spinal fracture may have been associated with previous metabolic bone disease or trauma.

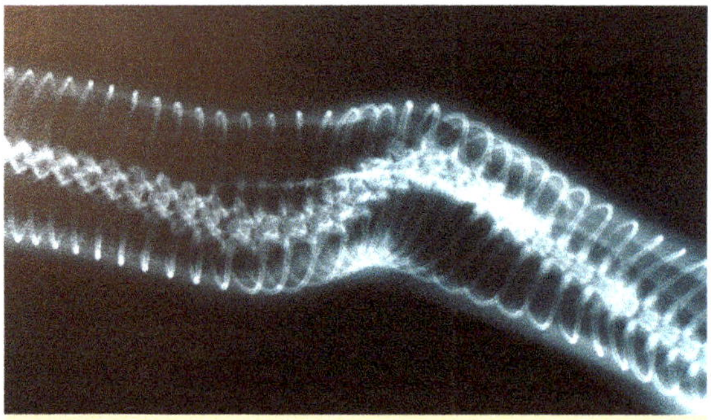

Figure 7.13
Radiograph of a grass snake showing fracturing of the spine.

If fractures are found on radiographs, this should immediately lead to the evaluation of the entire skeleton to check for any previous fractured and healed bones (Fig. 7.12). The spine can be difficult to evaluate in smaller species, and care should be taken to check all vertebrae closely for fractures (Raftery 2011).

Trauma

Although MBD causes fractures to develop without any history of blunt trauma, reptiles will develop a range of injuries without bone weakening being evident. While MBD may be associated with insidious onset of symptoms, trauma is likely to be acute. Environmental considerations such as enclosure size, the handler's age and experience, and the choice of furnishings are important in both diagnosis and treatment of trauma.

Superficial bruising and muscle damage is often associated with handler inexperience or inappropriate selection of enclosure furnishing. Bruising is very difficult to evaluate in any reptile species; shells, scales, and generally a hard integument mean that bruising is often overlooked. The practitioner will often find an area of sensitivity when palpating along a limb or the spine which on closer examination may be discolored. The reptile will almost always be less active than normal and withdrawn, making evaluation of lameness difficult. In these cases radiographs would be advisable (Fig. 7.13) to rule out MBD and ensure no deeper skeletal injury exists.

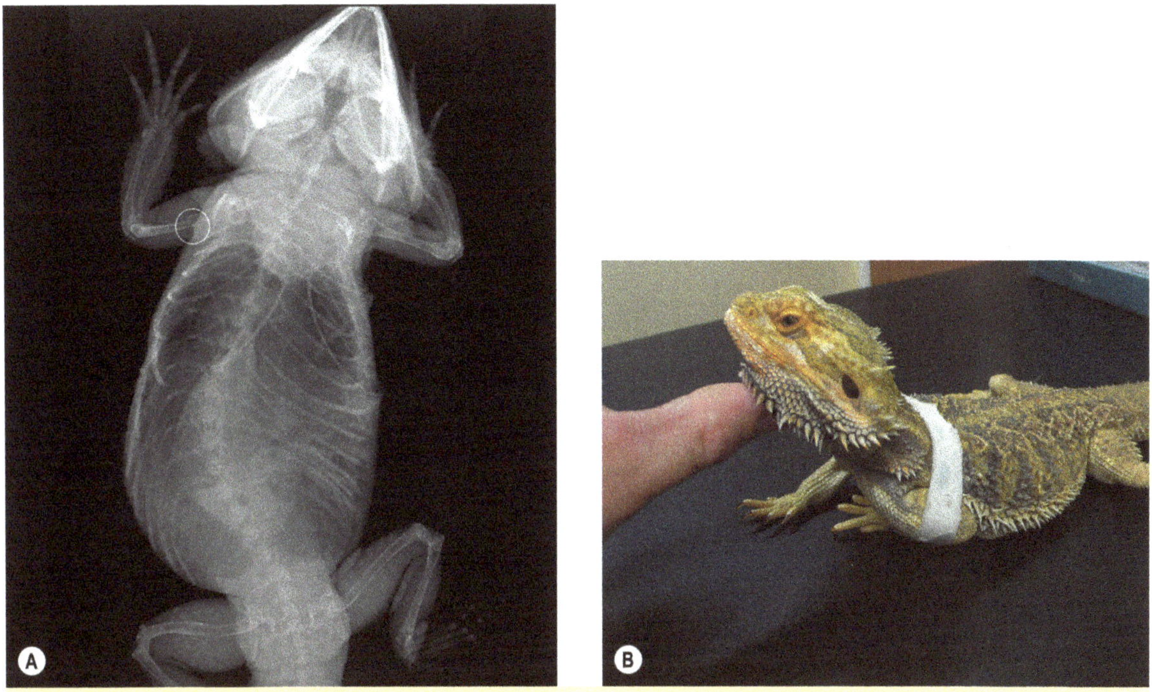

Figure 7.14
(A) A fracture to the mid-humerus caused by the owner dropping the animal. (B) The tape splint was left in place for four weeks. This bearded dragon was kept on calcium and vitamin D supplements to ensure no metabolic bone disease was present.

Moderate trauma may result in deep bruising and muscle tears, luxations, and damage to tendons and ligaments. The patient will have more marked clinical signs of lameness and pain. Chelonians are prone to coxofemoral luxations that can go undiagnosed for some time making treatment difficult. Damage to stifle joints and ligament injuries have been recorded, and these should be included in any differential diagnosis list.

Fractures are the most common presentation with or without the presence of MBD. Fractures can involve any part of the skeleton and may be accompanied by various levels of tissue damage and open wounds (Fig. 7.14A and B).

Osteomyelitis

Infections involving bones are a common presentation in reptiles. The insidious onset of symptoms means that cases are often advanced before presentation. The infections can be hematogenous in origin or arise as the result of local trauma and rubbing. In live fed reptiles, infections can occur as a result of being bitten by prey. Infection may occur local to an injury or result from hematogenous spread of bacteria. In lizards and snakes spinal osteopathy may be initiated when localized infection is present, and the osteopathy (not to be confused with osteopathic treatment) can spread infection further. In chelonians the shell rubbing on the limbs can result in localized and ongoing superficial infections that later lead to osteomyelitis. In some of the more active reptiles, repeated collisions with cage surfaces and furniture can lead to deep infections that persist until the cage environment has been changed. Mandibular infections may arise as a result of dental disease with characteristic swellings along the jaw line.

Diagnosis of osteomyelitis is most often made using radiographs which show classic lytic lesions in the affected bone without the periosteal reaction seen in mammals. This may easily be misinterpreted by the clinician as being neoplastic. These lytic lesions can persist for some time after the infection has been cleared. Draining sinuses, swellings, heat, and pain are not always present, and the absence of these may cause a clinician to miss an infection. Cytology and culture of affected sites may be helpful in planning treatment, especially with the selection of an appropriate antimicrobial. Bacterial culture can be challenging as dry swabs are unlikely to yield a good result. The best results are obtained from tissue samples submitted in saline or blood culture media. Samples from small sites may benefit from irrigating the site with saline and collecting the saline with a swab. Culture of the blood is often positive in septicemia, although false positives from contamination are common.

Spinal osteopathy complex

A syndrome in reptiles characterized by proliferative segmented spondylosis of the vertebrae has been described. Clinically this may present as deformation and swellings along the length of the spine. The etiology of the condition is unknown and may relate to several causes with similar clinical symptoms and outcomes. Sepsis, immune mediated disease, nutritional causes, viral disease, confinement, neoplasia, trauma, and vascular disease have all been postulated as the cause. Clinically, the animal presents with a varying degree of loss of mobility and neurological deficits. Swellings will be palpable along the spine. Radiography to highlight the areas of the spine that are fused is diagnostic, and further investigations such as biopsy, tissue and blood culture, and histopathology can be used to rule out possible etiological agents. Treatment is challenging and almost always unsuccessful. It relies on identifying an underlying agent as a cause and removing it with aggressive antimicrobials or treatment for nutritional deficiencies (Fitzgerald and Vera 2006).

Differential diagnosis

Reptiles are complex animals with very specific environmental requirements. When determining a diagnosis, in addition to the presenting complaint, it is important to consider the animal holistically to determine the other possible factors that may be contributing to a condition. Success in treatment is dependent on the clinician's ability to determine these contributing factors. The use of radiographs to rule out differential diagnosis is essential, with follow-up blood and tissue samples as required (Table 7.1). Recently the use of MRI and CT scanning has enhanced diagnostic capabilities. The most common differential diagnoses are shown in Table 7.2.

Lameness

All aspects of metabolic bone disease will lead to varying degrees of lameness, with bone demineralization and replacement with fibrous tissue. Pathological fractures, swollen and misshapen limbs, and spinal deformities are common presentations. Trauma from bites (from prey and cage mates) as well as neoplasia, cellulitis, and abscesses may all contribute to lameness. Joint disease will lead to swelling of the joints and a reduced range of motion; septic arthritis, degenerative joint disease, and ligament injuries need to be considered. Gout from uric acid deposits and pseudogout from calcium deposits may also present with swelling of the joints and variable lameness. Luxations from trauma, congenital deformity, or as a spontaneous event may go undiagnosed without radiography.

Reluctance to move

If a reptile is reluctant to move generalized disease, hypothermia or debilitation, and all the causes of lameness must be considered. Egg binding, constipation, large calculi, foreign bodies, and trauma can all mimic neurological or orthopedic abnormalities due to compression or damage to organs. True paralysis or paresis can result from spinal nerve compression by masses, organ enlargement, or disorders affecting the spine such as trauma, fractures, the spinal osteopathy complex (osteomyelitis, osteoarthritis, and osteoarthrosis), and neoplasia. Hypertrophic osteopathy has been recorded in lizards with the characteristic periosteal reaction on radiographs.

Musculoskeletal deformities

Due to the temperature-sensitive nature of incubation there is a wide range of deformities that may arise

Table 7.1 The most common orthopedic conditions and their main clinical features and interventions

Condition	Symptoms	Diagnosis	Treatment
Metabolic bone disease	Lameness Lethargy Anorexia Pathological fractures Joint swellings Weakness Neurological deficits	Radiographs Physical examination (blood tests)	Calcitonin Calcium supplementation (oral and injectable) UVB provision Supportive care
Trauma	Lameness Fractures Swellings Bruising Skin tears Pain	Radiographs Physical examination	Routine fracture management Environmental modification Pain relief Supportive care
Osteomyelitis	Swelling Pain Lameness Draining sinus or abscess formation	History Physical exam Radiography Culture and sensitivity	Antibiotics (based on culture results and species tolerance) Supportive care
Spinal osteopathy	Lethargy Gait abnormalities Neurological deficits Loss of normal range of motion of the spine (unable to climb or cling, falling off cage objects)	Physical examination Radiographs Identification of contributing factors	Treat contributing factors Pain relief Supportive care with osteopathic medicine

congenitally both in captive-bred and wild-caught specimens. Shell deformities may arise from historical and ongoing nutritional imbalances, trauma, or bacterial or fungal disease.

Tail deformities may arise as a result of incomplete autotomy, trauma from prey and cage mates, damage from external parasites, thermal injuries, and cloacal disease damaging adjacent tail structures.

Spinal deformities may arise from nutritional imbalances (both ongoing and historical), trauma, neoplasia, sepsis, and the spinal osteopathy complex.

Limb and head deformities may arise as a result of previous or ongoing metabolic bone disease, congenital deformity or previously healed fractures.

Swellings

Although swellings may be associated with all the conditions mentioned above, they may not be related to lameness or reluctance to move. In mammals there is consistent pain and heat in areas that have infection, but this is not always true of reptiles. Any single swelling on joints and bones needs to be evaluated for infection, neoplasia, osteoarthritis, trauma, previously healed fractures, and metabolic bone disease, and also gout and pseudogout. The animal needs to be evaluated for systemic disease if there is more than one site involved. Whole limb swellings may require evaluation of the lymphatic drainage from the limb.

Medical considerations

Trauma and fractures

All traumatic conditions require the practitioner to take a logical approach to treating the patient:

1. *Stabilize the traumatized area.* If fractures are present then apply splinting to prevent further tissue damage. Reptiles are very amenable to splinting either as a temporary fix for initial evaluation or as external support for healing. The options are only limited by the clinician's imagination.

Table 7.2 The most common differential diagnoses	
Bacterial	Osteomyelitis Abscess formation Cellulitis
Viral	Herpes virus
Trauma	Iatrogenic (from prey and handling) Inappropriate housing
Degenerative	Osteoathritis Spinal osteopathy
Developmental	Deformities relating to incubation temperature Other congenital deformities
Neoplasia	Osteosarcoma Soft tissue tumors or organ enlargement
Toxic	Cage disinfectants Cage substrate ingestion
Metabolic	Metabolic bone disease (nutritional secondary hyperparathyroidism) Hypervitaminosis D Visceral gout Pseudogout
Miscellaneous	Hypertrophic osteopathy Hypothermia Thermal injuries Egg binding Constipation Urinary calculi Autotomy

2. *Provide analgesia.* Although pain is difficult to evaluate in reptiles, all physical trauma is painful and the patient should be assumed to be in pain. There is now good pharmacological information on some of the more common nonsteroidal anti-inflammatory and opiate derivatives that can be used in reptiles.
3. *Start treatment for wounds.* Initially this will involve the irrigation and protection of open wounds (which can be carried out with the patient conscious). Warm saline should be used to flush wounds and remove debris followed by the application of dressings to protect the wounds.
4. *Evaluate for concurrent disease.* Initially this should involve a thorough assessment of management and clinical history, and then the obtaining of radiographs. Further blood and tissue samples for laboratory evaluation may also be required, and action should be started to correct any abnormalities found before starting further intervention.
5. *Plan further surgical intervention if required.* For animals with metabolic bone disease the use of surgical implants for fracture stabilization should be avoided if at all possible. Reptile fracture may take up to 50 percent longer to heal than mammalian bones, and this may lead to implant failure if the bones are not fully mineralized. The use of splints and other limb immobilization techniques is successful if applied with care, making sure that circulation is not compromized. Wounds need to be evaluated for contamination and surgery. Closure may be delayed to allow open drainage if required.
6. *Plan how recovery is going to take place.* The owner needs to be made aware of the need for changes to the environment that will be required for recovery. Initially it will be important to encourage eating and to maintain the patient's hydration while allowing the affected area to rest and heal. Monitoring splints and bandages for complications is essential, as is monitoring any changes in tissues in the surrounding areas. After the trauma or fracture has healed, the use of physiotherapy, hydrotherapy, and exercise regimens to encourage return to normal limb function may be required (Mitchell 2002).

Metabolic bone disease

The management required for patients with MBD will need to be based on the severity of the clinical signs and the degree of associated trauma.

Invasive treatment is reserved for patients with severe low blood calcium. These patients may present with tetany and neurological signs consistent with low blood calcium and will require calcium borogluconate (10 percent at 100 mg/kg) intramuscularly or intracoelomically. Beyond this the use of injectable calcium should be avoided. Once a patient is no longer at risk from tetany, and blood calcium levels have been restored, then treatment can move on to the replacement of bone calcium. Animals that have had bone calcium depletion for some time will have high levels of parathyroid hormone present and often hypertrophy of the parathyroid glands. Correcting this hormone level may take several months and can delay the replacement of bone calcium. The use of synthetic calcitonin (SCT) will accelerate the process but only if sufficient blood calcium is present. If the blood calcium is too low then the calcitonin will cause bone to take up too much calcium from the blood and may precipitate tetany. It is preferable to give several days of treatment with oral calcium gluconate and vitamin D_3 before administration of the SCT. If SCT is unavailable then the use of oral vitamin D_3 and oral calcium gluconate is acceptable, but it will take several months rather than weeks for bone mineralization to return to normal. As part of the treatment of the disease, evaluation of requirements for feeding, hydration, housing, and provision of UVB lighting should be made.

Osteomyelitis

The treatment of osteomyelitis requires appropriate antimicrobial selection and also management of predisposing factors to prevent recurrence. Selection of an appropriate antimicrobial can be challenging because of the unknown kinetics of antibiotics in some species and the difficulties of sample collection to identify the organism responsible.

Osteopathic evaluation

Introduction

The osteopathic evaluation of reptiles starts with taking the history, but forming a working osteopathic diagnosis is an ongoing process from history taking through osteopathic examination and treatment. The diagnosis should be constantly reassessed and modified throughout treatment, as the practitioner incorporates new findings into the existing framework of information in response to the tissue's reaction during manipulation. The osteopathic approach is therefore an ongoing dynamic process based on self-reflective practice (WHO 2010).

Case history

Questions about behavior, energy levels, appetite, weight loss, skin shedding, copulation, and bowel and urinary function will provide useful information about the animal's general health. The case history should explore anything reported by the owner as being abnormal for the specific patient. In addition, specific questions about previous surgery, trauma, past and current disease, and medication provide essential information when forming a prognosis and deciding on treatment. The husbandry, including caging, lighting, humidity, and diet, should also be investigated and assessed on the basis of needs specific to each species (McBride and Hernandez-Divers 2004; Wappel and Schulte 2004; Mitchell 2004).

General observation

The reptile's general behavior, awareness, and ability to explore the surrounding environment should be observed. Changes in feeding behavior and activity occur prior to ecdysis - the shedding of skin. Snakes in particular become more restless and start to rub against rough surfaces around this time (Fig. 7.15). They are more irritable than usual and cannot see clearly at this stage. Snakes tend to shed the whole skin during a process that may take up to two weeks - after which they may defecate, be very thirsty, and are susceptible to dehydration. Lizards and chelonians shed their skin piecemeal, and this makes them more vulnerable during ecdysis. Signs of dehydration include: decreased

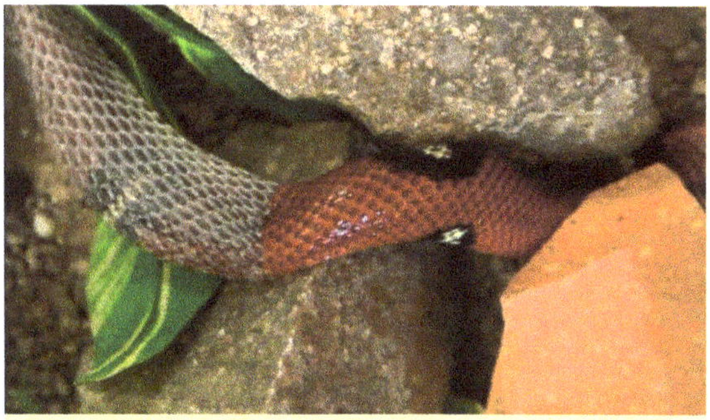

Figure 7.15
The normal shedding of skin in a snake.

skin turgor, presence of multiple skin folds, sunken eyes in lizards and chelonians, and shrunken and opaque spectacles (fused eyelids) in snakes and some lizards.

When sick, reptiles actively seek an external source of heat to enhance the immune system - an event known as behavioral fever (Firth and Turner 1982). This is because reptiles cannot raise the body temperature endogenously to fight infection as mammals do. In cases of severe respiratory disease snakes will show mouth breathing.

Finally, the presence of abnormal odors, burns, abrasions, wounds, abscesses, discharge, swelling, and audible respiratory noises (sneezing, wheezing, gasping, etc.) should be noted. When observing the animal's stance, check the skin, symmetry of bony landmarks, and muscle development.

Observation during movement

This part of the examination assesses the general balance of the animal when weight-bearing together with the range, quality, and symmetry of motion during weight transfer between limbs. In particular, the position and symmetry of movement of the head and neck are observed, together with the range and freedom of movement in the forelimbs and hind limbs. Any dysfunction or pathology in the latter may result in an asymmetrical gait, limping, impaired balance or inability to coil on branches or logs. Gait and general reptile movements should be observed in the respective natural or captive environment (Fig. 7.16). Each species has its own pattern of locomotion.

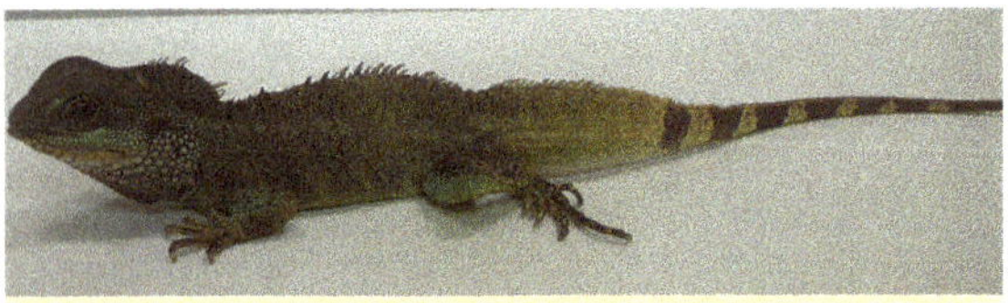

Figure 7.16
Observing a reptile's general movements in its environment allows key information to be gathered about its behavior, weight-bearing, balance, mobility, and quality and symmetry of movement.

Despite the weight of the shell, terrestrial chelonian species support all their weight on their legs, can move at great speed, and are generally bright, alert, and responsive when handled. The plastron (the flat ventral surface of the shell) bears no weight and should not touch the ground during locomotion (Fig. 7.17).

Freshwater turtles swim with a paddling motion, and some can even walk along the bottom. This is different to marine turtles which move the forelimbs like flippers while using the rear limbs like rudders for steering (Walker 1973). The swim should be assessed and should be evenly balanced in water. Altered buoyancy may suggest a respiratory or gastrointestinal disorder (for instance, pneumonia or foreign body).

Snake locomotion involves undulating and sidewinding. The former occurs when the snake wriggles laterally, thrusting itself forward when in contact with a rough surface, while adjusting the movement to the local terrain; the latter involves moving laterally by throwing the body sideways in loops (Fig. 7.18A and B). In addition, large snakes such as pythons use the ventral skin and attached segmental muscle to pull themselves forward in a straight line using their ribs causing a wave effect known as rectilinear locomotion (Pough et al. 2002). Any unusual coiling, twisting motions, weakness of the distal body or decreased constriction should be noted.

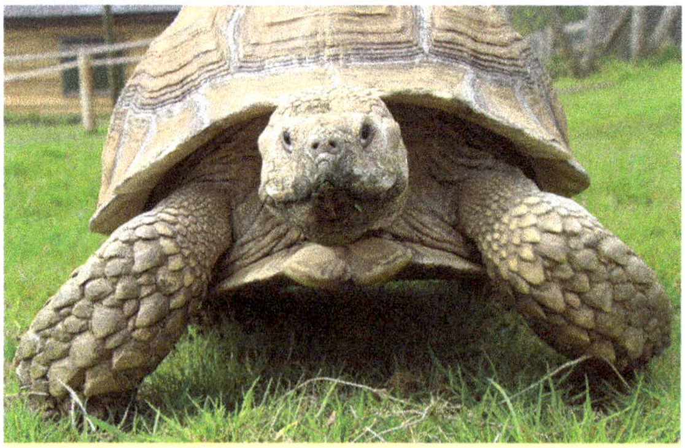

Figure 7.17
In normal conditions terrestrial chelonians support all the weight on their legs thus keeping the plastron off the ground.

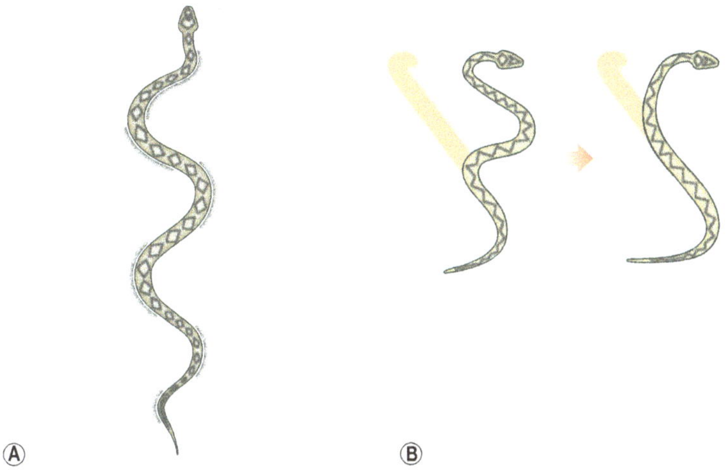

Figure 7.18
(A) Lateral undulation. The snake grips the surface with some of its ribs and pulls itself along in sections, creating an undulating effect. (B) Sidewinding. The snake throws part of its body in loops sideways, grips with its ribs, and pulls the rest of the body so that it follows.

Safety and handling

Washing the hands before and after touching reptiles is good practice to limit the spread of disease, but also to remove any kind of scent that a snake may mistake for food. Reptiles can carry infections such as salmonella that are infectious to humans.

Before and during handling, the practitioner should always be aware of possible sources of stress for the reptile and should always be monitoring the surroundings closely. Even tame reptiles can react badly to loud noises or other stimuli they may find upsetting. Surprising the reptile by touching it unexpectedly should be avoided; use a combination of sound and touch (such as gently tapping the cage) to make the animal aware of your presence. The handler should always move slowly and, if possible, should not approach the animal head on. Also approach at its level, rather than from above. The reptile should be allowed to get comfortable with the operator's hold before starting treatment. The operator should provide full and secure support of the reptile's body weight and length (Fig. 7.19). Dangling a reptile in the air, turning it upside down, sudden movements or looking too closely at its head are practices that should be avoided as they can stress or startle the animal. The reptile will give warning signs whenever it is uncomfortable, agitated, or in pain (Table 7.3). These should be immediately recognized and responded to by the operator in order to avoid injury to the animal or to themselves.

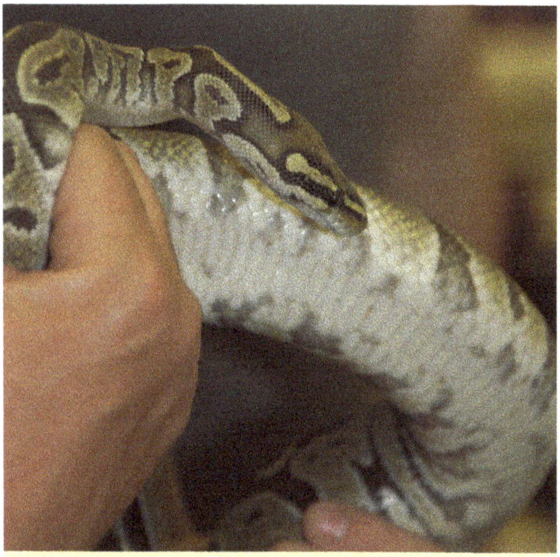

Figure 7.19
Regardless of its size and species, the reptile should always be supported fully and securely throughout its length. Also, allow time for it to get comfortable in the osteopath's hands.

Table 7.3 The most common warning signs of stress when handling reptiles

Warning signs	Type of reptile
Repeated attempts to escape Unnatural fussiness Heavy breathing Squirming	All reptiles
Hissing Thrashing around	Snakes and lizards
Clawing Flailing legs Opening or gaping mouth	Lizards and tortoises

It is generally a good idea to handle reptiles during a time of day when they are lethargic. However, they should not be overhandled, especially small lizards and snakes, for up to three days after eating (due to the risk of regurgitation). Handling snakes and lizards should be avoided or kept to the absolute minimum during ecdysis.

Regardless of how much a given species is known to be docile and easy to handle, the practitioner should always remember that reptiles, just like any other live animal, have individual personalities, and handling should be adapted to each individual case.

Most pythons, boas and many of the American rat snakes are easy to handle, but they can still bite and constrict. Nonvenomous species, such as water pythons, racers, and whip snakes remain untrustworthy throughout their lives. It is recommended that only experienced reptile veterinarians examine and treat venomous species. These may need to be sedated before proceeding with the osteopathic palpation and treatment. Generally, the younger the snake is, the more active and "jerky" it will be during handling. Never pin a snake or lift it by its neck; the cervical vertebrae are susceptible to damage and the animal is apt to be permanently disabled. Although it will struggle if restrained, the head will tend to relax if the body alone is gently supported (Fig. 7.20). If the snake is over six feet long, the assistance of another person is generally needed, especially if the animal gets scared and may constrict. If it is a constrictor snake its full weight should be supported, and it

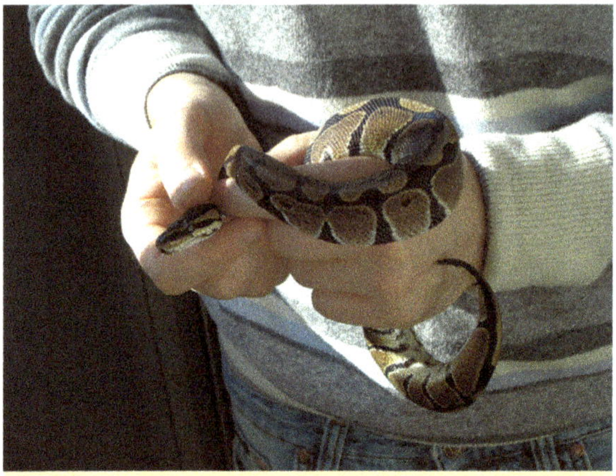

Figure 7.20
If held gently, the snake's head can be safely handled while the rest of the body is fully supported.

is likely to wrap its tail around the operator's wrist and forearm. The animal should be allowed to move freely through the operator's hands rather than being grabbed and held tightly. If the reptile coils around the handler's hands, neck or chest, it should be supported underneath its body and repositioned for the handler's safety. After treatment, the snake should be returned to its cage by slowly lowering it in, either onto a branch or the cage floor.

Lizards can be safely picked up by cupping the hands under their bellies, with a finger between their forelegs, while the rear end rests on the operator's wrist or arm (Fig. 7.21). Large lizards, such as iguanas, should be picked up with one hand holding the front of the body and the other hand supporting the lower abdomen, hips, and the base of the tail. If the lizard has a whippy tail, it is recommended that the length of its body is supported along the handler's forearm, with the palm up supporting the animal's sternum while the tail is tucked loosely between the operator's forearm and rib cage. The larger skinks such as blue-tongued lizards (*Tiliqua helonian*), shingle backs (*Tiliqua rugosa rugosa*), and bearded dragons (*Pogona vitticeps*), but not the eastern species (*Pogona barbata*), are normally docile and used to handling, although they can still bite. They

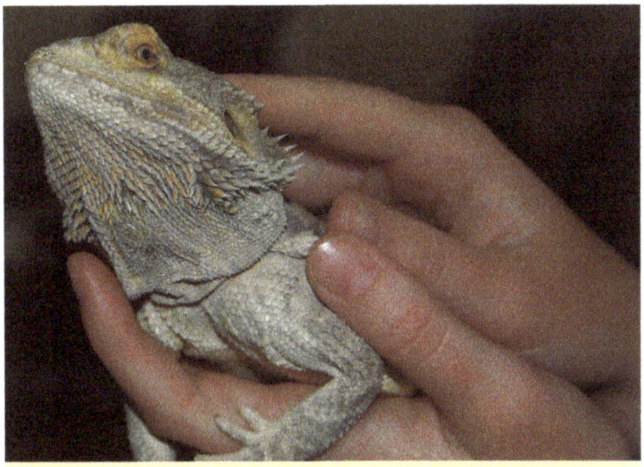

Figure 7.21
To pick up a lizard safely, cup both hands under the belly, with a finger between the forelegs, while the rear end is resting on the operator's wrist or arm.

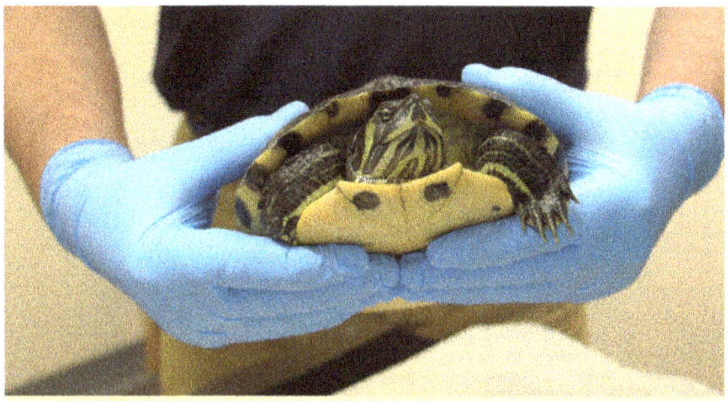

Figure 7.22
To hold a terrapin safely, hold it by the sides of its carapace behind both forelimbs.

have powerful snapping jaws, with the adductor jaw muscles originating from the temporal fossae at right angles to the open jaw (Johnston 2014). Eastern water dragons (*Physignathus leseurii*) are flighty and can be aggressive as adults, but youngsters may be "hypnotized" by being laid on their backs while the handler gently strokes their abdomen (Cannon and Johnson 2015). Other species such as varanids may scratch and flick their tail.

When palpating lizards remember that some species have a superficial parietal gland or third eye just beneath the skin between the parietal and frontal bone. This organ has a lens, cornea, and retina, but it does not form images. It is thought to aid thermoregulation by sensing changes in the intensity and wavelength of light (Solessio and Engbretson 1999).

Chelonians have glands on either end of the bridge between plastron and carapace that may discharge a pungent fluid. The turtle should be approached from the side or rear and held by its carapace behind both foreflippers (Fig. 7.22). Although most of the common freshwater turtles can be restrained manually without much danger, due to their small size, some of them (the red-eared slider and painted turtle) will readily bite. Others such as matamata (*Chelus fimbriatus*) and snapping turtles (*Chelydra serpentina*) are aggressive with powerful jaw muscles that can cause severe damage. When handling the latter, the operator can lift the rear end of the turtle by grasping the base of the tail with one hand and slipping the other hand under the plastron for support (Moon and Hernandez Foerster 2001).

Palpation

A thorough palpation is performed while exploring the entire reptile body from head (from frontals to occiput and from temporals to submandibular region) to tail, including the body (from cervical to sacral region), limbs (from proximal to distal), and shell if present.

The reptile's skin is dry and has far fewer glands than either amphibians or mammals. It is heavily keratinized, generally thicker dorsally than ventrally, and contains a lipid layer to prevent water loss. The scales are an integral part of the skin and provide protection from abrasion, besides their role in permeability. During palpation of this tissue any sign of dehydration, congestion, abrasion, inflammation, or altered tissue texture should be detected.

The epaxial muscles lie dorsally, whereas the hypaxial muscles are usually lodged ventrally and between the ribs, forming an interlocking system of muscle chains and tendons that should show a homogenously firm tone on palpation. In snakes, the hypaxial and intercostal muscles not only help in locomotion but also in respiration and in the passage of prey for digestion. Therefore, during any of these functions, different muscle groups may develop an altered ability to contract and relax. Consequently, palpation of these structures should be performed very carefully, feeling for any sign of increased muscle tone, including reactions to pressure (Fig. 7.23). Abnormalities in muscle tone and posture, muscle fasciculation, and fitting may indicate metabolic bone disease that can lead to hind limb and tail paresis (especially in small lizards).

When palpating chelonians, particular attention should be addressed to the strong retractor muscles that extend from the supratemporal fossae and supraoccipital crest to the base of the neck enabling the head retraction. Whereas the trunk is fused with the shell (and lacks a sternum), the neck and tail are highly flexible with well-developed epaxial and hypaxial muscles (Evans 1986). These allow for bending of the neck sideways (Pleurodira) or inside the shell (Cryptodira). The largest muscle mass is present in the limbs, with powerful fan-shaped pectoral and pelvic muscles connecting the respective bony girdles to the carapace and plastron (Nagashima et al. 2009). All of these structures should be carefully palpated to detect any sign of dysfunction at the head, neck, and limbs (Fig. 7.24). The author (PT) has found that a useful technique to encourage most tortoises to bring their head and limbs out of the shell is to hold the tortoise facing downward toward the floor and then bring it through a quick U-shaped motion to face upward to the ceiling. It can be useful to apply a series of gentle pressure tests along the margins of each scute, on both the carapace and plastron (Fig. 7.25). This can help to identify the equivalent of intraosseous strains along the shell structure or a corresponding dysfunctional visceral pattern, since most of the organs are anatomically related and connected with the shell (Fig. 7.26).

With regard to palpation of bone tissue, it is important to remember that flexibility of the spine is crucial to reptiles for locomotion, rather than a rigid backbone supporting weight. As they have no diaphragm, and consequently no division between the thorax and abdomen, the terms thoracic and lumbar are replaced by the term presacral region, which is divided into sacral and caudal segments. The number of presacral vertebrae varies from 18 in Chelonia (of which eight are cervical vertebrae and 10 are trunk

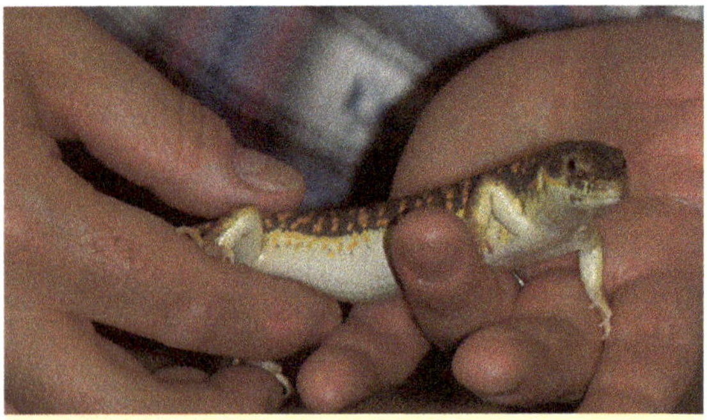

Figure 7.23
Accurate palpation of the epaxial and hypaxial muscle groups allows the operator to detect any signs of dysfunction, such as altered muscle tone, and avoid causing pain reactions by applying pressure to the area.

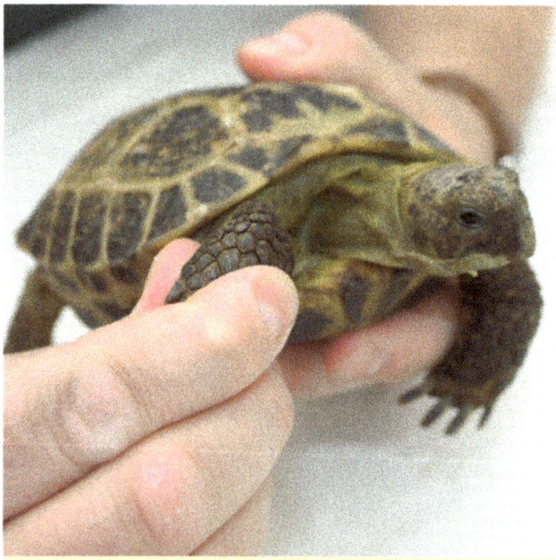

Figure 7.24
A thorough examination of the limbs can be performed by carefully palpating the bony structures and related muscles.

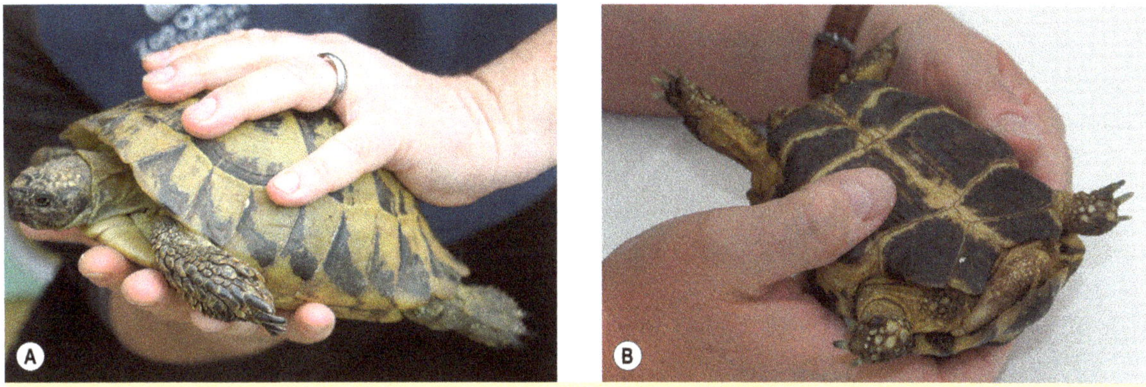

Figure 7.25
Gentle pressure tests can be performed along the margins of each scute on the carrapace (A) and the plastron (B) to identify areas of dysfunction in the shell and of corresponding visceral structures.

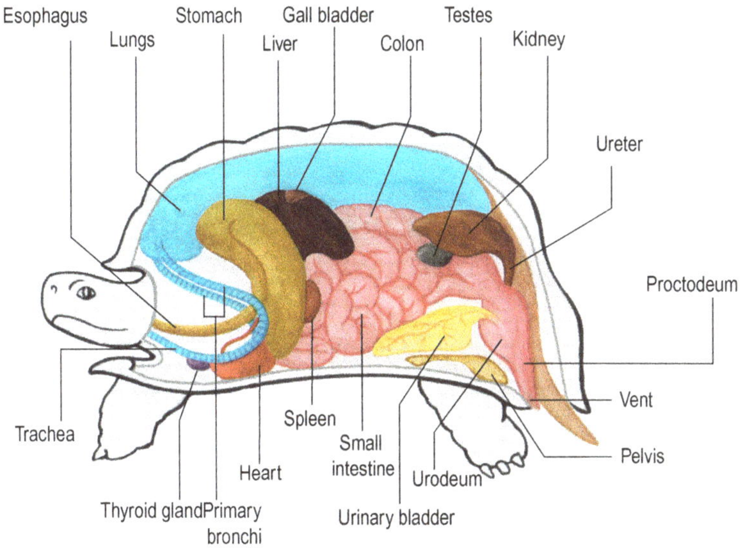

Figure 7.26
A midsagittal view of the internal anatomy of a chelonian.

vertebrae), 24 in some lizards, and up to 200–400 in snakes (Hoffstetter and Gasc 1970). Unlike mammals, reptiles do not have a cauda equina since the spinal cord extends down to the tail tip. Snakes do not have a mandibular symphysis; instead, flexible skin allows the jaw bones to move apart and forward or backward. In addition, snakes do not have a distinct cervical region but the first two vertebrae lack ribs. The ribs attach by muscles to the inner surface of the ventral scales since both the sternum and costal cartilages are absent. Apart from Chelonia, the ribs of reptiles are well-developed and, in addition to supporting the body wall, they perform the function of respiration and locomotion. The whole of these bony structures should be carefully assessed during gentle palpation from head to tail in order to feel for the presence of bony landmark asymmetry, abnormalities, loss of integrity, and protective reactions to pressure.

Finally, the ventral coelomic cavity between the ribs should also be gently palpated, feeling for the resilience of the organs and for the presence of any altered tissue texture, including fluid accumulation (Fig. 7.27). Pressure should be applied gently, especially if the animal has recently been fed, in order to avoid regurgitation. Reptiles should not demonstrate pain with gentle abdominal palpation. Any abnormal finding should lead to a veterinary examination to differentiate between tumors, granulomas, intestinal impaction, retained eggs or fetuses, foreign bodies, etc.

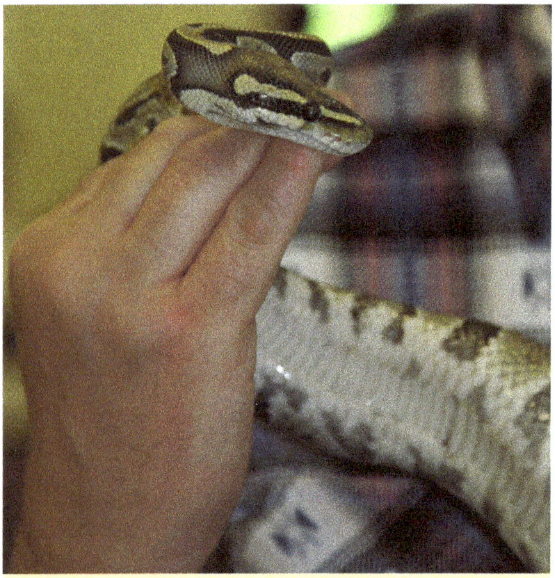

Figure 7.27
The ventral cavity should be carefully examined by gentle palpation to detect any sign of altered tissue texture.

Mobility testing

Osteopathic mobility testing should aim to identify any restriction of motion and functional asymmetries in the head, neck, spine and rib cage, forelimbs, rear limbs, and tail. The operator should gently assess each segment, constantly feeling for tissue response and adapting the hold according to the animal's position and reaction.

Reptiles have a well-developed neck, which enables them to scan the horizon (a marked difference to amphibians). The osteopath assessing this region may gently use the head as a lever and should find a high degree of freedom and range of motion. Particular attention should be addressed to the occipitoatlantal joint (Fig. 7.28A and B). There is a single occipital condyle, articulating with the atlas, which in turn is firmly connected with the axis, so the occipitoatlantal joint is the main center for neck movement (O'Malley 2005). All the vertebrae except the cervical ones bear ribs, leaving little flank area. Ventrally the ribs either join the sternum, the opposite rib, or end free in the muscular body wall. Lizards in particular have a flexible backbone. Their presacral segments can be assessed through a double-hand contact on the spine, with one

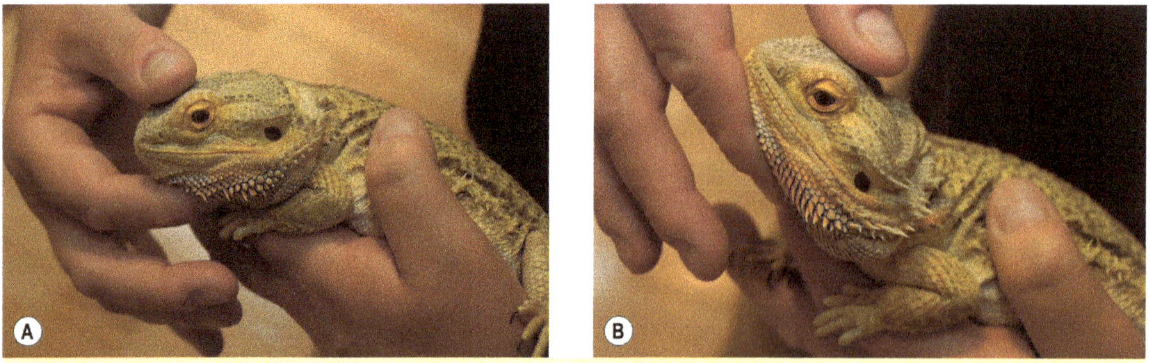

Figure 7.28
The occipitoatlantoaxial complex can be examined by gently using the head as a lever to induce flexion (A) and extension (B).

hand fixing the vertebrae and the other hand mobilizing the next caudally situated segment while using the rest of the body as a lever (Fig. 7.29).

For snakes the author has found it extremely useful to use a gentle pressure test along each region of the spine, using a double-hand contact to assess the tissue's viscoelastic response to the force being applied. In the presence of somatic dysfunction, the tissue will show an increased density and resistance to pressure, together with an inability to return to the original tension once pressure is released. In addition, vertebral group mobility testing can be performed along the snake's spine using the same hold as described above, gently inducing motion in all directions (particularly laterally).

Lizards have well-developed legs and a long tail for counterbalance. In lizards, as well as in chelonians, these structures deserve particular attention during mobility testing. Girdles should be gently tested by fixing the proximal end while using the humerus or femur as levers (Fig. 7.30). The same principle can be applied to the rest of the limb, with the proximal segment being stabilized and the joint tested by using the distal segment as a lever. It is quite common, especially in chelonians, that the animal retracts the limb strongly

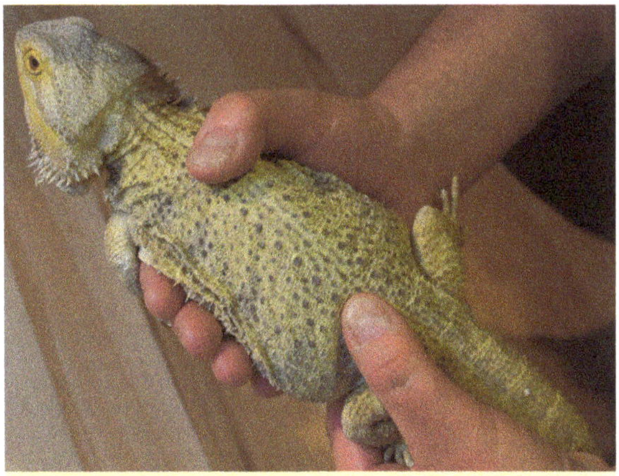

Figure 7.29
The presacral segments in lizards can be easily assessed using a double-hand contact on the spine, and by using the body as a lever during segmental mobility testing.

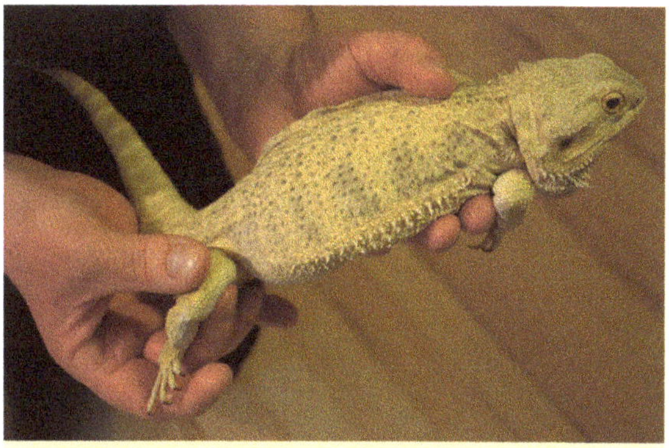

Figure 7.30
To test the pelvic girdle, fix the pelvis and use the femur as a lever for mobility testing.

during testing. If this occurs with a moderate force, the operator may offer mild resistance in an attempt to keep the hold and continue the procedure. If, however, the reptile reacts strongly to the operator's restraint, it would be advisable to change the hold, or trigger the head and neck to come out (as described in the palpation section), or carry on the routine, assessing a different area and then coming back to the difficult limb. If clear signs of distress are present then interrupt the examination (see Table 7.3). Finally, mobility of the tail should be assessed; stabilize the proximal segments and induce motion in all directions using the caudal end as the lever (Fig. 7.31).

Further osteopathic examination

Palpation of the cranial and fascial rhythms may offer the osteopath further information about the animal's dysfunctional pattern, also offering the opportunity of a different perspective on the findings identified up to this point in the examination (Fig. 7.32A and B). Many reptiles (like snakes and lizards) have a kinetic skull, which means a large part of it fails to ossify, and elastic cartilage allows for movement between cranial bones (O'Malley 2005), but the perception of any intrinsic involuntary rhythms (such as the cranial rhythm) is extremely difficult to achieve in reptiles (but not in varanids). The author's hypothesis is that, as an expression of the body's metabolic activity, these rhythms in reptiles may be easily dissipated into the environment, rather than resonating strongly through the tissues and thus being easily appreciated by the practitioner. This may be related to the fact that reptiles are ectothermic and rely on external sources to regulate their body temperature through behavioral and physiological processes (Espinoza and Tracy 1997). The most widely accepted theory about the nature of involuntary rhythms in humans is based on cyclic frequencies in blood-flow velocity (0.10 to 0.20 Hz, 6.0 to 12 cpm) linked to oscillations in activity of the autonomic nervous system (Glonek et al. 2005). In reptiles these oscillations are presumably absent, or at extremely low frequencies, as there tends to be a constant vasomotor dilation of peripheral blood vessels during the day in order to aid thermoregulation (Pough et al. 1998).

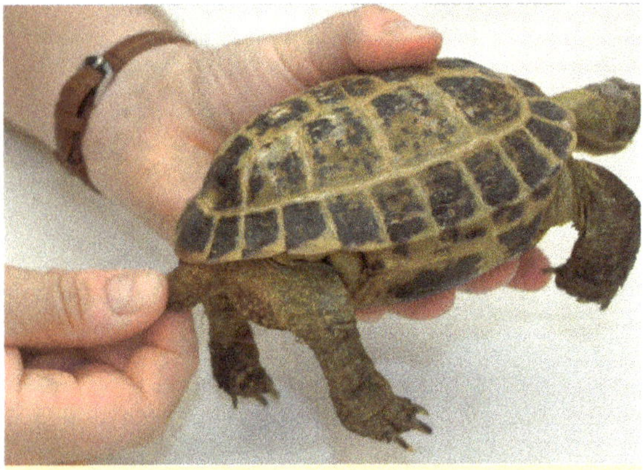

Figure 7.31
To test the tail take a firm contact on each caudal segment and apply gentle mobility testing in all directions feeling for any restriction of motion.

Visceral testing can be performed by gently palpating the organs and assessing for dysfunctional texture, mobility, and motion (Fig. 7.33). It is possible to test the viscera by exploring the reptile's ventral region from the cervical area (trachea and esophagus), cranial body half (heart, lungs, and liver), to the caudal half (stomach, small intestine and colon,

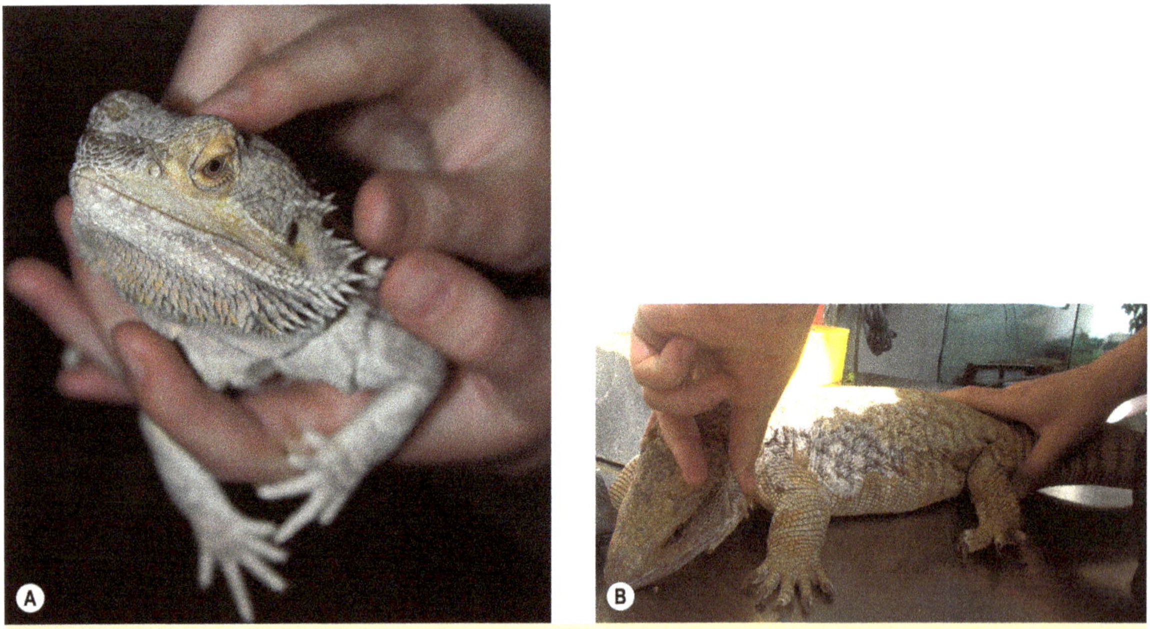

Figure 7.32
Palpation of the craniosacral rhythm on a bearded dragon (A) and a varanid (B).

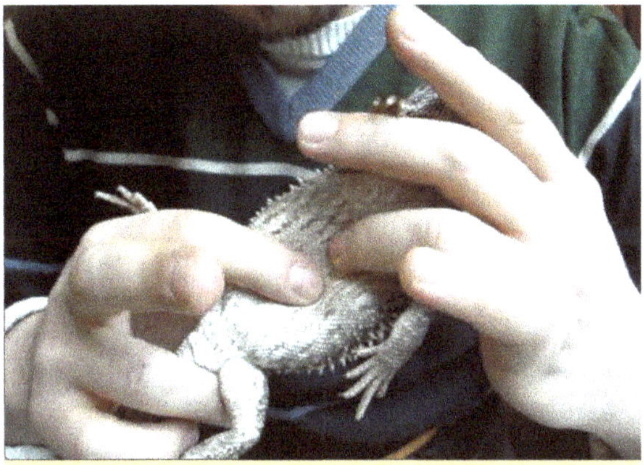

Figure 7.33
Osteopathic visceral testing can be performed while holding the reptile's head and forelimbs with the index and middle fingers of one hand and holding its tail and rear limbs with the fourth and fifth fingers of the other hand.

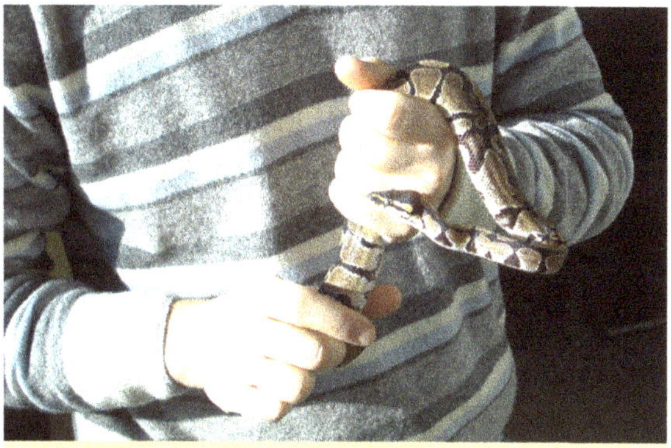

Figure 7.34
Articulatory techniques can be efficiently applied both sideways and in a dorsoventral direction, or in a combination of both if needed, using a double full-hand contact on the snake's body.

cloaca and bladder). In chelonians, the author assesses the viscera indirectly by applying a series of pressure tests along the margins of the corresponding shell scutes. Any increase in tissue density and loss of resilience may indicate the presence of related visceral dysfunction.

Osteopathic treatment

Reptiles are generally very responsive to osteopathic manipulation. However, it is not always easy to adapt a technique to their body size, shape, and reactions. The osteopath will need to constantly adjust the hold or change the technique according to the animal's response for reasons of safety and in order to deliver effective treatment. Even the most tame reptile can react badly if under stress or in pain. It is recommended that before starting treatment, the operator should have a clear plan of which areas need treatment and how it may best be delivered. The period of handling should be limited to the correction of dysfunctional areas only. The type and duration of techniques being applied will vary depending on the species and the conditions being treated; however, the author (PT) has found he rarely administers treatment to a reptile for more than 10 minutes. In most cases, a double-hand contact is recommended to control the animal's reactions, to feel for the tissue response, and to direct the forces applied more precisely during a given manipulation. If a stroking action is ever employed during manipulation, the direction of stroke should always be in the direction of the scales, from head to tail. In some species scales may be lifted and can be injured, together with the underlying skin, if stroked backward. Jerky movements should be avoided as they are likely to trigger a protective response from the animal. If the reptile shows any sign of stress or pain (see Table 7.3) at any point during treatment, the osteopath should recognize this immediately and possibly end the treatment within a few seconds. In any event, never take an unreasonable risk - there will always be another or a better day for treatment!

Snakes can best be handled and approached starting with treatment of the body, leaving the head and tail to the end. Gentle slow articulatory techniques can be effectively applied to these reptiles, especially in lateral directions, along the dysfunctional vertebral and costal groups (Fig. 7.34). Dorsoventral movements may also be integrated into the technique. This will often lead the operator to detect a spiral-like motion when feeling for the tissue tension, and the treatment forces should be adjusted accordingly. Usually the snake will move through the operator's hands once the release is achieved! The author has found snakes respond well to a sort of viscoelastic approach. This means administering a gentle but progressive compression to the dysfunctional part of the animal's body, following the "lines" of tissue response to such pressure, until the density of the dysfunction is felt to be enclosed within the resulting hold. The end hold needs to be maintained until the release is achieved, usually within a few seconds (Fig. 7.35). When moving toward the cranial cervical region it is advisable to avoid any direct technique as this part of the snake's spine is generally quite sensitive, and direct techniques are likely to trigger a reaction if used with too much pressure or force. Instead, a more functional technique is better suited to this area, gently positioning it in a tension neutral point, and holding this until the release is felt (Fig. 7.36). The head can be approached by applying a gentle inhibitory pressure on any cranial sutures found in dysfunction.

The author commonly finds a tensional pattern in the submandibular region in the associated soft tissue. This may be because of the considerable amount of stretch these structures undergo during ingestion of prey. This area can be released using gentle slow craniocaudally directed strokes while holding the top of the snake's head with both thumbs and thenar eminences. If the animal's head struggles during the technique, treatment should be promptly interrupted and, if necessary, it should be performed under sedation. Surprisingly, visceral mobilization in snakes can produce dramatic changes in the related tissue motion. In particular, the area corresponding to the passage of the esophagus, stomach, small and large intestine, and rectum can be freed through a gentle inhibitory pressure, or through the equivalent of direct myofascial work, using a ventral contact and a laterolateral hold of the rest of the body (Fig. 7.37).

As mentioned previously, the author finds it extremely difficult to feel involuntary rhythms in snakes, and it is therefore unlikely that these can be effectively used during treatment. In contrast, lizards and, in particular, large lizards such as iguanas are highly responsive to the engagement and balancing of involuntary rhythms. Involuntary rhythms are usually one of the first systems available to the operator when treating lizards, which will rapidly go into a "parasympathetic state" as the cranial rhythm is felt (Fig. 7.38). This certainly helps the practitioner to perform the rest of the treatment effectively and safely. Most cranial techniques, including CV4, V-spread techniques and occipitosacral balancing, can be successfully performed especially in large lizards, given

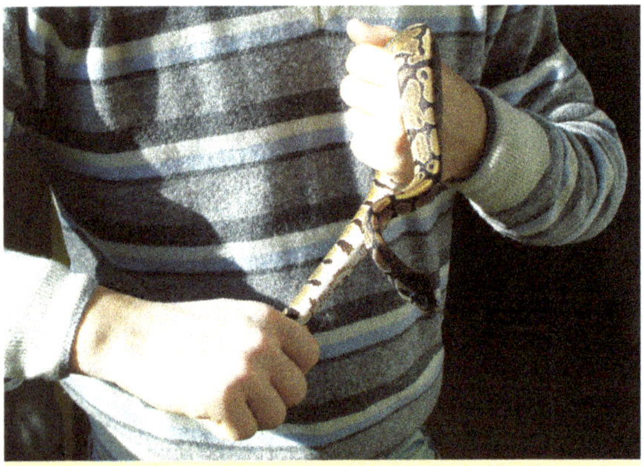

Figure 7.35
It can be particularly useful to apply a viscoelastic approach in snakes by administering a gentle but progressive compression to the dysfunctional area and enclosing the denser feeling part until the release is felt. This is a modified version of the sustained positional release technique.

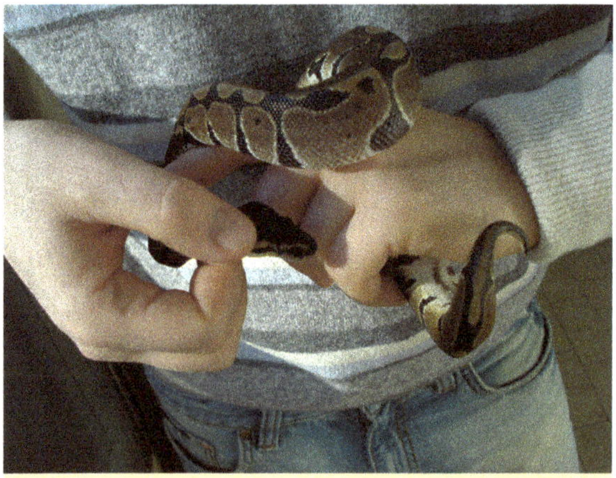

Figure 7.36
Indirect approaches, such as positional facilitated release (functional release) or balanced ligamentous tension techniques, are particularly suitable for treating the snake's sensitive cranial cervical area.

that the hand contacts must adapt to the animal's size and body shape (Fig. 7.39). This kind of intervention may produce effects on the reptile's thermoregulation, which is controlled by the hypothalamus, pineal gland, and in some species by the parietal eye (Pough et al. 1998). This in turn will cause changes in behavior and physiology. Articulatory techniques may follow where needed, and usually have very good results in lizards, whether applied to the spine or on the extremities. To work on the spine the proximal end of the reptile's body is supported and held by one of the operator's hands while the animal's distal end is mobilized with the other hand (Fig. 7.40). A combination of movements can then be applied in all directions using coordinated movements of both hands, focusing the forces applied on the dysfunctional vertebral group. The same principle can be applied to the tail and to the limbs and related joint (Fig. 7.41).

Small lizards appear to be extremely responsive to fascial work and in particular they readily unwind any inherent myofascial tension. The whole body can be supported through a craniopelvic hold. Gentle traction or compression can then be administered to induce the unwinding process. The operator should examine the full pattern of any inherent myofascial tension,

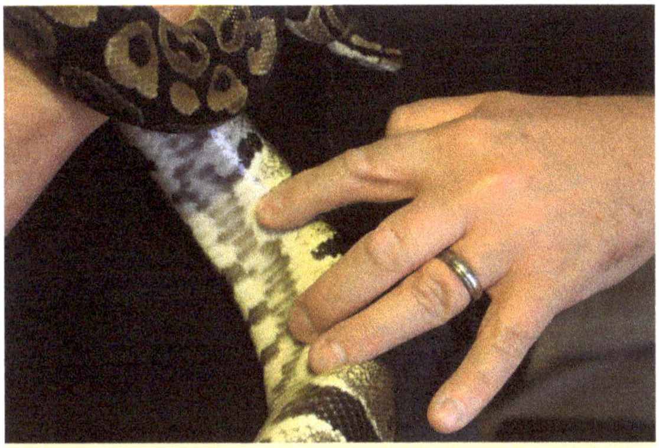

Figure 7.37
Visceral release can be performed in snakes through gentle inhibitory pressure, or the equivalent of direct myofascial work, by taking a ventral contact and holding the animal with both hands.

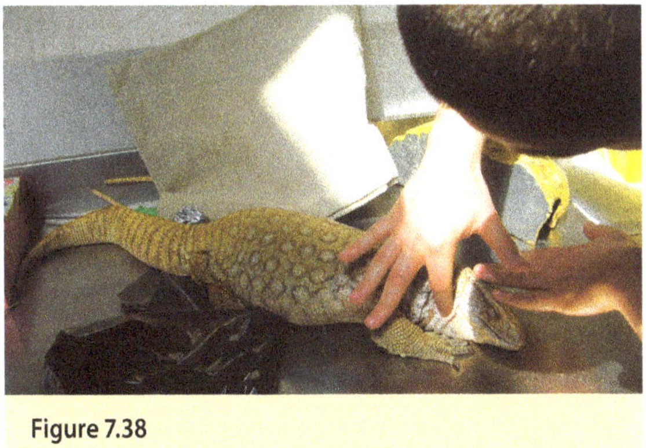

Figure 7.38
Quite often lizards and iguanas will fall into a very relaxed state as the craniosacral rhythm is engaged and balanced.

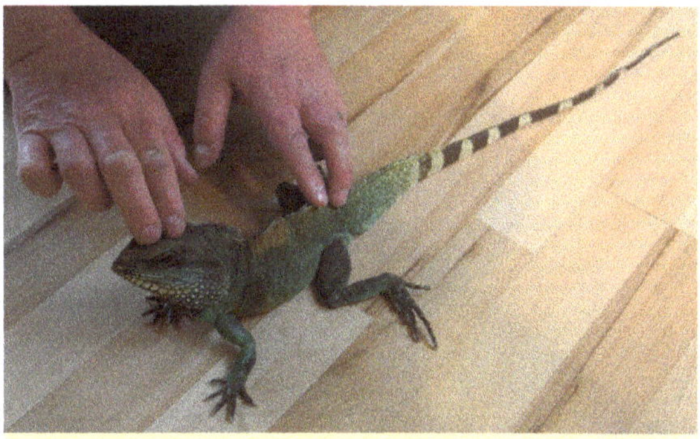

Figure 7.39
Occipitosacral balancing performed on a water dragon.

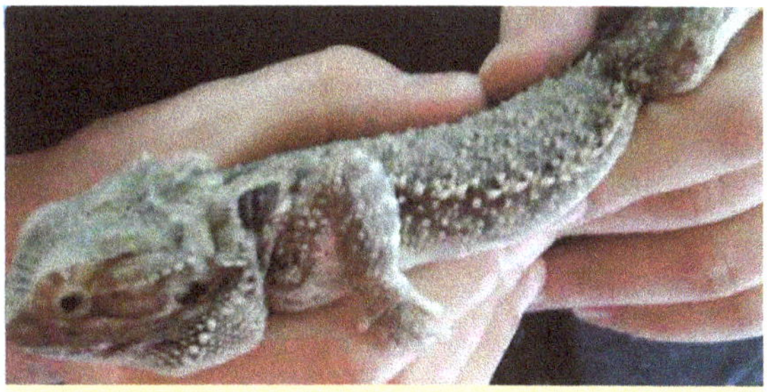

Figure 7.40
Articulatory techniques can be successfully applied on a lizard's spine by holding the proximal end of the dysfunctional vertebral group with one hand while using the distal spine as a lever to focus the corrective motion in any direction needed.

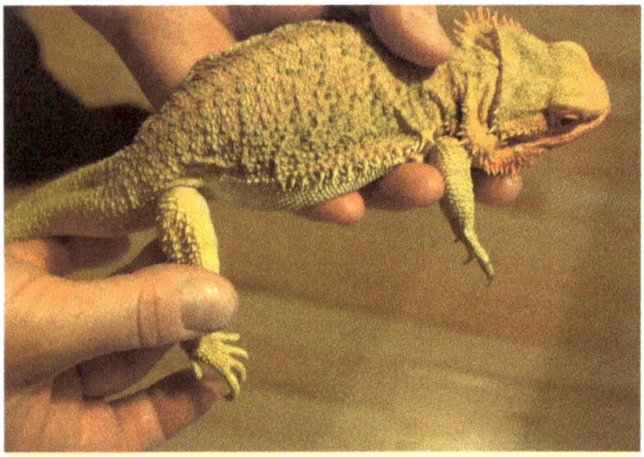

Figure 7.41
Using the same principle applied to the spine, articulatory techniques can be efficiently delivered to the lizard's limbs, tail, and related joints.

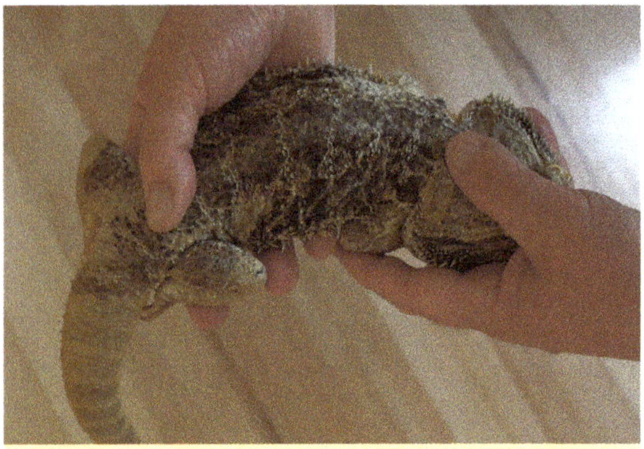

Figure 7.42
Total body myofascial unwinding is particularly suitable for lizards displaying a total-body dysfunctional pattern. The inherent myofascial tension is followed and amplified through a craniopelvic hold until a full release is achieved.

following directions of ease, without forcing or resisting any directional alterations (Fig. 7.42). This is continued until sufficient soft tissue release is gained.

Chelonians are highly responsive to treatment of their carapace or plastron. The dysfunctional areas found in these structures can be approached through slow inhibitory pressure or quick recoil or toggle techniques (Fig. 7.43). This is probably one of the few cases of osteopathy applied to animals

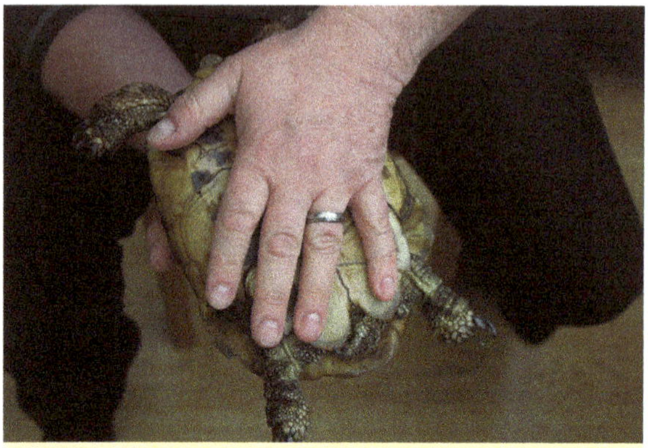

Figure 7.43
Inhibitory pressure, a recoil, or a toggle technique may be performed on a chelonian's carapace and plastron (although the latter requires less force to be used), resting the animal on the operator's lap if needed.

where quick movements are not only safe but also very effective. When performing a recoil, it is best to rest the animal on a hard stable surface (such as a table), whereas for a toggle the author finds it easier to rest the animal on his lap. When these approaches are performed on the plastron, less force should be administered than when applied to the carapace. It should be noted that these techniques addressed to a dysfunctional scute will often also have a direct or indirect effect on the corresponding viscera. The head and neck can be gently worked through mild traction and articulatory induction of motion (Fig. 7.44), although it is likely they will be retracted within a few seconds of being contacted. The treatment must, therefore, be quick, precise, and effective. In addition, the occiput can be held with the index fingers while the middle fingers slide into the cranial opening of the shell to approach the base of the neck. Gentle pumping maneuvers can then be applied to the neck and thoracic "inlet." This is particularly valuable in species like the European pond turtle (*Emys orbicularis*), which have a lymphatic ring around the base of the neck that anastomoses with both thoracic ducts (Ottaviani and Tazzi 1977). With turtles the author has found it best to work with the patient in the water, where each movement produced from the animal or applied by the operator will be more natural and smooth, with better results

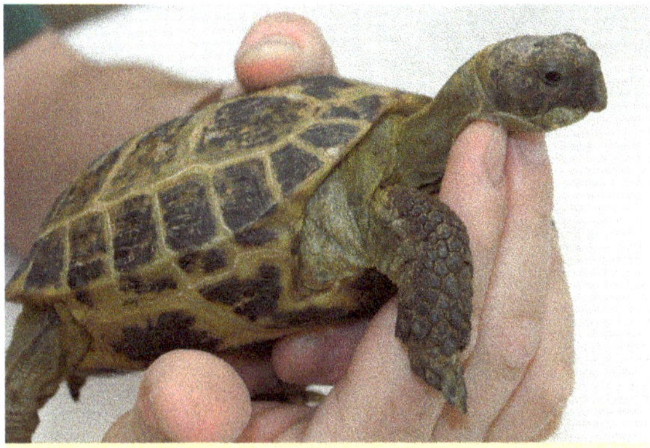

Figure 7.44
Gentle traction can be provided using a two digit contact while holding the animal from both sides just behind the forelimbs.

and less stress for the reptile. All four extremities can be treated by traction and articulation, as can the tail (Fig. 7.45A-C). The focus of the traction can also be moved centrally to have an effect on the anatomically related viscera. In tortoises, the serratus muscle inserts onto the coracoid in the forelimbs while the obliquus abdominis inserts on the skin of the hind limb. Both of these muscles originate from the shell and play a major role in active inspiration by creating negative pressure during limb movement resulting in lung expansion (Pough et al. 2002) (Fig. 7.46). By restoring mobility in the limbs, therefore, the pulmonary function can be optimized, with a consequent impact on blood oxygenation levels and fluid dynamics. Using the same principle, the tail can be used as a lever to approach the proctodeum, urodeum, and urinary bladder.

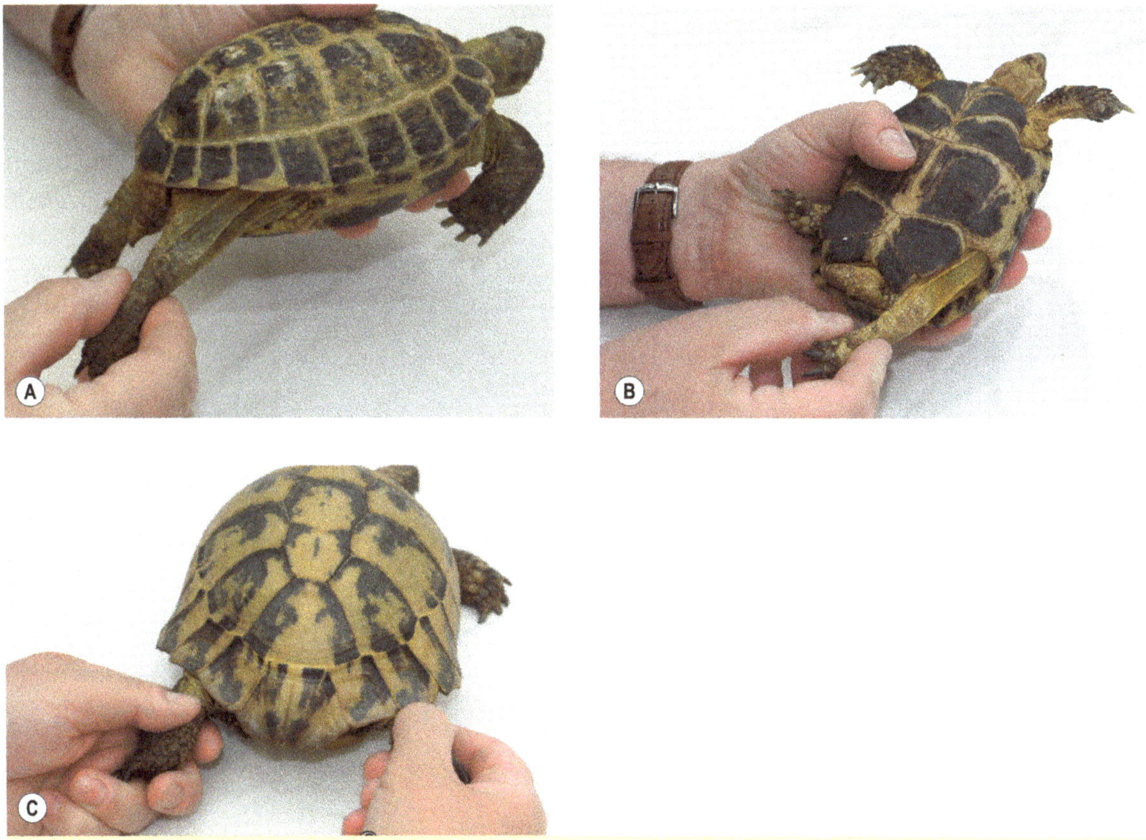

Figure 7.45
Traction and articulation can be applied on each limb with the animal held ventrally (A) or dorsally (B). A release by traction can also be achieved on both limbs simultaneously (C).

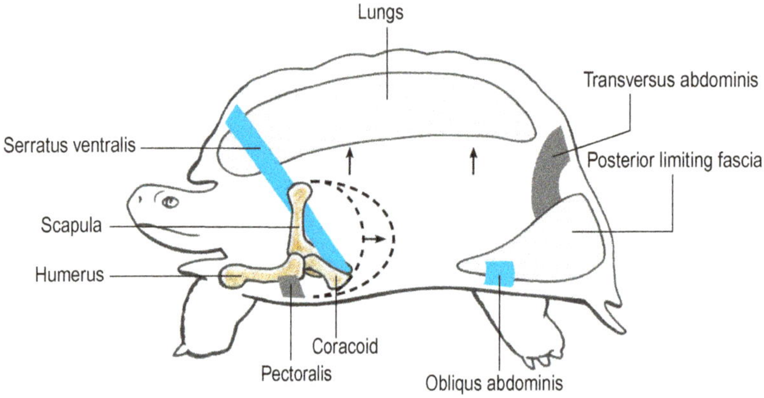

Figure 7.46
Lateral view of a tortoise showing the muscles of respiration. *Blue* shows the position of the muscles of inspiration and *gray* indicates the position of the muscles of expiration.

Management

The health of captive reptiles is intrinsically linked to suitable husbandry practices (Divers 1996). The eight "H"s of husbandry (heat, humidity, hygiene, healthy appetite, habitat, hide, handling, and health) should be regularly checked and appropriately provided by the owner.

- Reptiles should be housed at temperatures similar to field conditions. As a general rule, the best temperature variation is the range that allows the reptile to choose its thermal environment - and adequately thermoregulate - as well as achieve optimal metabolism. This varies with species.
- Ultraviolet light is essential for the synthesis of vitamin D_3 and calcium metabolism. It should be provided to species such as bearded dragons and eastern water dragons when they are kept indoors.
- Humidity requirements vary with species (40-80 percent). For example, the environment of an inland bearded dragon needs to be much drier than that of a green python. Regardless of the degree of humidity, however, vivaria should be adequately ventilated and furnished with a large water bowl for drinking and bathing.
- Good hygiene is dependent on proper disinfecting and cleaning practices and the use of an appropriate substrate. The latter will vary according to the needs of the species. For instance, newspaper is suitable for arboreal species, whereas bearded dragons thrive on a mix of substrates and also suitable rocks or logs for basking. Gravid females need a suitable substrate for digging and ovipositing. Good hygiene also implies provision of optimal water quality for captive turtles. Water should be tested and, if necessary, treated daily using a standard aquarium kit to measure pH, ammonia, and nitrite levels.
- Usually reptiles should be fed no more than 20 percent of their body weight at a time (Cannon and Johnson 2015). Small species and young lizards need to eat daily whereas most adults are usually fed every two to three days and hatchlings every four to five days, with the feeding area being in a separate container. An adult python may be fed every one to two weeks (never in the same vivarium as other snakes), and preferably with prefrozen prey to limit parasitism and preserve animal welfare. Failure to eat may occur if vision is inhibited due to the spectacles not being shed. This can occur if the vivarium has low humidity. Increasing the humidity and

providing rocks or logs for the snake to rub against will prevent this problem.

- Cage furnishings and shelter should be adjusted for the species. For instance, it is good practice to provide places in the vivaria for reptiles to hide. Poorly furnished enclosures lead to stress-related behavior and may even lead to reptiles becoming unable to thermoregulate as they choose the coolest (rather than the warmer) area of the vivarium in which to hide.
- Ensure that handling is regular and appropriate for the species. This allows the animal to get to know and bond with its owner, and also allows the owner to assess the animal's body and its mental condition.
- If all of the above are in order then you should have a healthy, contented animal.

Suboptimal temperatures, excessive humidity, inappropriate substrate or poor hygiene may predispose reptiles to various kinds of disease, such as skin infections and stomatitis. In contrast, good husbandry is a valid support for osteopathic intervention as well as for patient health and quality of life.

Chapter 7

Case study 7.1

Bearded dragon (Pogona vitticeps)

Signalment

The patient was an 18-month-old, male bearded dragon.

History

In October 2014 the patient, who was kept in captivity, presented for veterinary consultation with lethargy and loss of appetite. The history revealed a progressive reduction in growth rate, vitality, and appetite in the previous two months, although the animal stood out as strong and energetic compared with other pogonae raised in the past by the same owner. Good environmental and nutritional management was provided, except that the dragon was not sharing the terrarium with another reptile.

Veterinary evaluation

On palpation the abdomen was globose, and there was a dilated lower intestinal tract (subsequently confirmed by X-ray investigation). Fecal examination revealed excessive numbers of oxyurids (nematodes).

Differential diagnosis

Constipation caused by parasites or ingestion of substrate or of idiopathic etiology.

Medical intervention

Treatment was with vegetable oil via the esophagus and rectum, administered through a probe. Daily baths in warm water were also provided to rehydrate the animal and stimulate intestinal peristalsis. The oxyurid infestation was treated with 50 mg/kg of febendazole (Panacur® 2.5 percent) for three consecutive days.

Initial results

The reptile began defecating and eating after three days of treatment.

Follow-up

During the following months, the animal presented with recurrent episodes of constipation and reoccurrence of lethargy and lack of appetite. Subsequent fecal examination was normal (to February 2015). The clinical evaluation found an absence of any abdominal palpatory findings of constipation. Instead, there was a reluctance to bear weight on the left hind limb, which was noticeable at rest and during movement. This was associated with a general loss of muscle mass in the left hind thigh. The knee was held in extension during most phases of the gait (Fig. 7.47). According to the owner, this

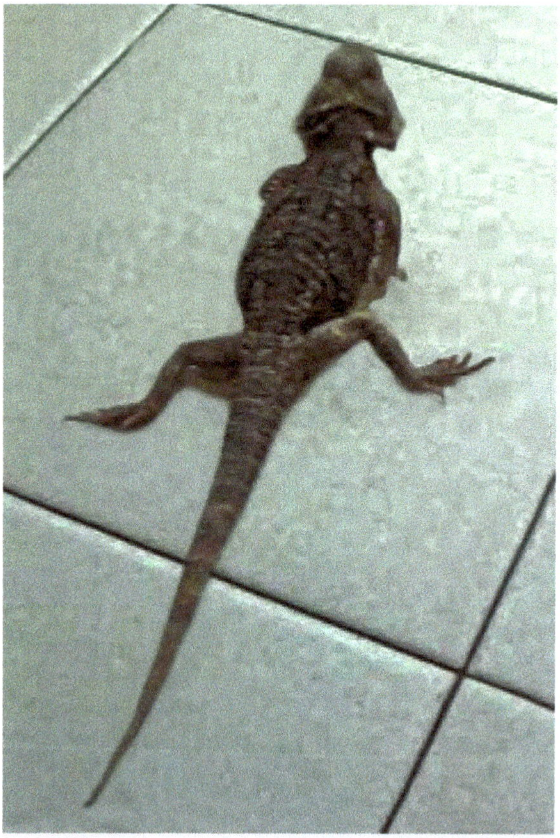

Figure 7.47
Dysfunction of the left posterior limb. The dragon kept the left stifle in extension both when standing and when moving. There was a general loss of muscle mass in the same thigh. The animal was unable to raise his weight on the hind limbs.

mechanical limitation of the limb was also preventing the animal from copulating, although it had made several attempts to rise on the hind limbs. Nothing abnormal was found on X-ray investigation (Fig. 7.48). The animal was then referred for an osteopathic assessment.

Osteopathic evaluation

A general reduction in vitality was found in most involuntary rhythms of the dragon, together with a palpable compression of the cranial base and a remarkable intraosseous strain of the left femur. In addition, the lumbar spine showed a general reduction in mobility associated with chronic changes in the surrounding soft tissues. Finally, areas of the colon were held in a hypertonic state of contraction in both the pelvic and lower abdominal regions.

Osteopathic intervention

The reptile underwent a weekly osteopathic manipulation for one month. Initially, treatment included a release of the cranial base and of the femoral intraosseous strain through cranial and fluidic approaches respectively. This was intended to balance and support the dragon's involuntary rhythms. Secondly, a series of articulatory and fascial techniques (Fig. 7.49) were applied to the spine and posterior limbs to enhance the arterial supply and venous drainage in the areas and to restore mobility where it was compromised. Finally, specific mobilization of abdominal and pelvic viscera was applied with an emphasis on the dysfunctional regions of the colon.

Follow-up

Fifteen days after the first treatment, the veterinary assessment was summarized as: "Animal awake, aware, in good general health, with a good ability to explore the surrounding environment and to follow his normal behavior. He uses the limbs equally and freely both when standing and in movement, showing balanced weight-bearing on all four limbs" (Fig. 7.50).

Twenty days after the third treatment, the left hind limb showed the same muscular mass as that of the contralateral limb. The owner reported a good appetite and a general increase in the reptile's weight and growth, which had been constantly within normal values for the

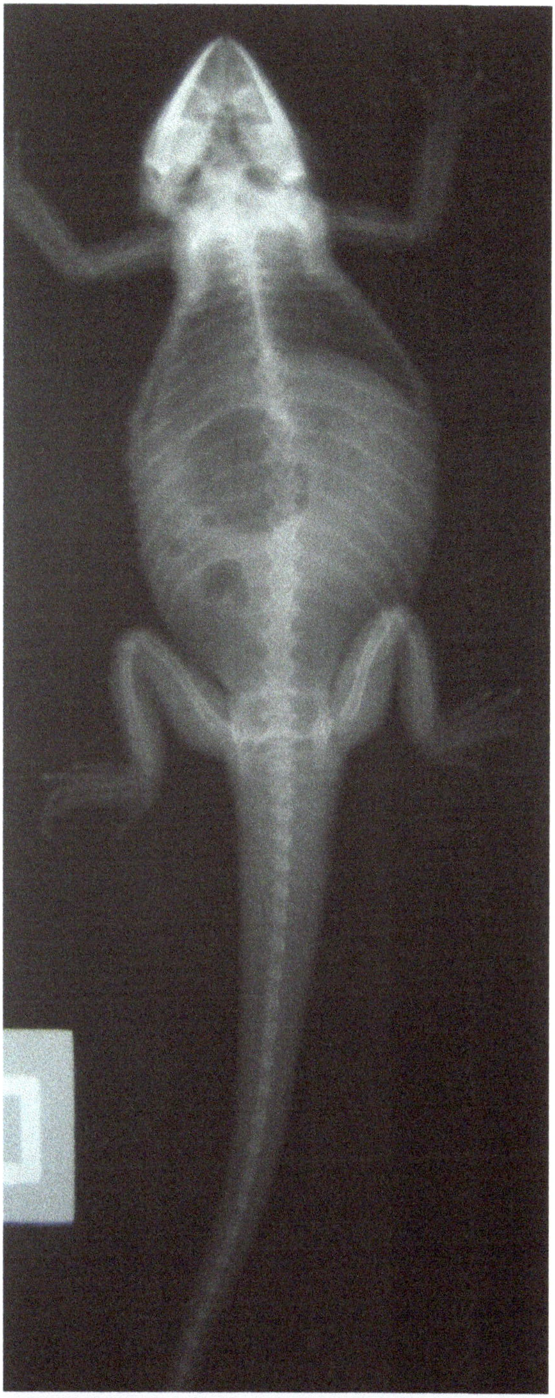

Figure 7.48
X-ray imaging. The dorsoventral radiograph shows normal bone mineralization and an absence of skeletal or gastrointestinal abnormalities.

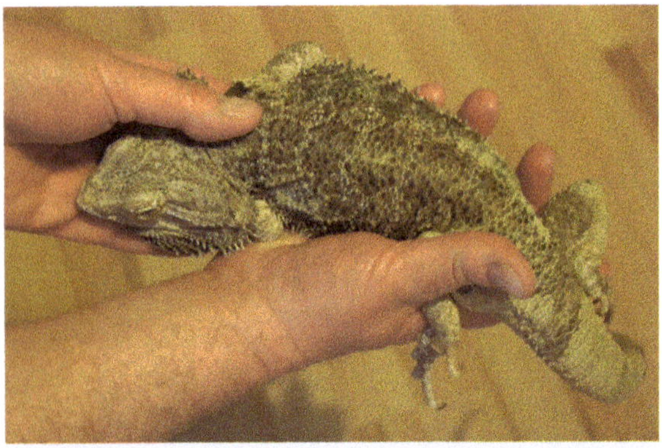

Figure 7.49
An articulatory and fascial approach to the spine. The reptile is held with a cranial and pelvic hold which will eventually engage the forelimbs and hind limbs respectively as levers during the technique. This hold can either be used to articulate the spine at different levels or to release myofascial dysfunctions along the trunk.

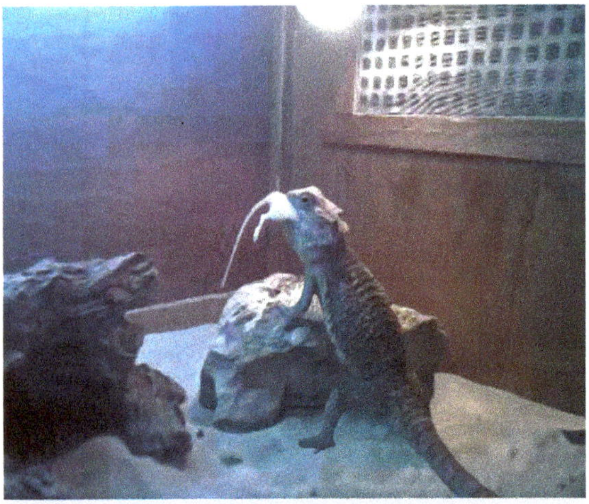

Figure 7.50
Restoration of function. Following osteopathic treatment, the dragon returned to its normal function and vitality, eating and growing appropriately, and regaining balanced hind limb mobility. This allowed the animal to feed and to copulate.

previous two months. Furthermore, the sexual activity of the dragon returned to normal, thanks to the restored function of the back limbs, resulting in the production of eggs by the female dragon and the birth of six baby dragons.

Conclusions

Traditional medicine and complementary medicine have their own strengths and limitations. An integrated treatment involving both approaches may offer a broader view in the evaluation of the patient as well as a more global and effective treatment

Case study 7.2

Hermann's tortoise (*Testudo hermanni*)

This case presented in the Drasi wildlife rehabilitation center in Thessaloniki, Greece.

Signalment

The patient was an adult female Hermann's tortoise.

History

A wild Hermann's tortoise presented with soft tissue trauma to the legs and head.

Veterinary evaluation

Fracture of the mandible and soft tissue laceration of the face and the left tibia.

Medical intervention

Treatment included cleaning and sterilizing the tibial laceration. Subcutaneous fluid was administered for 15 days. Antibiotics were given for seven days (enrofloxacin 10 mg/kg subcutaneously). The patient was unable to eat, and so nutritional support was given by stomach tube.

Follow-up

The lacerated soft tissue and the mandible started to heal. Walking was limited. The tortoise was referred to the osteopath to improve limb function.

Osteopathic examination

Examination revealed limited walking, soft tissue laceration, and hypertonic connective tissues of the left tibia and mandible. There was reduced extension and abduction of the left hip and reduced extension of the left knee.

Osteopathic treatment

Osteopathic manipulation was performed for a few minutes every two weeks on three consecutive occasions. Treatment included gentle articulation (Figs 7.51 and 7.52) and functional techniques in order to reduce fascial and articular restrictions, improve drainage, and improve movement of the injured limb and cervical spine.

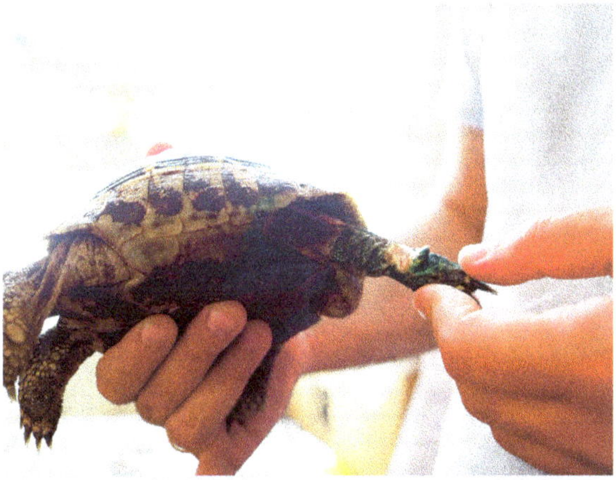

Figure 7.51
Articulation of the hip, stifle, and tarsal joints into extension.

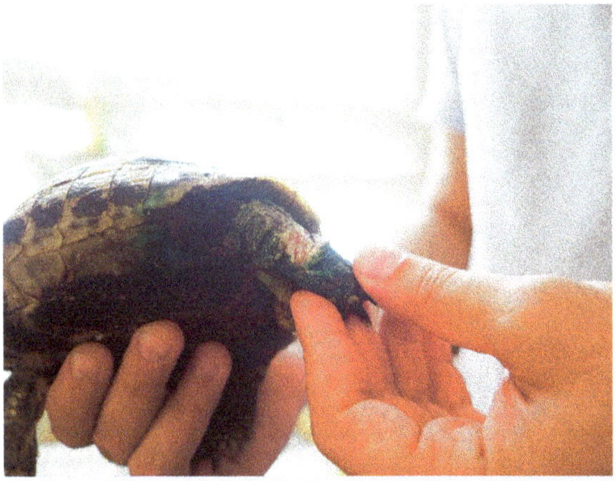

Figure 7.52
Articulation of the stifle and tarsal joints into flexion.

Initial results

Hip and knee movements increased to full range of motion after the first treatment.

Follow-up examination

Osteopathic examination in the second week revealed improved healing of the soft tissue lacerations and walking. A degree of hip restriction had again developed in the left limb. In the fourth week, osteopathic assessment revealed normal range of movement in the hips and knees. Release to the wild had to be postponed until the mandible was functional and the tortoise was able to feed herself.

Conclusions

Soft tissue restrictions can remain after trauma limiting joint mobility, walking and optimal vascular drainage of a limb. In this case osteopathic manipulation together with proper husbandry was successful in returning full mobility and function to the hind limb.

References

Antwis RE, Browne RK (2009) Ultraviolet radiation and vitamin D_3 in amphibian health, behaviour, diet and conservation. Comparative Biochemistry and Physiology Part A: Molecular and Integrative Physiology. October; 154 (2) 184–190.

Cannon M, Johnson R (2015) Handling and Nursing Reptiles (What's Normal & What's Not). Available: www.ava.com.au/sites/default/files/Handling%20and%20Nursing%20Reptiles_MCannon.pdf [July 15, 2018].

Divers S (1996) Basic reptile husbandry, history taking and clinical examination. Practice. February; 18 (2) 51–65.

Espinoza RE, Tracy CR (1997) Thermal biology, metabolism and hibernation. In: Ackermann L (ed.) The Biology, Husbandry and Healthcare of Reptiles. Volume 1: The Biology of Reptiles. TFH Publications Inc. pp. 149–184.

Evans HE (1986) Reptiles – Introduction and anatomy. In: Fowler ME (ed.) Zoo and Wild Animal Medicine. 2nd edn. Saunders, pp. 108–132.

Firth BJ, Turner JS (1982) Sensory, neural and hormonal aspects of thermoregulation. In: Gans C, Pough FH (eds.)

Biology of the Reptilia, Volume 12. London: Academic Press, pp. 213–259.

Fitzgerald K, Vera R (2006) Spinal osteopathy. In: Mader DR (ed.) Reptile Medicine and Surgery. 2nd edn. St. Louis, MO: Saunders Elsevier, pp. 906–912.

Glonek T, Sergueef N, Nelson KE (2005) Physiological rhythms/oscillations. In: Chila A (ed.) Foundations of Osteopathic Medicine. 3rd edn. Philadelphia, PA: Lippincott Williams & Wilkins, pp. 162–190.

Hoffstetter R, Gasc JP (1970) Vertebrae and ribs of modern reptiles. In: Gans C (ed.) Biology of the Reptilia, Volume 1. London: Academic Press, pp. 201–302.

Jacobson ER (1993) Exotic pet medicine I. Snakes. Veterinary Clinics of North America: Small Animal Practice. November; 23 (6) 1179–1212.

Johnston P (2014) Homology of the jaw muscles in lizards and snakes-a solution from a comparative gnathostome approach. The Anatomical Record (Hoboken). March; 297 (3) 574–585.

Klaphake E (2010) A fresh look at metabolic bone disease in reptiles and amphibians. Veterinary Clinics of North America: Exotic Animal Practice. September; 13 (3) 375–392.

Mader DR (2006) Metabolic bone diseases. In Mader DR (ed.) Reptile Medicine and Surgery. St. Louis, MO: Saunders Elsevier, pp. 841–851.

McBride M, Hernandez-Divers SJ (2004) Nursing care of lizards. Veterinary Clinics of North America: Exotic Animal Practice. May; 7 (2) 375–396, vii.

Mitchell MA (2002) Diagnosis and management of reptile orthopedic injuries. Veterinary Clinics of North America: Exotic Animal Practice. January; 5 (1) 97–114.

Mitchell MA (2004) Snake care and husbandry. Veterinary Clinics of North America: Exotic Animal Practice. May; 7 (2) 421–446, vii–viii.

Moon PF, Hernandez Foerster SH (2001) Reptiles: aquatic turtles (Chelonians). In: Heard D, Caulkett N, Deem S et al. (eds.) Zoological Restraint and Anesthesia. Ithaca, NY: IVIS.

Nagashima H, Sugahara F, Takechi M et al. (2009) Evolution of the turtle body plan by the folding and creation of new muscle connections. Science. July; 325(5937) 193–196.

O'Malley B (ed.) (2005) Clinical anatomy and physiology of exotic species. Elsevier Saunders, pp. 17–39.

Ottaviani G, Tazzi A (1977) The lymphatic system. In: Gans C and Parsons T (eds.) Biology of the Reptilia, Volume 6. London: Academic Press, pp. 315–458.

Pincheira-Donoso D, Bauer AM, Meiri S, Uetz P (2013) Global taxonomic diversity of living reptiles. PLoS ONE. March; 8 (3) e59741.

Pough FH, Andrew RM, Cadle JE et al. (1998) Herpetology. Englewood Cliffs, NJ: Prentice Hall, pp. 137–172.

Pough FH, Janis CM, Heiser JB (2002) Vertebrate Life. 6th edn. Englewood Cliffs, NJ: Prentice Hall, pp. 294–341.

Raftery A (2011) Reptile orthopedic medicine and surgery. Journal of Exotic Pet Medicine. April; 20 (2) 107–116.

Solessio E, Engbretson GA (1999) Electroretinogram of the parietal eye of lizards: photoreceptor, glial, and lens cell contributions. Visual Neuroscience. September–October; 16 (5) 895–907.

Uetz P (2000) How many reptile species? Herpetology Review. 31 (1) 13–15.

Walker WF (1973) The locomotor apparatus of testudines. In: Gans C and Parsons T (eds.) Biology of the Reptilia, Volume 4. London: Academic Press, pp. 1–99.

Wappel SM, Schulte MS (2004) Turtle care and husbandry. Veterinary Clinics of North America: Exotic Animal Practice. May; 7 (2) 447–472, viii.

World Health Organization (WHO) (2010) Benchmarks for training in osteopathy. Geneva: World Health Organization, p. 12.

Further reading

Chinnadurai SK, DeVoe RS (2009) Selected infectious diseases of reptiles. Veterinary Clinics of North America: Exotic Animal Practice. 12 (3) 583–596.

Chitty J, Raftery A (2013) Chapter 20 Lameness. In: Essentials of Tortoise Medicine and Surgery. Wiley-Blackwell, pp. 225–228.

Educational Council on Osteopathic Principles (ECOP) (2011) Glossary of Osteopathic Terminology. Chevy Chase, MD: American Association of Colleges of Osteopathic Medicine (AACOM), p. 53.

Naylor AD (2013) Femoral head and neck excision arthroplasty in a leopard tortoise (Stigmochelys pardalis). Journal of Zoo and Wildlife Medicine. December; 44 (4) 982–989.

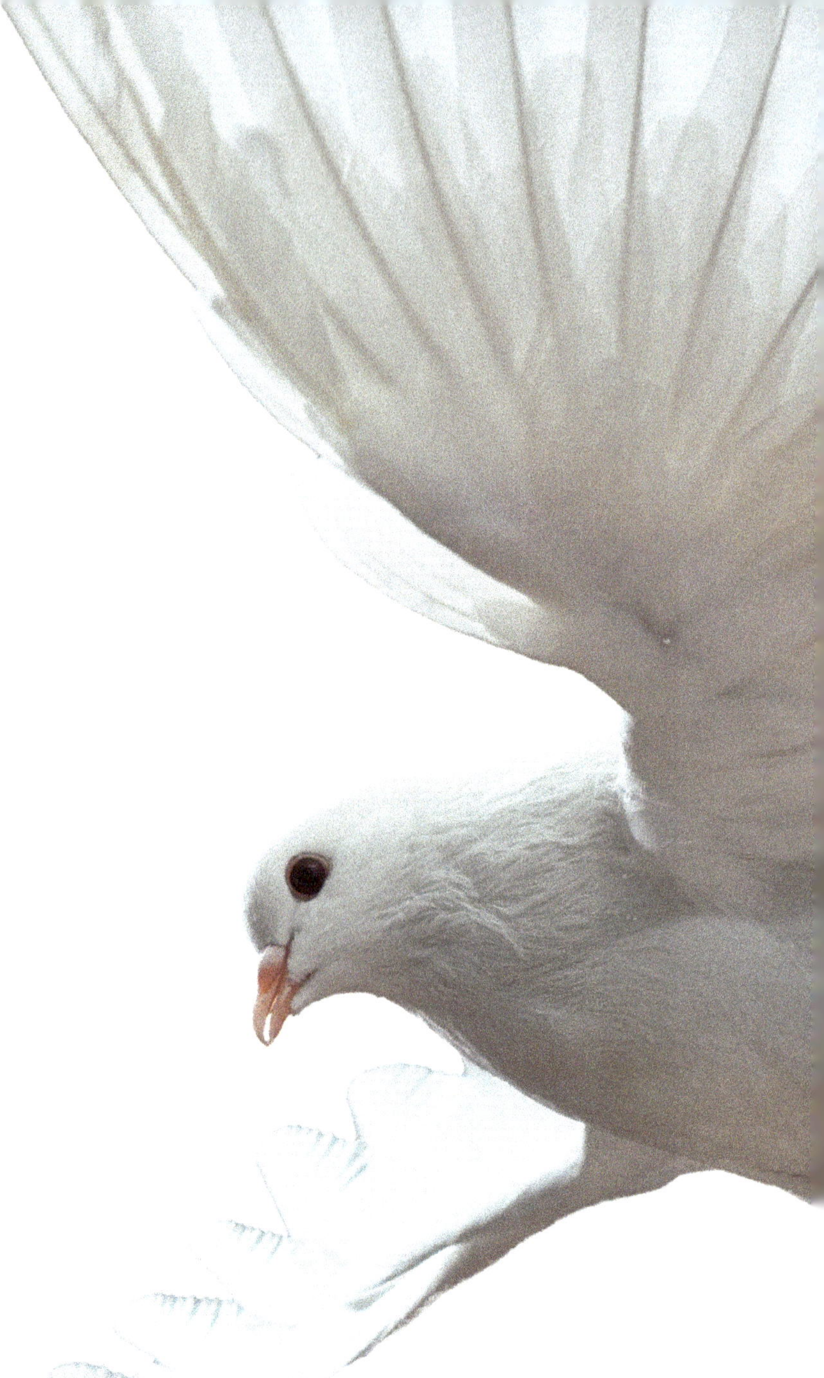

Chapter 8 BIRDS

Tony Nevin, Andrew Routh, Leonidas Christodoularis, Caroline Gould

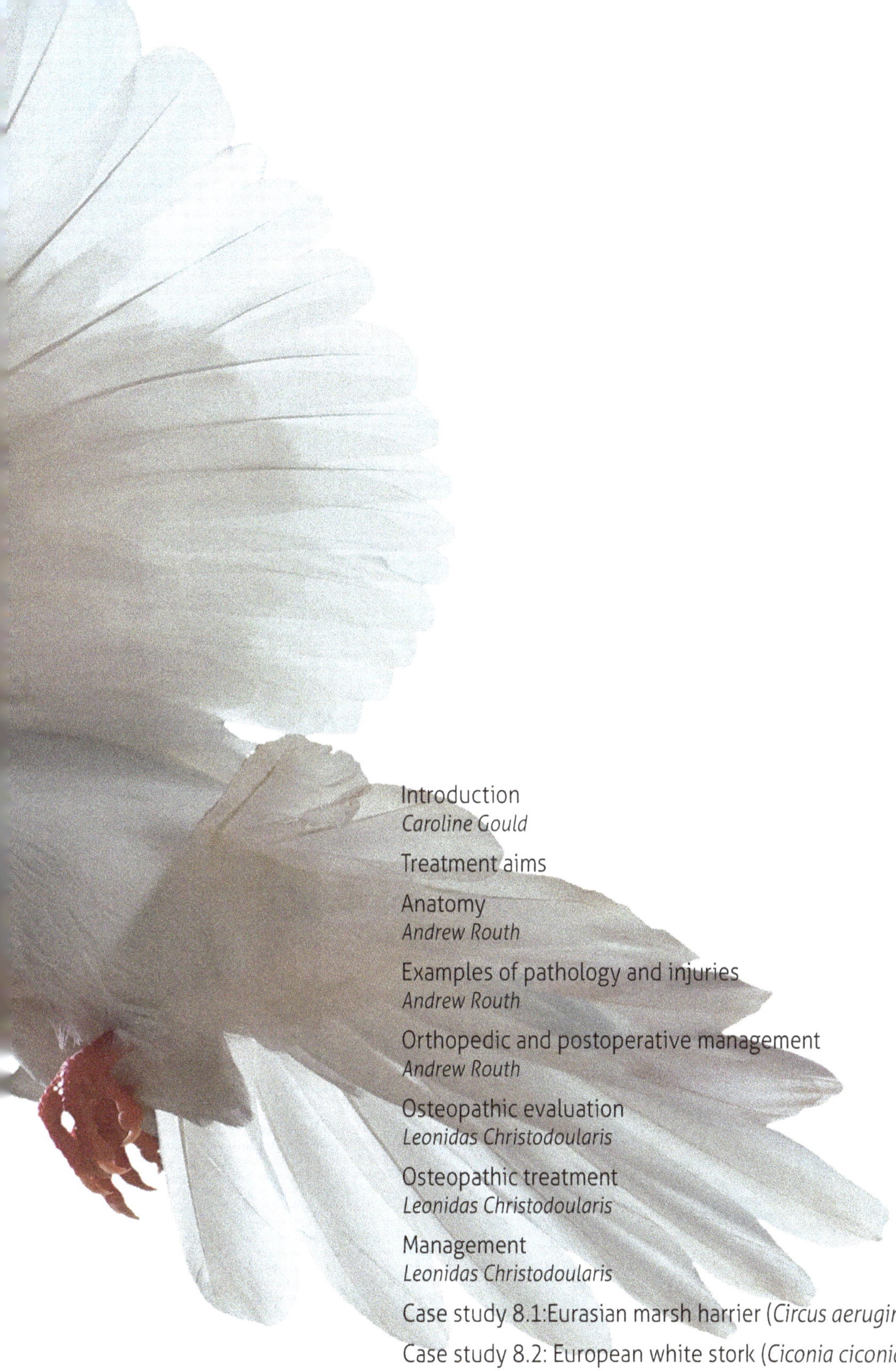

Birds

Chapter 8

Introduction

Applying osteopathic principles to the treatment of birds requires specific knowledge of avian anatomy and physiology in order to avoid catastrophic results. There is very little published material to help the osteopath, and that which does exist was written several years ago and was aimed very much at the wildlife rehabilitation community (Nevin 1999). Two papers were presented at the First International Congress on Animal Osteopathy (Christodoularis 2012; Nevin 2012). This chapter aims to introduce the concept of avian osteopathy and help reduce the possibility of future generations making the same mistakes that the authors inadvertently made in the earlier parts of their careers. The advice given in these pages needs to be taken seriously. Bird physiology allows very little margin for error. Osteopaths are renowned for wanting to be hands on. With avian patients they must practice patience. The most important factors to assess before treatment are the case history and observing the patient while it is calm and relaxed. By the time the hands are placed on the avian patient, the osteopath should have a treatment plan in his head, involving the minimum amount of handling needed to ensure a positive outcome.

Handling guidelines

There are many important differences in the avian structure and how it functions when compared with mammals. From a handling point of view, extreme delicacy needs to be used to avoid causing feather damage. Care also needs to be taken from a safety aspect with regard to birds' talons and beaks (Fig. 8.1).

Birds host some rather unpleasant parasites, which are often more frightening than harmful to the osteopath. The most bizarre of these are flat flies. They can move over your body and limbs so fast that getting them off you is not easy! Although blood feeders, flat flies will rarely bite you. However, some parasites can and do carry extremely dangerous infectious diseases and this must be taken into consideration.

Avian osteopathy is a challenging area in veterinary osteopathy. Birds generally have a higher rate of metabolism than mammals as well as some unique anatomical and physiological adaptations. All of these differences make it essential that treatment sessions are tailored to the higher metabolic rates, kept short, and the techniques are applied in such a way as to avoid trauma to any of the structures. This sounds obvious on paper, but can easily be overlooked in practice.

When being treated wild bird casualties rarely give any visible feedback that indicates pain or their general state. Some birds when stressed will gape their mouths (Fig. 8.2). Delicate palpation is vital to ascertain the patient's condition and any improvement that has taken place. Where possible it is also important to view any radiographs, looking especially for fracture

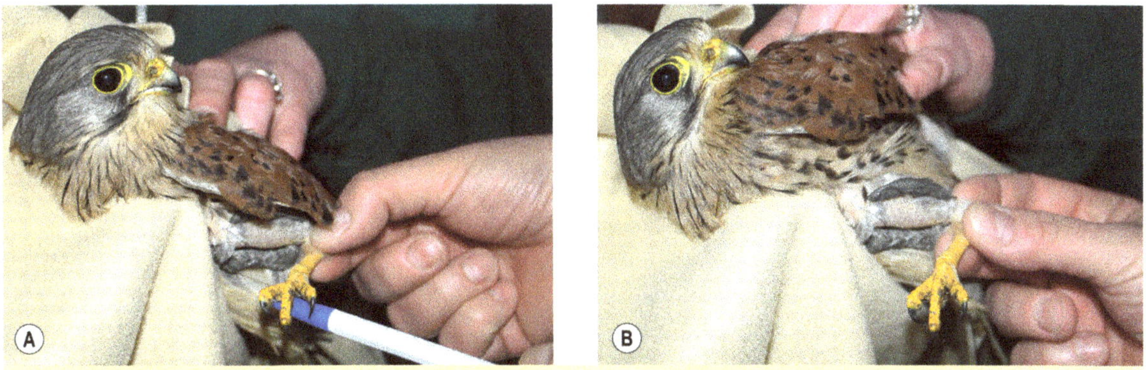

Figure 8.1
(A) Using a pen to avoid talons on a male kestrel (*Falco tinnunculus*) with external fixator to stabilize a tibial fracture. (B) With the leg secure, functional treatment can be administered safely.

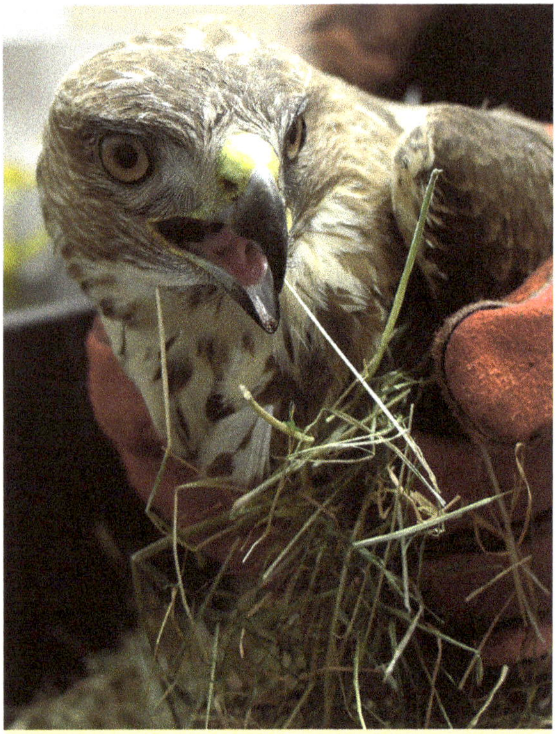

Figure 8.2
A buzzard showing signs of stress by mouth gaping during assessment.

sites as the location of these can have a massive impact on the prognosis for rehabilitation (see the section on Fractures under Orthopedic and postoperative management). Many wildlife hospitals now have CCTV fitted to aviaries, so in these situations it is possible to view the patient while it is unaware of your presence. A study, carried out at Gower Bird Hospital, Wales, UK, has shown that a wild bird will often react differently when it knows it is being watched (BWRC 2010). Buzzards (*Buteo buteo*) will try to behave as if they are 100 percent fit, whereas a red kite (*Milvus milvus*) will usually adopt a dead posture and throw itself onto its back. The first time the author (TN) experienced this was quite a shock.

Safety issues

Some wild species need particular knowledge when being handled. Some vultures (Accipitridae and Cathartidae) will regurgitate any food in their stomachs when handled. Fulmars (*Fulmarus*) will vomit food as a defense mechanism, whereas herons (*Ardea*) will strike at your eyes with their beaks if unrestrained. Some sea birds, such as gannets (*Morus*), have serrated beaks, which cut like a knife if they grab hold of you. Gannets also have internal nostrils (an adaptation that allows them to dive into open water at great speed), which must be remembered when handling in order to avoid suffocation. Most wild raptors are more likely to use their talons to defend themselves rather than their beaks, and there are clever ways of extricating your hands and fingers if this happens. These techniques are covered in the section on health and safety in avian rehabilitation later in the chapter. If your skin is pierced there is a high risk of infection setting in if untreated. It is essential therefore that you follow strict hygiene protocols if this happens.

Some species are very susceptible to the heat from the human hand. This is especially so with passerines. Their small size and high metabolic rate predisposes them to suffer heat stress when handled. This is another reason why osteopathic treatment time must be limited to an absolute minimum (Fig. 8.3).

Knowledge of different avian species is essential - not only of their basic habits but also what they really need in order to survive and thrive in the wild. Apart from the captive species that an osteopath will be asked to treat, the majority of avian cases will be wild casualties. Their problems will range from colliding with man-made structures such as stock fencing and glass windows to more violent trauma such as illegal shooting of raptors, which in certain parts of the world is an extremely common factor.

Health and safety in avian rehabilitation

The author (CG) of this section has been working in the treatment, care and rehabilitation of sick and injured wildlife for over 30 years, initially with no knowledge or experience whatsoever. The first few years were a huge learning curve, not only in how to capture a casualty, but how to keep it, what to feed it, how to treat any injuries, and how to prepare it for release back into the wild.

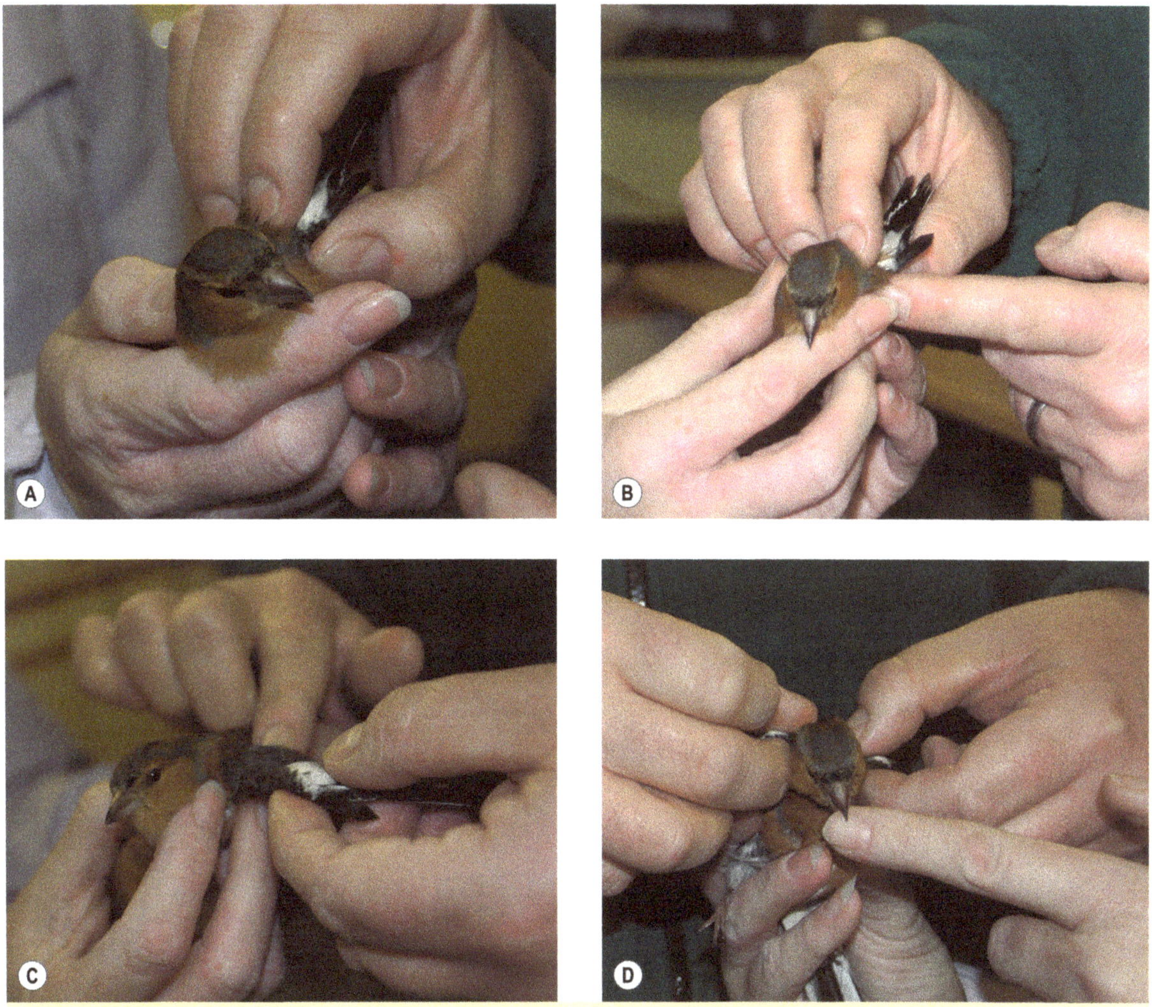

Figure 8.3
Male chaffinch (*Fringilla coelebs*). (A) Glenohumeral joint examination. (B) Glenohumeral joint articulation. (C) Functional treatment of the left wing. (D) Comparing glenohumeral ROM bilaterally after osteopathic treatment.

The author quickly learned that health and safety needed to be paramount. Her own health and safety had to come first, but she also had to consider other people who might be involved in, present at, or even travelling past a rescue situation. The well-being of the casualty itself, of course, must not be forgotten.

The handling of wildlife casualties, even though many are small and look harmless, is the first subject that needs highlighting (see Table 8.1). Learning the hard way, as the author did in the early days, is not recommended.

A harsh lesson involved an emaciated and very weak heron which was brought to Vale Wildlife Hospital by an RSPCA inspector. It was the first heron that the author had ever dealt with and she had no knowledge of how they reacted to being handled or what their method of defense was. The bird was so weak that it offered no resistance to being handled and appeared

Table 8.1 Health and safety precautions for the handling of avian patients			
Species or type of bird	**Capture guidelines**	**Methods of transportation**	**Defenses to be aware of**
Small or garden birds	Small net Towel or tea towel	Covered box with air holes Pillowcase, cloth bank bag	No major risks
Medium-sized birds (corvids, pigeons, etc.)	Suitable net Towel or tea towel Wear gloves for corvids	Covered box or pet carrier with air holes Pillowcase	Beaks and feet – corvids in particular Wings – mainly wood pigeons
Seabirds (gulls, cormorants, gannets, etc.)	Large net Blanket or large towel Restrain head and beak**	Covered box or pet carrier with air holes Vari Kennel® or similar	Strong beaks Gannets stab at face – wear goggles Restrain head
Other water birds (ducks, geese, swans, herons, etc.)	Large net Swan hook Large towel or blanket Immobilize head and wings	Suitable sized Vari Kennel® Large towel or blanket Swan bag (swans and geese) Deep box (herons)	Beaks (herons, grebes, etc.) Wings (swans and geese) Beware of protective group members (swans in particular) Herons stab at face – wear goggles
Birds of prey	Suitable net Towel or blanket Restrain legs and wings Wear gloves	Covered box or pet carrier with air holes	Strong talons and in particular beaks

**Note: the beaks of gannets should not be held shut for long periods as they have no external nostrils and therefore risk suffocation.

hardly to have the strength to hold its head up. As the author lifted it up to examine it, she was struck in the face with the dagger-like beak at lightning speed. Blood started running down her cheek from a puncture wound about one centimetre from her eye. Always wear goggles when handling birds such as herons, cormorants, gannets, or any other mainly fish-eating birds. You may look ridiculous, but you only have one pair of eyes and you do not want to lose one. You need to protect your eyes at all times - renowned wildlife photographer Eric Hosking lost an eye when a tawny owl flew at him and a talon pierced his eye.

Consideration must also be given to the health and safety of casualties when they are being captured and transported. Ensure that appropriate aids are used to catch them without causing further injury and that suitable carrying cages are used for each species.

When handling any bird care must be taken to restrain it safely (Fig. 8.4).

Should an osteopath be unfortunate and become impaled by a raptor's talons there is a simple method to extricate oneself. A sudden extension of the raptor's hind limb(s) will create an involuntary extension to the digit joints and their associated talons. Care must be taken to ensure that the impaled part of the osteopath

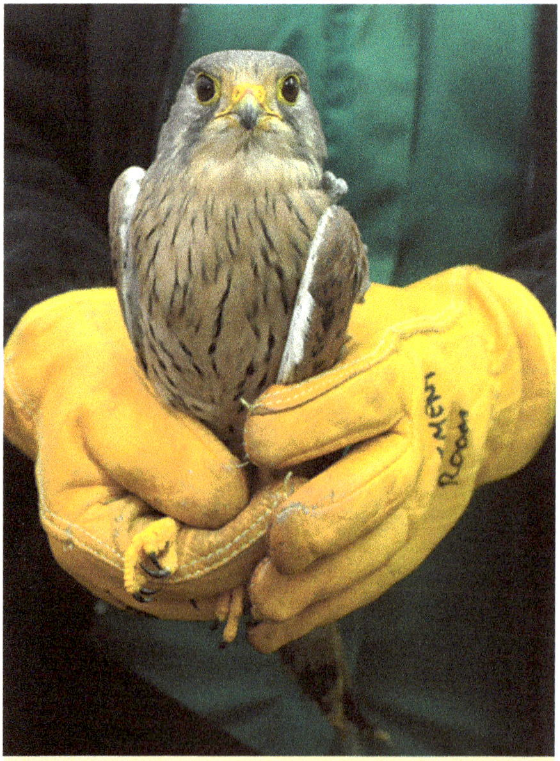

Figure 8.4
Male kestrel (*Falco tinnunculus*) with external fixation to the left wing, showing the safe way to hold and restrain.

is moved swiftly away from the patient, rather than the patient lifted off the osteopath. The latter will create a negative situation as the bird is likely to increase the flexion and grip on the osteopath. Clear communication is required if the raptor is held by a second operator.

- **Note: the beaks of gannets should not be held shut for long periods as they have no external nostrils and therefore risk suffocation.
- A suitable, nonslip floor covering such as towelling or AstroTurf® should always be used to line carriers.
- Never use mesh cat baskets or similar for transporting birds due to the risk of feather damage.
- There is a potential risk from zoonotic diseases and infections when handling *any* wildlife.

Treatment aims

Certain species have particular requirements for their lifestyle which must be met if treatment is to be successful. Raptors in particular require the ability to fly with enough agility to catch living prey. This is an area where the osteopath's skills are tested to the maximum. Another testing problem is with the long-distance migratory species where a minor disability becomes a matter of life and death. The ability to work closely with wildlife veterinary surgeons can often make all the difference with what are often endangered species. This is where osteopathy really takes on a whole new level of importance (Figs 8.5–8.9).

In the majority of cases the osteopath will assess and treat an avian patient while it is fully conscious, however, there will be occasions where treatment is best carried out under general anesthetic. It is at this point that a major difference presents itself when compared to treating any mammal patient, humans included. Birds do not have a diaphragm. Their respiratory system is very different in its makeup and physiological function when compared to humans. The osteopath must therefore remember that an anesthetized bird will need much more specialist monitoring than any mammal patient. This is yet another reason why the osteopath should stick to the four Fs rule (see below) and only spend the absolute minimum time required to assess and treat during any one session.

Find the problem

Feel the problem

Fix the problem

Free the patient

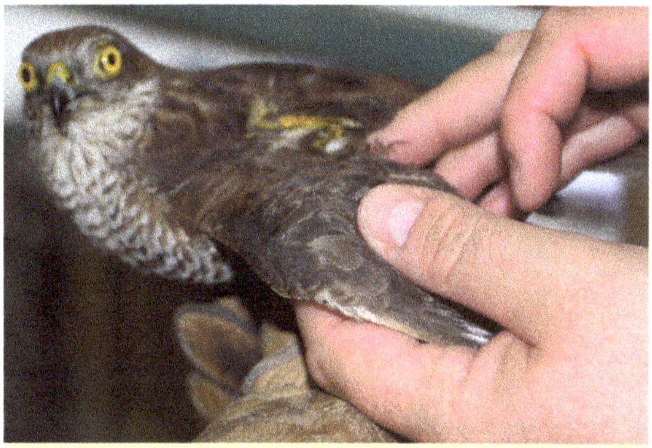

Figure 8.5
Assessing joint condition in the left wing of an injured sparrow hawk (*Accipiter nisus*).

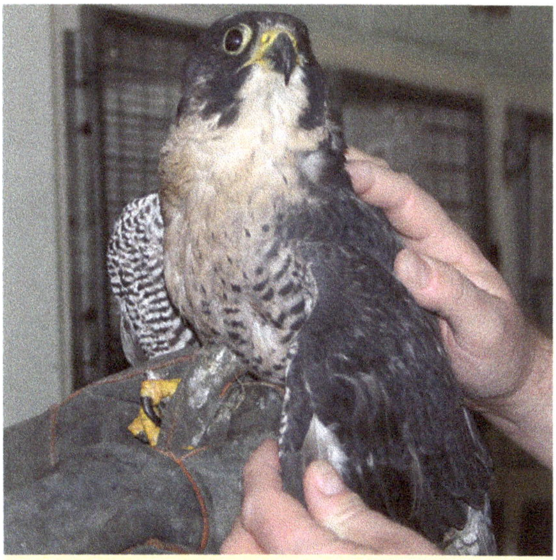

Figure 8.6
Testing joint mobility and motility through the left wing of a peregrine falcon (*Falco peregrinus*).

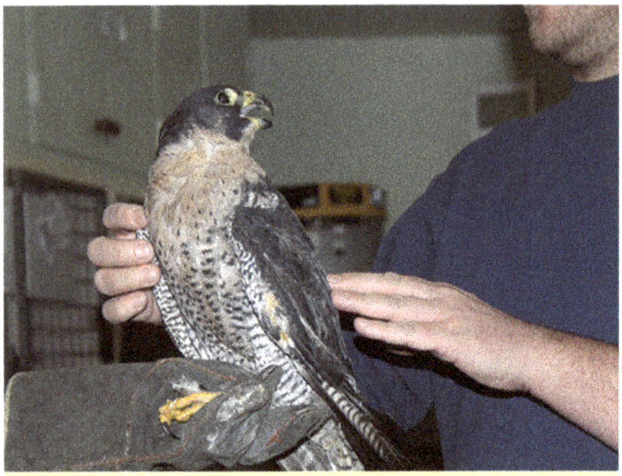

Figure 8.7
Checking the alertness of a peregrine falcon during initial palpation.

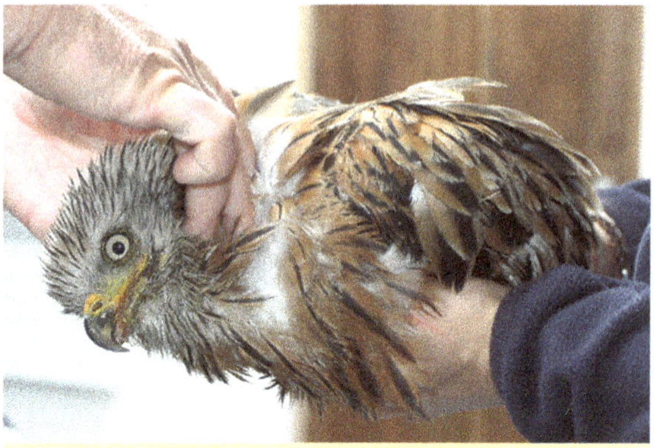

Figure 8.9
Assessing joint mobility in the cervical spine of a red kite (*Milvus milvus*).

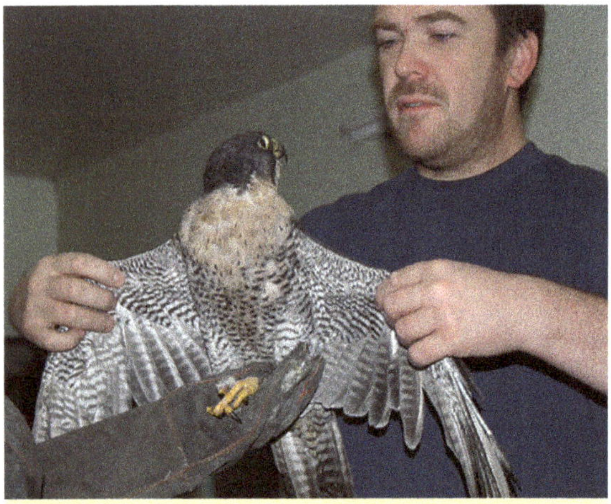

Figure 8.8
Examining wing articulation bilaterally on a peregrine falcon.

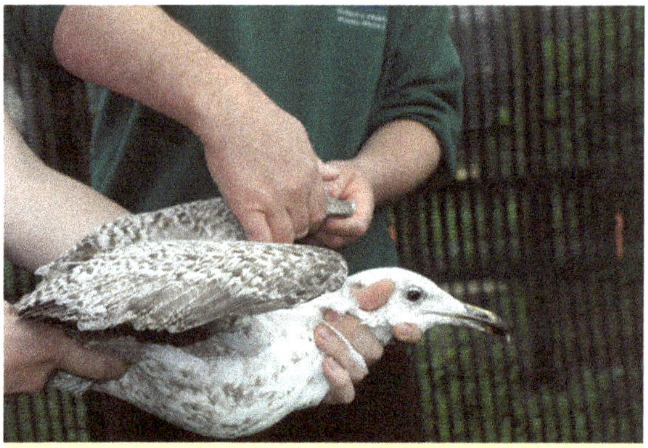

Figure 8.10
Restraint method allowing safe osteopathic examination of a juvenile lesser black-backed gull (*Larus fuscus*).

It is also worth noting at this point that when handling a bird that is trying to peck you on no account cover the nostrils on the dorsal aspect of the upper bill while restraining it. (Fig. 8.10). This may sound obvious, but you would be amazed how easily it can be done, especially if surgical tape is used to keep the beak closed. Remember not to tape gannets' bills shut, due to their internal nostrils, as mentioned earlier.

As with all nervous species it is important that noise and sudden movements, along with bright lights, are kept to a minimum. Careful, secure handling, along with a well-thought-out treatment plan - involving the shortest possible hands-on time for treatment to be achieved - are essential.

Captive birds, whether ornamental or those used in falconry, are usually easier to handle, except for parrots. Parrots will often bond with a single person and can be rather aggressive toward other people. They can be very adept at luring you to within striking distance by imitating human speech and presenting themselves as if they wish you to stroke them, and then they will peck you!

Anatomy

Avian anatomy and physiology differs in many important aspects from the mammal. While many of the adaptations observed derive from the ability of birds to fly, some are common to both volant and nonvolant species. The differences between birds and mammals have to be considered not only for the treatment of any conditions, but also in the way in which a bird is approached, handled, and restrained. Some adaptations will determine that the avian patient requires a fundamentally different approach. These essential changes in management strategies are not only for mutual safety but also to ensure that any treatments do not leave short- or long-term residual damage. It is essential to consider the health and safety of the avian patient and any workers or handlers in the approach to avian physical restraint and manipulations.

Metabolic rate

Firstly, all birds have an elevated metabolic rate when compared with mammals, particularly the passerines (perching birds). A benefit of this can be that healing can take place more quickly than in a mammal of a similar weight. However, diseases and physiological catastrophes also progress more rapidly. For the prescribing veterinary surgeon, any drugs used may need elevated doses to achieve therapeutic levels. This can be achieved by increases in dose rate, dose frequency, or a combination of both.

Respiratory system

All birds lack a diaphragm. They rely on excursions of the rib cage to move air through their respiratory system. The respiratory system itself differs from the mammalian system, having relatively fixed lungs attached to the dorsal thorax (rib cage). In addition, there are a series of membranous air sacs in the thorax and abdomen. (The air sacs also extend into several bones and this varies between species.) Though often compared to a series of bellows, the air sacs similarly rely on movement of the body wall to move air to and fro through the respiratory system. Unlike the lungs, which are highly efficient at gas exchange, the air sacs have no capacity for gas perfusion (Fig. 8.11).

It must be appreciated that any restraint that prevents normal thoracic movement can lead to asphyxiation and death. Bird deaths that occur during mishandling and restraint are often wrongly attributed to "cardiac arrest." Almost invariably these will have been due to respiratory compromise. Furthermore, periods of restraint in an abnormal posture, in particular dorsal recumbency, can lead to the viscera compressing the air sacs and a resultant reduced respiratory tidal flow.

Feathers and the integument

All birds, whether they fly or not, have feathers. Feathers differ in structure and function between species and on different areas of birds. At a simplistic level, the elongated wing feathers are designed to enable flight and the feathers of the body to retain heat. Many species carry additional feathers that play a role in courtship and display. In sexually dimorphic species it is the males that often have the more spectacular plumage.

The function of all feathers is maintained by the integrity of their macro- and microanatomy. All of this can be adversely affected by contamination, be it of spilt crude oil or topical preparations applied for veterinary reasons. The secretions of the preen gland do not per se render the feathers waterproof but enhance feather pliability and extend the life of a feather.

If handled inappropriately then feathers will become damaged or broken. As feathers are moulted to a set pattern this damage will have consequences through to the next moult. This could be up to 12 months away. Conversely feathers that are plucked, intentionally or inadvertently, will regrow over a period of weeks. (Plucking of feathers to initiate regrowth may be seen as an option, but any plucking should be considered as being a painful procedure, especially so for the primary [distal or flight] feathers of the wing. These have physical attachments to the periosteum).

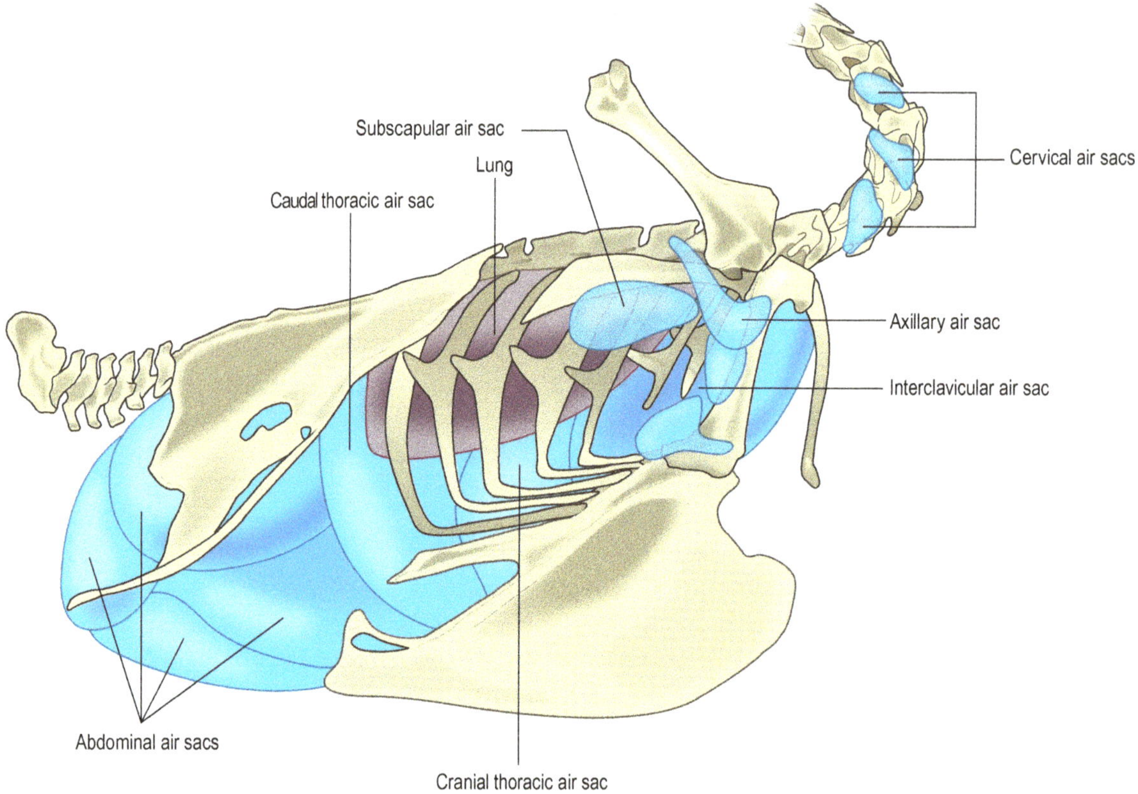

Figure 8.11
The air sacs of a bird.

There are featherless tracts of skin, known as the apteria. These are perfectly normal and lie between the feathered areas or pterylae. The apteria present potentially suitable areas for direct manipulation of the bird without feather involvement or compromise. However, it will be apparent on inspection of the apteria that the skin of the bird is relatively thin and poorly attached to the subcutaneous tissues. The delicate nature of the skin makes it very susceptible to iatrogenic physical damage. Pulling or shearing forces will result in tears to the skin.

The integument changes markedly, however, when one looks at the nonfeathered skin of the distal legs and feet. The epidermis is much thickened and scaled and is known as the podotheca. It is much less pliable and less mobile relative to the underlying structures.

Some species, primarily swimming species, have lateral projections to the epidermis, with this adaptation being at its most extreme in the waterfowl where there is complete interdigital webbing. These adaptations result in a more pliable epidermis that is more susceptible to damage, in particular if substrate is unsuitable and opportunities to swim are reduced.

The skeleton

The avian skeleton differs in a number of aspects from the mammalian skeleton (Figs 8.12 and 8.13).

Growth

Bone growth, most obviously of the long limb bones, differs in that they grow through a process of ossification of terminal plates of cartilage, both distally and

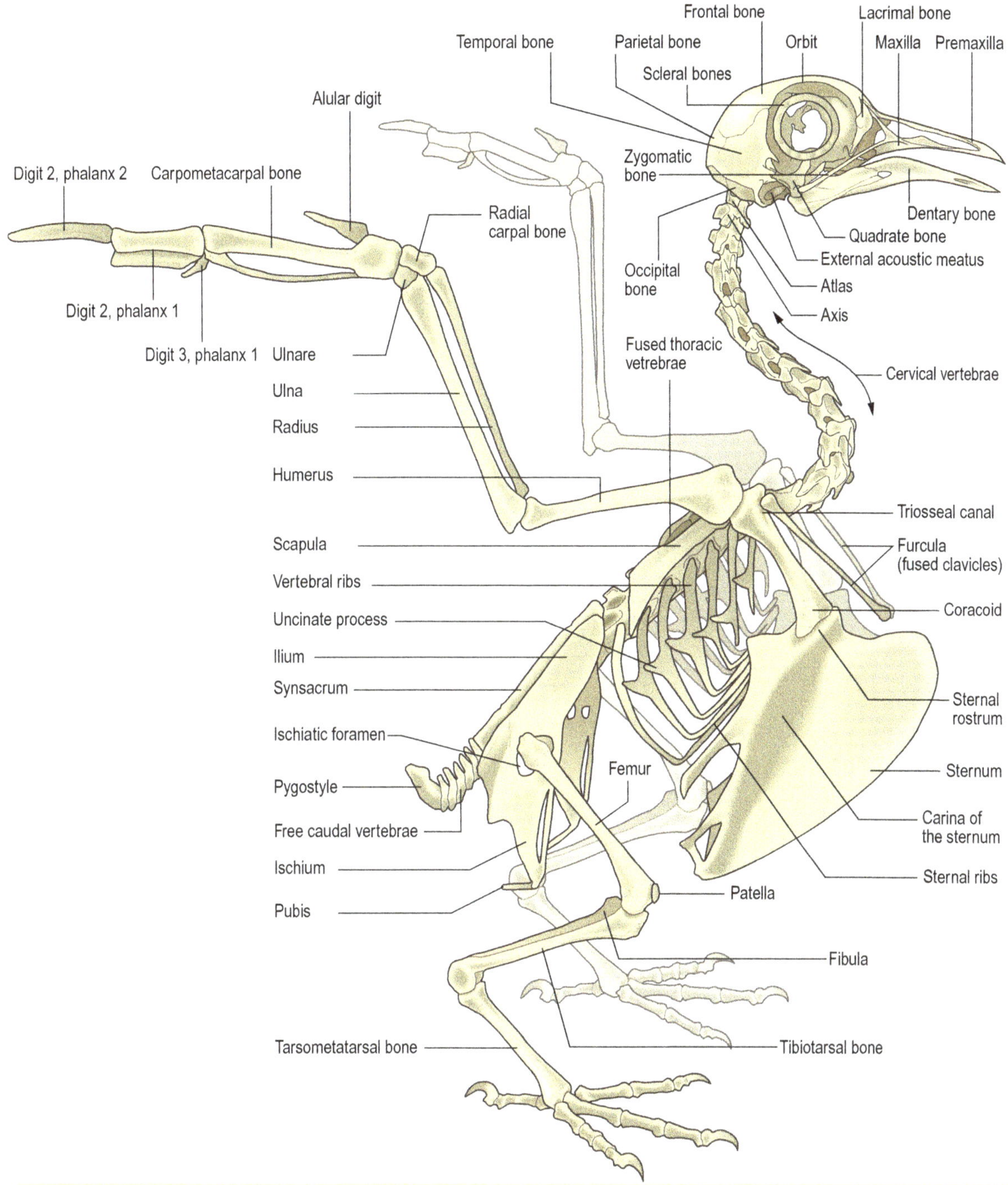

Figure 8.12
Skeleton of a flight-capable bird.

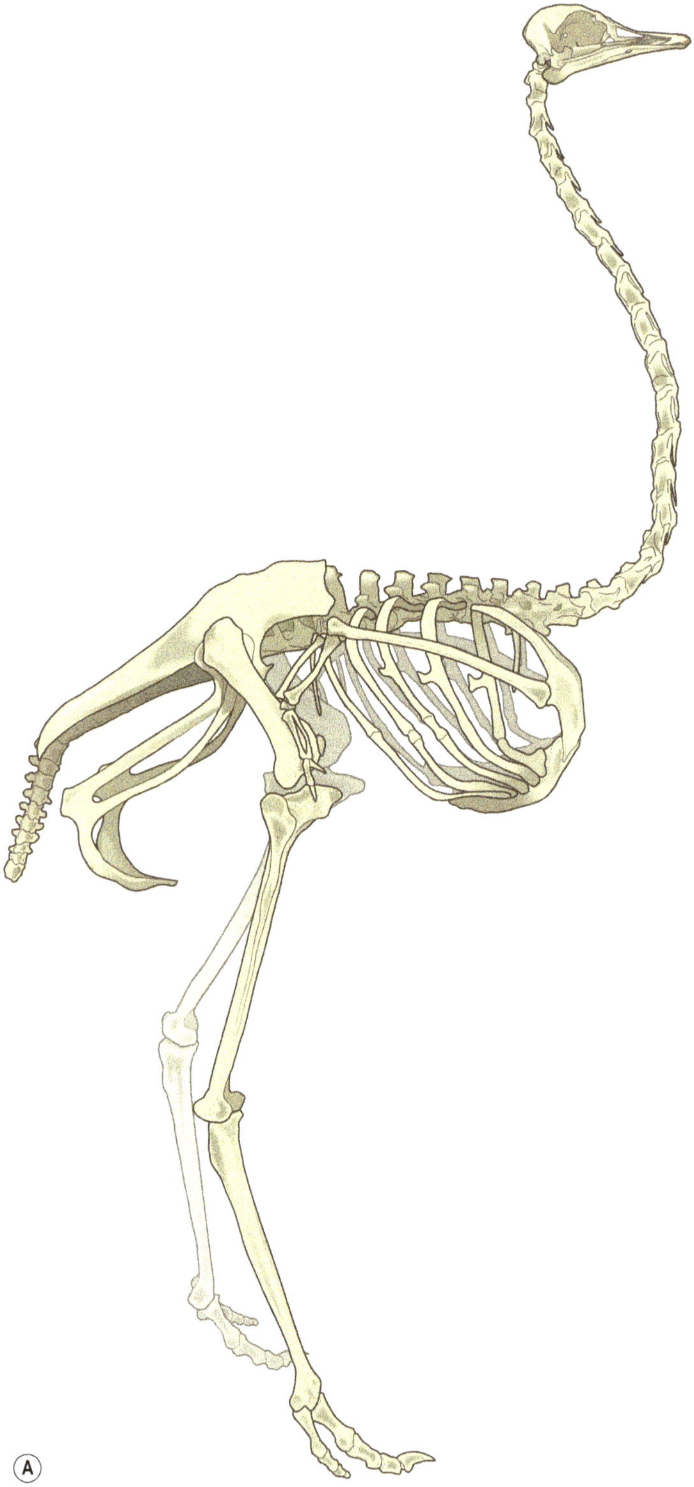

Figure 8.13
Skeletons of flightless birds.
(A) Ostrich.

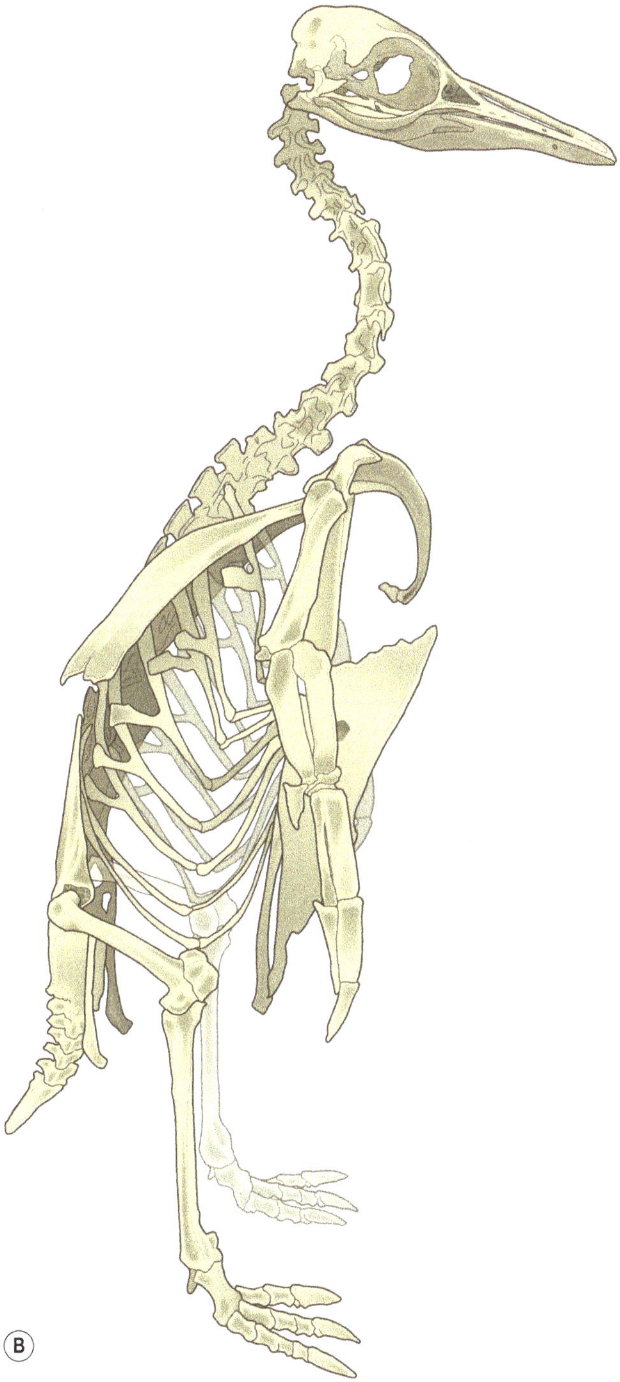

(B)

Figure 8.13—*Cont'd*
Skeletons of flightless birds.
(B) Emperor penguin.

proximally. In birds there are no centers of ossification and therefore no growth plates. At the end of growth the bone is completely ossified with the only cartilage remaining being that of the articular surface, as seen in mammals.

Pneumatic and nonpneumatic bones

Bone type can be categorized as either nonpneumatic or pneumatic. The nonpneumatic bones constitute the larger part of the skeleton. Some, as a weight-saving measure, may be thin and delicate and have relatively thin cortices but they are, essentially, similar to mammal bones.

It is the pneumatic bones that differ substantially from mammal bones. By definition they contain air sacs and thus are contiguous with the rest of the respiratory system. There is variation between Orders and Families but within this variation there are broad principles. Some bones of the axial skeleton may be pneumatic, for example the clavicle, but it is in the proximal appendicular skeleton where the pneumatic bones are more apparent and, for the purposes of this publication, more relevant. Both the humerus and the femur are pneumatic bones. These can be characterized by having very thin cortices and marked medullary cavity, often bridged with reinforcing bony struts or trabeculae. Simple fractures of pneumatic bones can lead to leakage of air into adjacent structures. If the fracture is compound, then the exposed bone can act as a portal for foreign material and infection into the respiratory system. (It also represents a site for leakage of anesthetics gases during surgical anesthesia.)

Anatomical variations

In comparison with mammals, elongation of the neck is achieved through the addition of vertebrae. This adaptation is, in part, driven by the fact that the avian eye is fixed in the orbit and a change to the field of vision is achieved by moving the head rather than just the eye. For example, the neck of the giraffe contains only the standard seven vertebrae seen in almost all other mammals, whereas the similarly elongated and highly flexible neck of the swan has well in excess of 25 vertebrae (Fig. 8.14). The cervical vertebrae vary in number between Orders and Families.

Progressing caudally, there are substantial differences between the avian and mammalian spine. Similarly, there are variations between avian Orders and Families. Generally speaking, however, in birds the spine is fused into two units (the notarium and synsacrum; see below).

Cranially the thoracic vertebrae (deemed to be four in number in the domestic fowl) are fused to form a single structure: the notarium. The ribs originating from

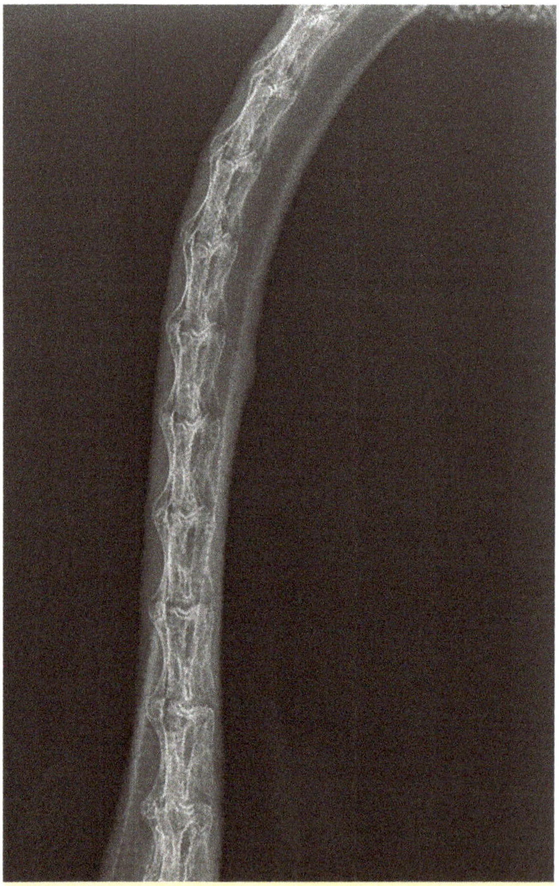

Figure 8.14
A lateral-view radiograph showing part of the cervical spine of a mute swan (*Cygnus olor*).

the vertebrae of the notarium all attach to the sternum. This provides a relatively rigid framework for the flight muscles.

Immediately caudal to the notarium there is an articulation that may or may not include a free, usually single, vertebra. Thereafter the spine fuses again, with, for example, in the domestic fowl, some sixteen or seventeen vertebra, which form the synsacrum. This structure is extensively fused with the ilium to form the pelvic girdle.

Finally, varying in number between species, there are free caudal vertebrae.

The bones of the wing follow the standard mammal pattern, with a humerus and paired radius and ulna. Based on this standard design there is variation between the Orders, with the wing being relatively truncated and rigid in the blade-like structure of the nonflying Sphenisciformes (the penguins). In the volant birds there is a reliance on rotatory movement to facilitate flight, with the smaller radius moving relative to the adjacent, larger, ulna. For those more accustomed to dealing with mammals the greatest difference is seen from the carpus distally. There is fusion of bones, with reduction, modification, and loss of metacarpal bones and phalanges (Fig. 8.15).

At first sight it may be thought that the leg follows the standard mammalian pattern. This is not the case. The femur articulates with the proximal tibia to form a stifle joint (containing, in many species, a patella). However, the tibia fuses with the proximal tarsus to form the tibiotarsal bone. There is then, to all intents and purposes, a conventional joint within the tarsus. The distal tarsus then fuses with a single metatarsus to form the tarsometatarsal bone (Fig. 8.16).

As would be anticipated through the wide range of ecological niches occupied by birds, there is great variation in the anatomy and function of the feet. Though there are generally four digits, reduction in number is seen in, for example, the cursorial, terrestrial

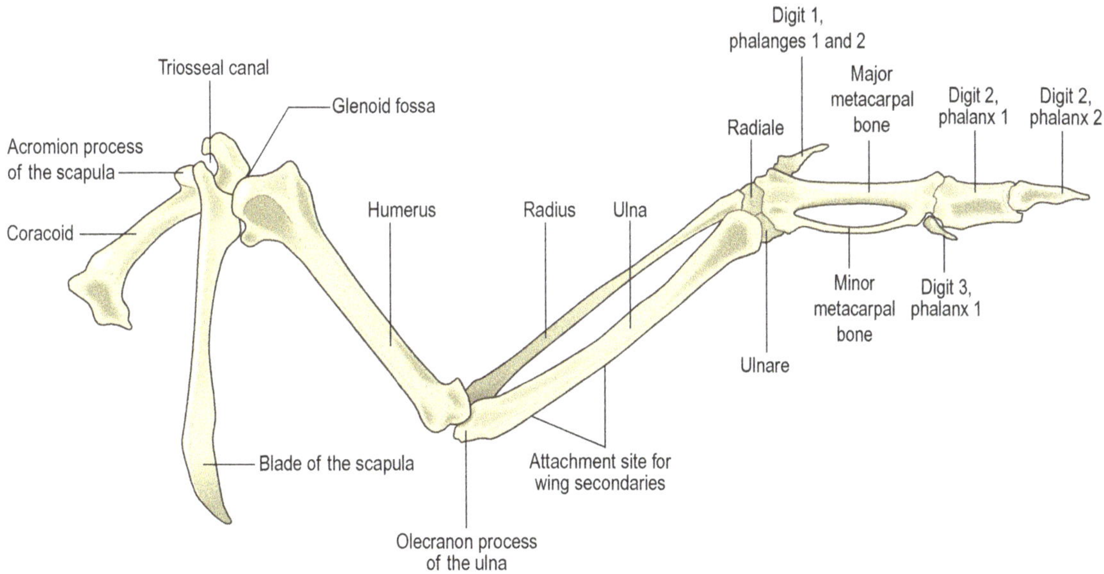

Figure 8.15
View from above (dorsal view) of the skeletal structures of the right wing and pectoral girdle.

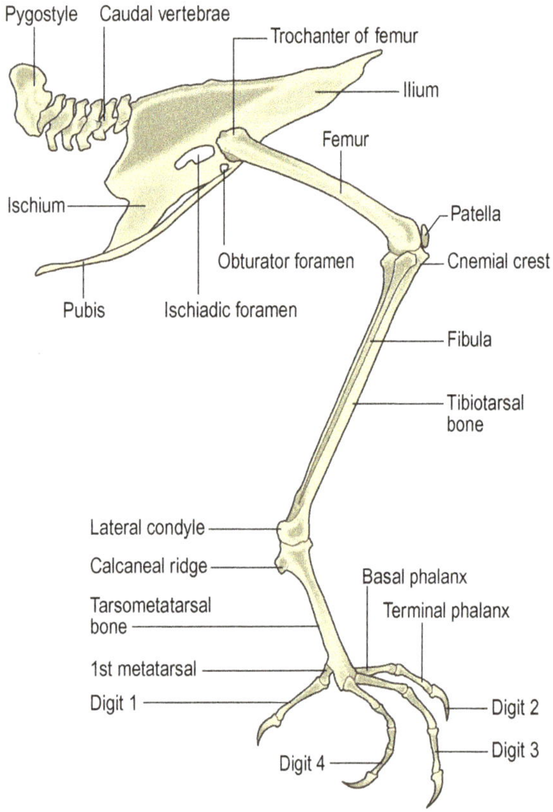

Figure 8.16
The skeletal structures of the pelvic limb.

Struthiformes (ostriches). Of the four digits the general pattern is to have the first digit (the hallux) directed caudally and digits 2, 3,and 4 directed cranially. This differs in the commonly seen Psittaformes, where digit 4 is also rotated caudally giving a zygodactyl foot. The zygodactyl foot has evolved convergently in other species, of which the more likely encountered ones include the Strigiformes (owls) and the osprey (which has a digit that can rotate to the more conventional position when perching).

In all the birds, but most markedly in those that perch, flexion of the proximal leg joints will produce a reciprocal flexion of the distal joints, including those of the feet. This generates a passive grip allowing birds to roost on branches with little conscious effort or expenditure of energy. Many species, in particular the raptors, can more actively generate a lethal grip with their feet as the digital flexor tendons insert at the distal tip of each respective distal phalanx, i.e., at the base of each talon.

Musculature

The muscle character in birds varies according to its function. This is readily appreciated in table poultry, with the very familiar white meat on the breast and the darker meat on the legs, with the latter containing far higher levels of myoglobin. Intratendinous ossification is found in the legs of a number of species of birds, with those most likely to be encountered including some raptor species and some Galliformes, for example, the turkey. While often not palpable, they can be visualized radiographically and need to be recognized as such (Figs 8.17A and B).

The largest muscle masses tend to be on the body of the bird or the proximal limbs. Limb movement is generated and modified through the actions of tendons and ligaments. This is particularly the case in the forelimb, the wing, where the muscles for flight are essentially all situated centrally on the body as the pectoral mass. (The muscles found on the wing itself are generally either for fine-tuning maneuvers during flight or for holding the wing in place when at rest) (Fig. 8.18A and B).

The sternum in flying birds is the anatomical origin of the flight muscles. As such it has been modified to accommodate this actual and physiologically large mass of muscle, having a prominent keel or carina for their attachment. While it may be anticipated that the breast muscles are those that are involved in the downstroke of the wing, the muscles that generate the upstroke are also found in the pectoral mass. It is the superficial and deep pectoral muscles that generate the downstroke whereas it is the supracoracoideus, via the triosseal canal which redirects the tendons, which provide the upstroke. The triosseal canal is formed by the convergence of the scapula, corocoid, and clavicles, with these three bones forming a collective unit often referred to as the pectoral girdle (Figs 8.19A and B, and 8.20).

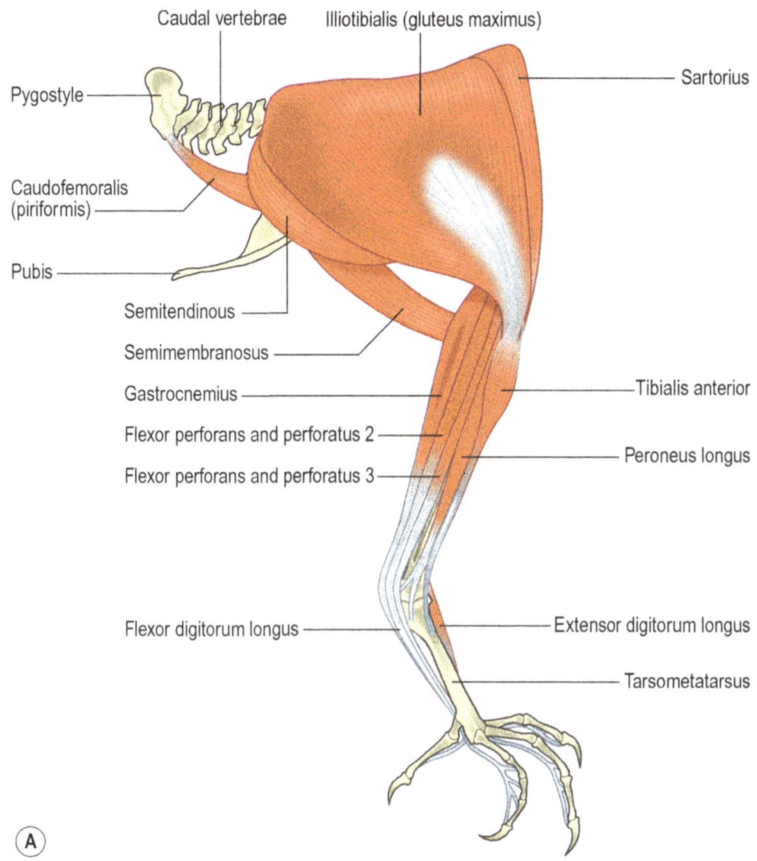

Figure 8.17
Musculature of the right leg.
(A) Lateral view.

The pelvic girdle, in nearly all species, is incomplete ventrally: an adaptation presumed to allow the passage of relatively thin-shelled eggs.

Examples of pathology and injuries

Masses: lumps and bumps

During any hands-on manipulation or examination, nonyielding, circumscribed, sometimes painful masses may be palpated. These need some consideration.

Bony exostoses are found in birds. These may or may not involve joints. Not only is radiography needed to determine the veterinary management of such cases but also to ascertain the cause of the swellings. The pathogenesis of these masses may not be due to bony changes but may be due to conditions rarely seen in mammals.

For example, the normal excretory product following protein digestion in birds is uric acid. In mammals it is the water-soluble urea. Kidney conditions (renal failure) in birds can lead to a build-up of blood uric acid and its deposition in tissues, (often in or around joints). These are often described as "tophi" but may also be termed "gout." Gout in humans is reported as being painful, and one must assume that this is also the case in birds. A blood sample for assessment of kidney function and radiography would be regarded as aids to diagnosis by the veterinary surgeon.

Typically, avian pus is hard rather than liquid as seen in mammals. Thus a hard mass associated with muscles or bones may essentially be an abscess.

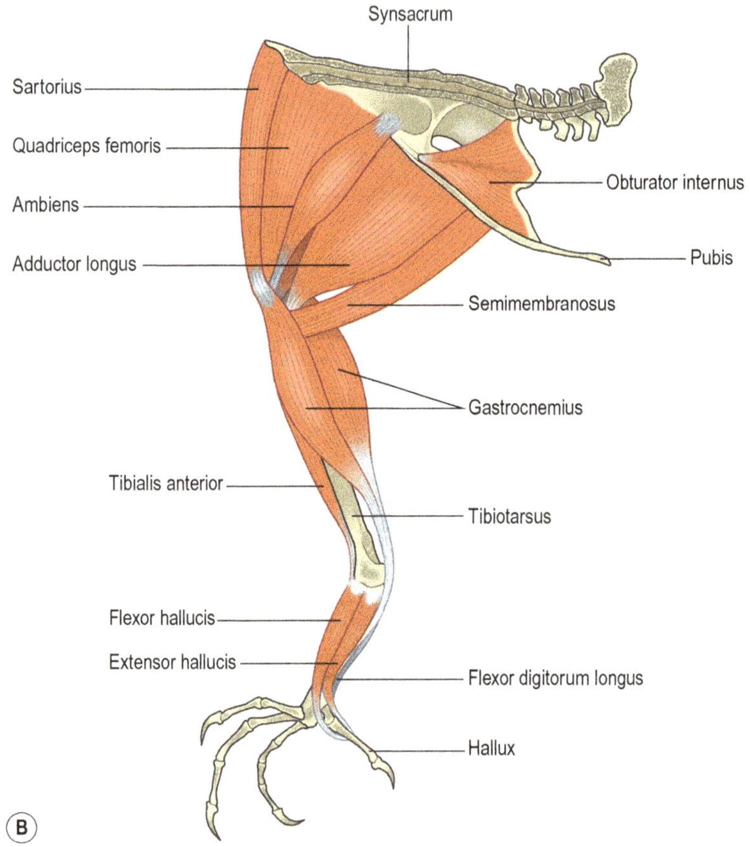

Figure 8.17—*Cont'd*
Musculature of the right leg.
(B) Medial view.

This abscess may potentially be either "cold" (where there are no remaining viable bacteria) or it may be active. In neither case would manipulation be appropriate. A fine needle aspirate taken by a veterinary surgeon with subsequent cytology would be diagnostic.

Swellings with infection

In one specific scenario an infection, and pus, can be relatively mobile. This is when the infection has gained access to a tendon sheath or joint cavity and is suspended in the physiologically or pathologically responding fluid therein. The infection therefore becomes more mobile, and manipulation of the swelling may spread the infection (Fig. 8.21).

There are several instances in which this may arise:

- Direct traumatic injury, penetrating a joint or tendon sheath with introduction of infection. The trauma may be caused by inanimate objects or by other animals, for example, penetration caused by the talons of a cage mate or bite wounds from a prey species. The initial injury broaches the tissues, with dirt and debris then being inoculated below the skin and into susceptible tissues.
- Where there is a build-up of debris on the ventral aspect of the tip of the most distal phalanx (in raptors this is often food and faeces). This build-up occurs at the base of the talon or claw and initially provides a microenvironment that leads to skin breakdown. Once the integument is broached, micro-organisms can enter. The tip of the distal phalanx is where the digital flexor tendon inserts. Infection can enter and track proximally along the tendon sheath. Resolution requires veterinary intervention and may ultimately be achieved only through the flushing of the tendon sheath under

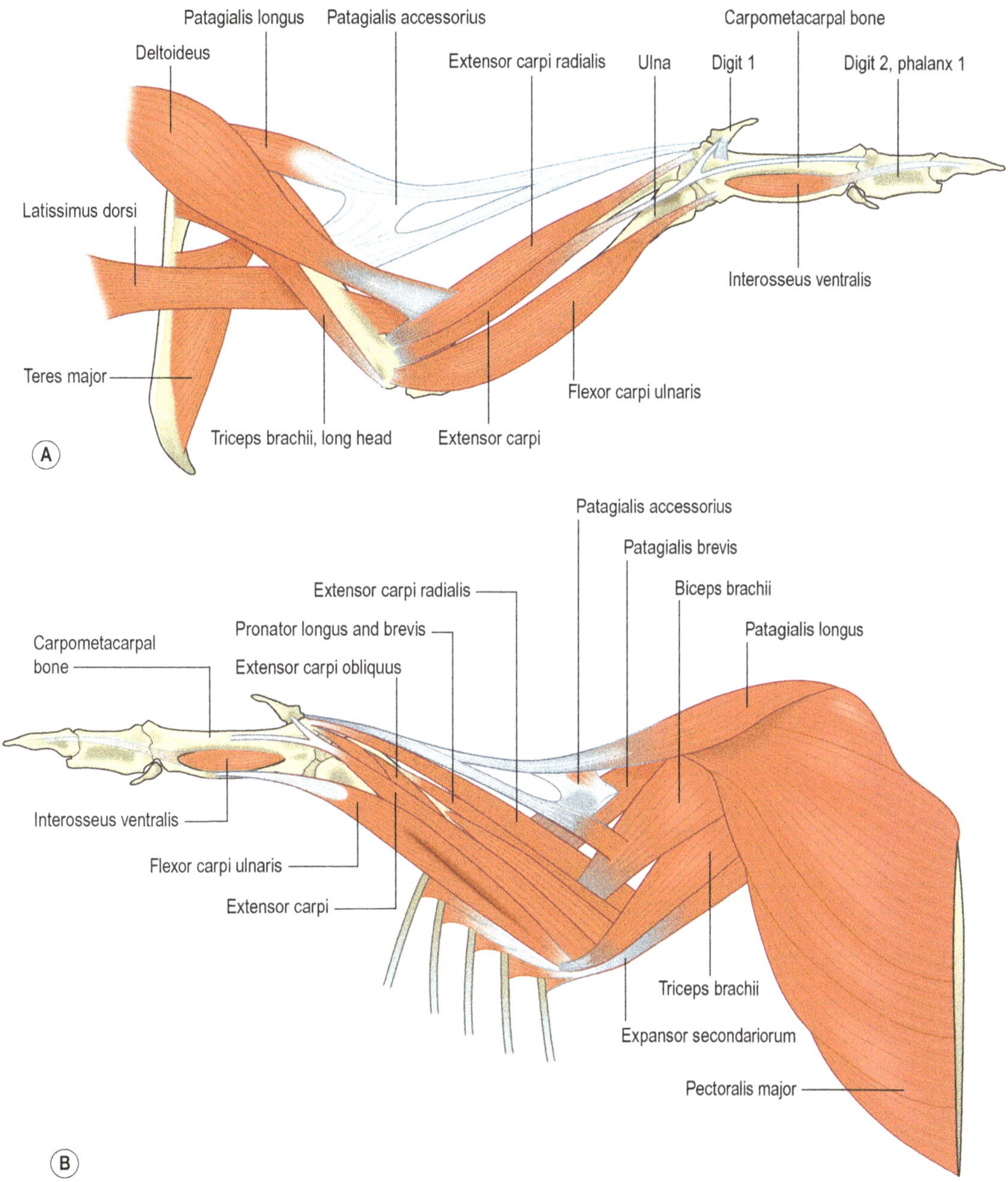

Figure 8.18
Musculature of the right wing. (A) Dorsal view. (B) Ventral view.

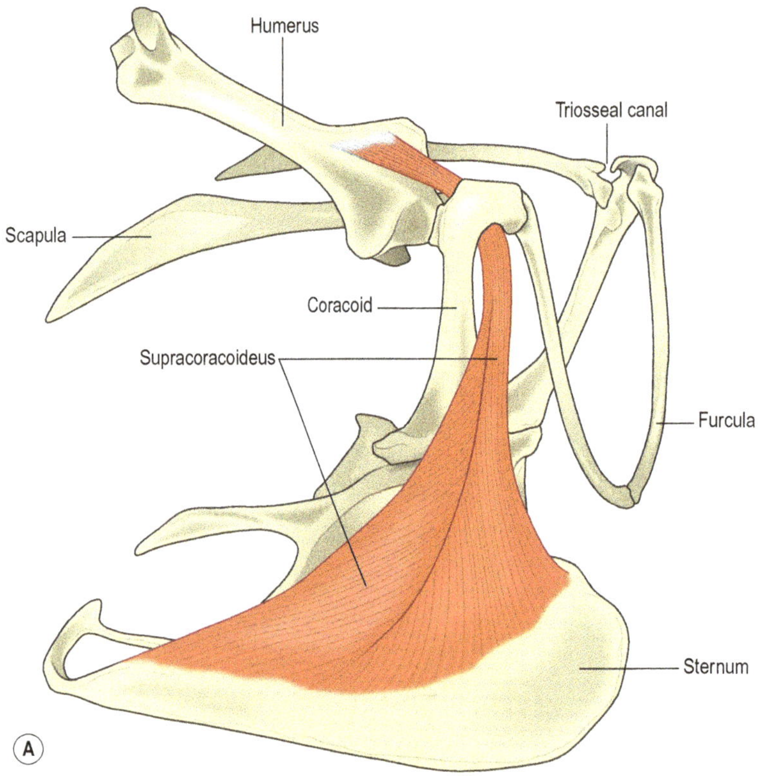

Figure 8.19
(A) Musculature of the pectoral girdle.

general anesthesia, in conjunction with appropriate antibiotics. Subsequent osteopathy could assist in preventing permanent restriction in movement of the digits should pathology develop, for example, scar tissue in the tendon or tendon sheath.

Bumblefoot

Taking this one step further is the condition referred to as bumblefoot. The specifics of the etiology and pathogenesis of this condition can be controversial, with it arising in different taxa due to different reasons. Bumblefoot can be graded according to its severity.

At the more severe end of the spectrum, there is a marked loss of tissues to the underside of the foot associated with infection. The primary driver of the disease is the ongoing devitalization of tissues, with progressive involvement of the skin, subcutaneous tissues, tendons, joints, and bones of the foot. Treatments at this stage need to be radical. Often robust surgical debridement of affected tissues, protective dressings, and appropriate antibiosis is required. The postdebridement coaptation and reconstruction of the foot where significant tissue deficits have been generated can lead to contracture of the digits in flexion. This contracture can be further compounded through the necessity of having to dress the foot, often with the digits intentionally flexed to allow healing, using techniques such as a "ball bandage." In these circumstances physiotherapy of the foot is beneficial in order to reduce the possibility of the foot healing with a degree of permanent digital flexion. Treatment sessions can be arranged with the veterinary surgeon to coincide with general anesthesia essential for postoperative dressing changes and diagnostic work, for example, follow-up radiography. Assessment of the site with reference to infection must

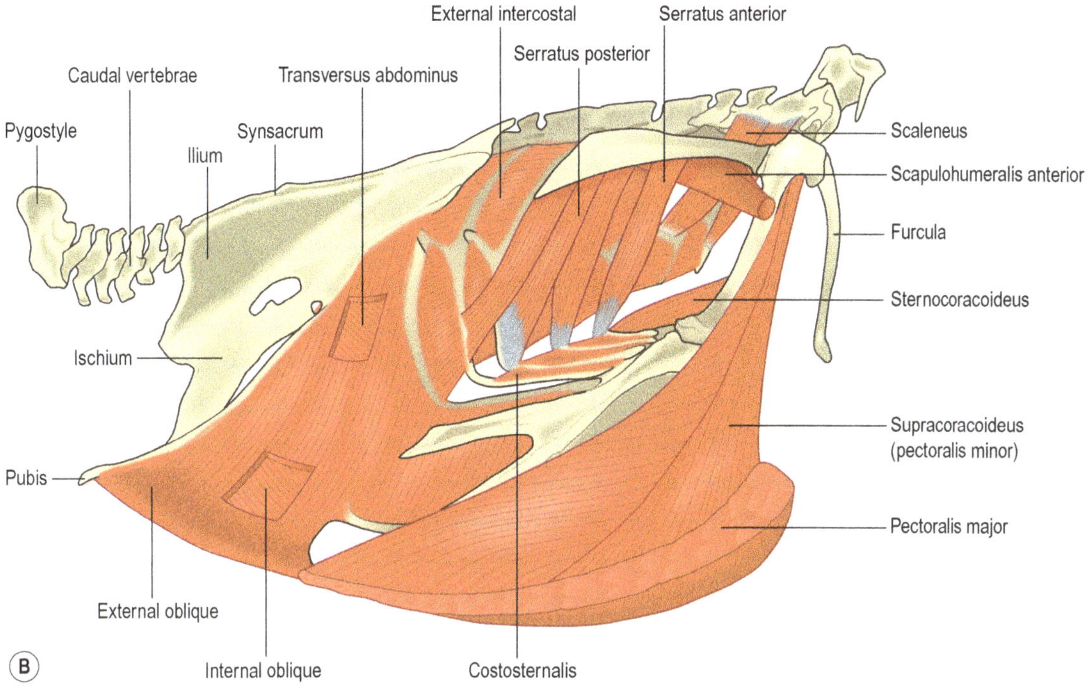

Figure 8.19—*Cont'd*
(B) Thoracic muscles.

be made in order to ensure that any manipulations do not disseminate infection.

The earlier stages of bumblefoot are less severe. They are caused by loss of the dermal papillae of the plantar aspect of the foot, giving the skin a slightly shiny appearance. Reddening of the area (erythema) and thinning of the skin are the next stages. There is no direct involvement of bacteria at these stages but deterioration can be rapid and marked. There are several causes that can initiate these low key changes, and they may act in a synergistic manner. All of these relate, to a greater or lesser degree, to a compromise of the circulation of the foot, specifically the weight-bearing area of the plantar foot. Resolution of the early stages can be achieved by addressing these underlying predisposing factors and enhancing circulation within the foot.

A harsh or dirty substrate or perch may be one factor. Perhaps counterintuitively a smooth perch may also be a factor as it often focuses weight-bearing onto the same, very restricted, areas of the foot and impedes circulation. Many birds that spend long periods of the day perching, for example raptors that are tethered when not flying, benefit from an irregular but yielding perch surface. Falconers make great use of AstroTurf® or similar surfaces to prevent foot conditions arising.

Increased bodyweight will also increase the pressure on the weight-bearing areas. This results in a local, discrete reduction in blood perfusion of the tissues of the foot. Added to this, an overweight bird may be less fit, so the tissue perfusion may be further reduced and the risk of local ischemia increased.

A unilateral presentation of bumblefoot is not uncommon. This may occur when there is a problem with one leg leading to increased weight-bearing on the other foot, which then develops clinical signs. The shift in weight-bearing can sometimes be the result

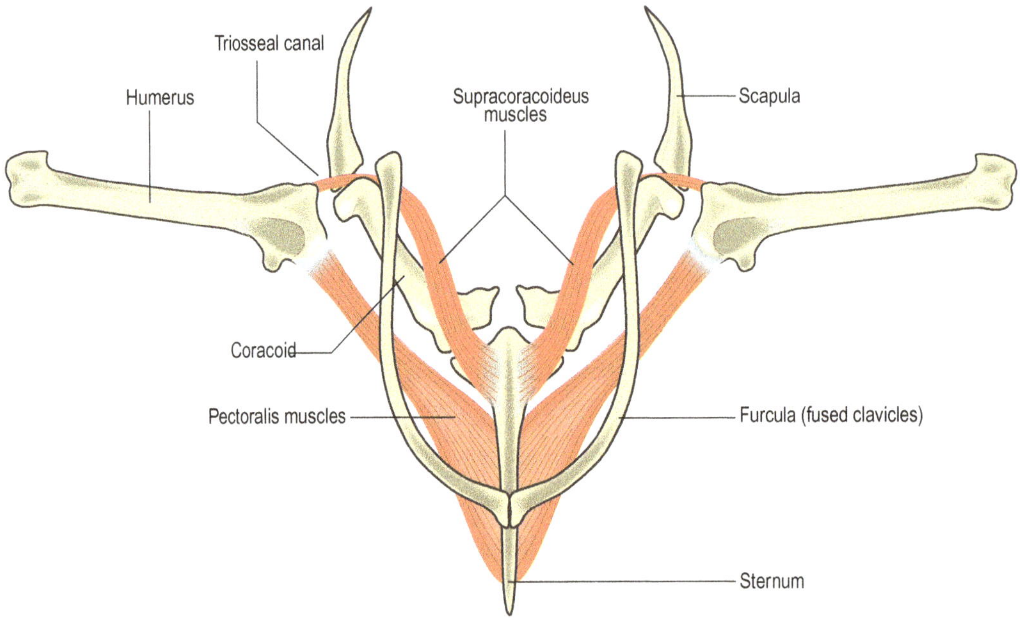

Figure 8.20
Transverse section through the pectoral girdle showing attachments for supracoracoideus (wing elevator) and pectoralis (wing depressor). Note the ventral origins that ensure muscle mass is close to the bird's center of gravity.

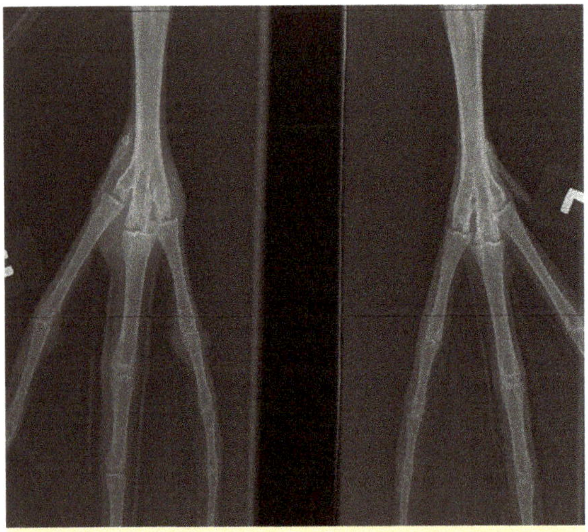

Figure 8.21
A craniocaudal radiograph of the tarsus of a mute swan (*Cygnus olor*). Note the soft tissue swelling in the image on the right, extending into the phalanges.

of an injury to the apparently healthy leg or it may be subsequent to a veterinary intervention, for example, where orthopedic surgery has taken place. The bird biases its weight onto the previously healthy leg which then develops bumblefoot. As the condition progresses both feet may become infected. The initial presentation of bumblefoot in one foot may therefore be indicative of a pre-existing pathology in the opposite leg.

Pulling all these elements together it can be appreciated that a bird postsurgery, held in a confined "hospital cage" with smooth perching, not exercising and additionally putting on weight, would be a prime candidate for the development of bumblefoot. An awareness of this allows one to factor in a regimen of manipulation, osteopathy, and exercise that will reduce or eliminate the possibility of bumblefoot developing.

A veterinary surgeon may diagnose a problem in the leg not showing the bumblefoot on first presentation.

Osteopathy to help the nonaffected leg may lead to improvement of the contralateral bumblefoot.

Growth and developmental conditions

Two growth or developmental conditions should be considered. Both are, by definition, seen in young, growing birds and have multifactorial causes. Certain categories of bird, often waterfowl, appear predisposed. Key factors appear to be rapid growth, a high protein diet, and suboptimal bone mineralization during the growing period. Correction of these factors may not on its own produce a satisfactory outcome as by the time of clinical recognition there is already a deformity of the bone present.

Angel wing

This condition has many colloquial synonyms and is seen primarily in waterfowl. It is often only recognized when the primary feathers start to grow. These are relatively heavy as the growing feathers contain blood and cause a rotation of the wing to develop distal to the carpus. Unless treated immediately, it leaves the bird with the rotated "hard-pinned" (fully grown) primary feathers perpendicular to the body, which results in a limited or nonexistent ability to fly. The condition does not resolve at subsequent moults. A support dressing in the very early stages in the growing bird may correct this deformity and stop its progression. To achieve this, the wing is held in the normal position with the carpus flexed and the feathers all correctly aligned. There are a number of soft, nonadhesive, self-gripping conforming bandages that can be used to achieve this. Despite the apparently yielding nature of such dressings, they can cause skin ulceration through exerting pressure on the soft tissuesand this risk increases as the bird grows (often very rapidly). Frequent redressing is essential. Not surprisingly this type of dressing, through its temporary restriction of movement, can also lead to soft tissue contracture and a reduced capacity for carpal extension.

Slipped hock

Slipped hock is seen in waterfowl, but also in poultry and allied Gallinae. The condition develops at the intratarsal joint, with deformity of the distal tibiotarsal bone and the proximal tarsometatarsal bone. Often the tendon of the gastrocnemius muscle becomes displaced, "slipping" medially. Initial presentation is generally of a young bird that appears clumsy. In more severe cases the bird can be unable to walk or stand. These cases do not respond to support dressings alone, as the degree of correction needed to reinstate the tendon alignment is not feasible. Some cases will respond to surgery, for example, replacement and fixation of the gastrocnemius tendon and subsequent support dressing. As with angel wing there has to be a balance in the application of any support dressing used for postoperative support to ensure it will not cause permanent restriction of joints or lead to pressure-induced soft tissue ulceration.

Both the above conditions require active manipulation of the limb between dressing changes to minimize any soft tissue contracture and to aid circulation. With the latter condition gentle, supported, swimming between dressing changes appears beneficial.

Metabolic bone disease

The decision to deal with angel wing and slipped hock as separate categories is somewhat arbitrary. A number of similar diseases fit under the umbrella of metabolic bone disease. These are, effectively, inadequate mineralization of the bone. Not surprisingly there is some overlap with the syndromes seen in growing birds but without solely involving the recognized predilection sites of the carpus and hock. Demineralization may occur throughout the skeleton, but it is the longer limb bones that more frequently demonstrate deformities or folding fractures or both.

Most commonly affected are hand-reared chicks of raptors, where the diet has too little calcium. The underlying problem is the diet being fed, which may be day-old chicks or simply meat. Meat fed without balanced supplementation has an inverted Ca:P ratio, producing a hyperphosphatemia and a hypocalcemia.

In psittacines, particularly the African grey parrot, there are believed to be roles played by UV light in healthy bone development. The diets fed in captivity (the worst being poor-quality sunflower seed) often lack calcium, have an inverted Ca:P ratio, and also lack the fat-soluble vitamins, critically vitamin D.

Clinically the impression is of delicate bones that may show gross deformity or may require radiography to demonstrate the extent of the problem. On radiography the bones may be less radio-dense than normal, indicating that they are poorly mineralized. The deformities are generally not as malleable as those seen in angel wing, being best considered as permanent. The prognosis therefore is poor. Some birds can survive with their deformities but rarely lead what could be regarded as a normal life.

Metabolic bone disease in older birds is almost exclusively a condition of female birds that have been laying eggs (often to excess) and not balancing the loss of calcium in the eggshells with calcium intake. The bones become demineralized and are subject to pathological fractures. Sometimes, particularly in caged birds, fractures may not be detected by the owner. These fractures, especially folding fractures, can heal when calcium homeostasis is re-established but the deformities become permanent. The affected limbs may benefit from osteopathy and exercise to strengthen muscles. Orthopedic surgery in these pathologically delicate bones is not usually indicated.

Orthopedic and postoperative management

Orthopedic management of avian cases can be complex. The choice of technique falls to the veterinary surgeon dealing with the case. Management of the cases postoperatively (including those that have been splinted or similar) fits into the usual pattern of needing to avoid soft tissue contracture and restriction of movement of joints.

Synostosis, where one bone fuses to another during healing, is relatively rare but is significant with reference to fractures of the radius and ulna. Fusion of these two bones can be critical. Their sliding movement relative to each other is essential for the distal wing to be "trimmed" during flight. A synostosis of these two bones can be a sufficient impediment to flight to prevent rescued birds being rehabilitated and released back into the wild.

Fractures

Other than those resulting from metabolic bone disease, fractures are the result of direct trauma, caused by collisions, shooting, or predation. The site of a fracture will determine the prognosis for the patient. Fractures very close to or involving a joint mechanism, as well as those in the shafts of the radius and ulna, will have less favorable outcomes than others (Fig. 8.22).

Legs and feet are common injury sites, but generally have less effect on the survival of an individual. Fractures through long bones are often stabilized using external fixation, followed by osteopathic treatment during the rehabilitation phase. Fractures in the foot are usually strapped to stabilize the site while healing takes place (Fig. 8.23).

Osteopathic evaluation

Case history

As in human practice, information from the case history helps to form a diagnosis and prognosis. It also helps to minimize handling of the avian patient. The age and type of species may determine differences in pliability and movement of skeletal structures. Anatomical and behavioral variations will give rise

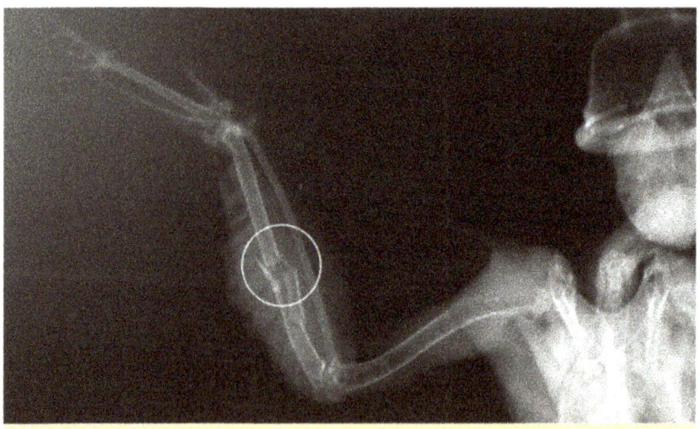

Figure 8.22
Dorsoventral radiograph showing a fractured ulna in a sparrow hawk (*Accipiter nisus*). Reproduced with kind permission from Vale Wildlife Hospital.

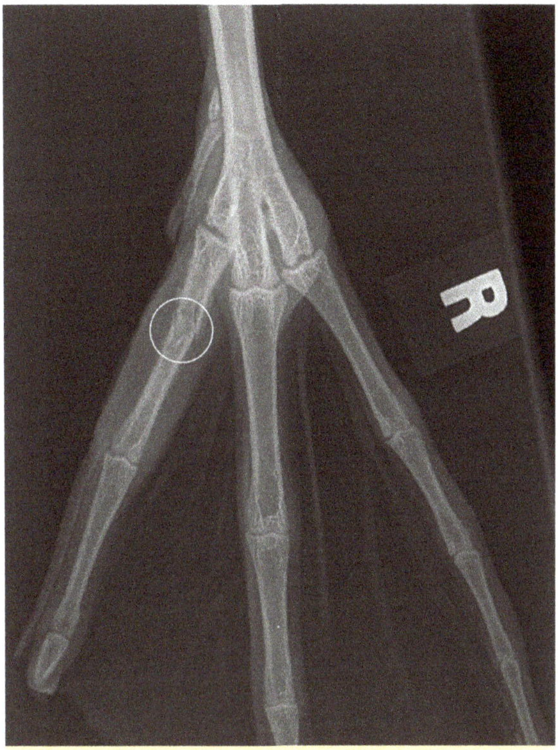

Figure 8.23
A craniocaudal radiograph showing a fractured medial proximal phalanx in a mute swan (*Cygnus olor*). Reproduced with kind permission from Vale Wildlife Hospital.

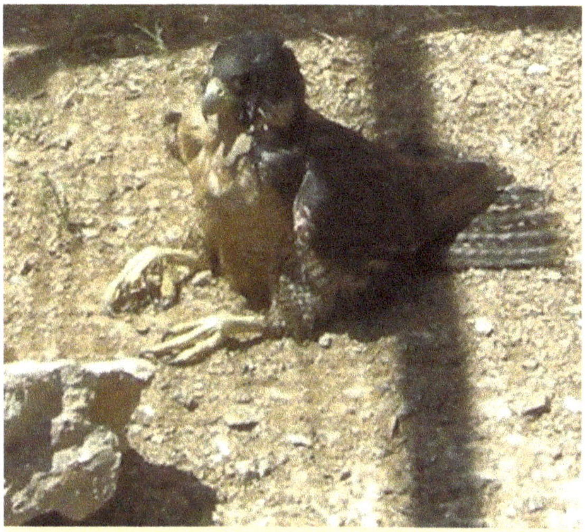

Figure 8.24
Digitigrade inability after spinal injury.

to defense mechanisms that must be considered. The injury site can determine areas of somatic dysfunction. The patient's previous living conditions must be noted and also the expectations of the owner or finder. Previous progress in the condition arising from factors such as veterinary diagnosis, joint stability and mobility, and response to any treatment administered (medication, surgery, vitamins, prescribed exercises, osteopathy) should be carefully assessed.

Observation and active movements

Observe the general appearance and breathing pattern of the avian. Is it agitated, aggressive or quivering? Are the movements and position of the head normal? Are there any pathological signs like torticollis, repetitive movements or asymmetry in limb position? A dropped wing may indicate neuropathy or musculoskeletal injury. Can the bird fly and, if so, is it symmetrical? Are pelvic limbs functional while standing, landing or catching a prey? See Figure 8.24 for an example illustrating digitigrade inability after spinal injury.

Palpation and mobility testing

An experienced bird handler can prove invaluable for immobilizing the bird, so that the osteopath may concentrate on their work. Proper attention should be given to the bird's defense mechanisms, which include the beak and talons. It is preferable to minimize both the patient's and the handler's stress before proceeding to any physical handling. Gentle articulation may be used for assessing quality and quantity of joint movement. Look for signs of somatic dysfunction like asymmetry, restriction of movement, and changes in tissue quality, such as hypertonic muscles. Size and mobility of skeletal structures differ among avian species. Proceed in testing limbs bilaterally for comparison. Vertebrae and ribs do not easily allow differentiating between individual joints, due to their minimal size. There should be a constant evaluation of the bird's general state and awareness of possible causes of pain, such as muscle or tendon laceration, osteoarthritis, luxation and fracture. It must be remembered that human handling is a stressful situation for wild birds, and they usually do not vocalize when they feel pain. Be alert to any signs of intolerance like fatigue, incoordination of movements, dyspnea, open-mouth breathing, and drooping wing (Martin et al. 1993). Stop if necessary and continue when the bird is less stressed.

Assessment of the cervical spine

The mobility of the cervical spine allows the head to be used like an extendable arm. Special characteristics of the upper cervical spine of birds includes lack of mobility of C1-C2 (when compared to mammals) due to connective tissue attachments and the dens of the axis extending through the atlas to contact the base of the skull (Kaiser 2007). The occiput, however, has a single condyle that increases head mobility, but it is also more prone to luxation. Evaluate for any hypertonicity of paraspinal muscles, which indicates areas of somatic dysfunction. Evaluate combined movement of cervical vertebrae by springing the posterolateral part of the vertebrae in a ventromedial direction (Fig. 8.25A). Translation can be assessed by mobilizing the lateral part of the vertebrae in a transverse direction (Fig. 8.25B).

Assessment of the thorax

Minimal movement exists in the thoracic spine due to the fact that most thoracic vertebrae are fused. The thorax expands and contracts during breathing and wing flapping. During the wing's downstroke the sternum tilts up, and with the upstroke the sternum tilts down (Videler 2005). The mobility of the sternum is due to the pliability of the ribs. This can be assessed by compressing together specific areas of the sternum and dorsal spine. The hand contact is explained in the treatment section of the thorax. Caution should be exercised so that only a mild pressure is applied to these delicate structures. Be aware that pressure on the thorax can impede lung expansion and breathing. Evaluating muscles of the thorax includes palpation of pectoral muscle (Fig. 8.26) which also indicates the bird's nutritional reserves (Coles 2007).

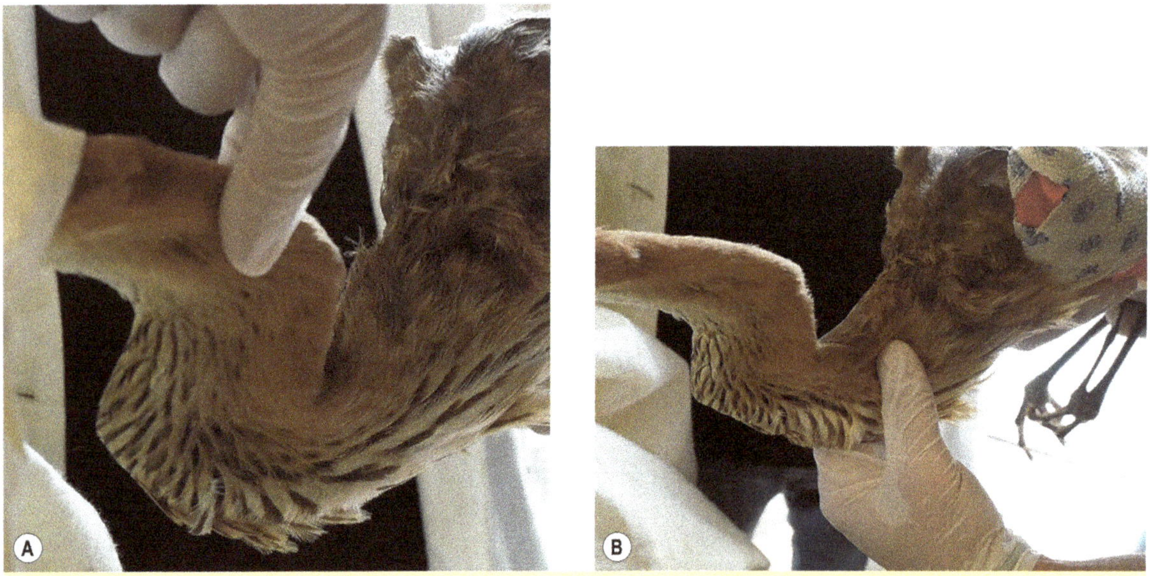

Figure 8.25
(A) Assessing cervical mobility and paraspinal musculature. (B) Assessing cervical mobility by translation.

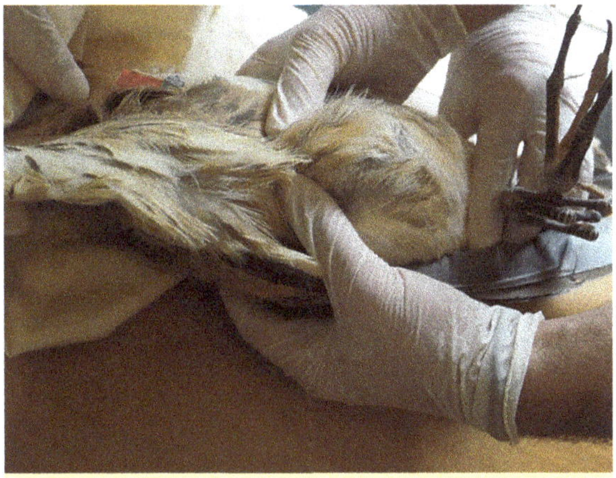

Figure 8.26
Assessing the pectoralis musculature.

Assessment of the caudal vertebrae

Only the last caudal vertebrae are mobile. They can be assessed as a group in flexion, extension, lateral flexion, and rotation (Fig. 8.27).

Assessment of the pectoral limbs

When the wing is closed the glenohumeral (GH) joint is placed in a depressed and retracted state while the elbow and wrist joints are held in flexion. When the wing opens, the elbow and wrist move together in flexion and extension. Skeletal and muscular elements allow the radius to slide along the ulna and produce synchronization of elbow and wrist joints (Beaufrère 2009) (Fig. 8.28).

Glenohumeral joint. The glenohumeral (GH) joint has a large amount of mobility. This includes movements of elevation, depression, protraction, retraction, and rotation. Check GH mobility and the integrity of propatagial (Fig. 8.29) and metapatagial membranes.

Elbow joint. Assess the integrity of the ulna and radius, and the myofascial tissue between the two bones (Fig. 8.30). Assess flexion of the elbow and the ability of the wings to close symmetrically. To assess elbow extension, hold the wrist joint and open the wing outward perpendicular to the torso, as explained later in the section on osteopathic treatment of the elbow. Wrist extension may enhance elbow extension and vice versa.

Wrist joint (manus). The wrist is a double joint. The two carpal bones are situated between the radius and ulna, and the carpometacarpal bone (Proctor and Lynch 1993). Evaluate wrist extension by unfolding the wing perpendicular to the torso from the carpometacarpal bone. The wrist joint in some species can rotate over 90 degrees when not in a fully extended position (Vazquez 1992). In full extension the wrist is locked, hindering any rotatory movements. This lock provides the necessary joint stability during flying.

Digits. There are three digits articulating with the carpometacarpal bone. Palpation of the digits (especially of the third) can be challenging due to the small size of the bones. Evaluate the integrity of the carpometacarpal bone and the mobility of the digits in abduction, adduction, and flexion and extension (Figs 8.31 and 8.32). The first digit, aside from the aforementioned movements, also allows supination in the up phase and pronation in the down phase of wing movement (Videler 2005).

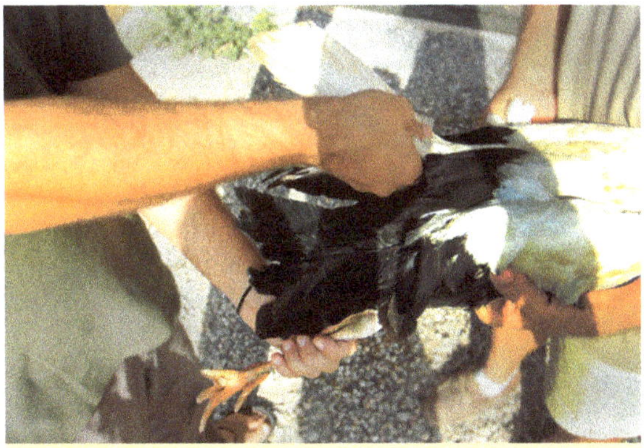

Figure 8.27
Evaluation of the tail extension.

Assessment of the pelvic limbs

The pelvic limbs are configured more similarly to mammals than the pectoral limbs. The movement of digits and tarsus joint are usually synchronized.

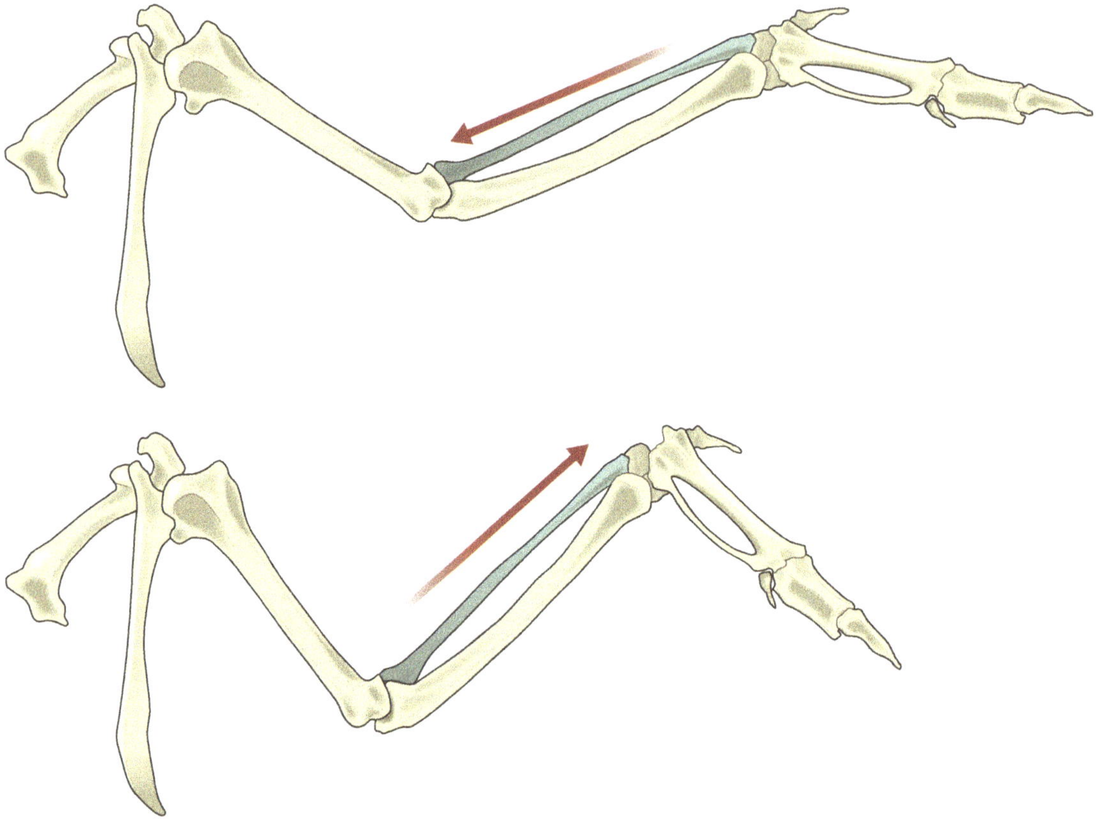

Figure 8.28
Synchronization of the elbow and manus in extension and flexion.

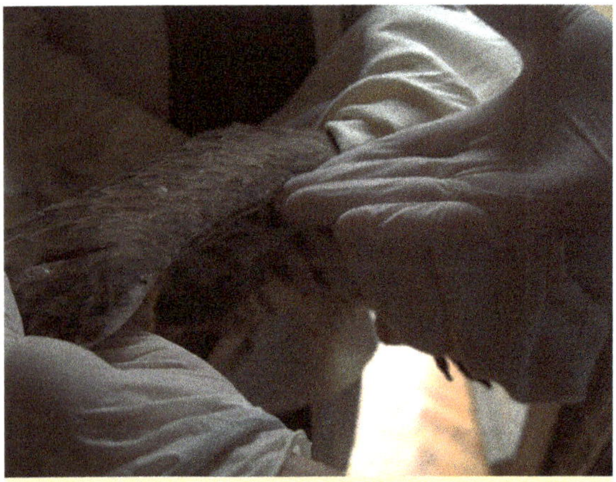

Figure 8.29
Assessing the integrity and tension of the propatagial membrane.

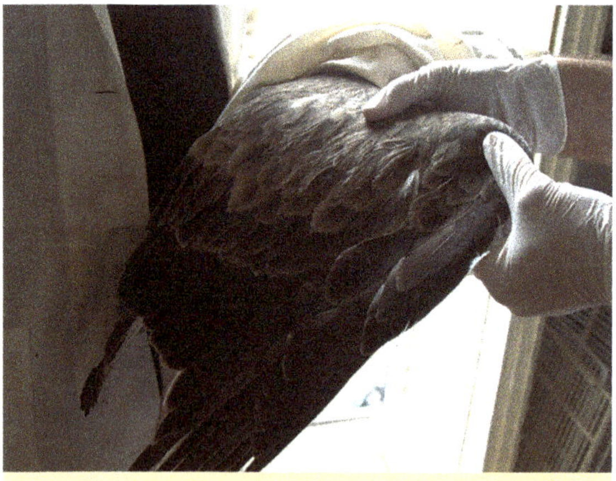

Figure 8.30
Assessing the integrity of the radius and ulna.

When the tarsus flexes or extends, the digits do the same. This action allows many avian species to hold and rest on branches with minimal muscular effort. Digits lock in a flexed position due to skeletal and tendinous structures (Einoder and Richardson 2007). Assess the general muscle tone and the integrity of musculoskeletal structures.

Hip joint. Evaluate the stability and mobility of the hip joint. The hemispherical shape of the femoral head gives the characteristics of a ball-and-socket joint. Assess joint mobility in flexion, extension, abduction, adduction, and rotation.

Knee, tarsus, and digits. Between the tarsus and digits tendons are noted running from attachments to muscles higher up in the limb. Assess mobility of the tarsus and knee in flexion and extension (Fig. 8.33). Assess the integrity of each digit and their mobility in flexion, extension, abduction, adduction and rotation. To extend or flex the digits, positioning of the tarsus in the same position may be necessary. Evaluation of individual interphalangeal joints can be carried out, but does depend on the size of the bird (Fig. 8.34).

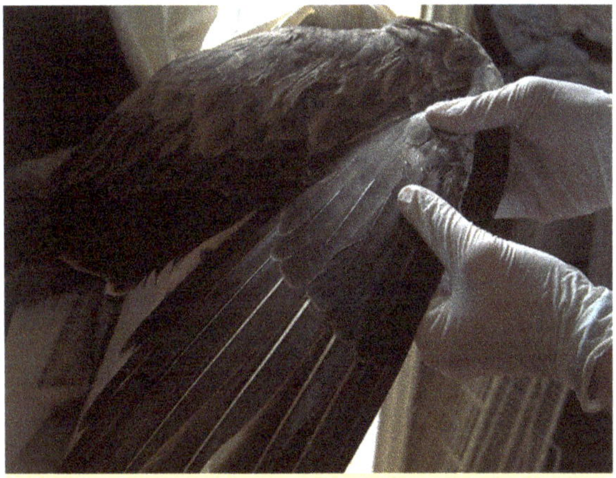

Figure 8.31
Assessing the integrity of the carpometacarpal bone and the mobility of the second digit.

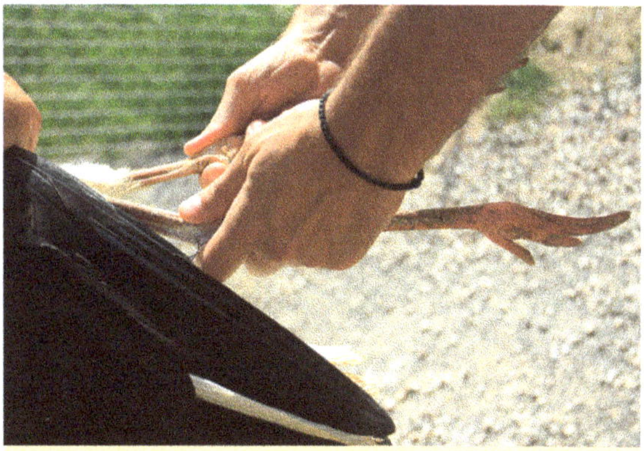

Figure 8.33
Assessing mobility and stability of the tarsus joints.

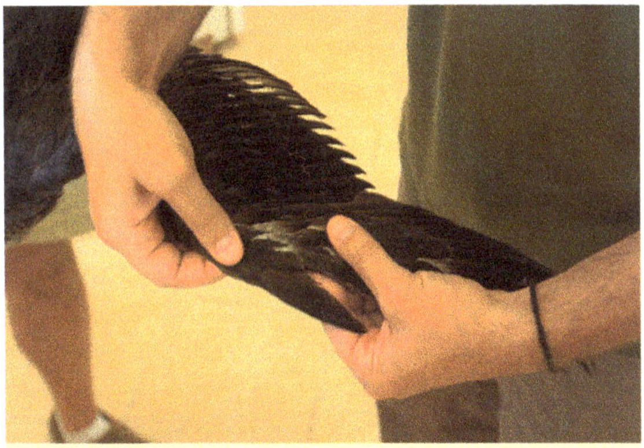

Figure 8.32
Mobilization of the first digit into abduction.

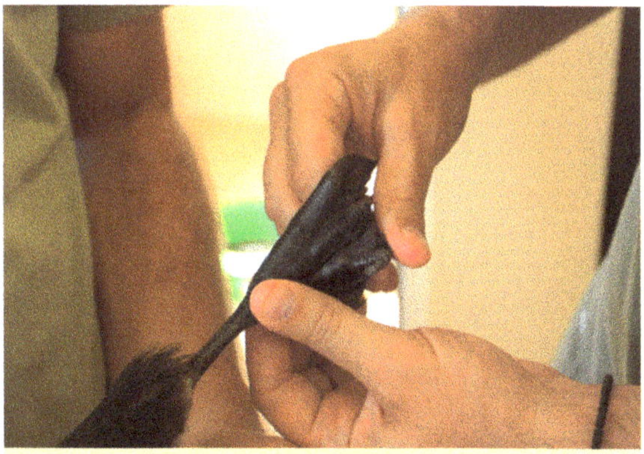

Figure 8.34
Evaluation of the interphalangeal joints into flexion.

Osteopathic treatment

Overview

It must be emphasized that it is in the nature of birds to respond with stress to any human contact so time for evaluation and treatment should be minimal. Thankfully, avian species respond fast to sessions of osteopathic treatment that usually last no more than a few minutes. Signs of tissue-softening, improvement in quantity or quality of movement reveal that tissue change has taken place and treatment is done. Different methods of osteopathic manipulation like functional technique and articulation often combine to provide better results. High velocity thrust technique is unnecessary and generally harmful due to the anatomical delicacy of most species. Always contact with care and avoid any unnecessary handling.

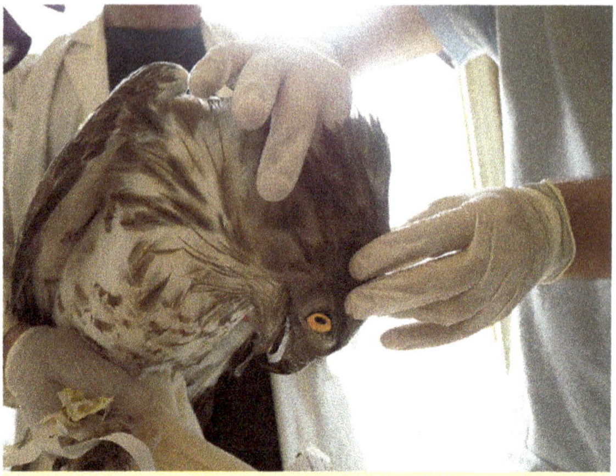

Figure 8.35
Articulation of the occiput.

Cervical spine

The cervical spine is commonly affected by collisions and trauma to the head. Addressing cervical restrictions can assist rehabilitation in cases with mild concussion, torticollis and eye injuries. Severe neurological damage will reduce the speed and degree of improvement.

Articulation and springing. To mobilize the cervical spine, apply springing to the posterolateral part of the vertebrae as explained in the evaluation section of cervical spine. To articulate the cranial cervical spine, you may stabilize the head and mobilize the cranial cervical complex or stabilize C1-C2 and mobilize the head (Fig. 8.35). Any mobilization to the cervical spine, especially of C1-occiput should be done with caution due to the possibility of luxation.

Soft tissue technique. Inhibition of tight cervical paraspinal musculature may be achieved with functional inhibition and during the springing technique phase.

Thorax

Thoracic cage restrictions may be related to conditions involving breathing difficulties, increased sympathetic tone and lack of exercise. Treatments like thoracic pump technique may help in the protection and treatment of aspergillosis, the most common fatal infection in captive birds. Supporting data from osteopathic literature provides evidence that lymphatic pump techniques (LPT) can protect the lungs in small mammals from pulmonary diseases, by increasing the number of circulating leukocytes into the lung (Hodge and Downey 2011). Although there are no data regarding this with avian patients, based on this author's (LC's) experience the technique does appear to help reduce recovery and rehabilitation times.

Thoracic pump technique. The thoracic pump technique can be applied while springing the thorax. At the same time you can test for soft tissue changes and restrictions in the thorax, and treat accordingly. Contact the dorsal spine and the dorsal ribs adjacent to the sternum. To mobilize the upper thoracic cage, spring each side of the cervicodorsal spine in a cranioventral direction while the rest of the finger pads contact the cranial part of the sternum (Fig. 8.36A). To mobilize the lower thoracic cage, contact the caudal part of the sternum with your finger pads and spring with your thumbs each side of the lower thoracic vertebrae, in a caudoventral direction (Fig. 8.36B). The thoracic pump should be rhythmic, fast, and well tolerated by the avian patient. About a

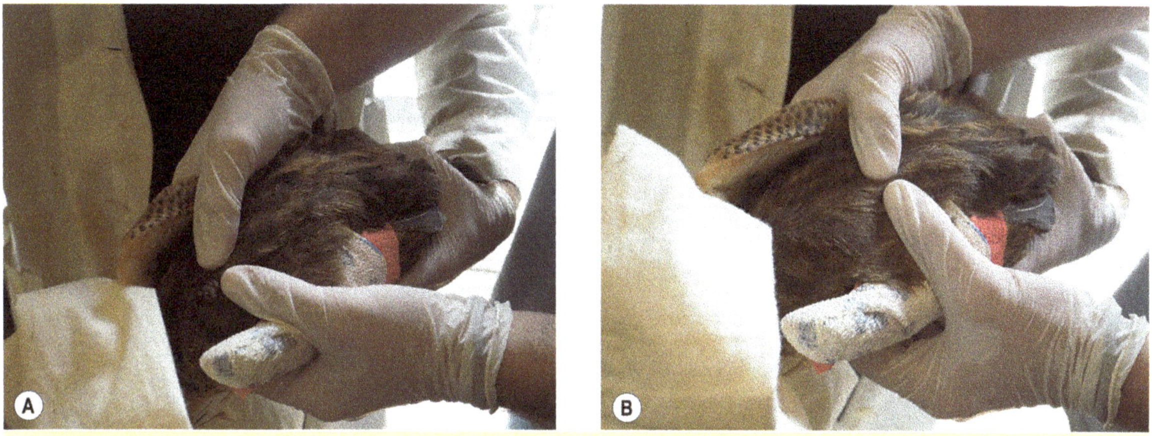

Figure 8.36
Hand position for evaluation and treatment of (A) the cranial thorax and (B) the caudal part of the thorax.

minute of pumping should be enough to improve the quality of restricted thoracic movement and to finish the technique.

Caudal vertebrae

The tail is involved in flight coordination. The caudal vertebrae are also involved with successful copulation and elimination processes.

Articulation. Stabilize the synsacrum and mobilize the last caudal vertebrae into flexion, extension, lateral flexion and rotation (Fig. 8.37). Care should be taken not to damage any of the tail feathers.

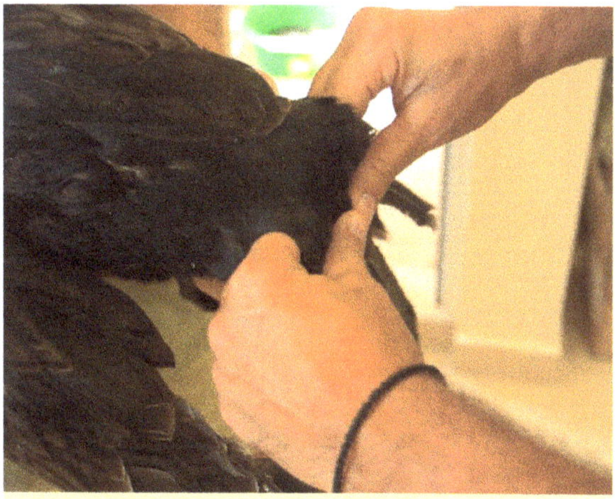

Figure 8.37
Articulation of the tail in flexion.

Pectoral limb

Wing injuries may present as asymmetric wing positioning, inability to fly, and reduced stamina. Any trauma resulting in damage to the musculoskeletal structures or nerves of the wing may render the bird unable to fly. Restrictions of the shoulder, elbow and wrist joint can occur post-traumatically or may be due to prolonged strapping. Remember there is synchronization of movements between pectoral limb joints. Due to this synchronization, any somatic dysfunction to a joint of the pectoral limb may ultimately restrict motion in other joints of the same limb.

Glenohumeral (GH) joint

Trauma and immobilization may cause shortening of pectoral muscles causing limitation of shoulder elevation. Adhesions of metapatagium or propatagium will affect movement of the GH joint and, hence, flight mechanics.

Articulation. Use the wrist joint as a lever to articulate the GH joint through elevation, protraction, retraction, and rotation (Fig. 8.38).

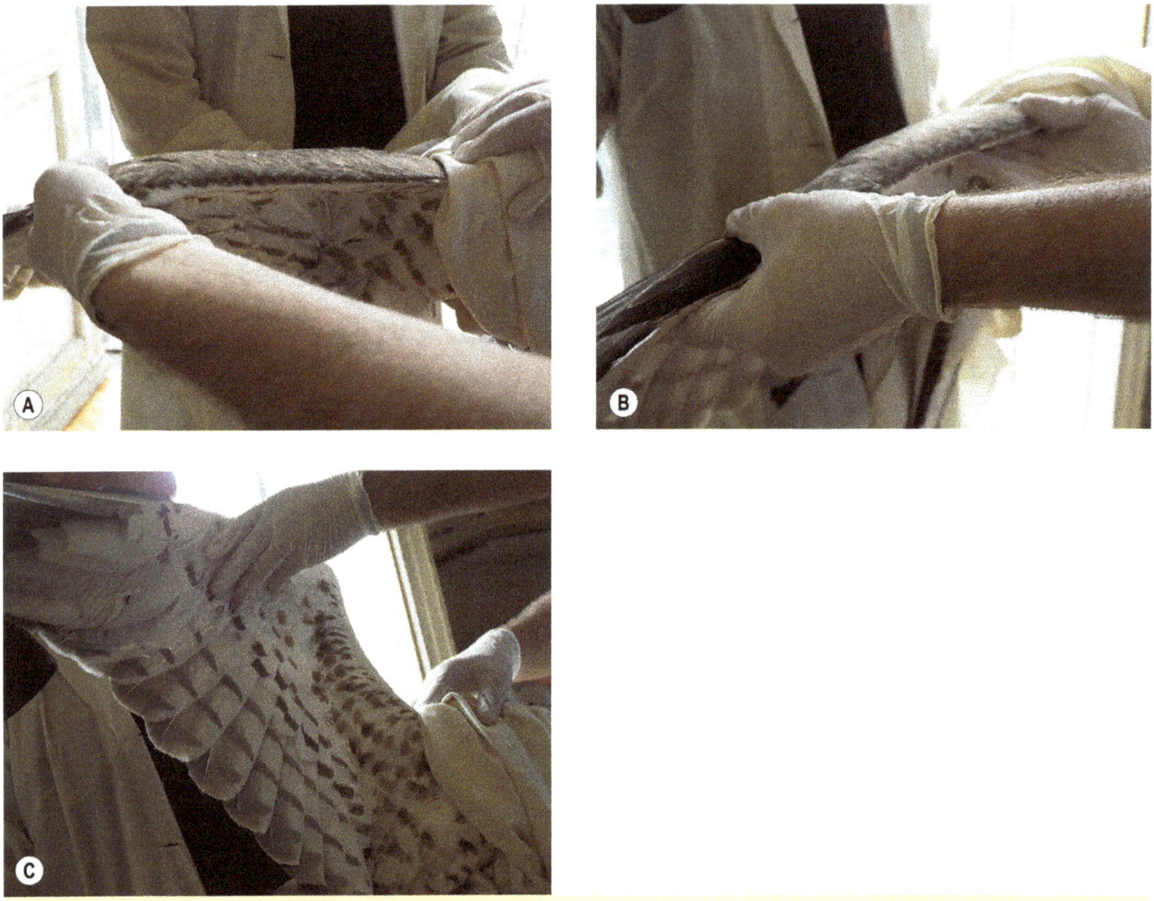

Figure 8.38
(A) Mobilization of the shoulder joint into retraction. (B) Protracting the glenohumeral joint while the other limbs and torso are stabilized by a second operator. (C) Wing elevation with hand contact at the glenohumeral joint and carpometacarpal bone.

Functional technique. Hold the wing at the wrist joint and functionally unwind the GH joint though wing movement.

Soft tissue techniques. Sustained stretch may be used in movement restrictions of the GH joint. When there is a recent injury it is safer to use this technique while the bird is under sedation. Care should be taken not to stretch from the carpometacarpal bone, to avoid damaging the primary feathers.

Elbow joint

Limited elbow extension may be related to functional conditions such as muscle contractures from prolonged strapping, trauma, adhesions of propatagium, and somatic dysfunction of the wrist or radioulnar joint.

Articulation. Hold the wing by the wrist joint or carpometacarpal bone to place the wing perpendicular to the torso. Stretch the wing outward while encouraging extension of the elbow joint (Fig. 8.39). Further elbow extension may be achieved by simultaneously extending the wrist joint.

Radioulnar joint

Myofascial restrictions found between radius and ulna can prevent the parallel gliding of the two bones and

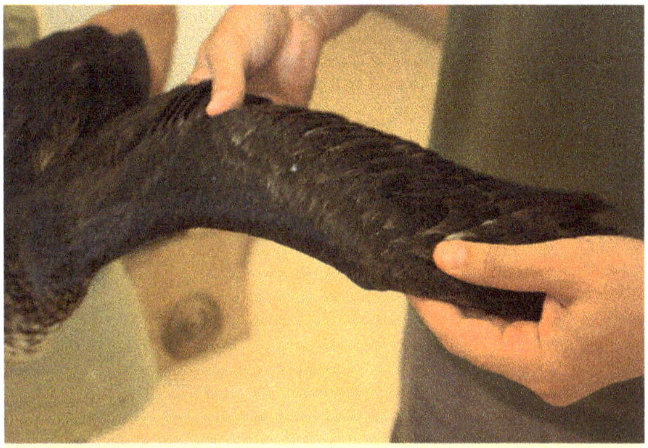

Figure 8.39
Full extension of the elbow joint. Note the hand contact on the elbow joint and carpometacarpal bone.

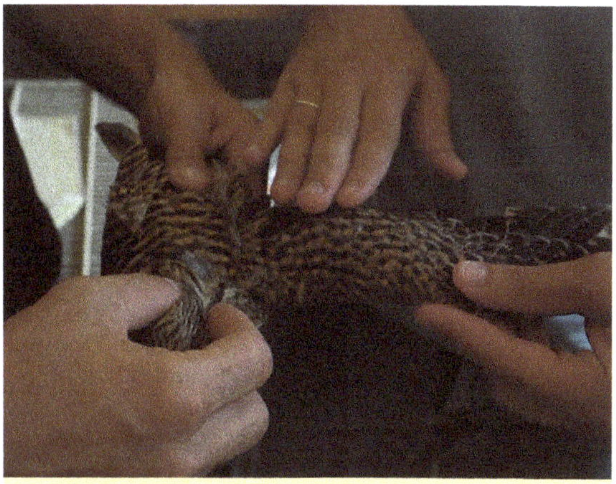

Figure 8.40
Full extension of the wrist and elbow joints. Note the pivoting of the manus with the index finger.

limit optimal elbow and wrist mobility. Synostosis of radius and ulna may occur after fracture and permanently limit optimal elbow and wrist motion.

Functional inhibition. Hypertonic myofascial tissue between radius and ulna can be treated with functional inhibition. Hold the wing by the wrist, moving the wing perpendicular to the torso, keeping the elbow joint in a semi-extended position. Then apply functional inhibition between radius and ulna, gently spreading the two bones apart.

Wrist joint (manus)

Limited extension of the wrist joint may be due to functional conditions like propatagial or metapatagial contractures and somatic dysfunction of the elbow joint and radioulnar interspace.

Articulation. To extend the wrist joint use the carpometacarpal bone to stretch out the wing perpendicular to the torso while simultaneously extending the elbow joint (Fig. 8.40). Rotation of the wrist joint can be achieved by rotating the carpometacarpal bone while stabilizing the forearm and keeping the wrist joint in a semi-extended position (Fig. 8.41).

Digits

Trauma to the digits will affect flight control.

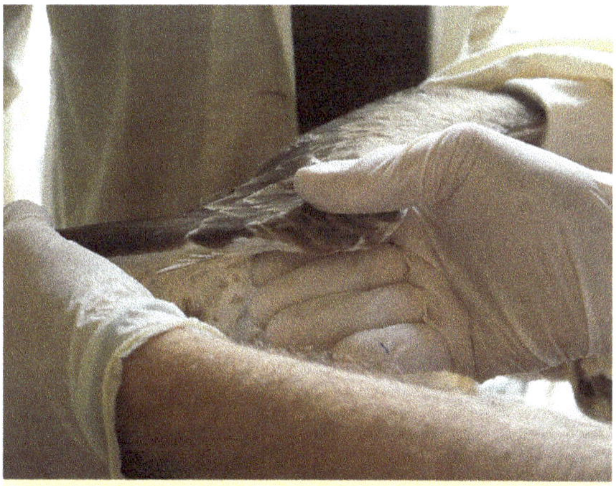

Figure 8.41
Stabilization of the forearm to rotate the wrist joint.

Articulation. Use the carpometacarpal bone to place the wing perpendicular to the torso. Articulate each digit through its physiological movements while keeping the wrist joint placed in a semi-extended position.

Pelvic limb

An inability to perch, walk or swim normally may indicate conditions like musculoskeletal injury, nerve injury, or metabolic- or mineral-related disorders. Malnutrition is a factor which is often seen affecting bone and tendon metabolism in young birds, leading to joint instability and bone deformity. Conditions of functional origin that may limit limb joint mobility include contractures and adhesions of the digital tendons and muscular shortening due to trauma or prolonged immobilization. Optimizing joint mobility increases vascularization aiding rehabilitation.

Hip, knee and tarsal joints

General limb articulation. To articulate the knee and tarsal joints in extension, stabilize the synsacrum and stretch the tarsometatarsal bone caudally (Fig. 8.42A). To articulate the hip, knee and tarsus into flexion, stabilize the synsacrum and elevate the tarsometatarsal bone (Fig. 8.42B). With some practice it becomes easier to focus between the three different joints and treat accordingly. Hip abduction and adduction can be carried out efficiently when combined with vectors of hip extension or flexion.

Sustained stretch. To extend the hip and tarsus (Fig. 8.43), use the tarsometatarsal bone to place first the hip joint in extension and then extend the limb at the tarsus. By locking the tarsus in extension you can extend the hip joint more specifically.

Functional technique. Hold each leg by the tarsometatarsal bone and articulate both legs at the same time but in different directions. When one leg is articulated into tarsal-knee-hip flexion, the other leg is articulated into tarsal-knee-hip extension (Fig. 8.44). This technique is characterized by a constant flowing movement that gently releases restrictions within the

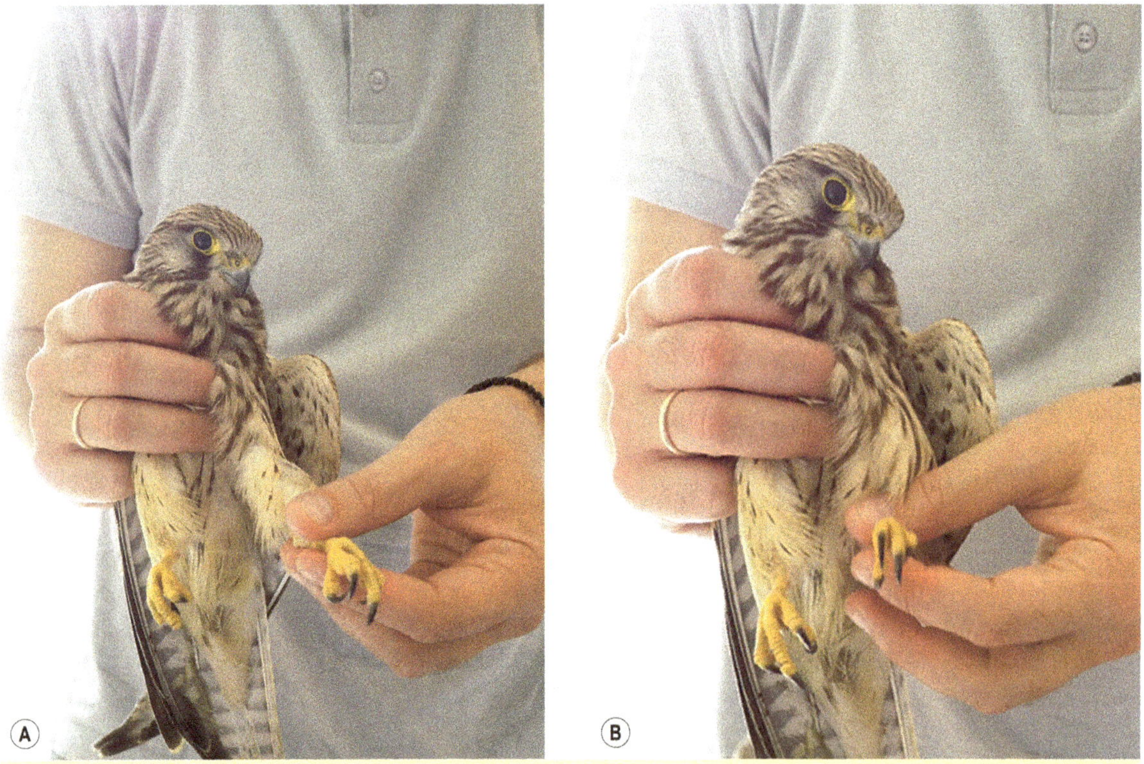

Figure 8.42
(A) Articulation of the tarsus and knee joints into extension. (B) Articulation of the tarsus, knee, and hip joints into flexion.

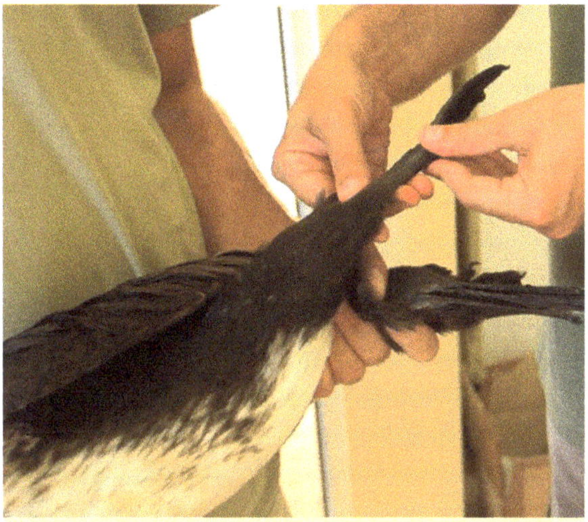

Figure 8.43
Articulation of the hip, knee, and tarsus into extension.

pelvic limbs. Note that this technique may be difficult to perform in large birds and that mobilization of digits is not maximal.

Digits

Restricted mobility in digits may be related to conditions like trauma, inappropriate floor coverings, calluses, and bumblefoot.

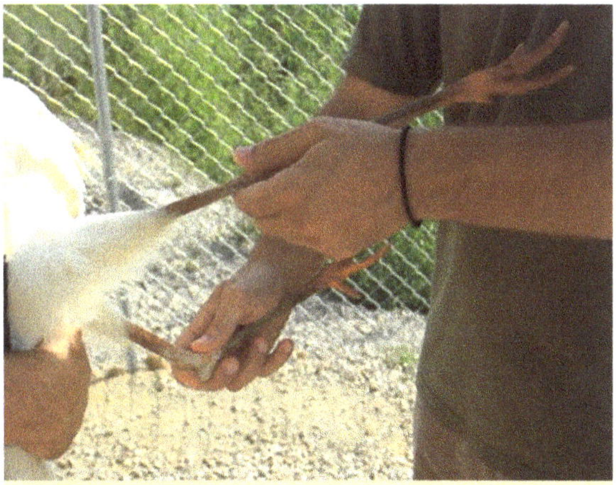

Figure 8.44
Functional technique applied to the pelvic limbs.

Articulation. Stabilize the tarsometatarsal bone and articulate each digit into abduction, adduction, rotation, flexion, and extension (Fig. 8.45). In order to articulate the digits in flexion and extension you may need to synchronize the tarsal joint in the same direction.

Management

Optimal care of wild species involves professional cooperation within a multidisciplinary team that includes veterinarians, technicians, biologists, and rehabilitators. Osteopaths working in the field of wildlife rehabilitation must build an affiliation with the staff and give assistance whenever appropriate.

Most admissions in Hellenic wildlife clinics are due to trauma (Action for Wildlife 2015). Any condition affecting the pectoral limb can lead to serious problems during flight (Beaufrère 2009). It must be remembered that wild birds do not fare well in captivity. Speeding recovery means reduced captivity-related problems like pelvic and pectoral limb trauma, infections, and human familiarization.

Passive mobilization and active exercise speed the process of rehabilitation by improving joint mobility and circulation. Lymphatic techniques may prevent infection or supplement treatment of certain

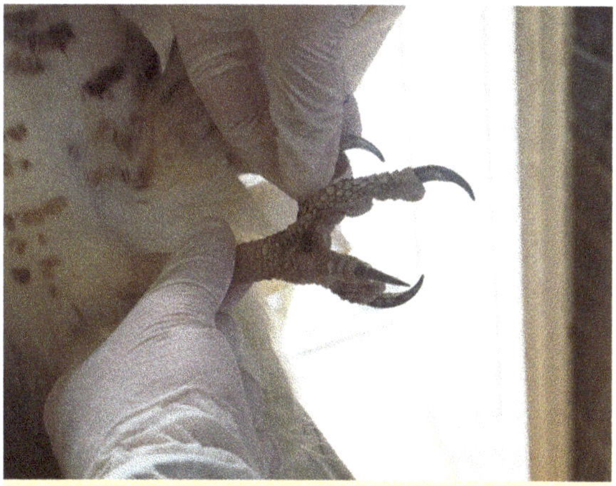

Figure 8.45
Stabilization of the tarsometatarsal bone to extend the third digit.

Table 8.2 Osteopathic treatment considerations and contraindications

Indications	Limitations	Contraindications
Joint restriction due to: musculoskeletal injury immobilization adhesions	Joint restriction due to: osteoarthritis synostosis surgical material	Joint instability due to: fracture luxation ligament rupture
Mild neurological injury: concussions torticollis brachial plexus bruising	Moderate and extensive neurological injury	Acute musculoskeletal injury
Infections: pododermatitis pulmonary disease	Moderate and extensive visceral pathology	Extreme animal stress
	Limited multidisciplinary team cooperation	Lack of veterinary diagnosis

infections. Articulation can be applied and tolerated after the bird has achieved biological stabilization, wound healing, and nutritional management (Table 8.2).

Conditions such as exhaustion, mild cases of soft tissue injury, concussion or nerve bruising can be successfully improved within a short time period. Casualties that are in captivity for only a couple of weeks do not lose significant fitness, but those staying longer require periods of exercise to regain strength and stamina. Flight enclosures provide space for improving proprioceptive control and strength via natural active movements and controlled flights. Fitness levels can be monitored from flight characteristics (length, height, speed) and breathing recovery rate after exercise. Blood lactate levels have also been used to assess fitness of raptors before being released (Chaplin et al. 1993; Holz et al. 2006).

Structural changes like osteoarthritis will limit treatment results. Osteoarthritis will have a detrimental impact on survival of wild birds since they need to be in top condition of fitness. Any fractures close to joints have a poor prognosis for full recovery due to permanent joint restriction. In most avian species the full functioning of both legs is probably not as important as that of the wings (Coles 2007), and a certain amount of leg impairment can be handled by some species.

If we want to prevent injuries, we need to remember that most avian casualties are due to human activities and related obstacles, for example, power cables, glass windows in buildings, car collisions, pollution, and heavy metal poisoning (ANIMA 2015). Various political actions and the educating of future generations are needed to improve the overall plight of avian wildlife.

Case study 8.1

Eurasian marsh harrier (*Circus aeruginosus*)

Signalment

This was a young adult female, with full flight plumage, in good health and condition (BWRC 2017).

History

The patient was found by a member of the public, caught in a barbed wire section of fencing bordering some arable farmland. It was assumed that the bird had been flying low to the ground in typical hunting mode, and that while performing this action she had struck the top wire of a barbed wire fence and become snagged by the right wing, causing a serious soft tissue wound distal to the elbow joint. The bird was examined by a veterinary surgeon at Weirfield Wildlife Hospital, Lincoln, UK. Conservative treatment was given in the form of cleaning the wound, before taping the wing to the bird's body to prevent any further soft tissue trauma to the injury site and placing the bird in a quiet, darkened cage to allow her to rest and recuperate.

Osteopathic treatment was advised once the taping was removed.

Presenting signs

The bird presented with increased resting tone in the cervical musculature, which was worse on the right, reduced extension to the elbow, and some soft tissue swelling around the glenohumeral joint. There was a mild fascial element with a pattern of recoil from the whole of the right wing, with a right rotational pull through the body of the patient (Fig. 8.46).

The bird was alert and showed very mild signs of stress when handled (Fig. 8.47). This was noted to ensure that examination and treatment contact time was kept to an absolute minimum.

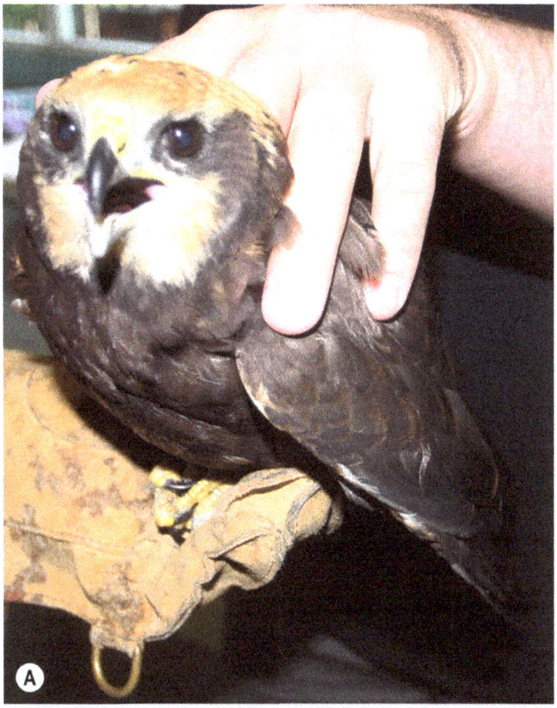

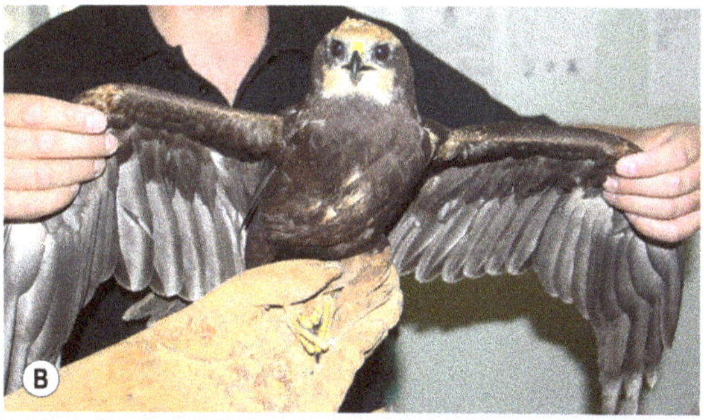

Figure 8.46
(A) Palpating the cervical spine. (B) Assessing wing symmetry.

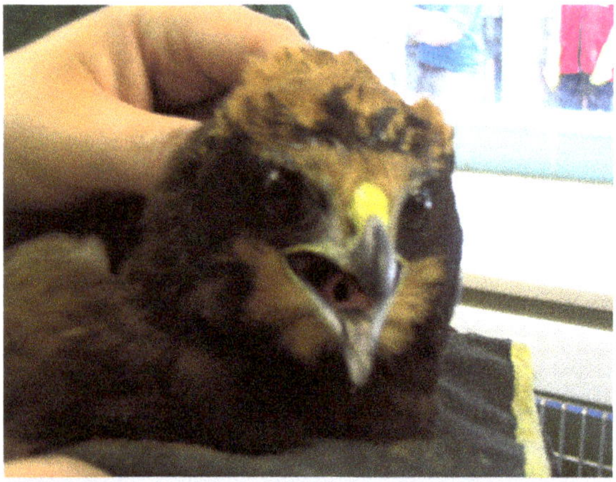

Figure 8.47
Mouth gaping – a sign of stress during examination.

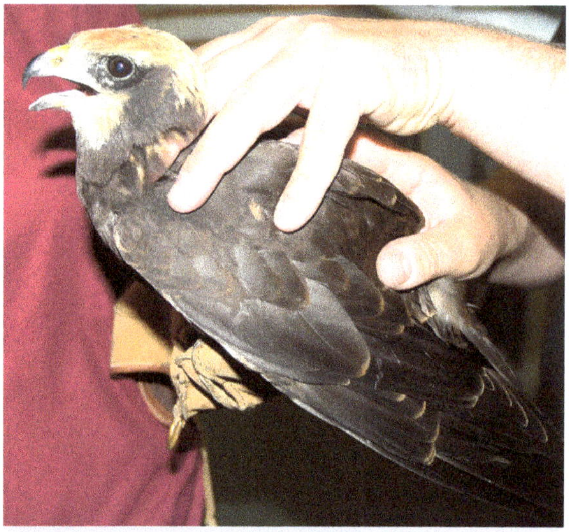

Figure 8.48
Applying a mix of functional and sustained positional release techniques.

Osteopathic treatment

Due to the need for any raptor to have pristine plumage in order to hunt, the author (TN) elected to use techniques that would minimize any disruption to feather integrity. Therefore a blend of functional and myofascial release work was combined with creating a temporary still point within the involuntary mechanism (IVM) of the patient (Fig. 8.48).

A second operator restrained the patient via its talons, while also ensuring that the healthy wing was controlled when the author was not handling it. Lighting in the hospital was dimmed and noise was kept to a minimum to help reduce any further stress to the patient.

This combination of osteopathic techniques allows for short, gentle treatment sessions that have been noted to aid recovery rates of wild raptor patients in the UK (BWRC [n.d.]). The initial session lasted around five minutes after which the patient was placed back in her cage with a towel placed over the front of the mesh door to give her further peace and quiet.

The next session was performed two weeks later. There was a marked increase in left elbow movement and the torsion pattern through the body of the raptor was greatly reduced. The soft tissues had a much healthier, elastic feel and the patient was not stressed when examined and then treated. Treatment followed the lines of the initial session, with the addition of some controlled wing-strengthening exercises. These were to be introduced prior to moving the patient to a prerelease flight aviary, to allow her to build up strength and stamina before her return to the wild.

The exercises involved a handler holding the patient via the distal parts of the legs and allowing her to extend and flap her wings. To encourage the wing movements, the handler was to move their extended and abducted arm (with the bird held in their grasp) up and down in a vertical plane of about 30 cm. The bird's instinct is to stabilize itself, and hence wing movement is initiated (Fig. 8.49).

Outcome

The author was only required to perform two osteopathic treatments, after which a member of the hospital staff was able to perform daily wing-strengthening exercises for a week. The patient was then transferred to a flight aviary where she spent a further week, before being successfully released back into the wild at a site where she could be monitored and where food was put out in the form of day-old chicks

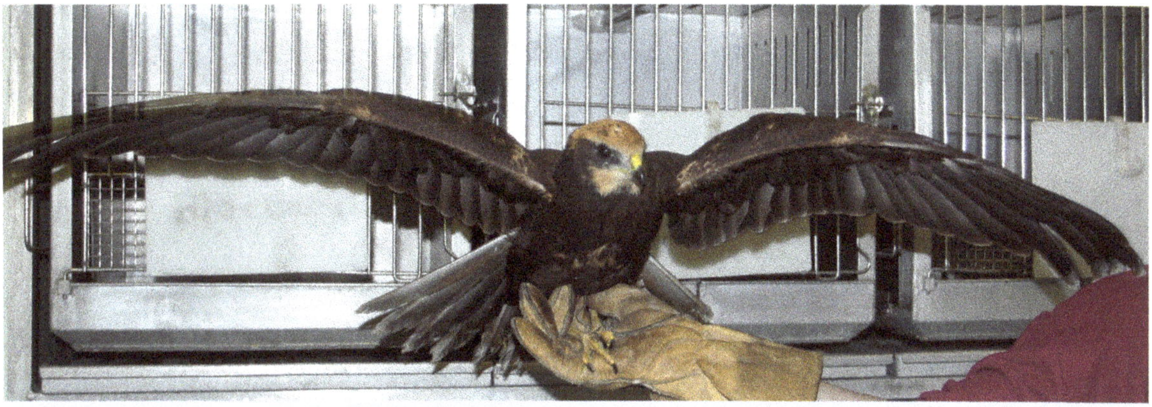

Figure 8.49
Encouraging wing use to aid balance in a rehabilitating marsh harrier prior to introduction to a flight aviary.

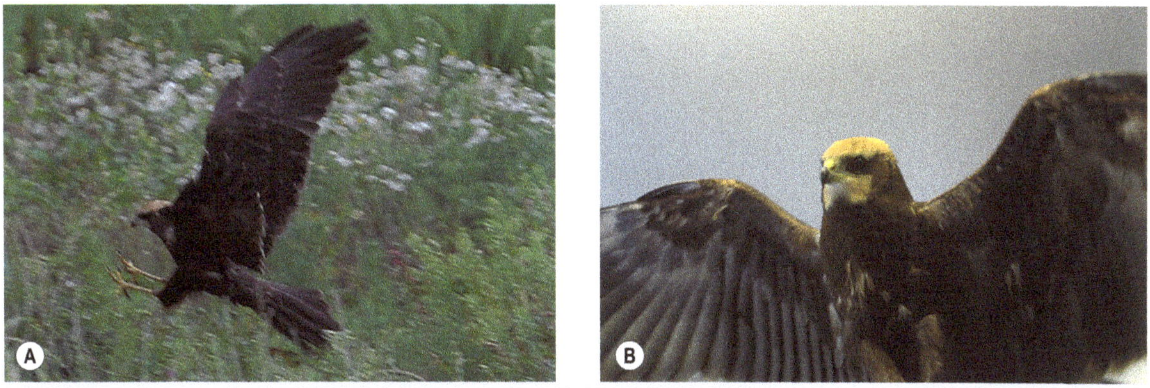

Figure 8.50
(A) A marsh harrier immediately taking to the wing once released into the wild and (B) gaining height once released back into the wild.

until she no longer returned for these. The monitoring ceased after seven days, as food was not being taken; however, there was a marsh harrier spotted in the area regularly during and after this period, and it was assumed (due to their relative scarcity at the time) that this was the patient (Fig. 8.50).

Conclusions

Osteopathic intervention can be used to assist recovery and rehabilitation of certain avian patients. It is best used in collaboration with other professionals such as veterinary surgeons and the all-important wildlife hospitals. These cases are time-consuming and, due to the complexities of flight dexterity that raptors require, can involve complex and intricate treatment programs. This has to be weighed up against the need to keep stress to the wild patient minimal. Osteopathy is justified when stress can be minimized and treatment can reduce the overall rehabilitation time frame.

Case study 8.2

European white stork (*Ciconia ciconia*)

Signalment

Adult male.

History

An adult male white stork presented with an inability to fly.

Veterinary evaluation

Closed fracture of right humerus.

Veterinary intervention

Surgery was performed with external fixation. Antibiotics were given for seven days (marbofloxacin 10 mg/kg IM and clindamycin 50 mg/kg per os). Anti-inflammatory drugs (meloxicam) were administered for three days starting on the day of surgery. The wing was put in a splint and the bird placed in a box to restrict wing movements for three days. On the third day the splint was removed and the patient was referred for osteopathic treatment to reduce soft tissue contractures.

Osteopathic evaluation

Mobility evaluation revealed pronounced restriction of extension of the elbow and manus of the injured limb. This is not usual as a humerus with external fixation should not affect elbow and wrist joint mobility.

Osteopathic intervention

Gentle articulation and stretching of elbow, manus, and shoulder joints was performed twice a week for six weeks, lasting approximately two to three minutes. In order to stretch the tissue more effectively, articulation and stretching may be carried out under sedation, reducing the bird's agitation and possible disarrangement of the external fixation (Fig. 8.51).

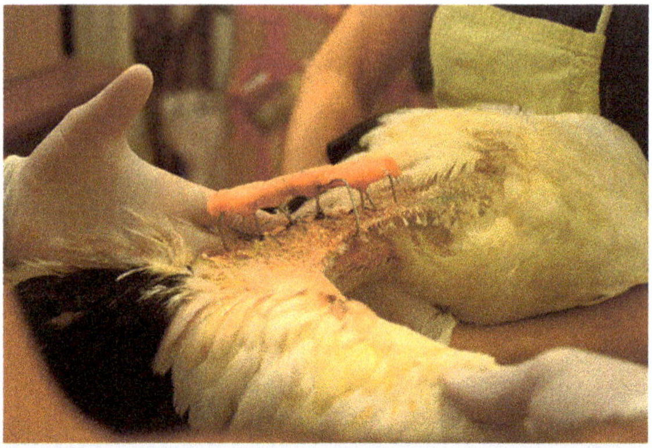

Figure 8.51
Articulation of the glenohumeral joint in protraction and elbow joint in extension.

Initial results

After initial treatments pectoral limb movements improved. The manus and elbow joints still showed marked restriction in extension.

Follow-up

Further change was not evident after the first two weeks of treatment. Radiographs acquired at the third week showed callous formation at the site of the fracture and the external fixation was removed after a few days. Evaluation of mobility still revealed markedly restricted extension of the elbow and manus - about 60 percent of normal joint motion. The bird was placed inside an open-roof aviary, close to wetland, for a soft release program. The bird was properly socializing with birds of the same species on the ground, stretching and strengthening his wings naturally. In the sixth week the mobility had greatly improved to about 90 percent of normal movement. In the seventh week the bird was able to jump out of the open-roof aviary and test his flying abilities around the wetland area (Fig. 8.52).

Conclusions

It seems the fracture had been present for some time, and the contracted tissues were not maximally

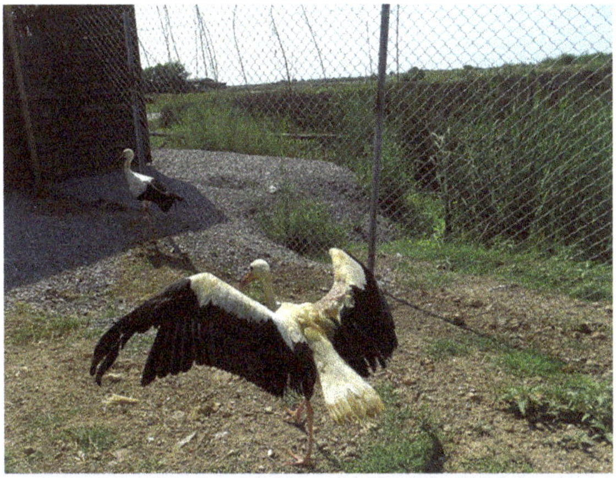

Figure 8.52
Socialization and active movement inside an open-roof aviary.

released before the surgery. In this case the patient did not respond with marked soft tissue release following osteopathic manipulation. Active movements in the open-roof aviary, however, allowed the bird to stretch his elbow and wrist almost to the maximum and fly off the ground. He will need 100 percent mobility, fitness, and reserves in order to have a good chance to migrate successfully, although the wetland where he has been released is a natural habitat where he can stay and breed.

Summary

- This is an area of osteopathic medicine where very small amounts of treatment can result in huge changes to a patient - for better or for worse.
- Birds come in all shapes and sizes. They have very different anatomical structures and internal organs, which make them very challenging to treat.
- Many species of bird are so shy that handling of any kind must be weighed up against the possibility of causing death by stress. This is true of most wild vultures (Accipitridae and Cathartidae).
- Species such as owls have specialized feathers (that are very quiet when the bird is in flight), but can be easily damaged during handling or by getting them wet. This is in stark contrast to waterfowl, which have evolved methods of waterproofing at the expense of noise reduction. These factors all make avian work much more interesting and rewarding for the osteopath.
- Feathers pose an incredible problem when palpating and require the osteopath to exert extreme care so as not to damage the intricate matrix within each feather and the layers of feathers that are essential to a bird's survival and well-being.
- The same applies to any hands-on treatment given. Primary flight feathers can take several months to grow back when damaged, and if the patient is a wildlife casualty this may spell the end of them if they need to be kept in captivity for a very long period of time.
- Osteopathic principles can be applied successfully and have been shown to dramatically reduce recovery times in wildlife casualties (Nevin 1999, 2012). They have also proved to be useful with domestic and exotic pet species, with specialist avian vets using the skills of a competent osteopath.
- In the zoo world, in the author's (TN's) experience, there have been modest inroads made, especially when assisting problem chicks in captive breeding programs and with certain postoperative rehabilitation cases (Figs 8.53, 8.54).

Most data regarding the osteopathic treatment of birds has been collected from wildlife casualties treated at wildlife hospitals in the UK and in Greece (authors' own data). Treatment efficacy has been compared with similar cases that did not receive osteopathic treatment but were treated in standard ways according to wildlife casualty protocols (BWRC, RSPCA, and ANIMA [Greek wildlife protection agency] guidelines).

As with all aspects of osteopathic medicine please remember that less really does equal more when it comes to applied treatment (Fig. 8.55).

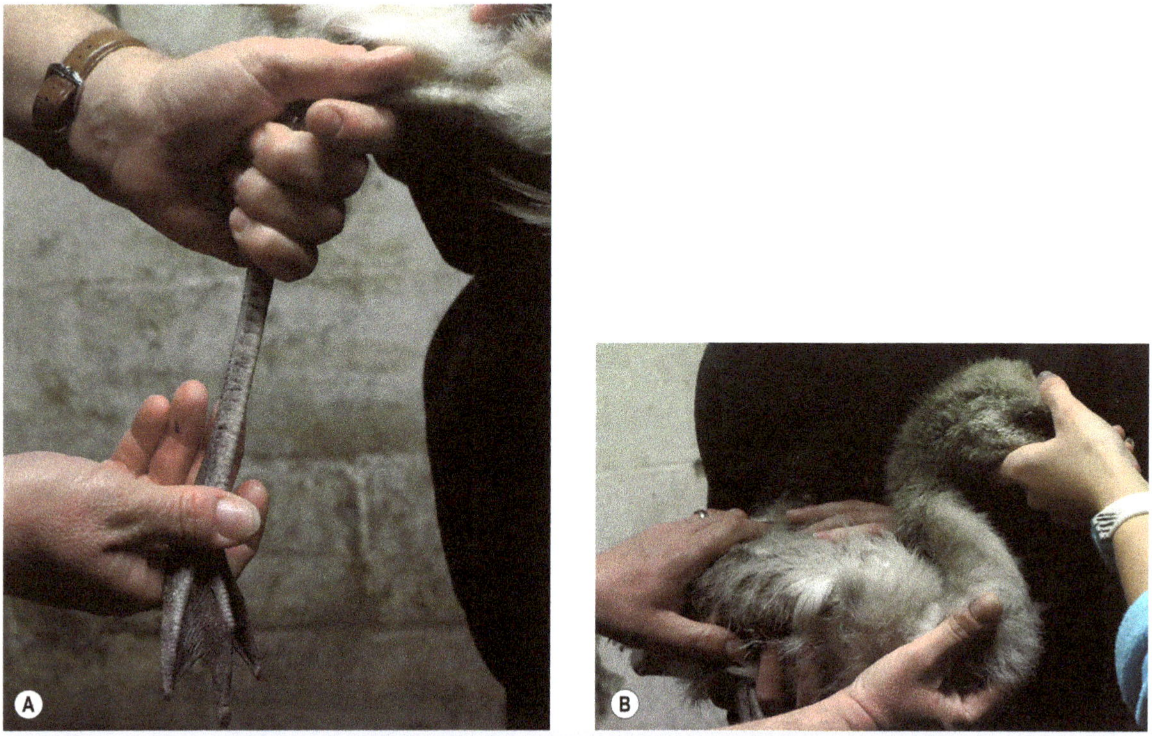

Figure 8.53
Assessing torsional deformity in a juvenile flamingo (A) and applying functional release work through myofascial lines (B).

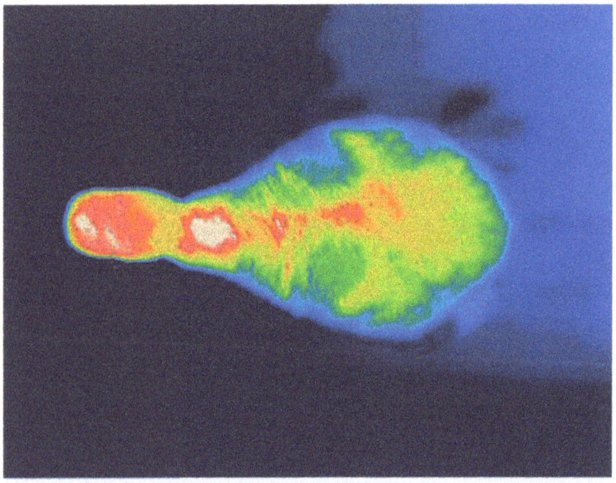

Figure 8.54
An infrared thermal image viewed from above of a flamingo chick.

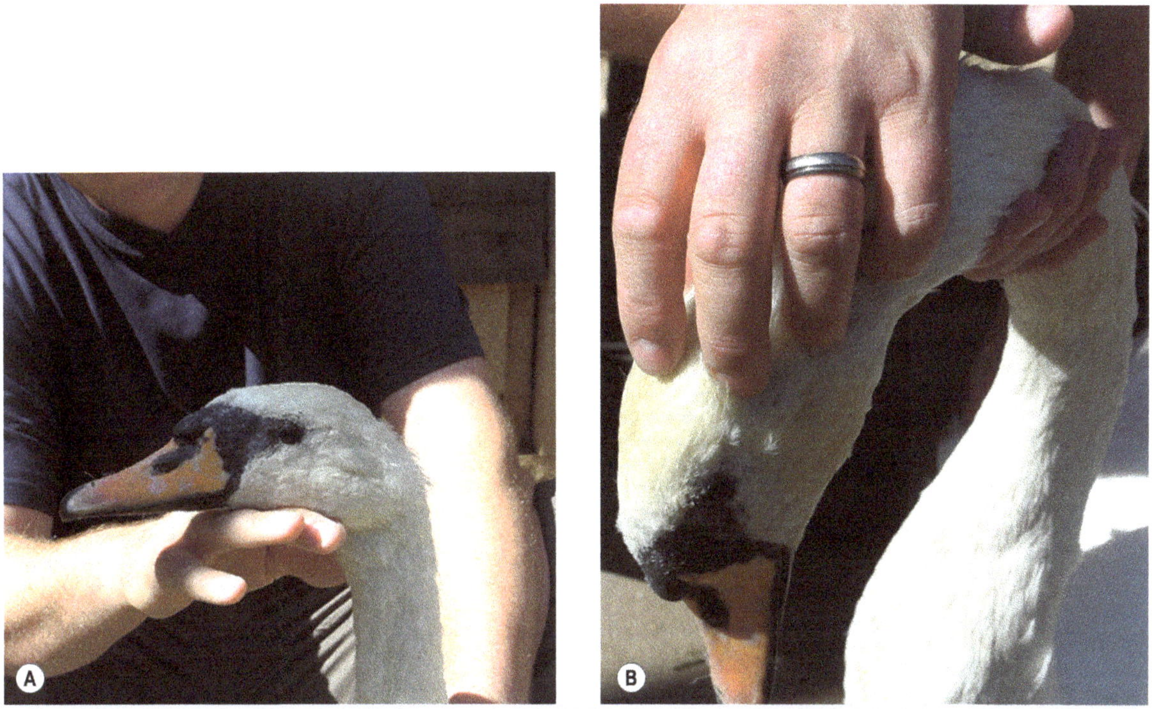

Figure 8.55
(A) Using minimal contact to apply functional release technique through the cervical spine of a rehabilitating mute swan (*Cygnus olor*). (B) Engaging with the involuntary mechanism (IVM) of an injured mute swan.

References

Action for Wildlife, Thessaloniki, Greece (2015) Discussion on citation and referencing. Personal communication [November 30, 2015].

ANIMA [Greek wildlife protection agency] At: https://www.wild-anima.gr/synergasies/elliniki-ornithologiki-eteria/ [May 16, 2018].

ANIMA [Greek Wildlife protection agency] (2015) Discussion on citation and referencing. Personal communication [November 12, 2015].

Beaufrère H (2009) A review of biomechanics and aerodynamics considerations of the avian thoracic limb. Journal of Avian Medicine and Surgery. September; 23 (3) 173–185.

BWRC – British Wildlife Rehabilitation Council [n.d] Unpublished symposium presentation. Data available on request from: http://www.bwrc.org.uk [May 16, 2018].

BWRC – British Wildlife Rehabilitation Council (2010) Gower Bird Hospital Study. Unpublished symposium presentation. Data available on request from: http://www.bwrc.org.uk [May 16, 2018].

BWRC – British Wildlife Rehabilitation Council Guidelines for Wildlife Rehabilitation Units. Available: http://bwrc.org.uk/#/guidelines/4549073116 [May 16, 2018].

Chaplin S, Mueller L, Degernes L (1993) Chapter 29 Physiological assessment of rehabilitated raptors prior to release. In: Redig, P, Cooper J, Remple J D, Hunter B (eds) Raptor Biomedicine. Minneapolis: University of Minnesota Press, p. 167.

Christodoularis L (2012) Osteopathic contribution in the well-being of raptors. The First International Congress of Osteopathy in Animal Practice, Rome. Available: http://www.congressodiosteopatia.it/congresso_osteopatia_veterinaria/eng/program.html [May 16, 2018].

Coles B (2007) Essentials of Avian Medicine and Surgery. 3rd edn. Oxford: Blackwell Publishing, p. 52, p. 213.

Einoder L, Richardson A (2007) The digital tendon locking mechanism of owls: variation in structure and arrangement of the mechanism and function implication. Emu. January; 107 223–230.

Hodge L, Downey H (2011) Lymphatic pump treatment enhances the lymphatic and immune systems. Experimental Biology and Medicine. August; 236 (10) 1109–1115.

Holz P, Naisbitt R, Mansell P (2006) Fitness level as a determining factor in the survival of rehabilitated peregrine falcons and brown goshawks released back into the wild. Journal of Avian Medicine and Surgery. March; 20 (1) 15–20.

Kaiser G (2008) The Inner Bird: Anatomy and Evolution. Vancouver: UBC Press. Chapter 2, p. 69.

Martin H, Ringdahl C, Scherpelz J (1993) Physical therapy for specific injuries in raptors. In: Redig P, Cooper J, Remple JD, Hunter B (eds) Raptor Biomedicine. Minneapolis: University of Minnesota Press, Chapter 36, pp. 207–210.

Nevin A (1999) Osteopathy for birds. Wildaid Conference, Inverness.

Nevin A (2012) Osteopathy and birds – a global approach. The First International Congress of Osteopathy in Animal Practice, Rome. Available: http://www.congressodiosteopatia.it/congresso_osteopatia_veterinaria/eng/program.html [May 16, 2018].

O'Malley B (2005) Clinical Anatomy and Physiology of Exotic Species: Structure and Function of Mammals, Birds, Reptiles and Amphibians. Elsevier Saunders, Chapter 6.

Proctor NS, Lynch P (1993) Manual of Ornithology: Avian Structure and Function. Yale University Press, p. 136.

RSPCA – Royal Society for the Prevention of Cruelty to Animals. At: https://www.rspca.org.uk/home [May 16, 2018].

Vazquez RJ (1992) Functional osteology of the avian wrist and the evolution of flapping flight. Journal of Morphology. March; 211 (3) 259–268.

Videler J (2005) Avian Flight. Oxford: Oxford University Press, Chapter 7, p. 100.

Further reading

Chitty J, Lierz M (2008) BSAVA Manual of Raptors, Pigeons and Passerine Birds, BSAVA.

King AS, McLelland J (1989) Form and Function in Birds, Vol. 3. Academic Press Inc.

Mullineaux E, Best R, Cooper J (2003) Manual of British Wildlife Casualties. BSAVA.

O'Malley B (2005) Clinical Anatomy and Physiology of Exotic Species: Structure and Function of Mammals, Birds, Reptiles and Amphibians. Elsevier Saunders, Chapter 6.

Thompson EE (1996) Anatomy of Animals: Studies in the Forms of Mammals and Birds. Bracken Books.

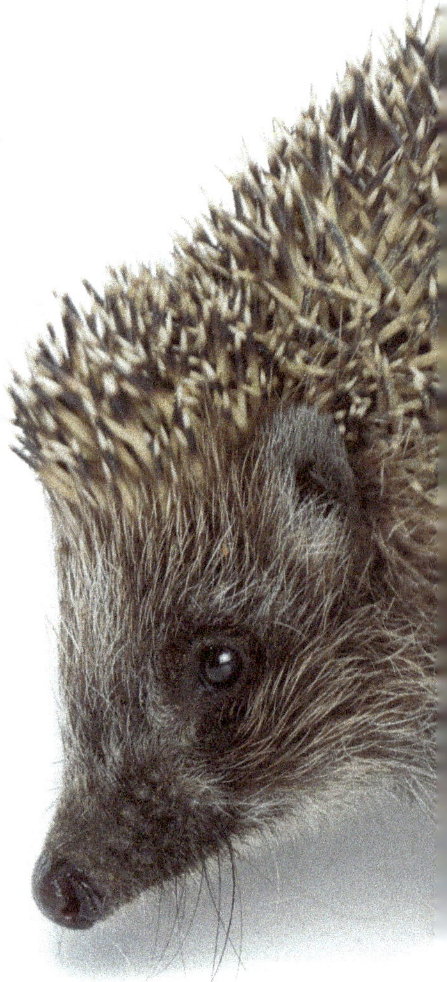

Chapter 9 SMALL WILDLIFE AND EXOTICS

Tony Nevin, Sophia Prousali, Caroline Gould, Leonidas Christodoularis

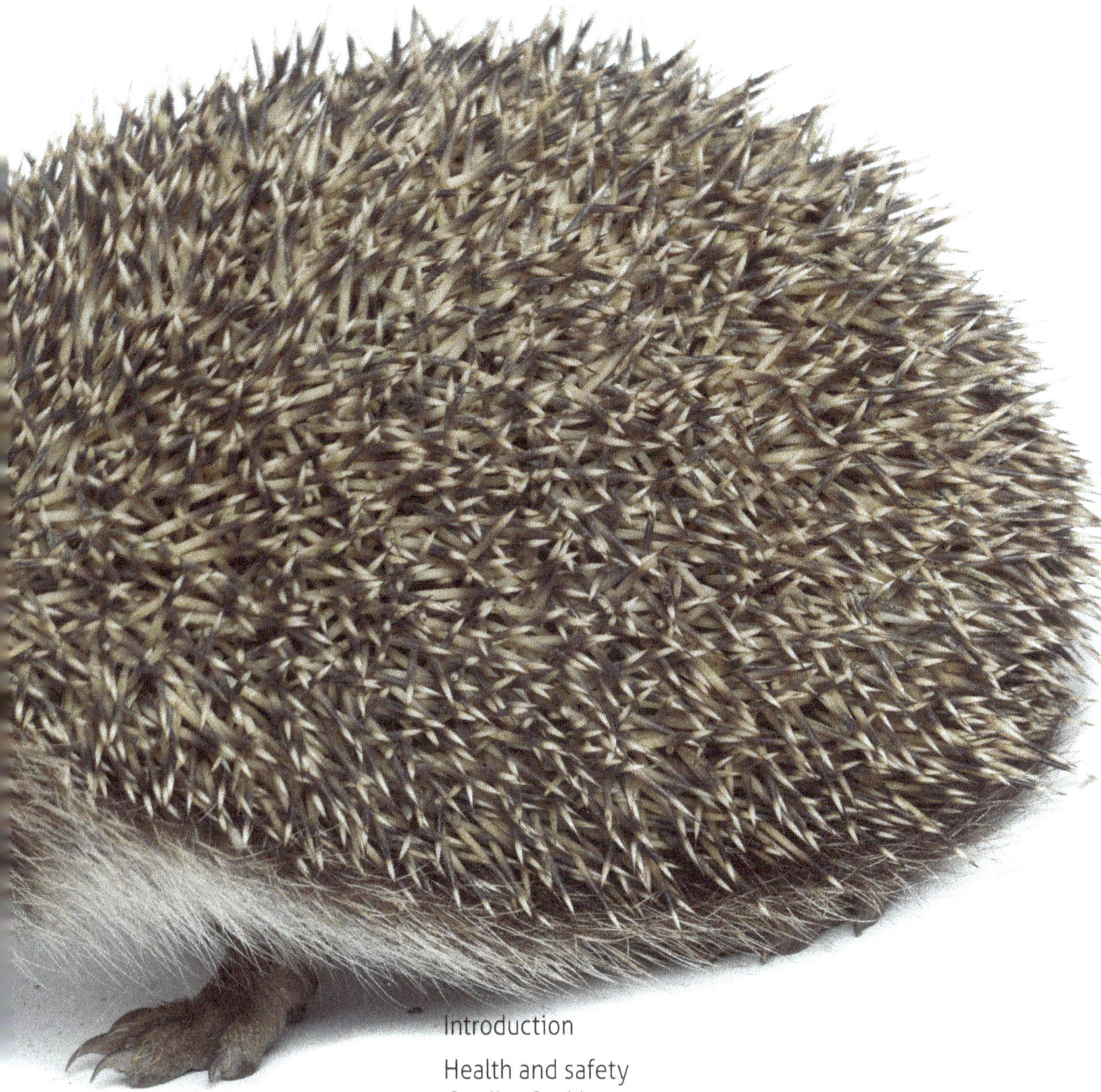

Small wildlife and exotics

Introduction

This chapter is aimed at introducing and helping the postgraduate osteopath to apply his or her skills to help injured and orphaned wildlife. There are certain aspects to this that pose challenges for the osteopath. One of the main differences to other animal treatment work is in the requirement to aid in the rehabilitation of these patients to a level that will allow them to survive and thrive once returned to the wild.

Many of these patients will have received veterinary treatment including surgical intervention. The role of the osteopath is to reduce the recovery and rehabilitation phase for the patient with minimal contact. This last statement cannot be overemphasized. Most wild creatures will soon become less afraid of humans if they experience repeated contact. Osteopaths therefore must be extremely careful not to spend any more time than is absolutely necessary in physical contact with or in close visual proximity to these patients. We need to consider our patients' acute senses. Sight, sound, and smell are very much more sensitive than our own therefore all noise, from speech to slamming doors and heavy footsteps, needs to be avoided. Allowing wild patients continuously to see humans is not good, and the use of perfumes and aftershave lotions that are scented really needs to be avoided, along with perfumed soaps, etc.

To avoid overlap with other chapters, this chapter does not cover reptile and avian patients. For guidance on working with reptile and avian wildlife see Chapters 7 and 8 respectively.

Except for a few cases most wildlife casualties that an osteopath is likely to see will fall into one of two categories:

1. *Physical trauma resulting in actual injury.* These can be man-made, such as those involving a road traffic accident (RTA), illegal shooting or poisoning. They may also be due to other animals, domestic or wild, or as a result of weather-related problems, such as floods, severe storms or drought.
2. *Nonphysical trauma resulting in psychosomatic or viscerosomatic problems.* This can be the result of human activity, such as noise or light pollution, destruction of suitable habitat resulting in man-wildlife conflict, or can be due to hunting or predation of their parents in the case of orphans. This includes poaching.

A useful mantra to remember when working with wildlife is that of the four Fs as outlined in Chapter 8 but worth repeating here:

Find the problem - observation.

Feel the problem - palpation.

Fix the problem - osteopathic treatment.

Free the patient - facilitate its successful return to the wild.

Health and safety

The handling of wild animals, even though many are fairly small and appear harmless, is the first subject that needs to be addressed (Table 9.1). Learning the hard way is not recommended.

Table 9.1 Guidelines for the capture, handling, and transportation of small wild animal patients

Species or type of mammal	Capture guidelines	Methods of transportation	Defenses to beware of
Small mammals (mice, voles, bats, etc.)	Small net Towel, tea towel or similar Wear strong gloves	Secure plastic tank (covered with towel or similar)	Teeth (rodent teeth inflict painful bites)
Polecats, weasels, and stoats (mustelids) Squirrels	Suitable net Towel Wear strong gloves	Secure plastic tank (covered with towel or similar) Wire carrier (small mesh)	Teeth (serious bites) Very fast, difficult to handle
Hedgehogs, rabbits, and hares	Blanket or towel Wear gloves Suitable net (rabbits and hares)	Covered box or pet carrier with air holes Vari Kennel® or similar	Bites and scratches Hind feet (lagomorphs kick)

Species or type of mammal	Capture guidelines	Methods of transportation	Defenses to beware of
Foxes, badgers, and otters	Grasper, bite stick Large net Large towel or blanket Wear strong gloves	Suitably sized, strong Vari Kennel® Large cat cage or crush cage Cover carrier with towel or blanket	Teeth (serious bites)
Deer	Minimum of two people needed Large net Towel, blanket or pillowcase to cover head Restrain legs and feet Control head	Large Vari Kennel® (for smaller deer) Stretcher (or blanket) May require sedation	Feet (powerful hind legs in particular) Antlers Teeth or tusks (muntjac deer)

Table 9.1 *Continued*

- A suitable nonslip floor covering such as toweling should always be used to line carriers.
- There is a potential risk from zoonotic diseases or infections when handling *any* wildlife.
- Some mammals may appear tame if in shock. Do not take any risks.

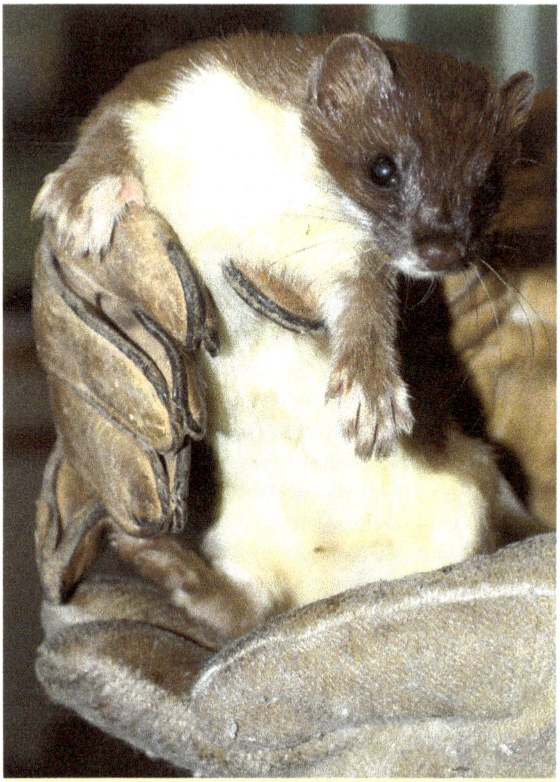

Figure 9.1
The use of stout gloves is recommended when handling and treating mustelids, even small ones like this juvenile stoat.

Another important consideration when dealing with wild animals is the risk of zoonotic diseases. A common-sense approach to minimizing risks is usually all that is necessary. Wear gloves whenever possible and practical, and always ensure that you wash your hands with an antibacterial handwash after handling or cleaning of animals and cages. Make sure that any existing cuts, grazes or breaks in your skin are completely covered, and if you do get bitten or scratched by an animal immediately wash the area thoroughly with an antibacterial solution and then cover it when handling or cleaning animals (Fig. 9.1).

Bear in mind that some diseases, for example, bovine tuberculosis (bTB), can be spread via droplets in the air expelled by infected animals. Badgers are not the only animals susceptible to bTB. Any mammal can catch the disease and it has been widely reported in deer and even hedgehogs. You may therefore want to consider the use of face masks if there is a risk of tuberculosis.

For those dealing with hedgehogs on a regular basis, ringworm is one of the most common diseases encountered. The wearing and subsequent disposal of disposable gloves is recommended when handling hedgehogs.

Anatomy

Introduction

The skeletal structure and basic physiological functions of wild animals do not differ significantly from those of domestic ones of the same taxonomic order or family. Minor differences do occur since every species is anatomically and physiologically adjusted to its own needs for survival.

In this chapter basic elements of biology, anatomy, and physiology of the smaller wild animals commonly seen as casualties are presented. Becoming familiar with the specific variations seen in these animals is essential in facilitating our efforts to help them. Some of the most frequent wild casualties seen in wildlife rehabilitation centers or veterinary clinics are hedgehogs, badgers, otters (and other Mustelidae), foxes, and deer.

Southern white-breasted hedgehog (*Erinaceus concolor*)

Hedgehogs belong to the order Insectivora which means that their main food source is insects. They do, however, occasionally eat other animal foods like eggs, small mammals, reptiles, and carrion (Step 1921). Other important elements of the hedgehog's biology are that it is a nocturnal animal and that it hibernates during winter months.

The dorsal surface of a hedgehog's body is covered by a spiny coat, but the abdominal surface is not. On the dorsal surface the hairs have been modified to spines (Vincent and Owers 1986). Fur still exists on the head, chest, belly, and limbs (Fig. 9.2). The spines are an adaptation to deter predators in conjunction with the hedgehog's ability to roll up. Spines (as well as hairs) are shed and regrow (Mullineaux et al. 2003, p. 50). Spines also act to absorb shock in case of a fall (Vincent and Owers 1986). The rolling ability is controlled by the panniculus carnosus – a muscle that envelops the hedgehog's trunk and is particularly well-developed in this species (Robinson 1918). The edge of this muscle is thickened in order to form the orbicularis – a "purse-string"-like muscle that also participates in the rolling mechanism (Carpenter and Lindemann 2017).

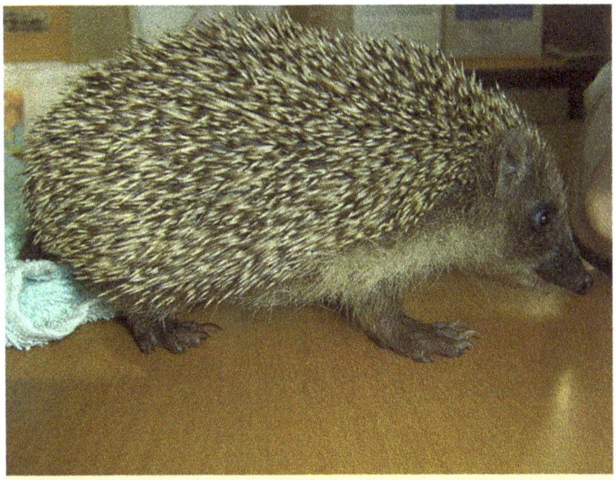

Figure 9.2
A hedgehog showing a spiny coat on the dorsal surface and fur on the rest of the body.

Reproduced with kind permission from Action for Wildlife.

The hedgehog's skeleton is similar to that of other mammals (Fig. 9.3). A noteworthy difference is the shorter neck which possibly facilitates rolling up. It should also be noted that the tarsal joint is quite flexible, allowing the metatarsal bone to turn toward the midline of the body (see the section on Differential diagnosis) when the animal rolls up (Fig. 9.4). Hedgehogs have five toes on each foot. The adult animal possesses 36 teeth.

Among the hedgehog's senses smell is the most developed sense followed by hearing. Vision is not well developed and it is possible for a blind hedgehog to survive if kept in a protected environment (Mullineaux et al. 2003, p. 50).

Eurasian badger (*Meles meles*)

Badgers belong to the order Carnivora in the family Mustelidae. They are, however, characterized as omnivorous since their diet consists of a variety of foods (e.g., eggs, insects, small mammals, fruits, seeds) (Neal and Cheeseman 1996). Like the hedgehog it is a nocturnal animal, but it does not undergo hibernation, especially in regions with warm climates (Kowalczyk et al. 2003).

The badger has a dense underfur and long sparse hairs that protrude. It has adjusted to live in underground tunnels, and has a powerful musculoskeletal structure needed to dig through the earth (Fig. 9.5). It has short, strong limbs and long claws, especially on the forelimbs. There are five toes on each limb. The badger's neck is short and its spine is not as flexible as that of most domestic carnivores (Mullineaux et al. 2003, p. 124). The adult dentition consists of 38 teeth.

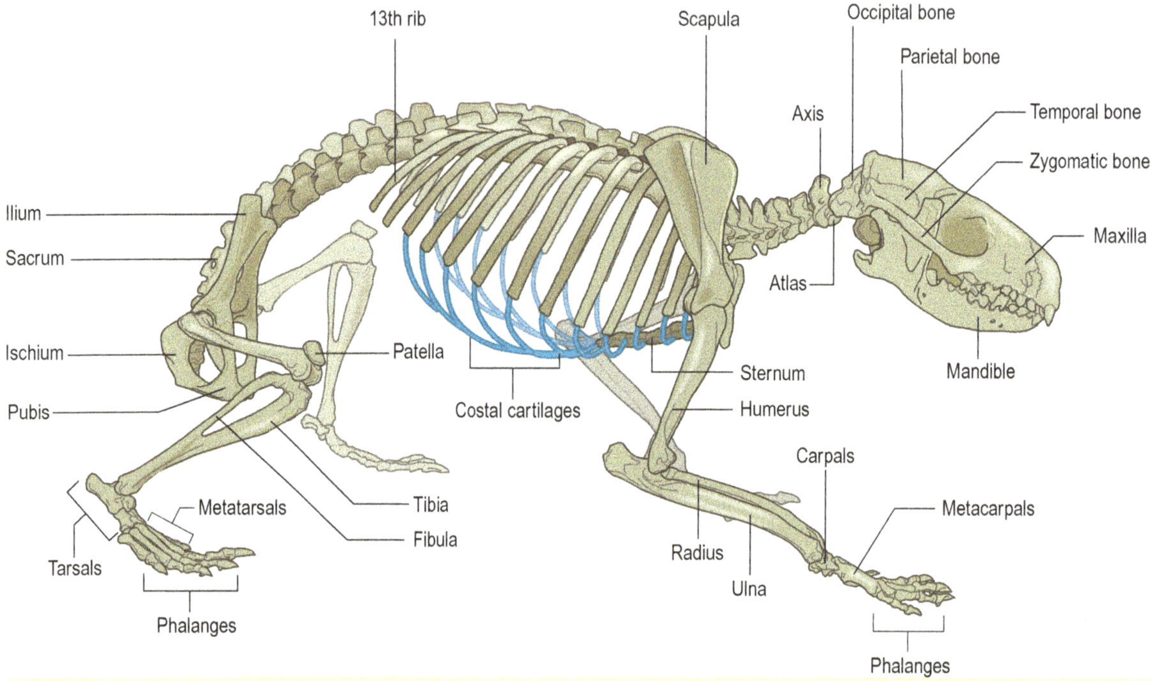

Figure 9.3
Hedgehog skeleton.

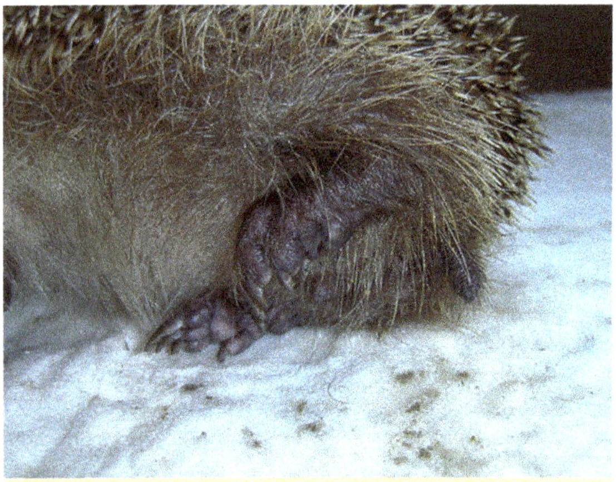

Figure 9.4
Hedgehog tarsal joint flexibility.

Reproduced with kind permission from Action for Wildlife.

The badger's best developed sense is smell. It has several glands that produce scent, which is used as a means of social communication. Hearing is well-developed, as is vision, although its eyes are relatively small. It is important to know that the badger can drop its body temperature from 37°C to 28°C in winter months (Fowler and Racey 2009).

Otter and other mustelids

In the same Mustelidae family as the badger are the Eurasian otter (*Lutra lutra*), weasel (*Mustela nivalis*), polecat (*Mustela putorius*), and marten (genus *Martes*).

The otter is predominantly nocturnal. It is an excellent diver, its prey consisting mainly of fish and amphibians. Otters live close to freshwater or the coastline (McCafferty 2005) (Fig. 9.6).

Otter fur is very dense, offering protection from cold water by trapping air in between its two layers. The otter has a long body and short limbs (Fig. 9.7). Its neck is strong and its tail thick. Each foot has five toes that have webs between them to facilitate swimming. The front feet are larger and with longer claws. In order

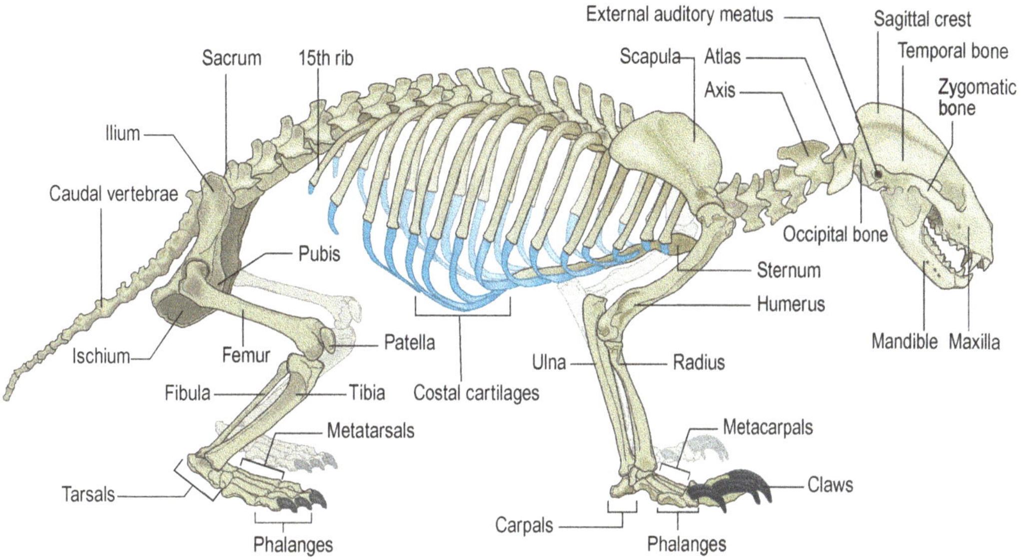

Figure 9.5
Badger skeleton.

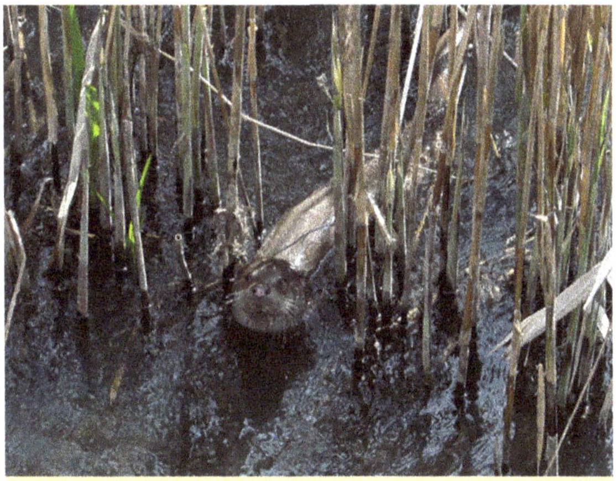

Figure 9.6
Otter swimming in fresh water.

Reproduced with kind permission from Christidis Aris.

to locate its prey the otter has long bristles on its muzzle called vibrissae. Similar bristles exist on its elbows (Mullineaux et al. 2003, p. 138). Adult otters have 36 teeth.

Other mustelids have similar body morphology to the otter but they are not adapted to swimming. Their chief characteristic is the elongated trunk and the short limbs (Fig. 9.8). They are agile and nimble, good at climbing, and have a long tail that serves well for keeping their balance (Step 1921, p. 64). They are mainly carnivorous with 32 (mustela) or 40 (martens) teeth.

Red fox (*Vulpes vulpes*)

Although of the order Carnivora the fox's diet is varied, ranging from fruits and insects to small mammals. As with all the above species, it is mainly nocturnal. Its fur is dense with a characteristically long bushy tail.

The fox's body structure is similar to a dog's since they belong to the same family (Canidae), but its figure is generally more slender (Fig. 9.9). It has adapted to the needs of hunting being fast with good endurance. Its hind limbs are relatively longer than those of other Canidae (Lloyd 1980), which is an advantageous feature when pouncing on its prey. The fox's forefeet have five toes each whereas its hind feet have four. The inner toe of the forefoot is not in contact with the ground.

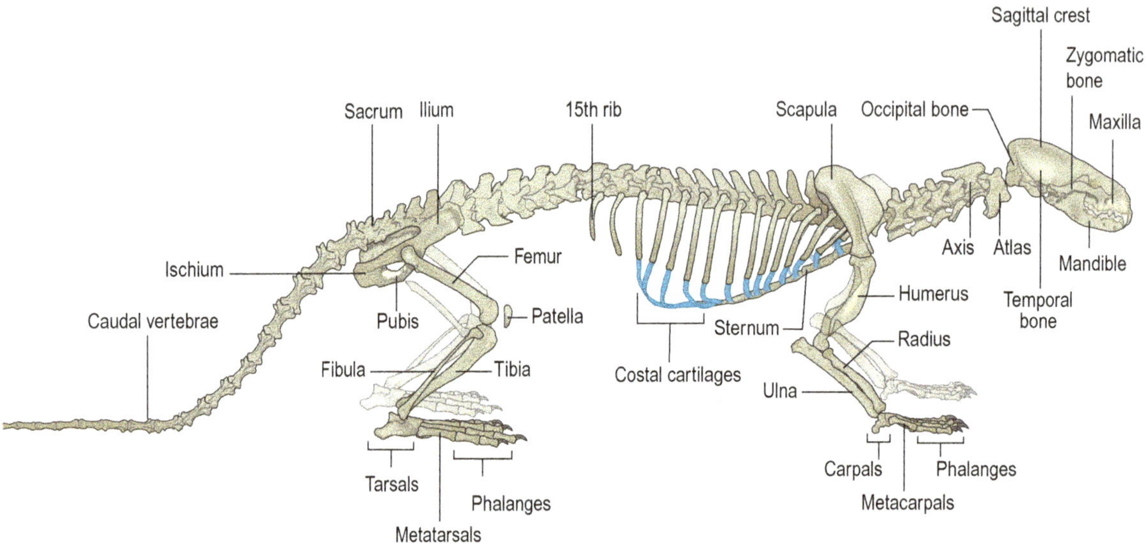

Figure 9.7
Otter skeleton.

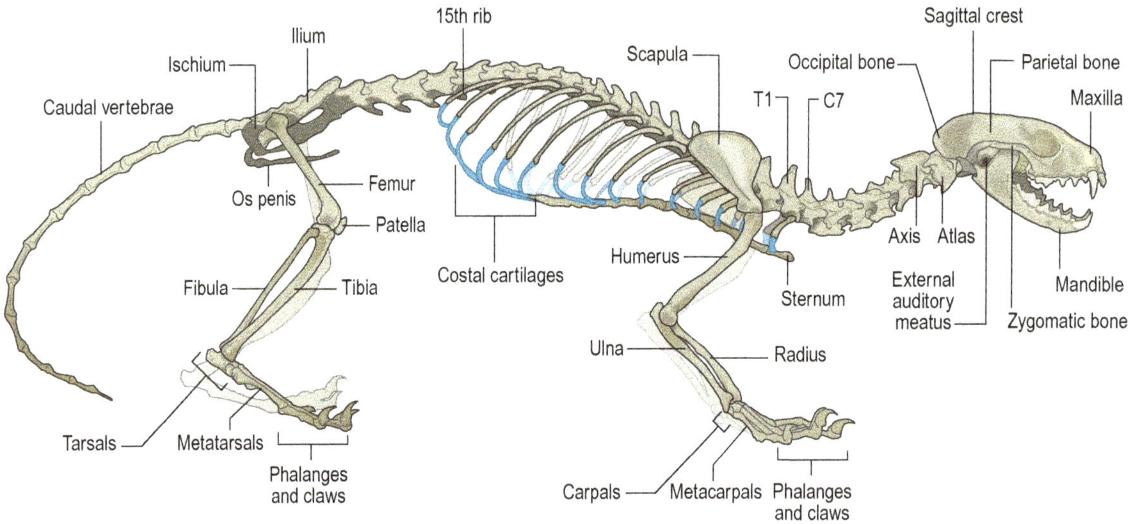

Figure 9.8
Weasel skeleton.

The fox's hearing is particularly well-developed, serving the need to locate its prey. The fox is myopic and is particularly sensitive to movement (Baldwin 2015a). The sense of smell is also well-developed. The fox's dentition consists of 42 teeth.

Deer (Cervidae)

There are ten species of deer living wild, either native or introduced, across the European continent. These are: red deer (*Cervus elaphus*), fallow deer (*Dama*

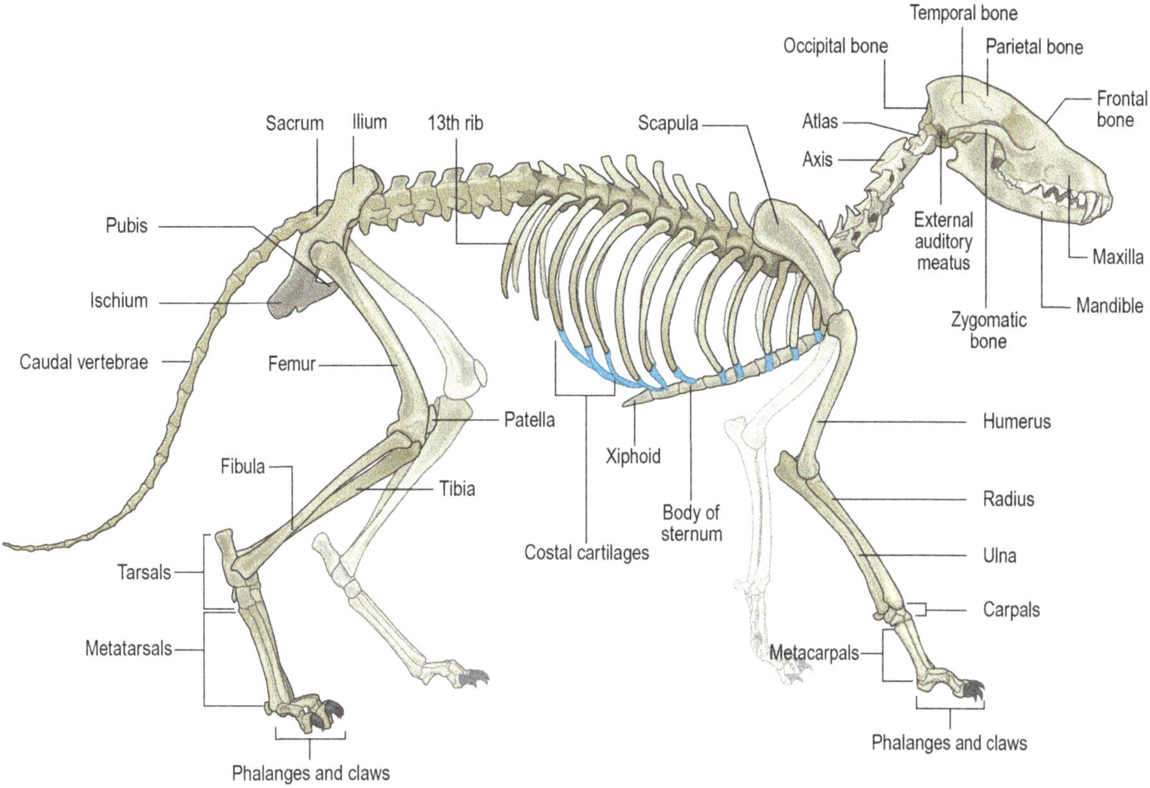

Figure 9.9
Fox skeleton.

dama), roe deer (*Capreolus capreolus*), sika deer (*Cervus nippon*), muntjac deer (*Muntiacus reevesi*), Chinese water deer (*Hydropotes inermis*), Eurasian moose (*Alces alces*), reindeer (*Rangifer tarandus*), white-tailed deer (*Odocoilens virginianus*), and axis deer (*Axis axis*) (Apollonio et al. 2010). Although there are differences between them, they all share the general anatomical and physiological features of the family Cervidae.

The anatomy and physiology of the deer is similar to that of the goat. Being herbivorous and ruminants their digestive system is adjusted to these functions. Their diet consists of grass, herbs, leaves, and fruits. They do not have a gallbladder. Antlers differ significantly from the horns of domestic ruminants. Antlers consist of bone tissue and are covered by the so-called velvet, which is a skin tissue full of nerves and vessels. Only males carry antlers, and testosterone levels control the antler's cycle of shedding and regrowing (Baldwin 2015b).

Deer walk on cloven hooves (Step 1920, p. 125) (Fig. 9.10). They have four toes on each foot but only the middle two touch the ground. As deer are a prey species all of their senses are well-developed to help them escape from their predators. Deer's upper jaws lack incisors, similarly to domestic ruminants. Their dentition consists of 32 teeth.

Common orthopedic conditions

Introduction

The most common problems that bring wild animals into care are anthropogenic. That is, they are caused by man's effect on, and modification of, the natural environment. The most common cause is accidental

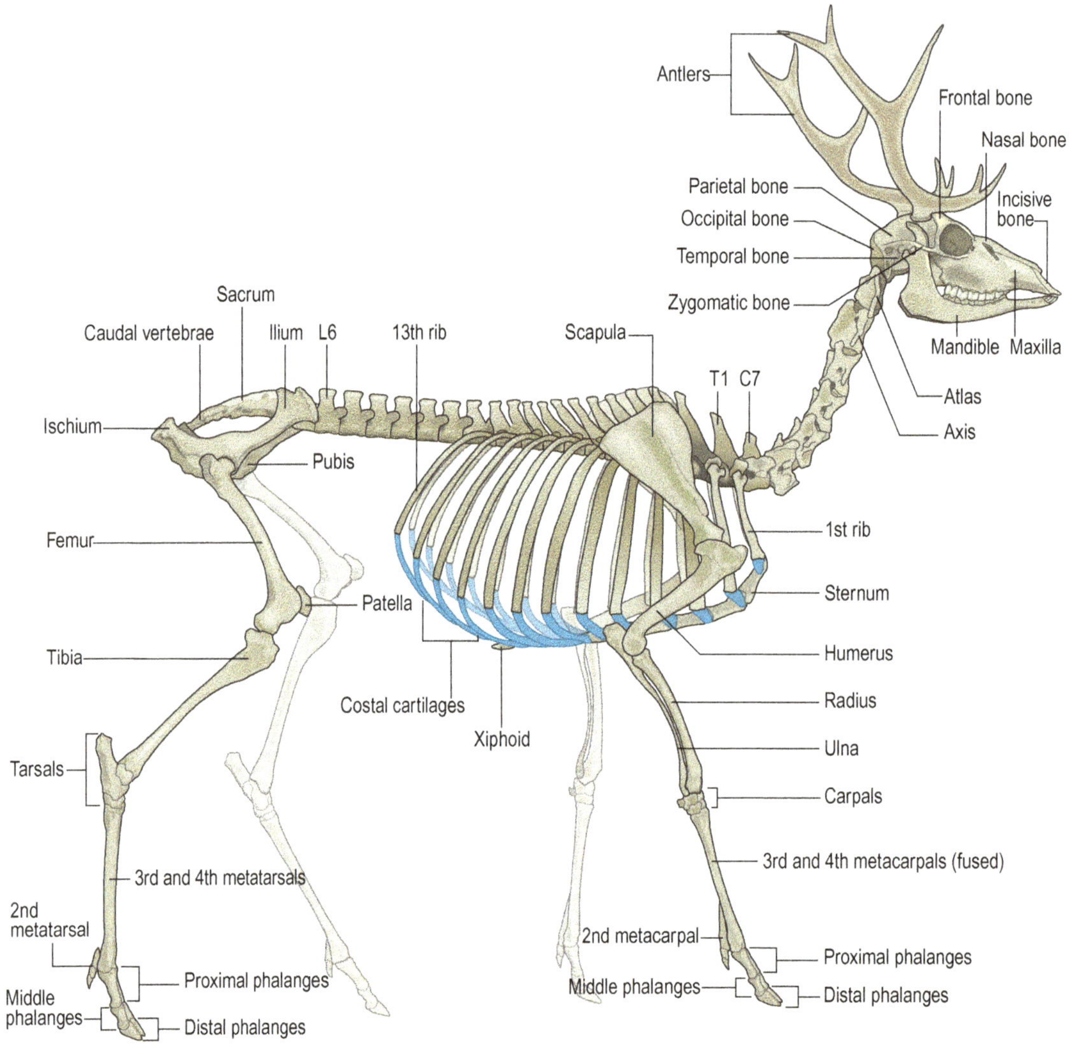

Figure 9.10
Deer skeleton.

trauma (Action for Wildlife 2015). Road traffic accidents are top of the list. For hedgehogs, badgers, otters, and deer this is the principal cause of mortality or trauma. For foxes the most common cause of trauma is trapping and getting caught in fences (Stocker 2005, p. 229). Other common causes of injury to wild mammals are snares, gunshots, territorial fights (especially between males), and bites from predators or domestic animals (mostly dogs).

All of these may cause orthopedic problems. The most frequent orthopedic conditions are fractures. Traffic accidents usually cause fractures to long bones of the limbs, the pelvis, and the spine. The most difficult to deal with are cases involving spinal cord injury. Some of these may lead to irreversible damage and the only solution is euthanasia. When treating wild animals we should always keep in mind that our aim is to return the animal to its natural environment fully capable and able to survive. The animal's welfare is our criterion for deciding what procedure to follow. Long-term captivity may be an option, but only if the animal will have a good quality of life in suitable facilities (e.g., a wildlife hospital).

The most frequently seen orthopedic injuries in wild mammals are discussed below.

Fractures

Limbs

Most commonly encountered are fractures of the long bones of forelimbs or hind limbs, that is, fractures of the humerus, radius or ulna, the femur and tibia, and the metacarpus and metatarsus (Fig. 9.11).

The clinical picture of such fractures is a "hanging" limb, which is often swollen. If during a proper clinical examination there are fragments of long bone that are visible the fracture is characterized as open or compound (i.e., part of the bone has penetrated through the skin) and comminuted (i.e., there are more than two pieces of bone resulting from the fracture). In cases like this the prognosis is very poor and euthanasia may be the best solution (Mullineaux et al. 2003, p. 159). When assessing possible treatments it is essential to know if a fracture is compound or comminuted or both.

Careful observation and palpation is the first step of the examination. The detection of movement at a point along the limb where there should normally be no movement in conjunction with crepitus

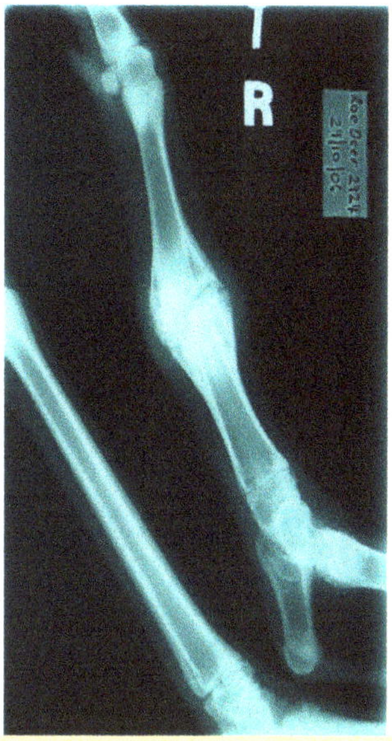

Figure 9.11
Lateral radiograph showing a healing fracture of the right metatarsus in a roe deer (*Capreolus capreolus*).

Reproduced with kind permission from Vale Wildlife Hospital.

(a characteristic grinding) are strong indications that the bone is fractured. The next step is to confirm the diagnosis by making radiographs.

The method chosen to stabilize the fracture will depend on the type of fracture as well as the bone involved and the species of animal (Table 9.2).

Table 9.2 Most probable immobilizing method and prognosis depending upon the location and type of fracture

Fracture location	Fracture type	Stabilizing method (fixation)	Prognosis
Humerus or femur	Open or compound	Internal	Poor
	Closed	Internal	Positive
Radius, ulna or tibia	Open or compound	Internal	Poor
	Closed	External or internal in badger	Positive
Distal limb	Open or compound	External or internal or no treatment in deer	Positive
	Closed	External or no treatment in deer	Positive
Pelvis	Open or compound (rare)	Surgical	Poor
	Closed	Cage restraint	Dystocia may occur in females
Jaw	Open or compound	Internal	Poor
	Closed	Internal	Variable

For hedgehogs simple fractures of the radius, ulna, and tibia, and those of the distal limb, can be stabilized with external fixation using immobilizing dressings. If the femur or humerus are involved, however, an operation (internal fixation) will be needed (Stocker 2005, p. 208). Rolling up is a natural function for hedgehogs, so care should be taken when choosing the stabilization method in order not to obstruct this function.

For foxes any attempt to use external fixation is doomed to failure as the animal will bite it off, even if an Elizabethan collar is used.

In the case of badgers external stabilization is difficult because of their anatomical structure (short limbs and limited free surface). It may, however, be used in some cases. Fortunately, badgers are rarely seen with compound fractures due to their muscular bulk protecting the bones.

In the case of deer a completely different approach may be recommended. Mullineaux et al. (2003, p. 174) suggest that fractures of bones above the carpus and tarsus, even compound ones, should be left without treatment. This is because deer are very susceptible to a condition called "capture myopathy," which occurs as a result of stress and the animal's attempt to escape and is life-threatening. Other workers do recommend stabilization and, if necessary, internal fixation of limb fractures (Stocker 2005, pp. 261–262).

The healing procedure will take at least three weeks depending on factors such as the nature of the fracture, the location, the stabilizing method, and the age and species of the animal. In badgers this process seems to take longer than in other animals (two to three months) (Stocker 2005, p. 239). Young animals show better and faster healing potentials than older ones. Hydrotherapy in warm water is suggested in the case of hedgehogs in order to stimulate them to use the healed limb (Stocker 2005, p. 209) (Fig. 9.12).

In all cases the goal is the complete functional restoration of the limb. It is very important to consider the natural biology of the animal and the functions that the limbs serve (e.g., digging, escaping from predators, preying).

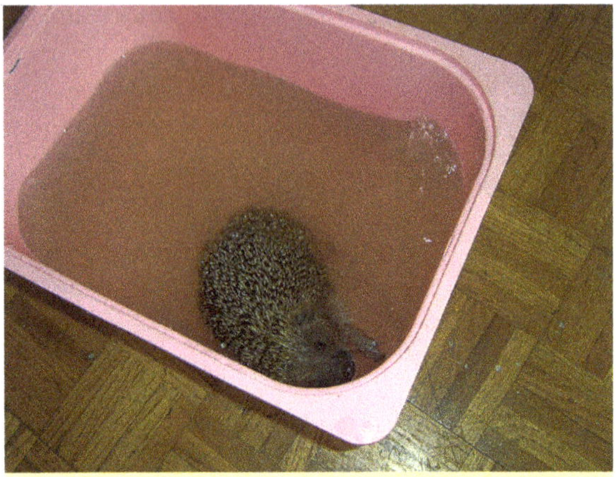

Figure 9.12
Hedgehog undergoing active hydrotherapy. Note that the water depth must be enough to ensure actual swimming.

Reproduced with kind permission from Action for Wildlife.

Pelvis

Pelvic fractures may often be observed as the result of traffic accidents, the function of one or both of the hind limbs being affected. Radiographs will confirm the diagnosis (Fig. 9.13). The healing of such fractures can lead to narrowing of the pelvic canal. In the case of females this may well result in dystocia, and thus euthanasia or spaying may be required.

Usually restricted mobility is quite sufficient for healing of pelvic fractures to occur. The animal should be kept in a relatively small cage as long as necessary. In a few cases surgical fixation may be required.

Jaw

Jaw fractures are particularly common in badgers and otters as a result of traffic accidents or territorial fights, but can occur in any species. In these cases surgical fixation should be performed; the function of the jaw should be fully restored so that the animal can catch, kill, and devour its prey or graze and ruminate (Figs 9.14 and 9.15).

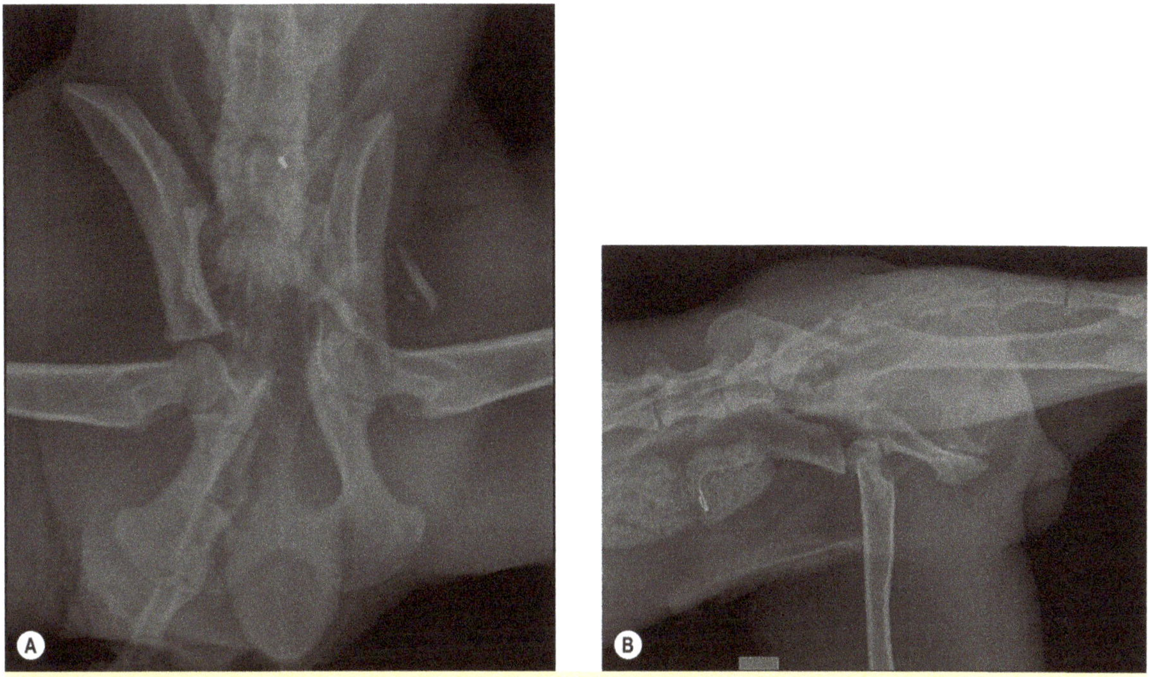

Figure 9.13
Lateral and dorsoventral radiographs showing a pelvic fracture in a young red fox.

Reproduced with kind permission from Action for Wildlife.

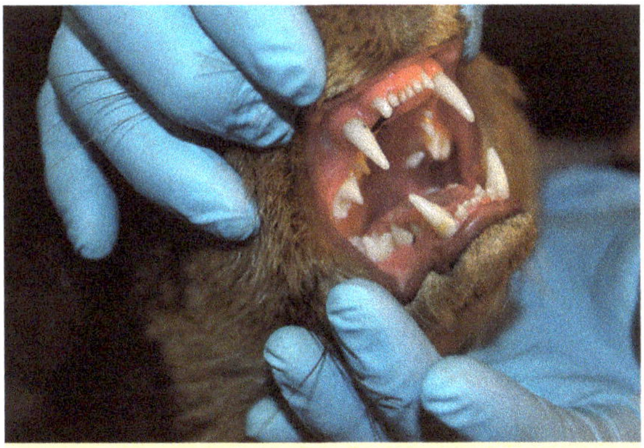

Figure 9.14
Checking dentition for trauma, and assessing temporomandibular joint (TMJ) mobility in an anesthetized European otter.

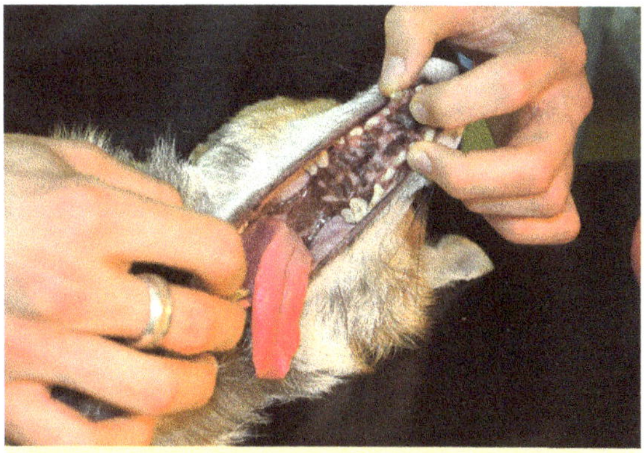

Figure 9.15
Assessing extreme range-of-mouth opening in an anesthetized European red fox.

Joint instability, ligament disruption, and dislocation

These situations usually affect limb joints. They are observed as a result of traffic accidents and trapping. Trapping in particular may lead to instability of a joint, to ligament disruption or to dislocation while the animal is trying to free itself. Such injuries are common in foxes (which in some countries are frequently caught in fences), but are also seen in deer trying to escape from hunting dogs.

The clinical picture may be that of a "hanging" limb depending on the joint that is injured. On palpation crepitus may be detected in the case of dislocation (and also with fractures).

Joint instability generally has a good prognosis. The joint should regain its function after a few days if the animal is restrained in a relatively small cage. Support dressing of the limb may not be necessary.

Ligament disruptions and dislocations may be difficult to deal with and often lead to joint ankylosis. The prognosis depends on the chronicity of the incident; if a dislocation took place shortly before the animal was examined the joint may be reduced easily. For any manipulation the animal should be under anesthesia. The limb should usually be stabilized in extension for one to two weeks to prevent redislocation (Olmstead 1995, p. 341). Surgical interference should be considered when the likelihood of redislocation is high. In chronic cases the development of scar tissue around the injured joint hinders joint reduction. In the latter situation the veterinarian should evaluate the chronicity of the condition based on the radiographic findings and should decide if an operation would be helpful. A nonfunctional joint cannot serve the essential needs of a wild animal, thus euthanasia or permanent captivity may be the only options.

Spinal injuries

Fractures or dislocations of the spine occur mostly due to traffic accidents. The clinical picture depends on the location of the injury and the severity of the damage induced (Fig. 9.16). Most frequently the hind limbs are affected, although when the injury is in the cervical spine forelimbs may also be affected.

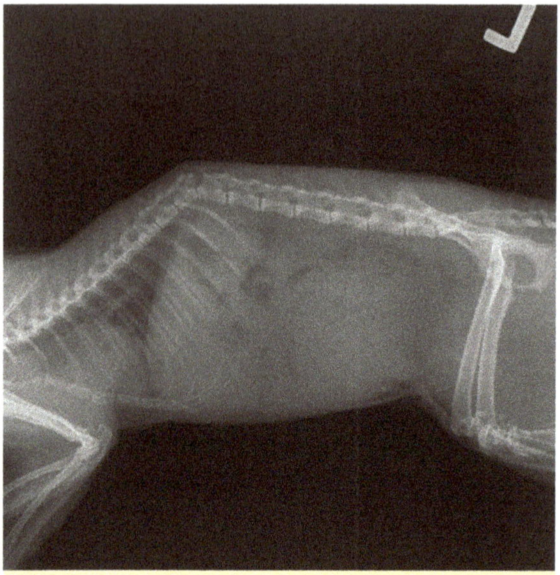

Figure 9.16
Lateral radiograph showing a caudal thoracic spinal fracture in a gray squirrel (*Sciurus carolinensis*).

Reproduced with kind permission from Vale Wildlife Hospital.

The usual clinical picture is inability to move the limbs, which is often misdiagnosed as paralysis. Shortly after the accident (within the first few hours) the clinical picture is that of shock and the temporary loss of function, but that can change within a few hours (Olmstead 1995, p. 183). Improvement of the clinical signs may be observed without any treatment in some cases.

Palpation of the spine may cause further damage and may not provide any significant information (Olmstead 1995, p. 183). A thorough neurological examination must be conducted in order to assess the level of the damage and the malfunction of the limbs. The inability to move the limbs should be graded in order to evaluate the possibility of recovery. The function of the bladder and large intestine should also be examined (Fig. 9.17). Radiology and other imaging techniques are essential to refine the final diagnosis.

Animals that suffer from spinal injuries should be restrained in a relatively small cage for several weeks so that moving is minimized. Surgery may be needed in some cases.

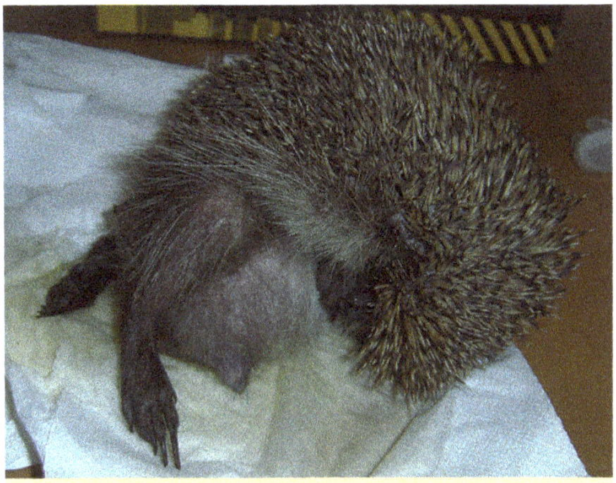

Figure 9.17
A male hedgehog with a spinal injury.

Reproduced with kind permission from Action for Wildlife.

Orthopedic injuries are common in wild mammals. In most cases the restoration of damaged structures must be complete if the animal is to return to the wild. Some treatments are time-consuming, and suitable facilities are needed for both treatment and rehabilitation (Fig. 9.18A and B).

Differential diagnosis

Introduction

The various orthopedic conditions that wild animals suffer from must be correctly diagnosed to allow for suitable treatment. There are specific orthopedic conditions that injured wildlife frequently suffer, but different conditions may have a similar clinical picture. It is essential therefore to differentiate the conditions and make a specific diagnosis in order to offer the animal the best possible treatment. History, symptoms, clinical examination, and findings from other diagnostic examinations are all necessary and should be taken into consideration.

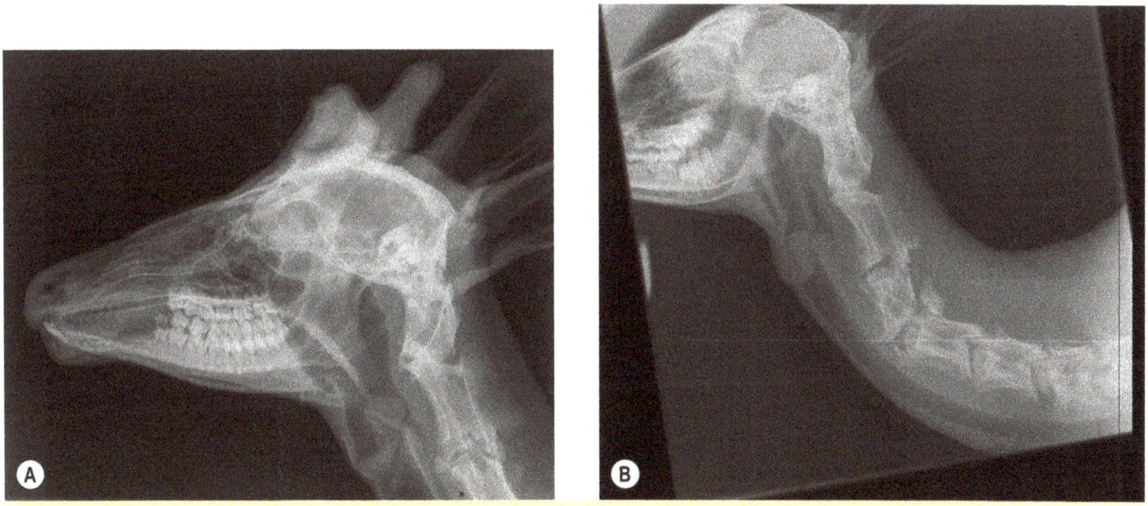

Figure 9.18
(A) Lateral radiograph showing the skull and occipitoatlantal joint of an adult roe deer road traffic accident casualty. (B) Lateral radiograph of the same deer showing an unstable fracture around C3–C4 vertebral joints.

Reproduced with kind permission from Vale Wildlife Hospital.

History

It is more difficult to collect history for wild animal cases than for domesticated animal cases. Occasionally the animal is found injured yet the cause cannot be identified. However, in other cases the cause is more obvious. For instance, in the case of an injured animal found at the side of a road the most likely reason for its injury is a traffic accident. There are cases where the rescuer frees a wild animal trapped in a fence or snare where again the cause of injury appears clear. All the obvious or suspected data should be collected in order to form a full history. Remember, however, an underlying problem may lead to a wild animal being injured. For instance, an infectious disease may cause changes to the animal's behavior, and that may subsequently lead to an accident. When examining wild animals be very aware of diseases that can be transmitted to humans. Rabies, for example, is life-threatening to humans as well as animals. All practicable safety measures should be taken when dealing with wild animals. As well as the cause the time of the incident should also be recorded. Although in many cases this might not be possible any information collected will be helpful. For instance, someone may report that a fox is wandering in his back yard and appears injured. The clinician should ask "for how long?" and record this information. The chronicity of the condition is important when considering the method of treatment. An open compound fracture has a very poor prognosis when it is a few days old. In such a case amputation may be the only solution rather than surgical fixation. In other cases the incident may be very recent and the prognosis may be more positive, for example, when the driver involved in a traffic accident is the one that brings the animal into care.

Clinical examination

The clinical examination will usually provide significant information for making a diagnosis.

The first step is to observe the animal carefully. Check if it can stand or if it is recumbent. If it can stand check if all the limbs are weight-bearing, and check the manner in which they contact the ground. It is necessary to know the normal physiological position of the limb for the species concerned. For example, in the hind limb the angle normally formed between the tibia and the metatarsal bone can be less than 45 degrees or more than 90 degrees depending on the species. Accordingly, there are three patterns of locomotion of the distal hind limb affecting which parts of the limb are in contact with the ground (Myers 2017) (Fig. 9.19):

Plantigrade: when the paw and metatarsal are placed on the ground during standing and walking. This category includes the hedgehog, the badger, the squirrel, and the otter.

Digitigrade: when only the paw is in contact with the ground, for example, the fox. Mustelids other than badger and otter are either digitigrade or plantigrade.

Unguligrade: when only the hoof is in contact with the ground as in the case of the deer.

A fractured limb must be differentiated from a dislocation and also from reduced motion caused by spinal injury. In all three cases the animal may hang or drag its limb. In the case of fracture of the femur, however, the picture may be different with the limb appearing bent due to the contraction of the associated muscles.

Only after careful observation should we move to the next step - examining the animal by palpation of the limbs. Always keep in mind that a wild animal, even if it seems to be in a coma, may react unexpectedly by biting, scratching or kicking. All safety precautions should be followed.

It is important to palpate the whole limb and not only the part that seems to be injured. A thorough examination may reveal problems that are not obvious by observation. Start palpation at the distal end and gradually move proximally (to the trunk). Crepitus may be perceived in both a fracture and a dislocation; in the case of a fracture, however, there is often abnormal mobility at a point along the bone, away from the joints.

A dislocated joint displays abnormal movement when performing flexion and extension, and the animal also shows signs of pain. In addition, with a recent dislocation the bone may be relocated and again readily dislocated (Piermattei et al. 2006). On the other hand, in joint loosening and ligament disruption the joint shows a wider range of lateral motion (Olmstead 1995). The flexibility of the joints differs between species. As mentioned before (see the section on Biology, anatomy, and physiology), hedgehogs have flexible

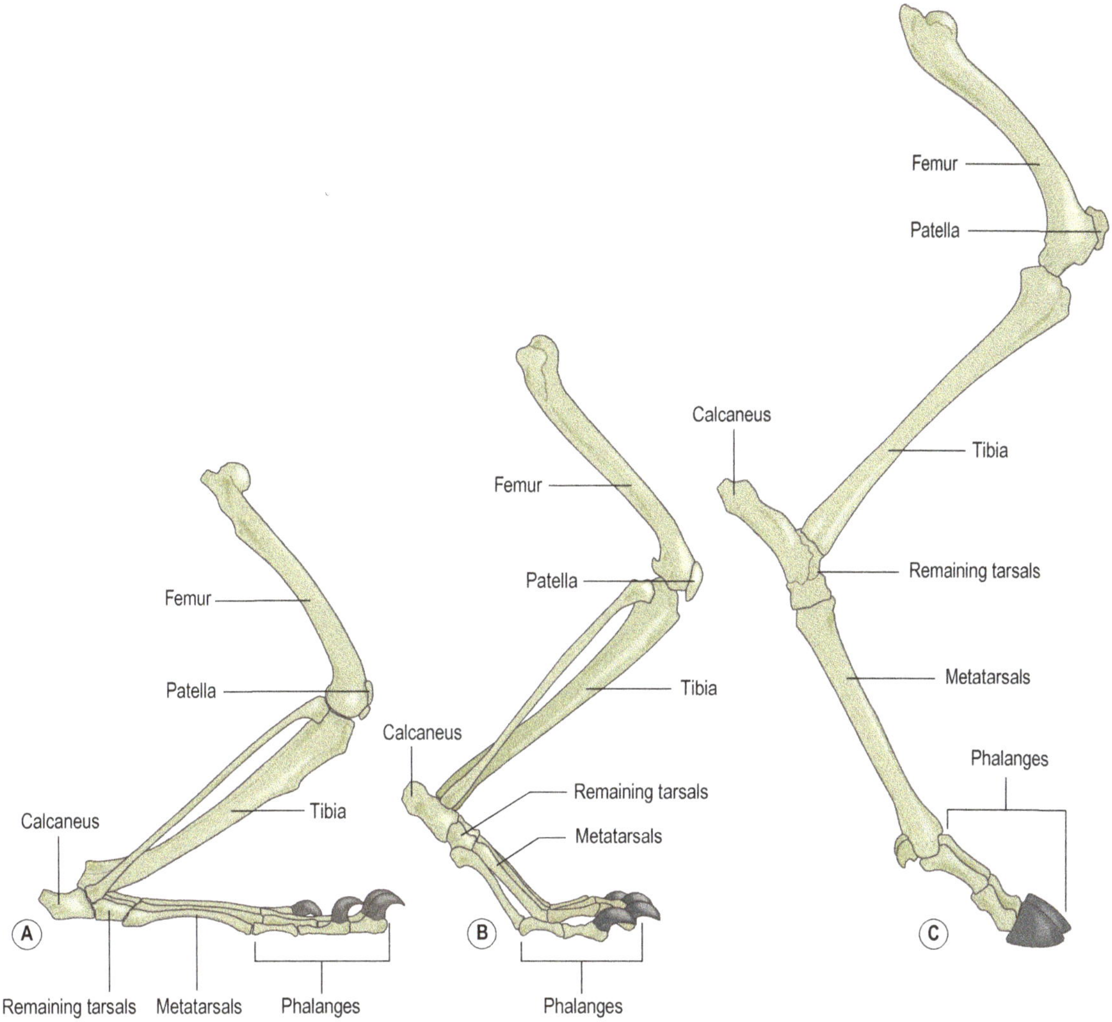

Figure 9.19
Distal limb evolutionary variations for different species (Myers 2017). (A) Plantigrade (squirrel). (B) Digitigrade (dog). (C) Unguligrade (deer).

Reproduced with kind permission from Professor Phil Myers.

tarsal joints that allow the metatarsus to rotate toward the belly when the animal is rolling up. Such species-specific movements should not be mistaken for joint loosening, ligament disruption or dislocation.

Pelvic fractures and spinal injuries may give a similar clinical picture. The hind limbs appear to be paralyzed. With a fractured pelvis the injury may be unilateral and the problem may only affect one limb. With a spinal injury, however, the damage is almost always bilateral. In pelvic fractures crepitus may be felt when palpating the bones of the pelvis, either externally or through the rectum, and lameness may be mild. On the other hand, spinal injury usually causes severe lameness (Table 9.3). If a spinal injury is suspected palpation should be minimal or completely avoided. Handling of the animal

Table 9.3 Findings of observation and clinical examination depending upon the type of orthopedic injury

Findings	Type of injury			
	Limb fracture	Dislocation	Pelvic fracture	Spinal injury
Lameness	Yes	Yes	Mild and usually unilateral	Severe and almost always bilateral
Crepitus	Yes	Yes	Yes	Palpation not recommended
Abnormal mobility along the bone	Yes	No	Yes (though difficult to detect)	Palpation not recommended

should be very careful and an accurate neurological examination needs to be performed.

In all cases, the final diagnosis will usually be confirmed by radiological examination or by other more sophisticated imaging techniques especially when spinal injuries are present.

Osteopathic evaluation

Observation

Prior to looking at any wildlife casualty it is essential to have a working knowledge of their habits, life cycle, and the abilities required to thrive and survive. This is before you perform any actual treatment.

Taking a case history has already been covered, but one thing this author (TN) would like to add is that historic data collected at wildlife hospitals can be invaluable for creating a benchmark for behavior patterns and potential prognoses of similar cases. There will also be a record of the patient's ability to move properly, feed, urinate, and defecate as expected. Wildlife hospitals are used to seeing thousands of casualties each year and keep up-to-date data on what is and is not normal. This is of huge use to the osteopath (BWRC [n.d.]).

Wildlife will often behave very differently if they know you are watching them. Most will behave as if they are 100 percent fit and healthy, but a few species will adopt a corpse pose. Some wildlife hospitals have CCTV fitted to their wards and enclosures. These have produced some interesting findings especially when members of staff walk past a patient. Unobserved viewing is of much more benefit here than with domestic species (Gower Bird Hospital 2018). Recorded footage is of great benefit when trying to formulate realistic treatment programs for each individual patient.

When observing a wildlife patient discreetly the author would adopt the same protocols as for domestic animal patients.

1. Start with the head. Look at how this is held. Look for any asymmetry. If the eyes are open and visible try to determine if either pupil is dilated. This is not always possible without the aid of a small torch, and can be performed with the veterinary surgeon once you reach the hands-on stage. If the animal has visible ear pinnae note their position and symmetry along with any movement, which should suggest that the patient can hear. Look at the snout and note any cuts, bumps, or discharge from the nostrils. If the animal opens its mouth try to see the condition of the teeth, gums, and tongue.
2. Look at the position of the neck and check for any asymmetry that might suggest trauma. As with other animal observation, compare the cervicothoracic junction and, in particular, where the neck appears to meet the forelimbs. In species like badger (*Meles meles*), and other mustelids, the sheer size of their muscling in this region can make this difficult to assess visually and is best done during the palpation phase of the consultation.
3. Compare the forelimbs for normal conformation and symmetry. Look at the condition of the feet, pads, and claws if visible. Pad wear can give an insight into the individual's gait, as can normal claw wear. Species like hedgehog can be difficult to assess this way.
4. Moving caudally from the thoracic sling look along the thoracic spine and around the rib cage. If the animal is standing or seated check for any roaching or dipping of the spine and any signs of

trauma. Check for scoliosis. Look along the ventral aspect of the chest and into the abdominal region. Look for any abnormal swellings or marks which might indicate trauma of both the musculoskeletal (MSK) system and internal organs.

5. Moving to the lumbar region and hindquarters again look for symmetry and a smooth transition from thoracic to lumbar regions. Look at the outline of the pelvis and, in particular, the tubera coxae and tubera sacrale. If the outline of the sacrum is visible check to see its position within the sacroiliac joints. Check the position and symmetry of the hip joints if possible. Compare with any radiographs, especially if an RTA is suspected.
6. Looking at the hind limbs check for normal conformation and orientation. Assess the feet and claws. If you can see the plantar aspect of the feet check for any signs of trauma, or pad wear, which can give you an idea of the animal's gait and general condition.
7. If the patient has a visible tail look at its condition, orientation, and any signs of trauma. If the animal is awake look for signs of tail movement. Some species will actively communicate this way (mustelids, deer), whereas others, such as foxes, will avoid giving any indication of what they are thinking.

Palpation

You will need to decide whether to examine a casualty awake, sedated, or anesthetized (see below). If it is to be handled while fully awake then certain methods can be adopted to reduce stress to it and to make handling safer for the osteopath and wildlife handler or veterinary surgeon. It is also worth noting that wildlife patients *will* have external parasites present such as fleas, ticks, and mites. This is in addition to internal ones such as nematodes, and most likely gut flukes, which need to be considered when handling each patient. Many of these parasites can live and thrive in or on humans. Many species can carry highly contagious infectious diseases and these are covered in Chapter 1 under zoonotic diseases. Note that in the UK several bat species are known to carry European bat lyssavirus (EBL), a form of rabies virus (*Rhabdoviridae*). At least one wildlife pathologist in the UK has died from contracting this disease from a dead bat he was handling without wearing suitable gloves (New Scientist 2002). It may seem trivial but these diseases are not discriminating as to whom they attack.

- *Fully conscious.* This is best reserved for species such as hedgehog, young orphans of most species, and also deer (these do not always fare well with anesthesia (BWRC [n.d.]). The use of soft fabric muzzles can assist in making examination and treatment safer with species such as large mustelids and fox, and in many cases the use of a soft cloth over the eyes will help to reduce stress to the patient (Fig. 9.20). Keeping bright light and sound levels to a minimum is also essential.
- *Sedated.* This is probably the least used method of restraint for wildlife casualties and is only really used when anesthesia is not an option.
- *General anesthesia.* Species permitting, this may be the only realistic option for examining and then treating certain patients properly (Fig. 9.21). Despite some opinions to the contrary, a patient that is anesthetized still gives excellent feedback through their soft tissues and joints as the autonomic nervous system should still be fully functional. These

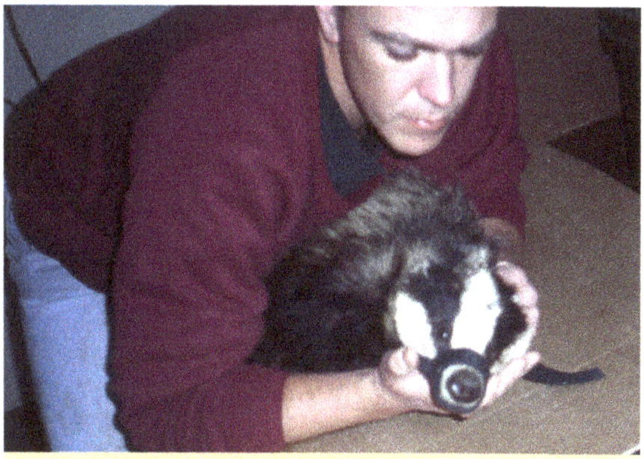

Figure 9.20
A fabric dog muzzle fitted correctly to a European badger (*Meles meles*).

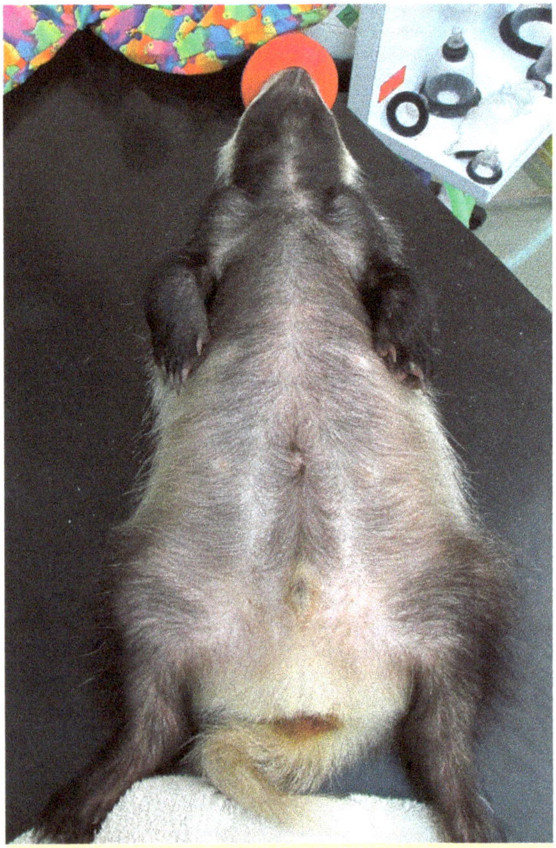

Figure 9.21
An anesthetized European badger ready for osteopathic evaluation.

smaller wildlife patients need to be closely monitored to keep them on a light plane of anesthesia. When choosing this method of restraint palpation is immediately followed by treatment as it is critical to keep anesthetic time to a minimum (Fowler 2008).

Whichever method of handling you choose for small wildlife casualties it is essential to keep all procedures to a minimum time. Being able to visualize their normal behavior, habitat, and gait will allow you to assess their present state and, therefore, what will be required to return it to a "normal state" for release back into the wild. It is at this stage that you need to be honest about whether you think you can achieve this result, along with the rest of the rehabilitation team. There is no point in treating purely for the sake of it.

The head

Taking care, use both hands to trace the outline and symmetry of the head and mandible. If the patient is conscious please ensure that a second operator secures the patient to allow you to perform this task safely.

If this is a suspected RTA casualty then be aware of common fracture sites to the mandible, orbits, and nasal bones. Feel for any increased heat and swelling that could indicate areas of trauma. Listen to the breathing and note if there appears to be any nasal restriction. If it is safe to do so you may smell the breath. This can indicate the general condition of the patient. Lung nematodes create a particularly nasty smell.

Feel for any wounds that may be hidden by fur or spines. If a casualty has been attacked by another animal or has been shot these wounds can be very difficult to palpate as they usually have very small entry holes. If in doubt take a radiograph.

Cervical spine and throat structures

Remember to check thoroughly along the ventral throat structures and especially around the cricoid, thyroid, and hyoid structures as any imbalances here with the soft tissue attachments will adversely affect the occipitoatlantoaxial articulations and therefore the overall gait mechanism (Pusey et al. 2010) (Figs 9.22A–C and 9.23).

With many small wildlife patients the ability to palpate individual cervical vertebrae is all but impossible. What you need to do is feel for asymmetry, scoliosis or any other abnormality as gently as you can. When palpating around the atlas please note that it can be easy to overstimulate the vagus nerve, which can cause a lightly anesthetized patient to wake up!

Try to make your assessment quickly as wildlife patients are much more likely to react adversely to

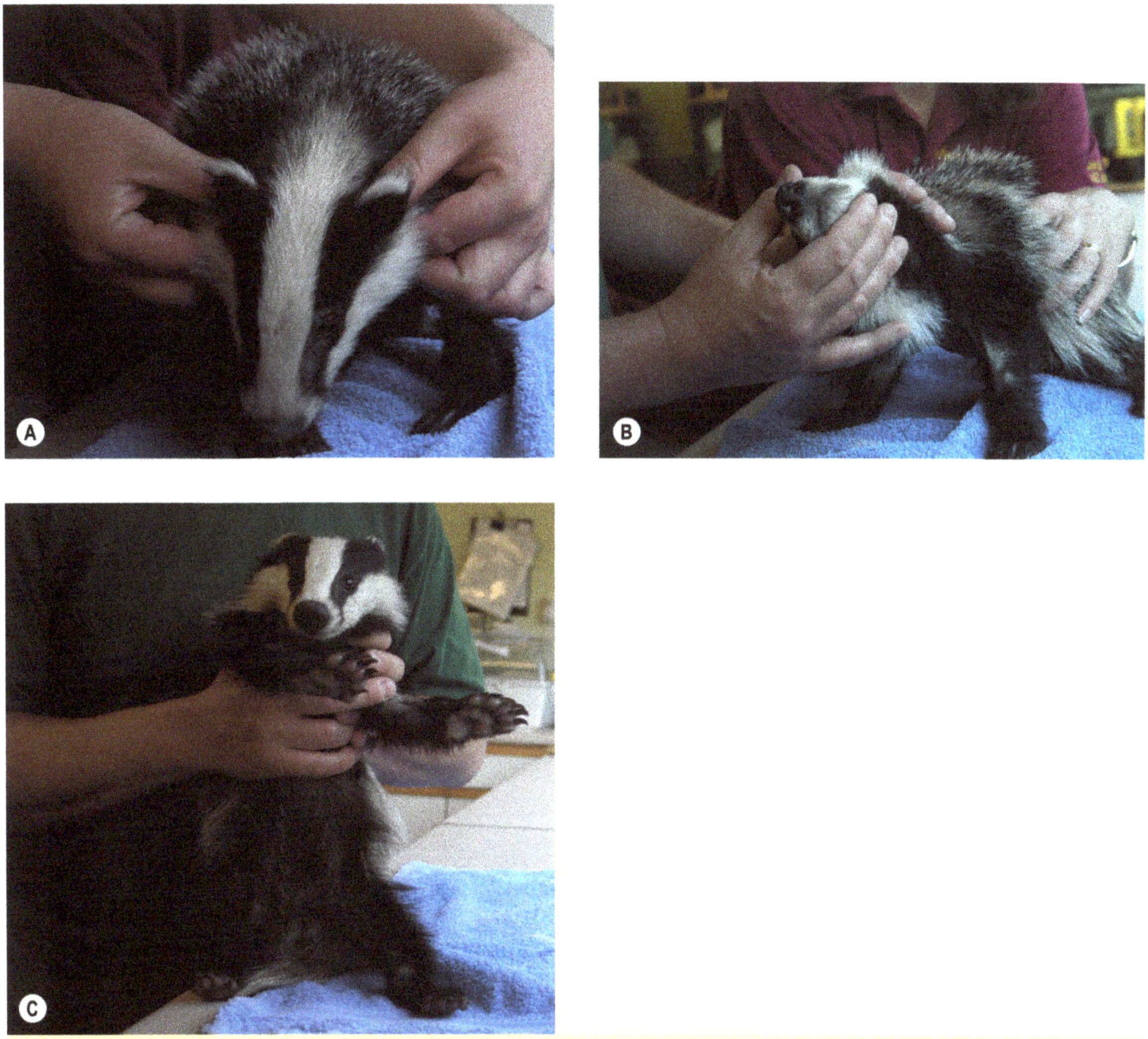

Figure 9.22
(A) Osteopathic evaluation of the occipitoatlantoaxial joint on a juvenile European badger. Note that this patient is not sedated. (B) Functional release work through the cervical spine and thoracic sling. (C) A functional lift, which releases tension through the axial skeletal and soft tissue structures.

handling even when you are using chemical restraint methods.

Shoulders and forelimbs

Feel for any heat, cold, swellings, fractures or dislocations (Fig. 9.24). Also note any skin lesions and be aware of possible infections such as bTB and ringworm. Working alongside a veterinary surgeon is essential here.

Try to elicit deep tendon reflexes via the triceps and biceps tendons. Examine the feet for any trauma, past or present.

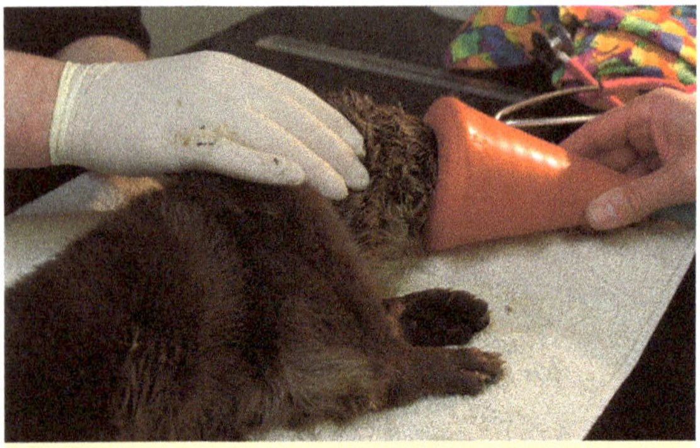

Figure 9.23
Initiating osteopathic palpation on an anesthetized European otter.

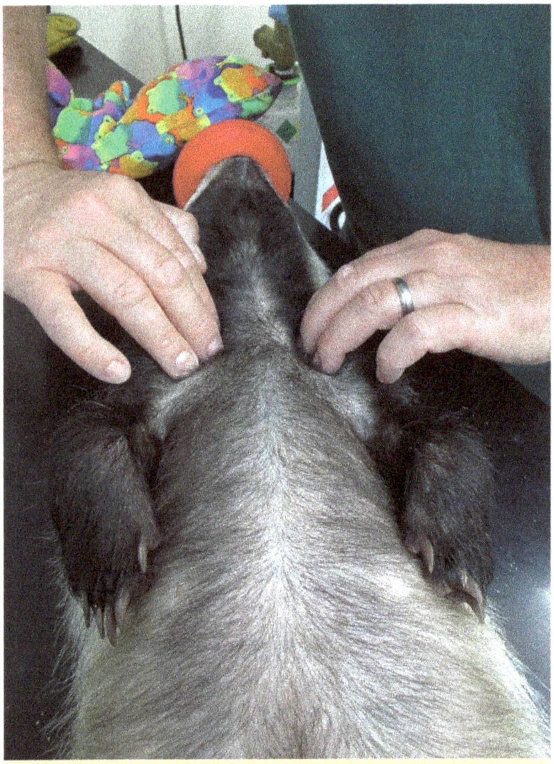

Figure 9.24
Osteopathic evaluation of the caudal cervical spine and thoracic sling structures in a supine anesthetized European badger.

Thoracic and lumbar spine

Depending on the species, note the shape and symmetry of the thorax. If trauma is suspected be very careful when palpating ribs as creating a pneumothorax is theoretically possible. Trace along the last rib to locate the thoracolumbar junction (Fig. 9.25). In many RTA victims this junction can be badly traumatized with spinal cord impairment (author's own experience with mustelid RTA casualties).

The lumbosacral junction is another key pivotal region and assessment of this, where possible, is required to form a suitable prognosis for osteopathic treatment.

Pelvis and hind limbs

Note the size, symmetry, and orientation of the ilia in relation to the sacrum. Note whether or not each innominate appears to sit normally. In many RTA victims one of the ilia can become shunted cranial or caudal to the normal sacroiliac joint position. The resultant muscle spasm often makes treating the conscious patient ineffective.

Most wildlife casualties will show no signs of pain when palpated, unlike a domestic animal. Therefore, extra care needs to be taken when assessing these patients.

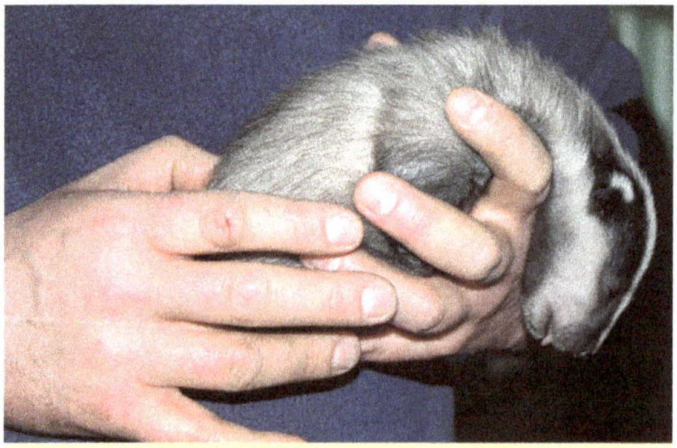

Figure 9.25
Osteopathic evaluation of the paravertebral musculature of an unweened European badger cub.

The hind legs should be assessed in relation to each other. Note any signs indicating trauma, and be aware of heat or cold. Feel for deep tendon reflexes and check for their symmetry (Fig. 9.26).

Tail

Feel for muscle tone, signs of trauma, and deep pain reflexes. The tail can be a common site for external parasites such as fleas and sarcoptic mange mites (especially in canids like the fox), so handle with care (Fig. 9.27).

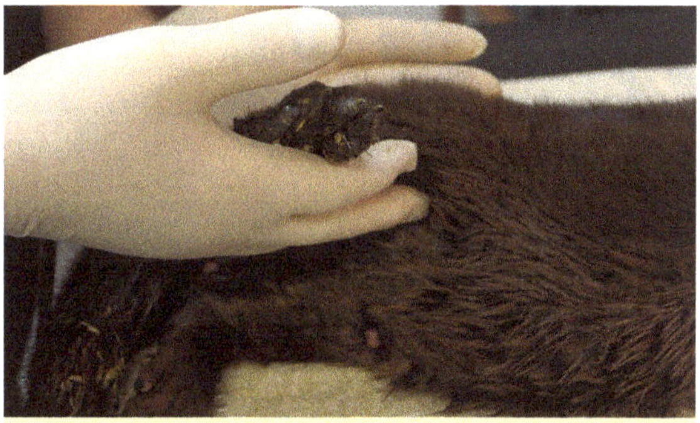

Figure 9.26
Osteopathic articulation of the right pelvic limb of an anesthetized European otter.

Osteopathic treatment

Wildlife patients do not respond well to lengthy treatment sessions. They can go into post-treatment shock and die. Plan what you hope to do before touching the patient and aim to execute the treatment within a period of two to five minutes maximum (TN's own experience).

Decide if the treatment is going to be performed with the patient awake or chemically restrained.

Techniques will vary depending on the species and conditions being treated. If the patient is awake the best techniques are those applied with continuous hand contact using slow, controlled movements. Where any high velocity, low amplitude thrusts (HVLATs) are used these are performed as a direct continuation of the full hand contact movements. At all costs try to avoid jerky hand movements and always think ahead as to what you want to achieve. These patients do not have the tolerance of a domestic animal to human contact.

More than in any other area of animal work you will need to combine your observations, case-history taking, palpation, and treatments so that they blend seamlessly from one to the other. Less is definitely more. Do what is absolutely necessary then leave alone. Think of your treatment as the catalyst to accelerating the patient's own healing and repair mechanisms.

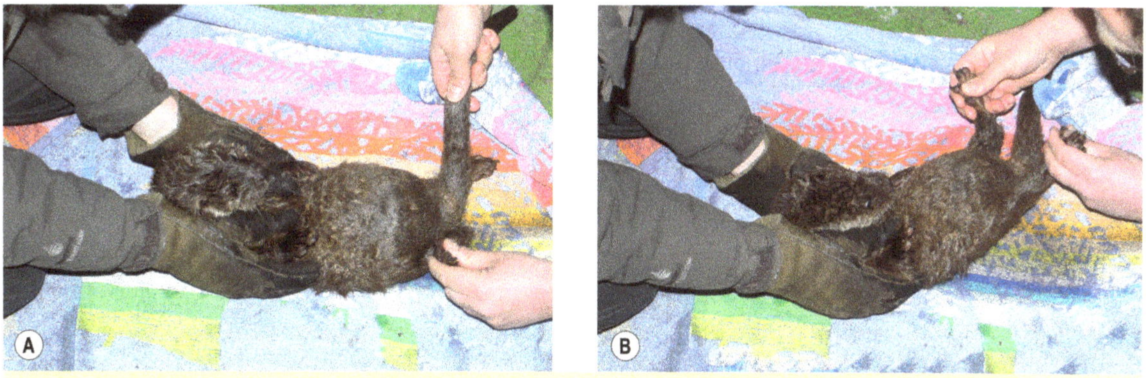

Figure 9.27
Applying a functional release technique to alter the resting state of the paravertebral muscles to a European otter cub with spinal injury.

Certain species appear to respond better to certain osteopathic modalities. Due to the fact that these patients must be able to fend for themselves once released, you should aim your treatment at achieving a survivable state in the minimum number of moves. Forget trying to create the perfect feel through the involuntary mechanism (IVM) or the perfect range of motion through each and every joint. Just ask yourself "Have I done enough for this individual to survive unaided?"

Every osteopath has preferred modalities that he or she works best with. The art is in knowing when you need to dust off one of your lesser used modalities for the greater good of the wild patient.

Osteopathic treatment considerations

When the author first started treating wildlife casualties he did not have the luxury of chemical restraint methods.

Badgers (*Meles meles*) and other Mustelidae

The most common badger casualties are those resulting from an RTA. Injuries suffered range from concussion, fractures, severe cervical muscle spasm, through to ruptured intervertebral discs (BWRC [n.d.]; Pearce 2011, pp. 74-77).

These patients are incredibly strong for their size. They possess a bite strong enough to amputate a human finger or fracture a forearm. Once they bite their jaws lock shut due to a clever evolutionary mechanism. If you try to pull free they will shake whatever they have got hold of, so it is best to avoid being bitten in the first place (Roper 2010).

Osteopathic treatment can be performed with the patient fully conscious with help from an experienced handler restraining the patient via the scruff of the neck and loose flesh over the dorsal lumbar region. A fabric muzzle is held in place due to the badger's neck being wider than the cranium. The front limbs also need restraining as the badger will use their long claws to pull the muzzle off - never a relaxing action for the osteopath! A small cloth covering the eyes and also the avoidance of bright lights and loud noises aid in securing the patient and keeping it calm (Clark 1992).

Osteopathic modalities that work best on adult badgers are very much more structural-based articulation, joint mobilization, and HVLAT work. If they are relaxed enough after these have been administered then finishing with a short cranial CV4 is fine, but only if you are sure there have been no central nervous system (CNS) bleeds.

Where possible the author would suggest treating badgers using anesthesia for restraint (Fig. 9.28).

Red fox (*Vulpes vulpes*)

Although red foxes are canids they have many feline characteristics, especially from an osteopathic point

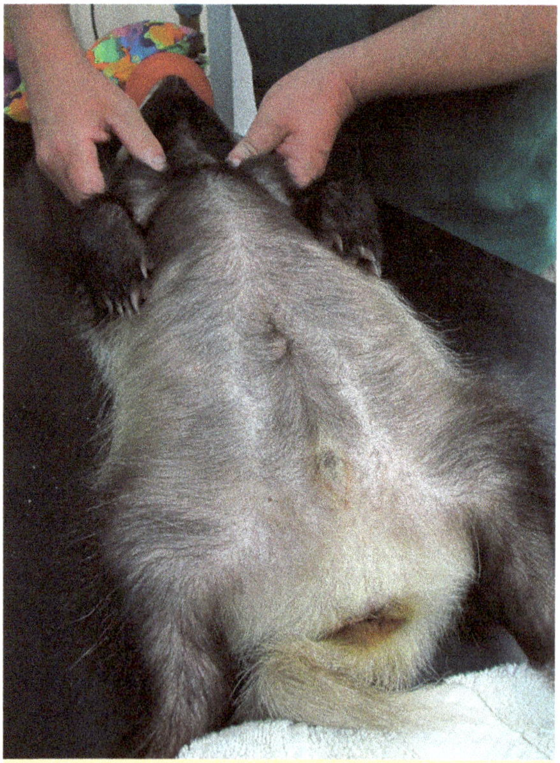

Figure 9.28
Osteopathic evaluation of the ventral throat structures, including the hyoid mechanism, of an anesthetized European badger.

of view. Anatomically their skeletons are finely boned, and the vertebral facet joints allow for much greater ranges of movement when compared to most domestic dog breeds. They are more agile and are better climbers than most other canids.

They are very quick movers and will give virtually no signs of pain or weakness when palpated. They can carry several highly infectious diseases (leptospirosis, sarcoptic mange, parvovirus, rabies) and need very careful handling to avoid being bitten (BWRC 2017).

They do respond well to most modalities of osteopathic medicine, but will not tolerate long treatment sessions. Again, less is more.

Deer (Cervidae)

Where possible try to avoid the use of chemical restraint as deer can react adversely. Quiet, low light, and gentle restraint are the best methods here. These creatures suffer stress and shock very easily so keep contact time to a minimum and use modalities that will release soft tissue tension and restore normal movement without triggering shock. Inhibition and functional and positional release work are good in this case, with only minimum use of HVLAT work if absolutely necessary. Sacroiliac and lumbosacral junctions which have been injured when deer have been caught by a back leg in a wire fence respond well to HVLATs. After treatment make sure that food and water are not available for about an hour to further avoid shock setting in (Fig. 9.29A and B).

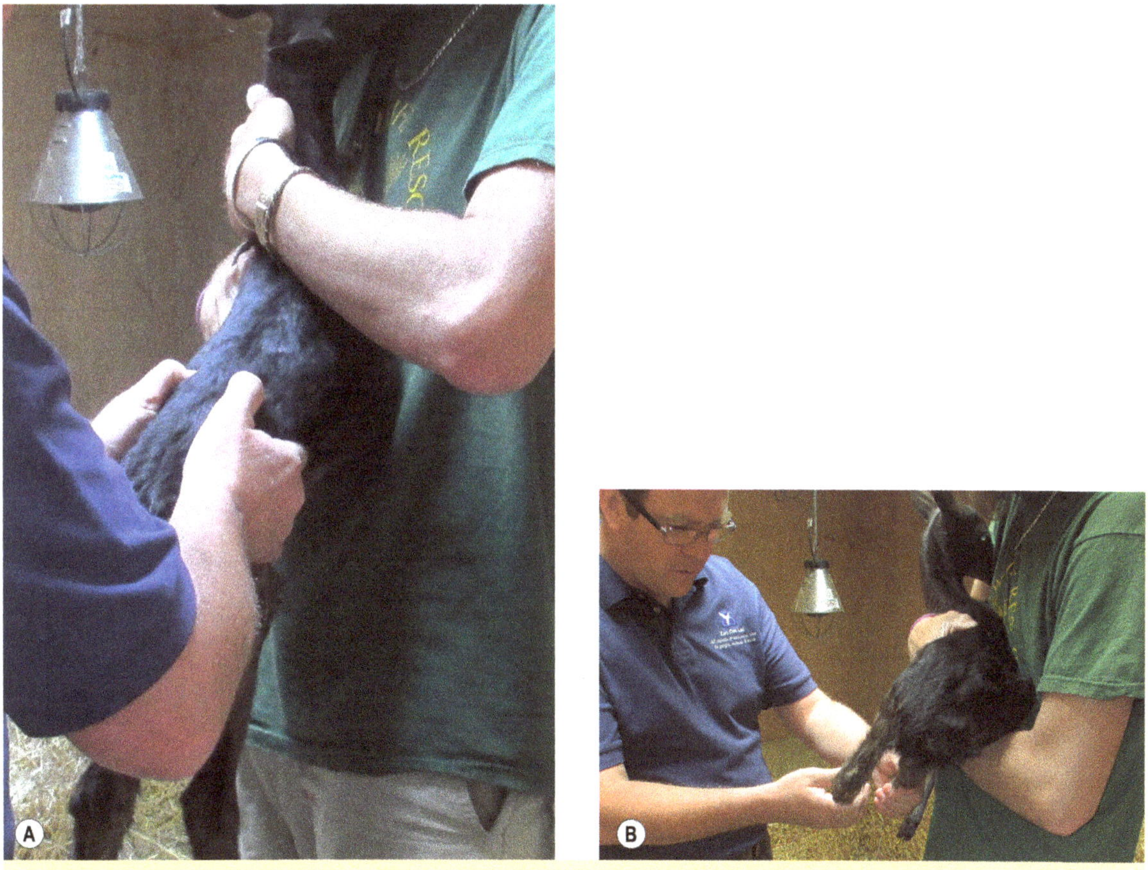

Figure 9.29
(A) Osteopathic evaluation of the lumbar spine of a fallow deer fawn road traffic accident casualty. (B) A comparison of hind limb flexion in the same patient.

European hedgehog (*Erinaceus europaeus*)

Most casualties the author sees have either lost a limb (caused by garden waste, and litter such as plastics, drinks cans, etc.) or have suffered poisoning. The former are treated to rebalance their bodies to function adequately on three legs and to be strong enough to remain curled up in the presence of a predator such as a fox or badger. With poison cases the aim is to stimulate their entire musculoskeletal systems to bounce back once the vets have medicated to neutralize the effects to their CNS and digestive systems.

When applying osteopathic treatment hedgehogs are incredibly sensitive to noise. Someone coughing or shutting a door will elicit a defensive activation of the spines, with those over the forehead pointing anteriorly via the fronto-cuticularis or preorbitalis dorsalis muscles. A more severe response involves contraction of panniculus carnosus muscle creating the classic curling response. This can prove painful for the osteopath if he or she is not wearing suitable gloves (Stocker 1992, pp. 109–110; Reeve 1997).

To uncurl a hedgehog a simple effective method is to place it on an examination table and then stroke the dorsal spines in a caudal direction several times Fig. 9.30). The hedgehog will uncurl and start to look around. You can now examine and treat.

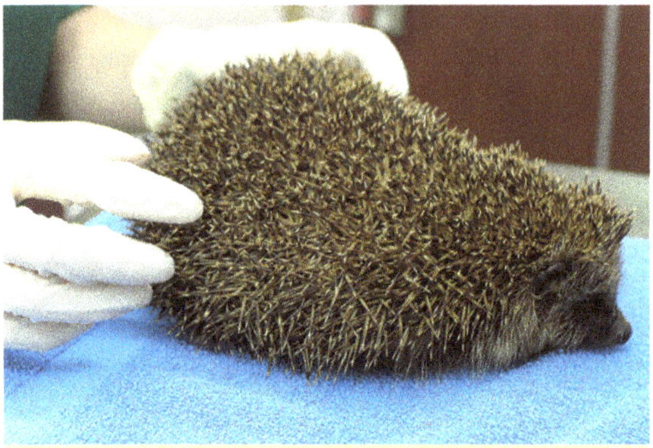

Figure 9.30
By stroking the dorsal spines in a caudal direction you can encourage a hedgehog to uncurl.

Unlike most wild animals, the hedgehog is pretty relaxed when handled quietly. The author has only been bitten once in 28 years (so far) and that was while being filmed.

Hedgehogs respond extremely well to functional and positional release work involving the whole body and also treatment of focal areas (Fig. 9.31).

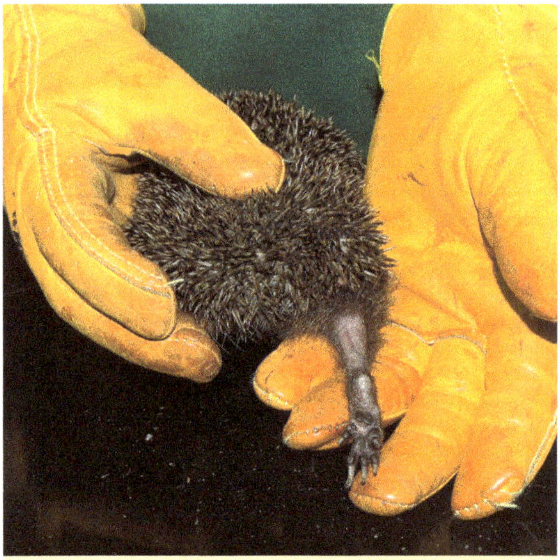

Figure 9.31
Applying a focused functional stretch technique through the right hind limb structures of a European hedgehog.

Most hedgehogs will be calm and relaxed, but do not allow more than five minutes for a treatment session from start to finish.

Bats (*Chiroptera*)

These can and do carry rabies, even in the UK. All UK species are insectivorous, which means they are armed with sharp shrew-like teeth. Their wings are incredibly delicate but extremely strong. Casualties tend to be orphaned youngsters or the victims of cat attacks (Richardson 1993).

Treatment of these fascinating creatures is minimalistic. Functional and positional modalities are the key here. Remember that bats have very fast metabolic rates, so keep treatment content and time to an absolute minimum.

Due to the small sizes of UK species these are best handled and treated by just the osteopath; however, do remember to wear gloves. Even a scratch from a tooth needs to be investigated due to the risk of rabies (Randerson 2002; Altringham 2003).

Wing injuries are common and if the wing is held up to a strong light, while shielding the bat's eyes, it is possible to see most fractures and dislocations (Robertson 1990) (Fig. 9.32).

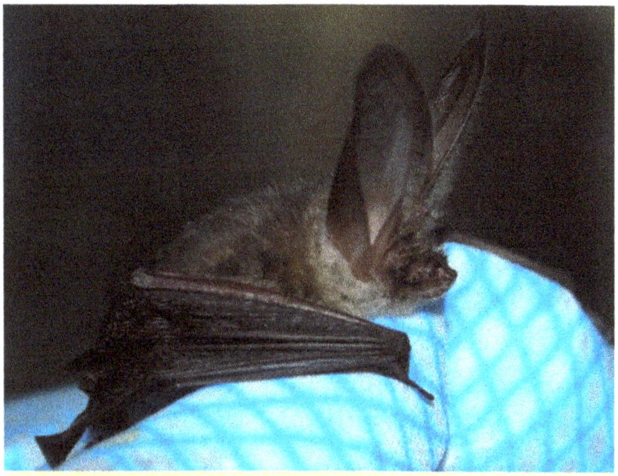

Figure 9.32
Using a cloth-covered hand to gently evaluate limb proprioception in a brown long-eared bat.

Case study 9.1

Golden jackal (*Canis aureus*)

Signalment and history

A young male golden jackal (*Canis aureus*) of about 4.5 kg was found in northern Greece inside the engine of a car. The animal had gone there to rest after being injured. The owner of the car found the animal and transported it to the Action for Wildlife animal clinic.

Veterinary evaluation

The jackal was unable to walk or stand. Radiography revealed epiphysiolysis in the distal end of the right tibia and a closed fracture of the left ulna and radius.

Veterinary treatment

Surgery was delayed for a few days while the nutritional status of the animal was corrected. The fracture site of the left radius was plated, and two surgical pins were used to stabilize the distal epiphysis of the right tibia. Painkillers (meloxicam) were prescribed for three days after the surgery, and antibiotics (amoxicillin, clavulanic acid) were administered for 15 days. The animal was constrained in a small cage to limit the movements of the injured limbs.

Follow-up

One week after the surgery the jackal was able to use his legs normally. Three weeks later a radiograph was acquired to evaluate the progress of the injuries. Bone healing was evident at the fracture sites. Mobility of the right hock joint was restricted in flexion, and so the animal was referred for osteopathic treatment.

Osteopathic evaluation and treatment

Evaluation and treatment was carried out under general anesthesia. The hock joint was extending properly but there was about 85 percent of normal flexion (Fig. 9.33A and B). The joint dysfunction had a "solid block" end feel indicating no functional component to the restriction.

Initial results

Articulation of the restricted hock did not achieve any improvement in joint mobility.

Follow-up

A few days after the second X-ray surgery was performed to remove the bone plate and the surgical pins. After the surgery, and while the animal was still under general anesthesia, the hock joint was evaluated revealing improvement in flexion to about 95 percent. The restriction again had a "solid block" end feel that resisted any improvement by the use of osteopathic means.

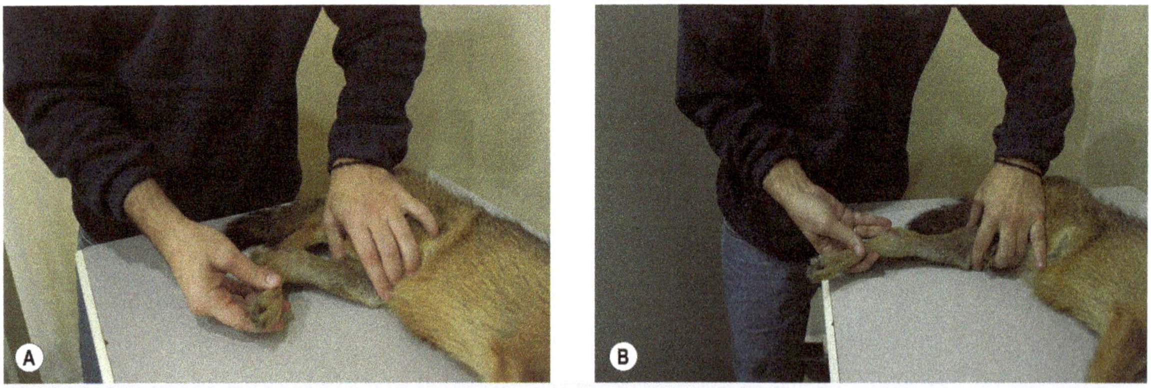

Figure 9.33
(A) Osteopathic evaluation of tarsal flexion in a young golden jackal. (B) Osteopathic evaluation of tarsal extension in the same patient.

The next day the jackal had recovered and was moving well. The animal was prescribed antibiotic treatment for three days and was placed in a large rehabilitation cage to improve his strength and stamina before being released into the wild.

Conclusions

Joint stability and mobility had returned to the limbs of the jackal. No changes in hock mobility were observed after osteopathic treatment due to lack of functional component to the restriction. Normal hock mobility returned after a four-week period influenced by the removal of surgical pins and the natural active movements of the jackal.

Case study *9.2*

European hedgehog (*Erinaceus europaeus*)

Signalment

The patient was an adult male European hedgehog.

History

The hedgehog was admitted to a UK wildlife hospital with a hind limb trauma injury. He had been found by a member of the public in their garden during the daytime, wandering around the lawn and dragging the right hind limb. The veterinary surgeon who examined the animal concluded that the limb had no viable vascular or nerve supply, and that the muscles were already necrotic around the stifle joint, which was unstable with an open fracture to the distal end of the femur proximal to the articular condyles. It was therefore decided that the limb should be amputated at the acetabulofemoral joint to ensure the patient could have a reasonable chance of being returned to the wild (Vale Wildlife [n.d.]).

Radiographs were taken to ensure that there was no other damage, especially to the pelvic girdle or spine. These showed no other injuries of a bony nature.

Surgery was successful, and osteopathic treatment was advised to aid recovery and rehabilitation (Fig.9.34A and B).

Presenting signs

The patient was placed on a clean floor in the examination room where the author (TN) was able to observe posture and gait. The patient was seen to move well, and there was good strength to the left hind limb, which he brought toward the midline in the cranial phase while walking. Proprioception and spatial awareness were all intact to touch and sound. There was obvious lameness, with a right lateral flexion bias

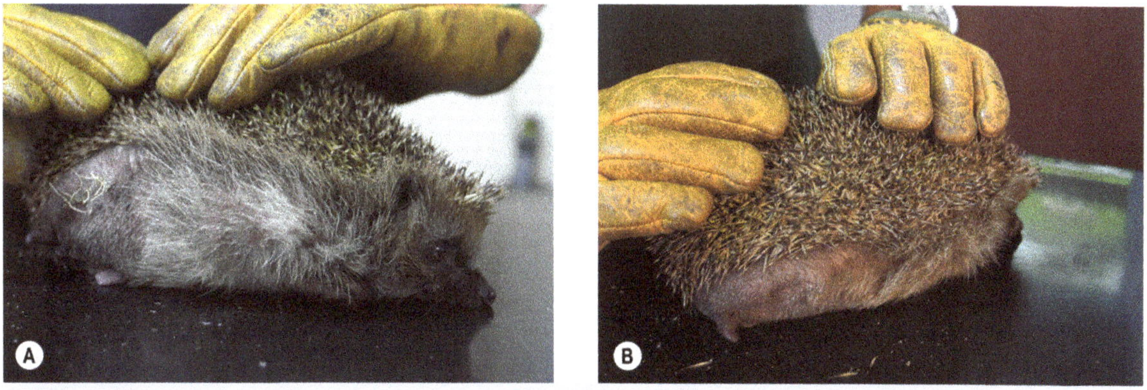

Figure 9.34
(A) Lateral view of a European hedgehog showing the surgical site after amputation of the right hind limb following irreparable trauma. (B) The same surgical wound now fully healed.

through the animal's trunk to allow the remaining hind limb to provide support and propulsion. The animal's center of gravity was also shifted cranially, with more weight pivoting over the forelimbs, and the nose was extended slightly when compared with healthy four-legged hedgehogs.

Osteopathic treatment

For the physical examination phase leather gardening gloves were worn and the patient was transferred to an examination table with a nonslip rubber surface. With the veterinary surgeon present, the osteopath first checked if the hedgehog was able to curl itself into a ball *and* if he had enough strength to keep curled even when moderate effort was exerted to try to open him up again. This hedgehog could withstand this and showed no signs of stress (Fig. 9.35).

The osteopath then used the standard method for encouraging the hedgehog to relax and open up again by stroking the surface spines caudally. The hedgehog uncurled and was then content to stand and walk about the examination table (Fig. 9.36A and B).

Using gentle, loose hand contact the osteopath was able to assess motility and overall mobility throughout the entire body and limbs. Care was taken around the suture sites and surgical areas before examination blended into a functional unwinding release through the entire length of the patient's spine, including the cervical structures ventrally as well as along the dorsal aspects. Gentle contact via the ventral aspect of the abdomen allowed the patient to release excess tension within the ventral spinal musculature, with the psoas in particular allowing the lumbar spine to dorsal flex and the left hind limb to extend at the hip.

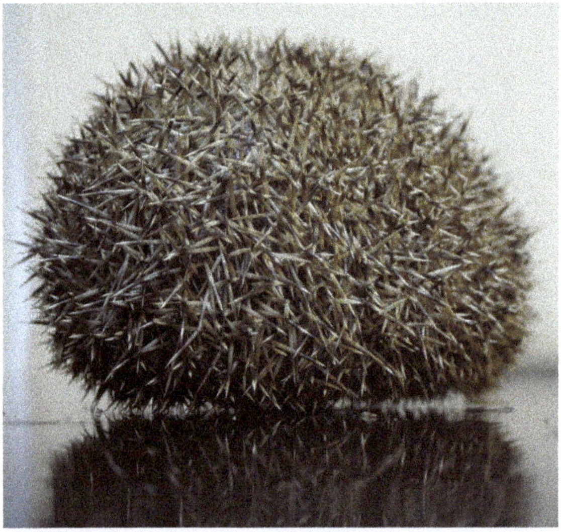

Figure 9.35
A fully curled European hedgehog. Note the asymmetry caused by right hind limb amputation.

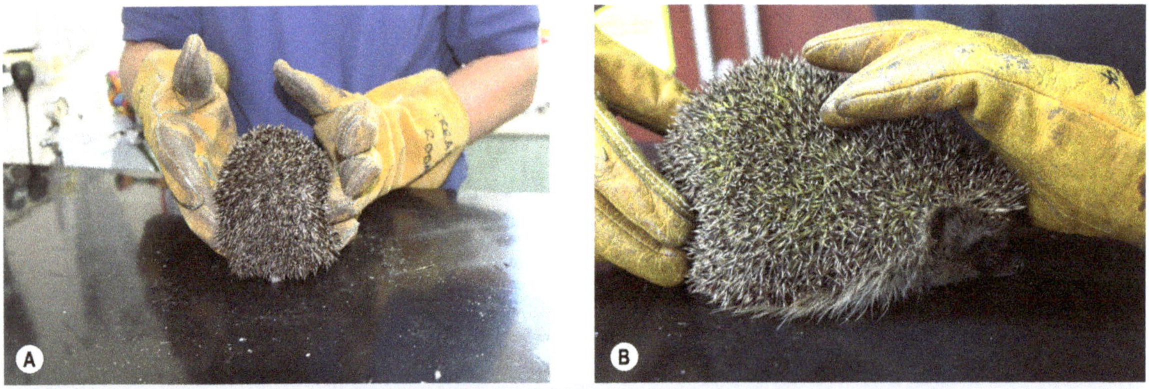

Figure 9.36
(A) Assessing muscle tone and spatial awareness in a European hedgehog. (B) Assessing muscle tone around the hips and pelvis of a hind limb in an amputee European hedgehog.

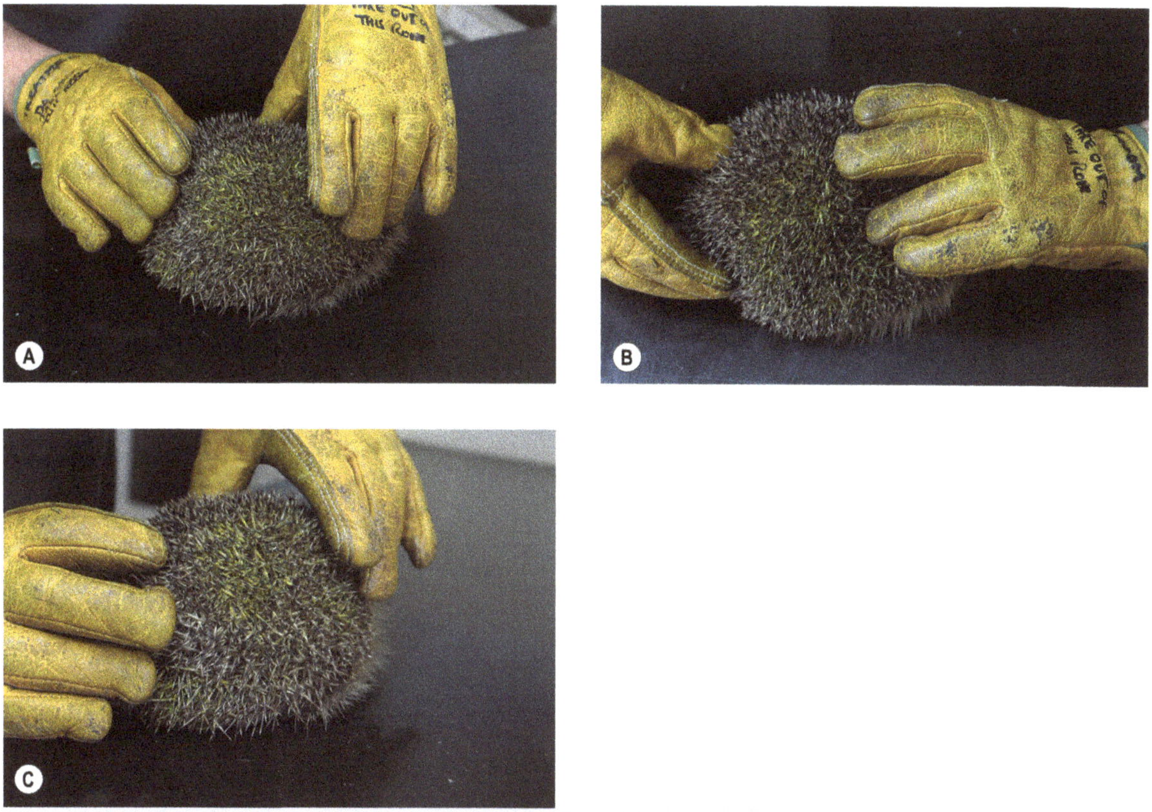

Figure 9.37
(A) Applying a functional release approach to a hind limb amputee European hedgehog. (B) Functional release work through the torso and pelvic structures. (C) Assessing the symmetry of soft tissue tone and joint mobility throughout the body of the same hedgehog following osteopathic treatment.

The strongest part of the myofascial pattern was the right lateral flexion through the core structures. The osteopath took these tissues further into this pattern and gently held them there until a lowering of the resting state was achieved. The patient indicated when this was happening by letting out an audible sigh and then physically relaxing (Fig. 9.37A–C).

Exercises were added to strengthen the patient's MSK system during these sessions (Fig. 9.38A–C).

Observation after treatment

Immediately after treatment had finished the osteopath was able to reassess the quality and symmetry of the patient's overall movement patterns before placing him on the floor and observing him walking around the room. There was less of an obvious bias in his movement, although the osteopath was fully aware that the patient would need to adapt muscling and movement patterns to accommodate the loss of the right hind limb.

Outcome

The osteopath performed a further examination and treatment seven days later, after which the patient was transferred to an outdoor rehab pen for further monitoring before a suitable release site was identified. Once this had been chosen he was released, along with another rehabilitated hedgehog, into a suitable garden equipped with a hedgehog box and a homeowner who

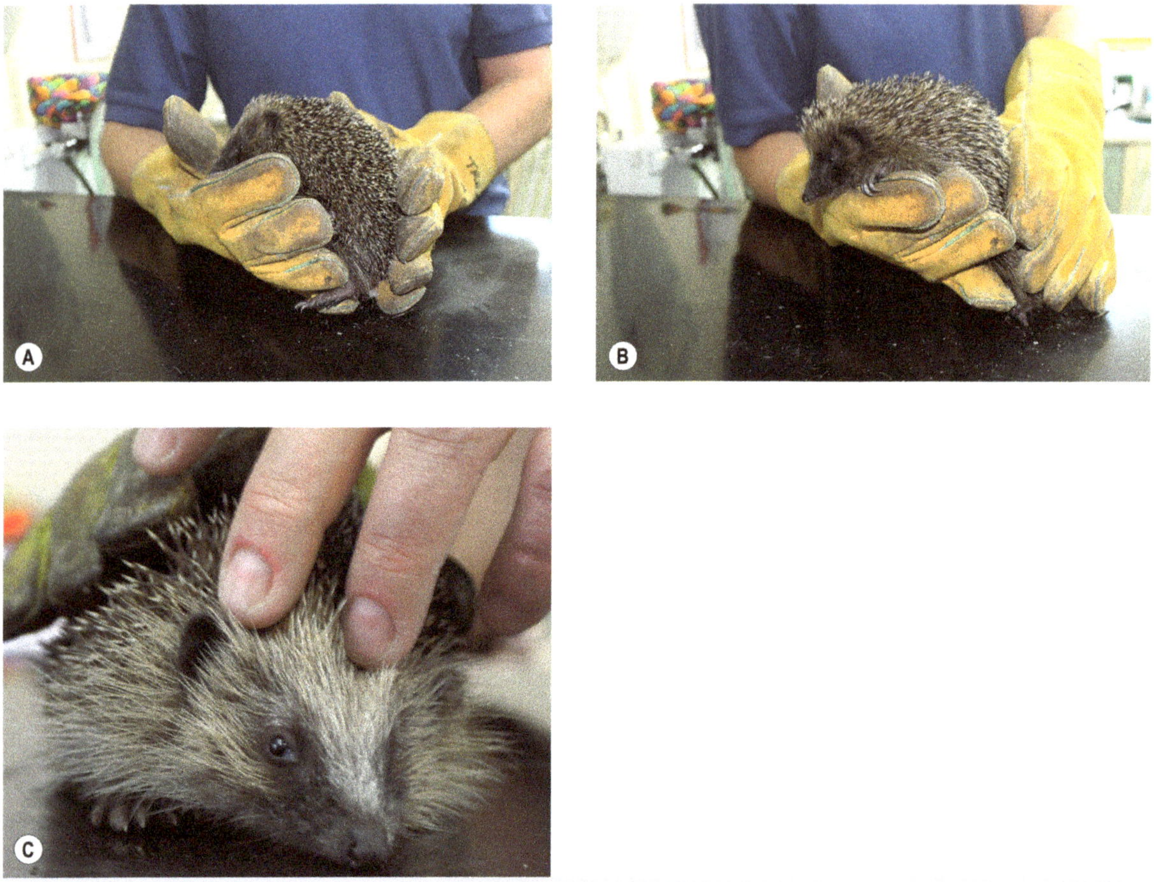

Figure 9.38
(A) Encouraging a European hedgehog patient to climb as part of its rehabilitation program. (B) Adding traction resistance to the same patient to help build muscle strength. (C) Engaging the involuntary mechanism of a European hedgehog.

was prepared to feed the animals until they either left her garden or no longer returned for the food.

The osteopathic patient was monitored for a further five nights before he moved away from the garden. He was not seen again for two months when he returned and was noted as occasionally being spotted in the garden, feeding on slugs and cat food over the following two weeks.

Conclusions

The majority of hedgehog patients that an osteopath is likely to see will have suffered trauma, and several of these cases will involve a limb amputation. The author has treated in excess of 150 different hedgehogs, with about 15 percent of these having received surgical amputation of a hind limb. These have not included any with a forelimb amputation, the assumption being that a hedgehog is not likely to be able to survive and thrive with the loss of a forelimb. See the British Hedgehog Preservation Society website for guidelines on rehabilitation.

Only viable wildlife casualties are referred for osteopathic intervention, as part of the overall rehabilitation program, as these are wild animals. Unlike domestic pets they must be able to survive and thrive on their own and in the face of predators such as badgers, foxes, and even brown rats (Stocker 1987, p. 129).

Those hedgehogs that the author has treated have responded well to osteopathic intervention where there is a purely MSK problem. The success rates fall when there are other internal disease processes present that can render any osteopathy useless. A strong individual is always more likely to recover. From data collected at various UK wildlife hospitals (BWRC [n.d.]) it has been noted that osteopathic treatment appears to reduce recovery and rehabilitation times, thus allowing individuals to be returned to the wild earlier than would have been expected and also reducing the financial burden to these charity bases.

Summary

Using osteopathy in the treatment of wildlife casualties is challenging. The rewards are great in advancing your core osteopathic skills, although you need to be fully aware of the dangers and potential pitfalls.

Working with other professionals and creating treatment programs are essential. Explaining what you propose to do prior to any hands-on contact will help to minimize stress and any adverse reactions.

Your own health and safety are paramount. Rarely is wildlife "owned." You are entirely responsible for your own actions and are rarely likely to get paid for this type of work; however, you will advance your skills and abilities to handle much tougher cases in your normal osteopathic work.

Above all you will discover just how effective small amounts of osteopathic intervention can be. The mantra is always *less is more*.

References

Action for Wildlife (2015) Personal communication with Action for Wildlife, Thessaloniki, Greece on data obtained from 2010 to 2014. Email: mail@drasi-agriazoi.gr [June 2015].

Altringham JD (2003). British Bats. Collins New Naturalist Library, Harper Collins.

Apollonio M, Andersen R, Putman R (eds.) (2010) European Ungulates and their Management in the 21st Century. Cambridge: Cambridge University Press, p. 618.

Baldwin M (2015a) Red fox (Vulpes vulpes). [Online] Available: http://www.wildlifeonline.me.uk/red_fox.html#vision [Sept 4, 2017].

Baldwin M (2015b) Deer. [Online] Available: http://www.wildlifeonline.me.uk/deer.html#antlers [Sept 4, 2017].

British Hedgehog Preservation Society. [Online] Available: https://www.britishhedgehogs.org.uk [Sept 4, 2017].

BWRC – British Wildlife Rehabilitation Council [n.d.] Data available on request from: http:\\www.bwrc.org.uk [Sept 4, 2017].

BWRC – British Wildlife Rehabilitation Council (2017) Guidelines for Wildlife Rehabilitation Units. Available: http://bwrc.org.uk/#/guidelines/4549073116 [Sept 4, 2017].

Carpenter JW, Lindemann D (2017) Overview of hedgehogs. [Online] Available: http://www.merckvetmanual.com/mvm/exotic_and_laboratory_animals/hedgehogs/overview_of_hedgehogs.html [Sept 4, 2017].

Clark M (1992) Badgers. Whittet Books.

Fowler M (2008). Restraint and Handling of Wild and Domestic Animals. Wiley-Blackwell.

Fowler PA, Racey PA (2009) Overwintering strategies of the badger, Meles meles, at 57oN. Journal of Zoology. 214: 635–651.

Gower Bird Hospital (2018) Increasing our knowledge. Data from: www.gowerbirdhospital.org.uk/research.asp [accessed January 10, 2018]. Email: admin@gowerbird-hospital.org.uk.

Kowalczyk R, Jędrzejewska B, Zalewski A (2003) Annual and circadian activity patterns of badgers (Meles meles). In: Białowieża Primeval Forest (eastern Poland) compared with other Palaearctic populations. Journal of Biogeography. March; 30 (3) 463–472. [Online] Available: http://onlinelibrary.wiley.com/doi/10.1046/j.1365-2699.2003.00804.x/abstract. [Sept 4, 2017].

Lloyd HG (1980) The Red Fox. London: B T Batsford.

McCafferty DJ (2005) Ecology and conservation of otters (Lutra lutra). In: Loch Lomond and the Trossachs National Park. Glasgow Naturalist. 24 29–35. [Online] Available: http://www.glasgownaturalhistory.org.uk/ll_papers/llproc_dmc.pdf. [Sept 4, 2017].

Mullineaux E, Best D, Cooper JE (eds.) (2003) BSAVA Manual of Wildlife Casualties. BSAVA Manuals, Gloucester: British Small Animal Veterinary Association.

Myers P (2017) Legs, feet, and cursorial locomotion. In: Myers P, Espinosa R, Parr C S, Jones T, Hammond GS, Dewey TA (2017) The Animal Diversity Web. [Online]

Available: http://animaldiversity.org/collections/mammal_anatomy/running_fast [Sept 4, 2017]

Neal EG, Cheeseman CL (1996) Badgers. Poyser Natural History, London: T & AD Poyser London.

Olmstead ML (ed.) (1995) Small Animal Orthopedics. St. Louis, MO: Mosby.

Piermattei DL, Flo GL, DeCamp CE (2006) Brinker, Piermattei, and Flo's Handbook of Small Animal Orthopedics and Fracture Repair. 4th edn. St. Louis, MO: Saunders.

Pusey A, Brooks J, Jenks A (2010) Osteopathy and the Treatment of Horses. Wiley-Blackwell.

Randerson J (2002) Bat enthusiast killed by rabies. New Scientist Daily News. [Online] Available: https://www.newscientist.com/article/dn3101-bat-enthusiast-killed-by-rabies/ [Sept 4, 2017].

Reeve N (1997) Hedgehogs, Poyser Natural History. London: T & A D Poyser London.

Richardson P (1993) Bats. Whittet Books.

Robertson J (1990) The Complete Bat. London: Chatto & Windus.

Robinson A (ed.) (1918) Cunningham's Text-book of Anatomy. 5th edn. New York: William Wood, p. 364.

Roper T (2010) The Badger. Collins New Naturalist Library. Harper Collins.

Step E (1921) Animal Life of the British Isles: A Pocket Guide to the Mammals, Reptiles and Batrachians of Wayside and Woodland. London: Frederick Warne.

Stocker L (1987) The Complete Hedgehog. London: Chatto & Windus.

Stocker L (ed.) (2005) Practical Wildlife Care. 2nd edn. Oxford: Blackwell Publishing, Oxford.

Vale Wildlife Hospital and Rehabilitation Centre [n.d.] Data available on request from: http://www.valewildlife.org.uk [Sept 4, 2017].

Vincent JFV, Owers P (1986) Mechanical design of hedgehog spines and porcupine quills. Journal of Zoology. September; 210 (1) 55–75.

Further reading

Jordan W, Hughes J (1982) First Aid and Care for Wild Animals and Birds. Care for the Wild Publication.

Kruuk H (1989) The Social Badger. Oxford: Oxford University Press.

Pearce EP (2011) Badger Behaviour, Conservation and Rehabilitation. Exeter: Pelagic Publishing.

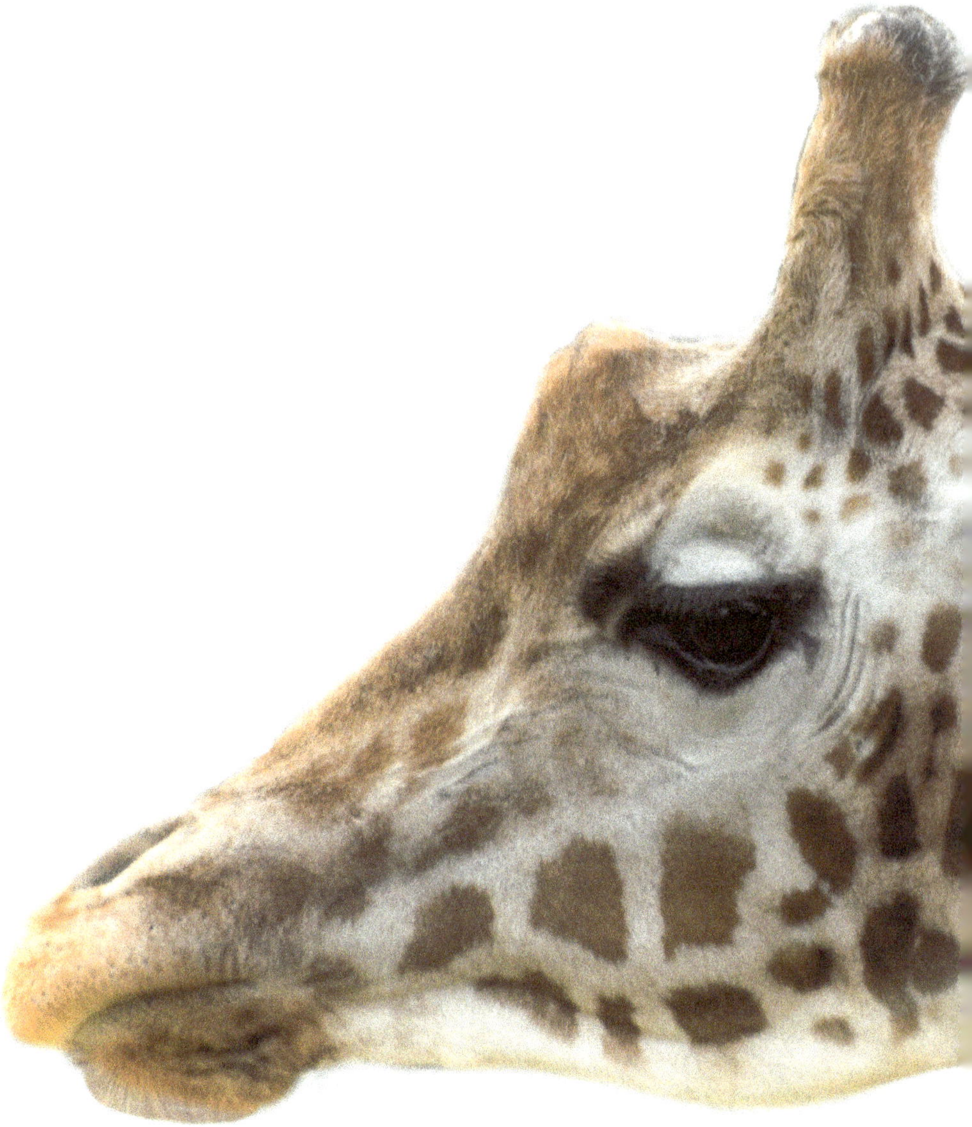

Chapter 10 MEGAFAUNA

*Tony Nevin, Jon Cracknell,
Nic Masters, Andy Hayton*

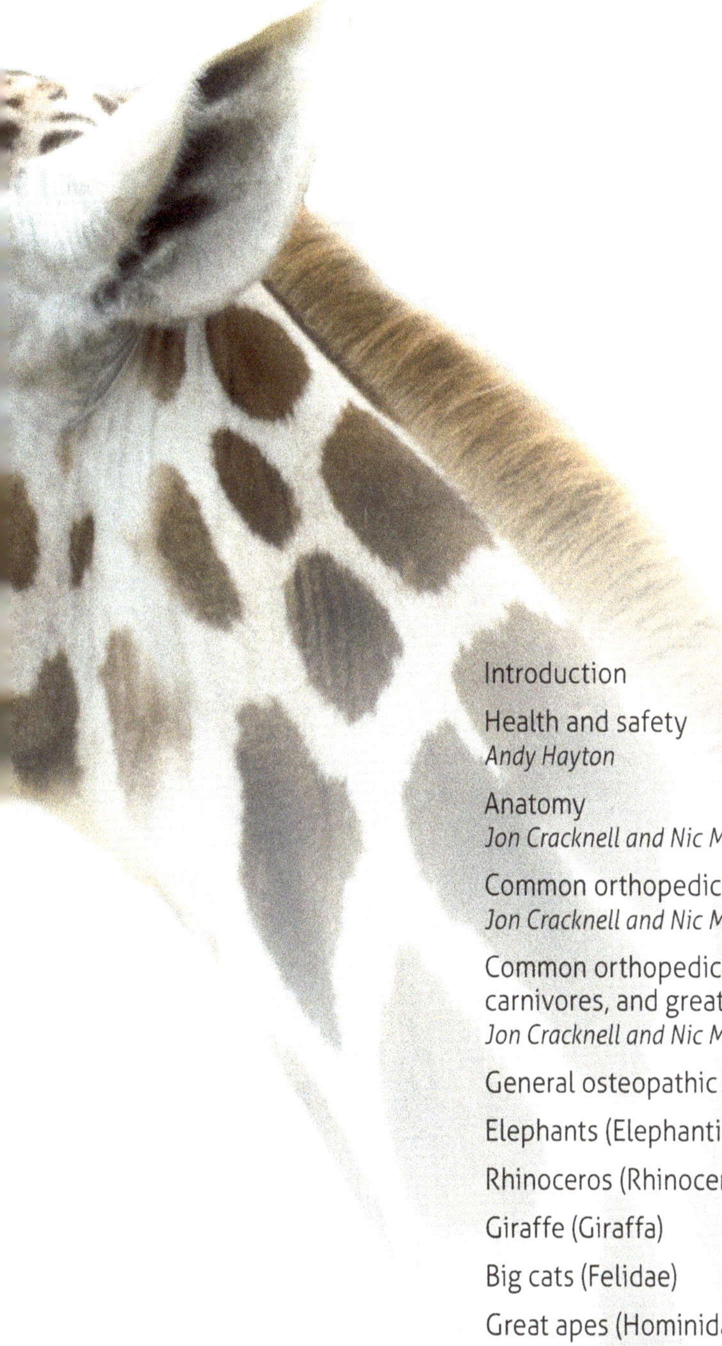

Introduction

Treatment of megafauna is an area of osteopathic medicine where there is little published research and knowledge available to help the osteopath, or those who might wish to elicit our help. Due to the sheer size and nature of these patients many people are unaware that osteopathy can have a beneficial effect on the animals' health and well-being. A concise description of what constitutes megafauna is found at the beginning of the anatomy section of this chapter.

Around 26 years ago the author (TN) successfully applied osteopathic principles to treat Asian elephants, southern white rhinos, and Rothschild's giraffe. Since then other species and subspecies of wildlife ranging from big cats to great apes have been added to the list. In some cases osteopathy has been used to intervene in situations where no other branch of medicine has been wholly effective.

At the time of writing some papers have been published (Nevin 2004, 2005, 2012), but these are mostly case studies, and it will be a while before data compiled thus far can filter through to peer-reviewed journals for future publication.

The osteopath wishing to work in this area must be able to work as an integral member of a team. Very often the osteopathic side of the work is not fully understood by those working on a daily basis in the zoo and wildlife world. The veterinary surgeons and key animal workers are our main allies here, and we have to explain thoroughly to these people what it is we are hoping to achieve and how.

Most of the cases an osteopath is called upon to treat will be of a musculoskeletal nature. However, once your skills are better understood you may well find yourself faced with anything from a psychologically traumatized elephant to a neurologically impaired lion.

There are textbooks covering the anatomy of certain species that are likely to be kept in collections, and these can be an invaluable aid to the osteopath. There is also a need to gain a working knowledge of the behavior of the species that you are going to treat. Usually the best people to speak to here are keepers and rangers. They know the behavior and individual habits of their animals better than anyone. Prior to any hands-on involvement it is necessary to have a meeting with all staff members who need to be involved to talk through what you hope to do and then to discuss with them the best, and sometimes only, way of achieving this. Realizing that you need an elephant on its other side after it has been anesthetized does not win osteopathy any new fans!

Please read the health and safety section of this chapter thoroughly prior to embarking on your first appointment.

Health and safety

The number of animals in a zoological collection that will readily submit to osteopathic treatment when conscious is extremely small. This is in no small part due to collections wanting the animals in their care to exhibit the most natural behaviors possible in the environment of a captive situation.

There are several main forms of large mammal that the author (AH) has personally dealt with in the past in addition to elephants. These are large carnivores and assorted hoofed animals. All these animals throw up behavioral issues and health and safety concerns that most people used to working around domesticated stock will not anticipate.

Elephants

The elephant presents many challenges that most osteopaths will rarely come across. Being in close proximity to an animal of their sheer size presents us with potential for harm even without any malice intended. Accidental injuries can occur just with an animal moving around and crushing unwary people against solid objects. This size, coupled with a huge intelligence and a fierce sense of right and wrong, can make for an incredible partner, who is willing and eager to work alongside a thoughtful and respectful team, or a terrifying and extremely dangerous prospect when treated lightly and pushed into a badly thought-out stressful situation with no prior planning.

There are two main recognized methods of handling and working with elephants, and both have their pros and cons.

Free contact

This is what most people would recognize as the traditional mahout–elephant relationship, where the two share the same space and work in very close confines with no barriers. The handler will use a number of tools to help guide and restrain the animal. Primarily these will include the ankus or elephant hook and, if needed for a more nervous animal, ropes or chains to offer some restraint.

Free contact allows unrestricted access to the animal for the team, allowing for different modes of manipulation. It includes the patient lying down on their side for treatment, which relies on very experienced handlers, a well-trained animal, and good communication and planning between the team. Free contact is losing favor in Europe and the US due to a number of accidents involving keepers and the public perception of "traditional" elephant training. It is still very much used in Asia where Tony Nevin has had great success in administering treatment to a wide range of animals.

Protected contact

Protected contact is a system gaining favor in zoos whereby keepers and elephants are permanently separated by a safety barrier and never share the same space. It is felt that this system has a far higher safety margin than free contact.

Elephants are trained to stand by a wall or barrier with access ports, where the animal will "present" parts of its body when asked. The animal can leave and end the interaction at any time of its choosing.

An elephant restraint device, or crush, where the animal's forward and lateral movement is restricted can also be used in protected contact. This method has a better safety value, due to the barriers present, but can still be dangerous to the unwary and unprepared. A patient can still grab a person with a trunk and pull them against the steel barrier, or an arm can be trapped between the barrier and the animal being worked upon. Protected contact also restricts the amount of contact that the osteopath has due to the nature of the barrier separating them.

Please also refer to the section on planning osteopathic treatment (page 421).

Hoofed animals

These animals range from the sublime to the ridiculous, from a 30 kg blackbuck antelope up to a 3,000 kg white rhino.

Rhinos are, on the whole, relatively amenable and will take to treatment fairly readily as long as slow movements are used and they are happy with the treatment. Rhinos have a very good sense of hearing but this, coupled with poor eyesight, can make them overreact and spook. We have always undertaken any treatment with a protective barrier separating us from the animal. Care must be taken not to get any part of your person between the animal and the barrier as crush injuries can easily occur.

Giraffe, antelope species, and wild equids have a very different take on life from rhinos. The flight response in the majority is strong, but in certain individuals and species of antelope and wild equids the reaction can be fight then flight. A bull eland weighs up to 1,000 kg and has horns 90 cm long. It is not something to start negotiating with when it is unhappy.

Certain collections have their giraffes trained to walk into restraint chutes or crushes. Treatment may be possible if taken slowly, but restricted space in the crush area and the type of manipulation required need to be considered. Giraffe have been known to decapitate lions with one kick when defending calves.

Smaller antelope almost invariably want to get away from you if in a confined space. This can easily lead to injuries being sustained by the animal. Horns can be broken off when running blindly into walls, and legs can be broken simply by the muscle power used in taking off from a stressful situation.

Wild equids such as zebra species, Somali wild ass and onager all differ in character and levels of aggression and flight responses. The author has always felt he is working on a knife edge with zebra, which can go from calm to disaster in the blink of an eye. Think of the spookiest thoroughbred and meanest Shetland pony bred into one beast.

With all these points in mind, the best and safest way for the animal and people involved in any treatment may be for the patient to undergo general anesthesia. Standing sedation has been used, but sedation can be unreliable. Adrenaline release caused by external circumstances can quickly turn the patient from a sedated state to excitation, meaning it could try to get away or take an aggressive stance toward anyone nearby. A semisedated, frightened animal is a danger to both itself and everyone around it.

This leads us to the question: how many people does it take to treat an animal? Obviously the difficulty of manipulating a very large antelope or a giraffe can be labor-intensive, but only the minimum number of people needed should ever be in attendance. If or when something unforeseen does take place, the fewer people there are to clear from an area the better. Speed can save injury to both animals and humans.

Carnivores

When undergoing treatment, carnivores by their nature invariably require general anesthesia to ensure human safety. There are some collections where keepers do enter big cat enclosures with specific animals that are bonded to their keepers, but these collections are the exception, and you may not want to be the first osteopath to try treating these animals!

Before starting work, all carnivores must be checked by at least two people to ensure they are fully anesthetized before any thought of opening a cage door takes place. If anyone has any reservations about safety in this situation they must speak up. Better to wait an extra five minutes than go in one minute too soon. A strong contingency plan must be in place when dealing with these animals. Doors must be kept secure to both the house and cages, and every unlocking and locking of cages and doors must be double-checked by keeping staff. Tasks must be clearly delegated to individual members of the team, such as monitoring reactions to treatment or anesthesia becoming light. All preparations must have been made to ensure either the quick return of the animal to a safe, locked area or the rapid evacuation of all people involved to a safe area. It must be in the forefront of everyone's mind at all times that 200 kg of teeth and claws is uncontrollable and will not be persuaded by anyone not to do what comes naturally to all carnivores.

Great apes

With great apes it is best if the osteopath keeps out of the way while darting and anesthesia are administered. When performing any hands-on assessment and treatment it is worth noting that treatment stimulates some patients, and they may begin to wake up. In this situation adhere to any instructions that are given. Once osteopathic treatment has concluded, ensure that you leave the patient to wake up quietly while they are monitored by a regular member of staff. This helps to keep stress and disorientation to a minimum.

When any megafauna are being treated, teamwork and good communication coupled with solid preparation for any eventuality are key to a happy outcome for both the animals and the humans involved. It must always be in the forefront of an osteopath's mind when treating nondomesticated exotic species that they never react in the same way as domesticated dogs, cats or horses when presented with a stressful situation. If the animal's keeper feels that something is about to happen, it is probably going to! During treatment the osteopath will probably have the best "feel" for any changes in the animal's demeanor when it is anesthetized and they must inform vets and keeping staff immediately. Better to stop for a false alarm than carry on into an irretrievable situation.

Anatomy

Introduction

"Megafauna" is a loosely applied term to include animals that weigh over 45-100kg. Where the cut-off is made is a matter of personal choice. Megafauna are not a specific taxonomic group, more a collective of the big land mammals. Typically, megafauna have evolved to have high longevity, slow population growth rates, and low mortality rates with few or no predators. As stated in the introduction to this chapter, there is a huge wealth of anatomical variation that the osteopath must be aware of before approaching the megafauna patient, and there is a range of sources of information that the osteopath can utilize to gather in-depth knowledge of specific species. Older sources such as the Victorian anatomists are very useful; there are a variety of texts available from the 1920s to the 1950s that are also useful. Surprisingly, modern papers and publications on the anatomy of the megafauna species have added little until the last decade or so when access to modern CT and MRI scanners has allowed a greater understanding of the mechanics and load properties, and sometimes even the anatomy, than was possible previously. It is outside the scope of this chapter to discuss in detail the specific anatomical variations found across the range of species, and readers are directed to the references for more specific anatomical consideration.

Due to the myriad potential species that may be presented to the osteopath, and the specific anatomical differences found within the range of patients, it is important that the osteopath knows which group of animals they are looking at. While there may be specific anatomical differences, most animals fit to a basic body plan that is related to the more common domestic cousins represented in their taxonomic groups. Knowing this allows the osteopath to overcome any fear or concerns when facing a new species and allows them to be able to make initial assessments based on what they know or have experienced with other more common species.

Classification of animals into similar groups is known as taxonomy. In simple terms, in the animal kingdom, the class *Mammalia* includes 19 orders that are then subcategorized into families, then genus, and species. All classes of animals have similar relationships, and often evolutionary development will be found in the family. The most similar animals may share the same genus. Understanding these relationships and the taxonomic grouping is critical to understanding new or similar patients. A good example is the common classification of hoofed stock. These are made up of two orders: the Artiodactyla, literally even-toed ungulates, and the Perissodactyla or odd-toed ungulates. The domestic cow, giraffe, all deer, camels, antelope, hippo and pigs all are artiodactyls. However tapirs, equids, and rhinoceros are perissodactyls (Groves 2011). Knowing this means that some assumptions can be made about similarities between say zebra and a domestic horse. Although comparing a tapir, with its almost trunk-like nose, to a horse or even a rhino appears at face value nonsense, these animals all share common ancestry and some extrapolation can be made across the shared taxonomic groups.

To rely solely on this basic foundation could result in disaster and it is imperative that additional species-specific knowledge is gained. When looking for the first time at any ungulate, however, simply grouping them into cow or horse anatomical variation is a good place to start.

The same basic principles can be applied to the carnivores and great apes; in many respects a lion is a large domestic cat and an orangutan's basic anatomy is not dissimilar to that of a human being. While there are obvious differences, this approach allows the osteopath to start on a sound basis. They must then build on these foundation principles with species-specific knowledge as they move forward with a case - understanding that the distal hind-limb anatomy of the gorilla is different to man, and that the cheetah is not a small tiger.

In general terms, the anatomical points outlined below are generally consistent within the taxonomic groups discussed.

Elephants

Asian (*Elephas maximus*) and African (*Loxodonta africana* and *Loxodonta cyclotis*) elephants have similarly massive skeletons comprising more than 200 bones (Fig. 10.1 A and B). Asian elephants have 19 pairs of ribs whereas Africans have 21 (West 2006) and the number of lumbar vertebrae varies from three to five (Montali 2006). There is, relative to other mammals, only a very small distance between the last rib and the hind leg,

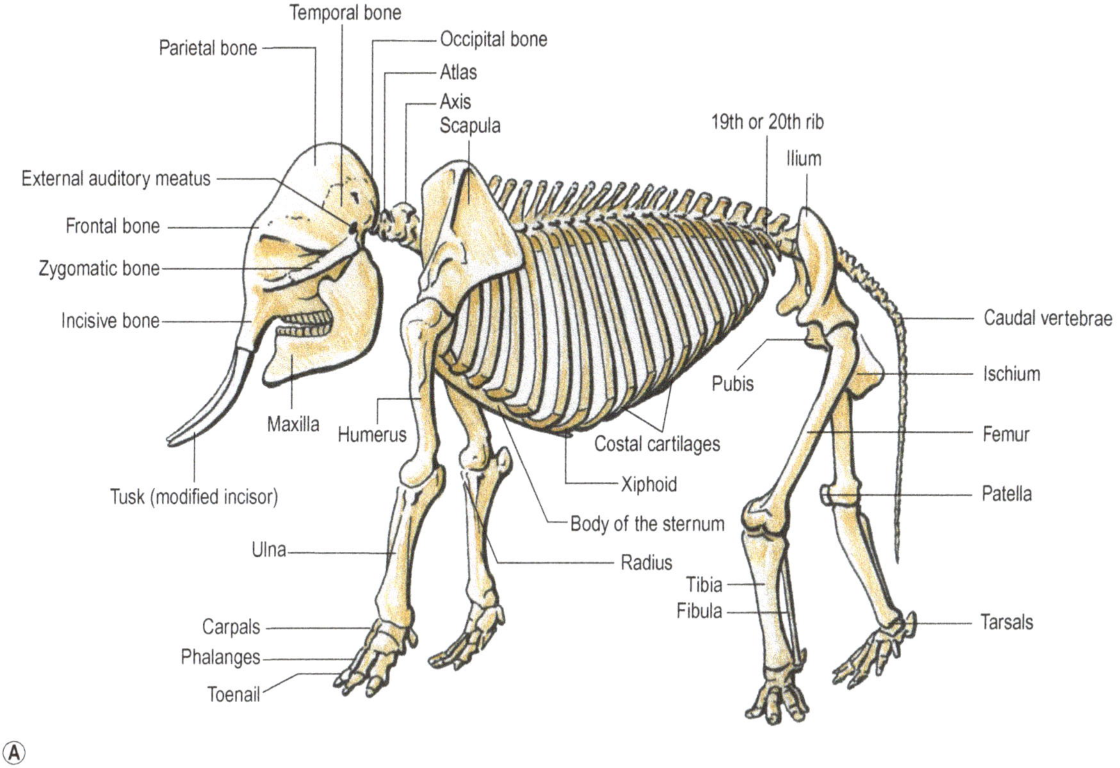

Figure 10.1
Diagram of the skeleton of (A) Asian elephant.

presumably to allow the axial skeleton to support the enormous weight of the internal organs. Appendicular limb bones lack a marrow cavity, which is replaced by a network of cancellous bone to provide additional strength as well as hematopoiesis (Shoshani 1992).

In African elephants the scapula, humerus, radius, and ulna, in particular, are massive compared to the relatively small bones of the manus. The front foot comprises eight carpal bones, five metacarpal bones, and five digits. Only digits 2, 3, and 4 comprise three phalanges (Fig. 10.2A and B). The distal phalanges of these central digits are very small and do not articulate with the middle phalanges (Smuts and Bezuidenhout 1993).

The femur is similarly massive and is the longest bone in African elephants, with the sturdy tibia and slender fibula only half as long. The patella is wedge-shaped and the femorotibial joint contains rudimentary menisci. The hind foot comprises seven tarsal bones, five metatarsal bones, and only four digits, with only digits 3 and 4 comprising three phalanges (Smuts and Bezuidenhout 1994).

The feet of African and Asian elephants are anatomically very similar but with minor differences in external shape and the number of toenails. The hind foot is smaller than the front foot and more oval. Not all digits have toenails; Asian elephants have five nails on the front feet and four on the hind feet, whereas African elephants have four nails on the front feet and three on the hind feet (Fowler 2006). Both feet have an unusual cartilaginous structure (called the prepollex in the front foot and the prehallux in the hind foot) that joins the first carpal and metacarpal bones (or the first tarsal and metatarsal bones) to the digital cushion, presumably stabilizing the digits over this structure of

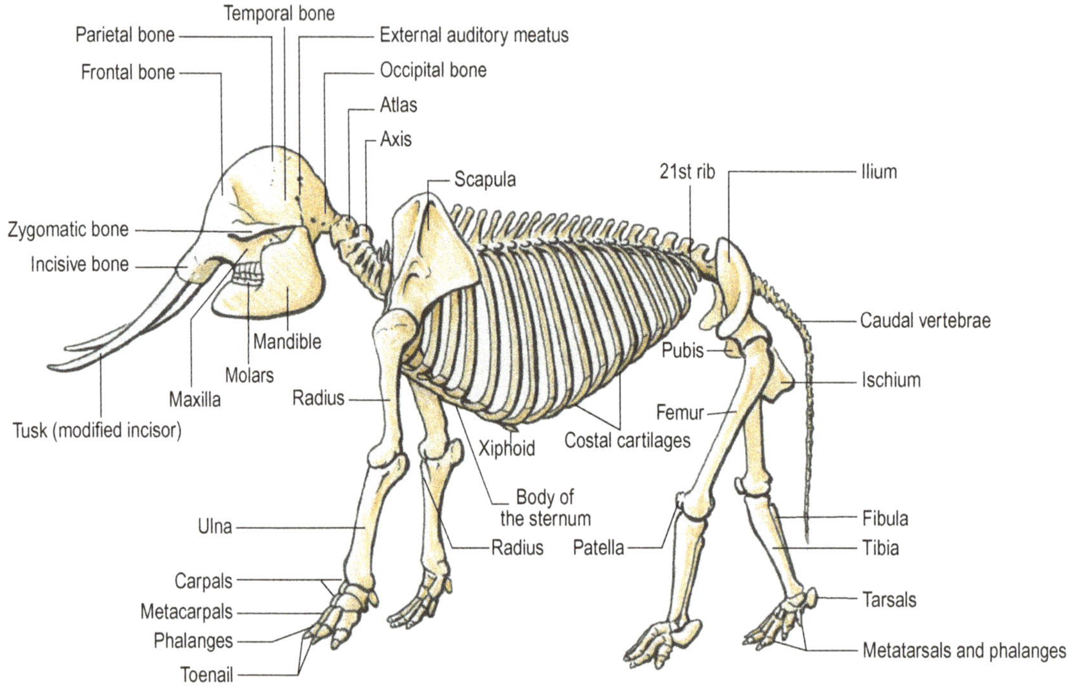

Figure 10.1 ***Continued***
(B) African elephant.

connective and elastic tissue. There are fascial sheets on the flexor surfaces of the metacarpals and metatarsals that bind the digits together. Extensor and flexor tendons insert onto the digits as in other mammals. All this combines to make elephants semidigitigrade in the front foot and semiplantigrade in the hind foot, so that during weight-bearing the metacarpals and metatarsals remain essentially vertical whereas the phalanges come to lie almost horizontal as they compress the digital cushion (Fowler 2006). This compression is an essential mechanism to manage the excessive pressures experienced by the foot (>1 kg/cm^2) (Alexander et al. 1979) and to maintain adequate blood circulation from these extremities back to the heart.

The order Proboscidea is so named because of the trunk (proboscis) - the feature setting elephants apart from all other land mammals - a tapering elongated upper lip and a nose that comprises only muscle and connective tissue and which in adults measures between 1.5 and 2 meters (Miall and Greenwood 1878). Four muscle groups (radial, longitudinal, and two oblique) are collectively responsible for the exceptional flexibility and strength that allows such diverse activities as the manipulation and carriage of loads weighing up to 300 kg, to the sucking and spraying of water (Rasmussen 2006). The trunk is a truly multifunctional organ, used for breathing, vocalizing, disciplining calves, triangulation of scents and their passage to the olfactory sensory areas, exploring the physical environment, snorkeling, and eating and drinking. The prehensile tip has finger-like projections dorsally and ventrally in African elephants, but only dorsally in Asian elephants. Unique and extensive sensory innervation and two sets of vibrissae are probably responsible for the elephant's ability to grasp tiny objects and to insert chemically active samples into the vomeronasal organ in the hard palate of the mouth (Rasmussen and Munger 1996).

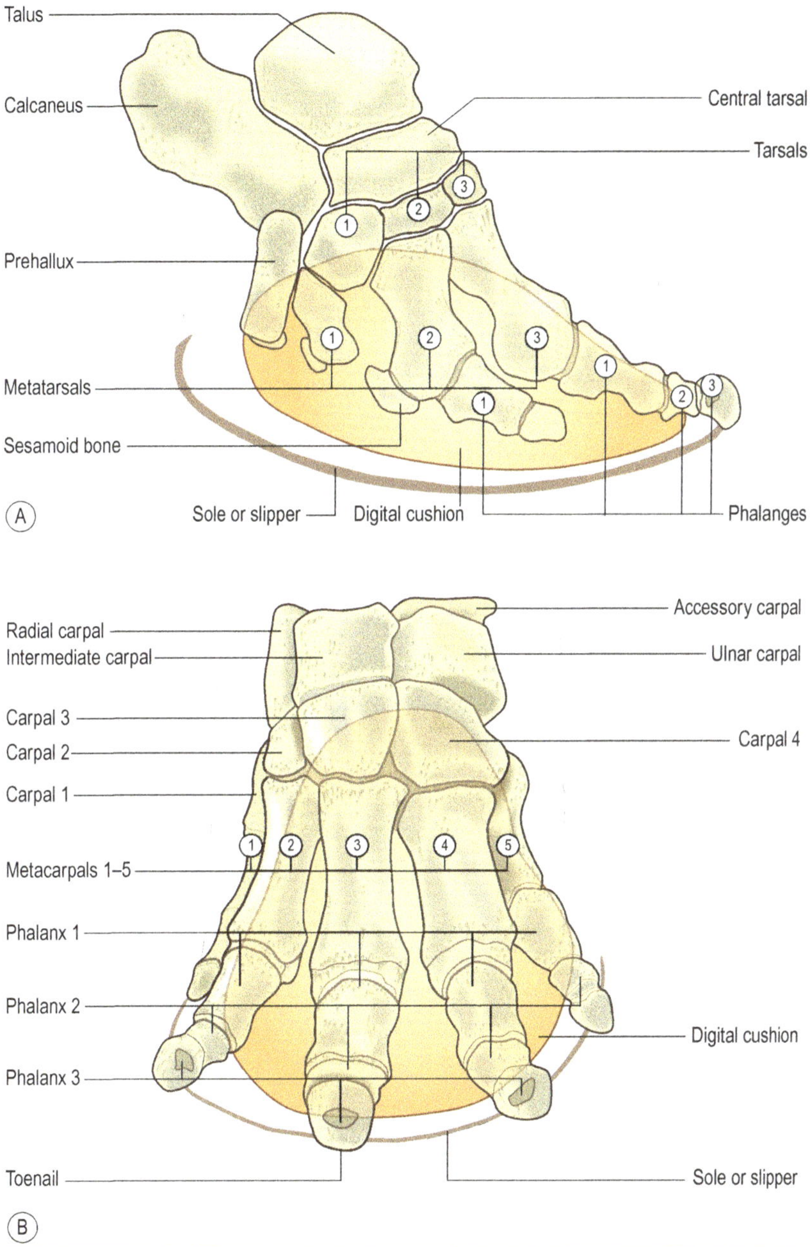

Figure 10.2
(A) Diagram of the lateral view of the bones of an elephant's hind foot. (B) Diagram of the front view of the bones of an elephant forefoot. Digit 1 has a toenail and occasionally a phalanx. Not all digits have toenails. Asian elephants have five nails on the front feet, whereas African elephants have four.

Ungulates (hoofed animals)

Artiodactyla

Artiodactyla is the order of mammals that contains the even-toed ungulates. Typically this includes the cow or deer-like animals, antelope, giraffe, camels, hippopotamus, and pigs to name a few. There are many families, often changing with modern techniques of classification, with the majority weight-bearing on the third and fourth toes. Basic anatomical consideration should be considered as outlined for domestic cattle in most cases (see Chapter 6).

Perissodactyla

Perissodactyls are the odd-toed ungulates, typically horse or pony forms. This group includes the equids, tapirs and rhinos. There is only a small number of families in this order, typically weight-bearing through digit 3, which is always the largest, although rhinoceros and tapirs have three toes in both the front and the hind feet (note that tapirs have a fourth toe in the front but typically this does not touch the ground when walking). The basic anatomy is similar to that of the domestic horse.

Carnivora

This diverse order contains over 280 species, all with considerable variation. The focus in this chapter is on the big cats, which is a small number of species of the Felidae family. The term "big cat" is not a specific term but refers to the tiger, lion, jaguar, leopard, and snow leopard: cats that can roar. Despite the variation in size the basic anatomy of the Felidae is extremely similar to that of the domestic cat (see Chapter 3). The only exception is the cheetah, which has species specific adaptations that make it very different to the other members of the family, including semiretractable claws.

Hominidae

This is the family of the great apes, which includes the four genera: *Gorilla* (gorillas), *Pan* (chimpanzees), *Pongo* (orangutans), and *Homo* (humans). The anatomy is similar in many respects in all four genera, with obvious differences being the adaptations of *Pongo* to a life in the trees with extended forelimbs and a more muscular countenance in all of the great apes when compared to humans. Their hind limb has adapted to function more like a hand, compared to the human foot. There is sexual variation, especially in the gorillas, where the males are often larger in build with some anatomical differences, such as the larger head and thicker neck muscles (Raven 1950).

Common orthopedic problems of elephants

Although in North American zoos the true prevalence of foot problems is unknown - there is no standard reporting system - it is estimated that more than 50 percent of captive elephants suffer from some form of foot disorder during their lifetime (Fowler 2006). Harris et al. (2008) reported that 80 percent of elephants in UK zoos had foot problems at some point during the course of their study. A more recent study undertaken on behalf of the Elephant Welfare Group (EWG) to assess elephants in British and Irish zoos found that 21.4 percent of the feet of Asian elephants had some form of disorder, whereas in African elephants 13.3 percent of feet were affected (BIAZA 2016). Both studies showed Asian elephants' feet were more affected than African elephants' feet, and front feet were more affected than hind feet; this was thought to be the result of anatomical differences between species and greater weight-bearing on front limbs respectively. Comparable data for free-living elephants is not available, but would be expected to show a much lower incidence. Foot problems include overgrown cuticles, nails, soles or pads, uncomplicated nail cracks, disfigured nails, and solar deficits, which may extend into deep tissue and can cause infectious osteitis of distal phalanges. Infected phalanges can be diagnosed using radiography, identified by bone lysis (Fig. 10.3A and B).

Degenerative joint disease (DJD) or osteoarthritis is generally accepted as a very common disease in captive elephants (West 2006), although evidence is largely anecdotal. A further study for the EWG that developed and validated a locomotion scoring system, found that only 26 percent of elephants in British and Irish zoos had a locomotion score indicative of

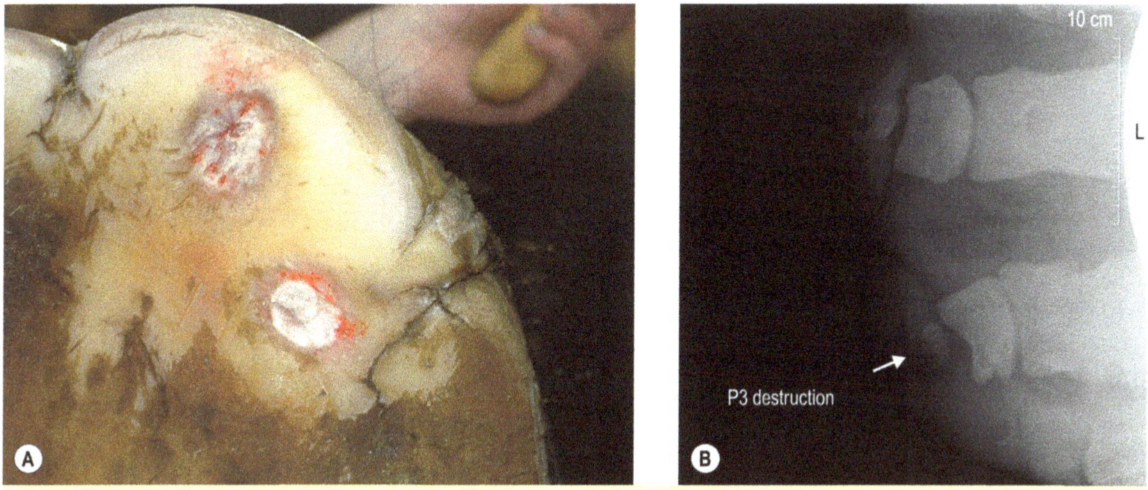

Figure 10.3
(A) Two typical full thickness solar lesions exposing soft tissue and possibly communicating with phalanx 3 centered over digit 4 of the left forefoot. (B) Radiograph showing lysis of the lateral portion of phalanx 3 of digit 4 of the same forefoot due to chronic infection. Courtesy of Nic Masters.

a completely normal gait (Masters et al. 2013). The remainder of the cohort demonstrated either a reduced range of movement in one or more joints ("stiffness"), abnormal tracking in one or more limbs, reluctance to weight-bear on one or more limbs, or any combination of these. Stiffness and reluctance to weight-bear were significantly more common in front limbs than hind limbs. Abnormal locomotion in elephants without obvious foot problems or other trauma could be a reflection of DJD (osteoarthritis). There are numerous examples of DJD (osteoarthritis) in preserved elephant skeletons (Fig. 10.4A and B).

Less common musculoskeletal diseases include:

- Trauma (to soft tissues including joint structures), as well as fractures and dislocations (West 2006).
- Trauma to the trunk (Caffee 1989).
- Metabolic bone disease in hand-reared calves (Ensley et al. 1994; Siegel 1973).
- Osteochondrosis in young elephants (Schmidt 1986).
- Reactive arthritis (Rothschild et al. 1994).
- Neoplasia (Brown et al. 1973; Liu et al. 2004).

The prognosis for these diverse diseases varies enormously. A summary is provided in Table 10.1.

Differential diagnoses

Lack of flexion in the foot indicates pain or ankyloses (Fowler 2006).

Tuberculosis should be considered in musculoskeletal disease with an unusual presentation or one that is completely nonresponsive to treatment; it can cause chronic osteomyelitis (West 2006).

Common orthopedic diseases of hoofed animals, carnivores, and great apes

Arthritis

Although there is widespread variation in body mass, body proportion, and limb loading within the families and across the various taxa, arthritis is a common finding in most species. The cause and the joints involved vary between species but the basic pathophysiology is similar (Miller and Fowler 2014). This is especially so in the primates which are commonly used as a model for humans.

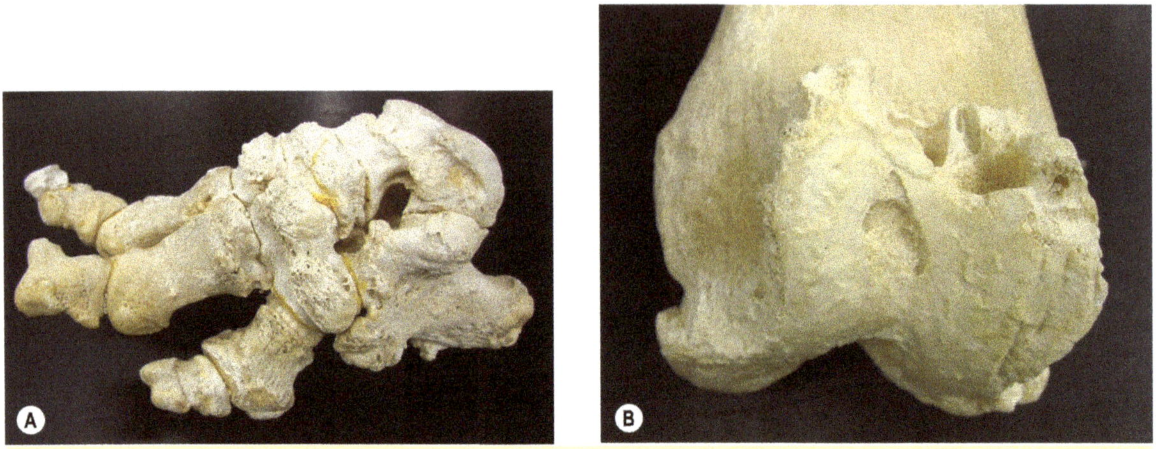

Figure 10.4
(A) An elephant foot showing extensive osteoarthritic changes. (B) An elephant femur showing extensive osteoarthritic changes to the distal condyles. Courtesy of Craig Pritchard.

Table 10.1 Common musculoskeletal diseases in elephants: their signs, causes and treatments

Disease process	Clinical and pathological signs	Etiologic factors	Therapeutics
Pododermatitis and other foot problems	• Lameness • Foot and or nail lesions • Radiographic changes (e.g., lysis of the distal phalanges)	• Often multifactorial • Repetitive mechanical insult, for example, hard floors • Lack of exercise • Excessive body weight • Poor conformation • Nutritional deficiency	• Flexible substrates • Weight loss if appropriate • NSAID therapy • Optimal exercise • Balanced diet • Preventive medicine to avoid DJD and conformational changes • Appropriate antibiosis
Degenerative joint disease (osteoarthritis)	• Lameness • Swollen joints • Long-term changes produce abnormal conformation and locomotion • Radiographic changes (e.g., proliferation, lysis) • Other imaging changes (e.g., scintigraphy and MRI)	• Often multifactorial • Repetitive mechanical insult (e.g., hard floors) • Lack of exercise • Excessive body weight • Poor conformation • Hyperextension of joints (e.g., while working or being restrained) • Reactive arthritis	Rest then gentle exercise Flexible substrates Swimming Weight loss if appropriate NSAID therapy (short-term therapy only to avoid proteoglycan suppression) Polysulfated glycosaminoglycan (IM) Chondroitin and glucosamine (orally) Acupuncture and/or osteopathy?
Trauma to carpal joints or other sites	• Lameness • Localized swelling and heat • Long-term conformational change	• Injury from working (e.g., in logging camps) • Injury from restraint method (e.g., chain or tether)	• Rest then gentle exercise • Cold water hydrotherapy • NSAID therapy
Fractures and dislocations (there are multiple examples of successful fracture management in captivity, but dislocations carry a poor prognosis)	• Acute and severe lameness • Conformation change	• Accidents in captivity while working or during loading • Aggressive encounters with conspecifics	• Rest • NSAID therapy • Topical and systemic antibiotics if appropriate

Table 10.1 *Continued*

Disease process	Clinical and pathological signs	Etiologic factors	Therapeutics
Metabolic bone disease in hand-reared calves	• Acute lameness • Radiographic thinning of long bone cortices and pathological fractures • Previous chronic diarrhea • Bone replaced by fibrous connective tissue	• Inadequate or inappropriate nutrition	• Correct nutrition • Orthotic braces
Osteochondrosis	• Joint disease • Subacute or chronic lameness	• Inadequate or inappropriate nutrition • Excessive amounts of dietary protein • Genetic predisposition	• Correct nutrition: reduce excessive protein, correct mineral imbalance • Check genetics
Reactive arthritis or spondyloarthropathy	• Lameness and joint swelling with concurrent infectious process (e.g., diarrhea)	• Hypersensitivity to infectious agents, for example, *Mycoplasma* spp. in the urogenital tract (Clark et al. 1980) or *Salmonella* spp. in the gastrointestinal tract (Chooi and Zahari 1988)	• Appropriate antibiosis • NSAID therapy
Neoplasia (e.g., fibrosarcoma)	• Dependent on site and extent	• Idiopathic • Carcinogenic insult	• Surgical resection • Chemotherapy
Trunk tip trauma	• Loss of prehensile (and other) function	• Enclosure injury • Predator or conspecific injury possible	• Surgical reconstruction (poor prognosis) • Cranial osteopathy

DJD = degenerative joint disease, IM = intramuscular, MRI = magnetic resonance imaging, NSAID = nonsteroidal anti-inflammatory drug

In captive wildlife there is a focus on extension of life, sometimes at the cost of quality of life, and palliative care is not uncommon with zoos often having aged animals. While age is not a disease itself, age-related pathologies are not uncommon. Arthritis is one such disease and is relatively common, with cases being found clinically, as incidental findings at postmortem, during health checks or simply identified on educational specimens of skeletons (Fig. 10.5A and B). The location, causal factors and impact on normal life vary by species. The level of support and management given to these cases varies, based on the perceived financial, logistical, and cultural value of the animal; for instance, elephants are supported much longer than, say, antelope species. Various forms of arthritis are reported across the different species, including degenerative arthritis, osteoarthritis, osteonecrosis-type lesions, calcification, periarthritis, and idiopathic skeletal hyperostosis (hyperostotic spondylosis). In addition, arthritic lesions can be associated with penetrating injuries such as horn or bite wounds, idiopathic darting injuries (Kock and Burroughs 2012), systemic infectious processes or sometimes as a result of neoplastic disease-related arthritis.

Often the causal agent is not identified and radiographic diagnosis is made either during routine health checks or as part of a clinical workup for lame animals. The clinical relevance of a lesion can be extremely variable and consideration must be given to the type of animal. For instance, animals that are typically herd species, often prey items for carnivores, will mask clinical signs until disease processes are well progressed (Greenough 2007), whereas lameness in a high-ranking predator may be associated with less severe pathology. An open mind is needed when approaching such a case, as it is not unheard of for fractures to be present in ungulates with minimal clinical signs of lameness.

In captivity, even subtle signs of lameness may be noted, allowing for early intervention. The osteopath may be called in after initial workups and diagnosis have already occurred. Radiographs, synovial fluid cytology, blood profiles and systemic assessments may all be available.

The ungulates with arthritis often present with mild to moderate lameness. If there is no history of trauma, and there are no obvious lesions, then arthritis must be considered as one differential. Lameness often responds to blanket therapy with analgesics, anti-inflammatories, and/or nutritional support, and

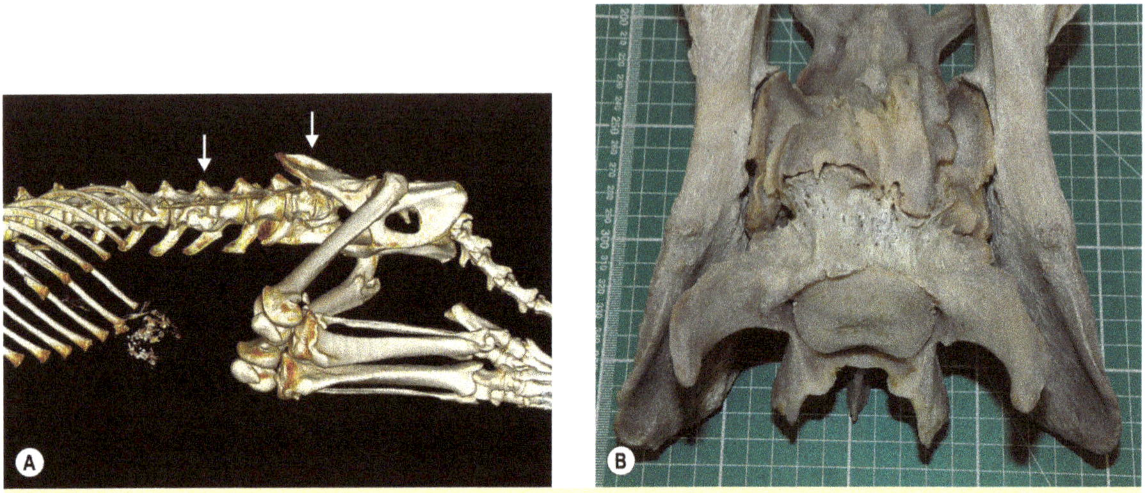

Figure 10.5
(A) A CT scan of an Amur tiger with severe spondylosis (indicated by the arrows). (B) Preparation following dissection of the lumbar spine and pelvis of the same Amur tiger.

only when refractory to such generalized treatment would full workup and diagnostics be undertaken. This means that an osteopath may be employed well down the pathological pathway where their job is much harder. It is prudent to develop a relationship with a practice to ensure early osteopathic support is given and to ensure optimal support and improved outcomes. Typically in artiodactyls, except with much older animals, individual cases of arthritis result from systemic or penetrating injury, i.e., septic arthritis. This needs to be treated with specific antibiotics, and any arthritic changes need to be managed. If groups of animals are noted with lameness or various levels of arthritis then the cause is likely to be an environmental challenge or nutritional problems. Reviewing the whole environment is critical as is reviewing the group of animals involved. Concrete flooring is one such example. Popular for cleaning and management, for most ungulates concrete leads to poor foot management. This is often associated with chronic insults to the supporting structures of the foot, resultant chronic lameness, abscessation, and arthritis (Fig. 10.6A and B). Equally important when considering the environment is drainage, cleanliness, substrate design (and frequency of access), paddock space, and knowledge of the adaptations of a species to their natural environment, for example, sitatunga cannot cope with dry environments.

Rhinoceros are particularly sensitive to being kept on concrete flooring, probably due to their weight. This type of management is still seen in some collections, however, and resultant arthritis and associated pododermatitis are often found in rhino (Dudley et al. 2015). Reviewing both rhinoceros and elephants is as much about the animal as it is about the environment being unsuitable for their locomotor needs.

Arthritis in great apes tends to fall into one of three groups: (1) nutrition-related arthritis (additional to secondary hyperparathyroidism), (2) traumatic arthritis or (3) age-related degenerative arthritis (Pritzker and Kessler 2012) although other causes do exist. Fractures and subsequent changes in loading are not uncommon in great apes and they are often noted to fall, sometimes long distances. Idiopathic skeletal hyperostosis is not an uncommon finding at postmortem examination, and is a condition osteopaths should be aware of before manipulating the lumbar spine. A particularly fine example of this was seen in Guy the gorilla at London Zoo.

The big cats also suffer from idiopathic skeletal hyperostosis and varying degrees of spinal pathology

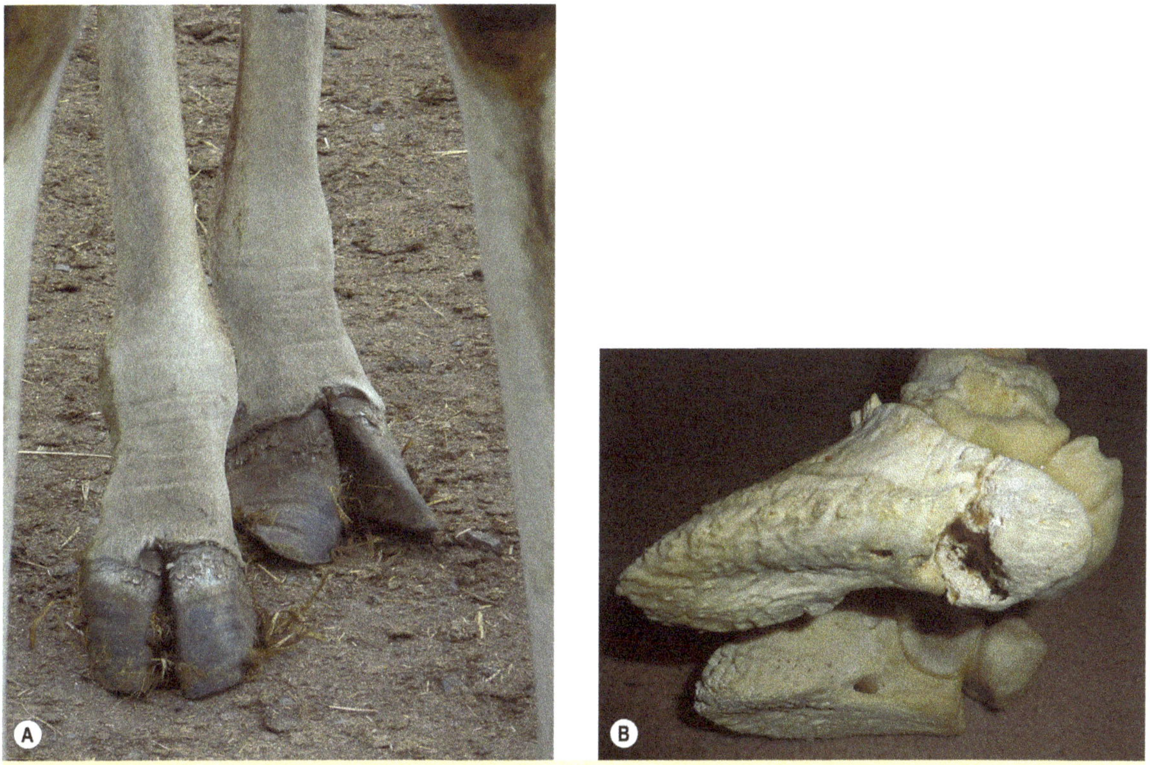

Figure 10.6
(A) A female Rothschild's giraffe with overgrown hooves. (B) A giraffe with a P3 abscess.

can be noted on radiographs. This is particularly common in elderly tigers which often suffer from hind limb ataxia and wasting, although this is more often associated with neurological disease. Spondyloarthropathy is a relatively common finding in large cats, with an incidence of 3.7 percent being reported (Kolmstetter et al. 2000). Arthritis resulting from other causes is common in aged carnivores, not just felids but also canids and ursids (bears).

Interdigital dermatitis

Interdigital dermatitis is specific to the artiodactyls and is caused by mild superficial infection and subsequent ulceration between the two principal digits. It can be very painful and is an extremely common cause of lameness (Fig. 10.7A and B). It is important that this is assessed as part of the general workup and that action is taken to cure it. If left it can become more extensive and spread to the bulbar horn at the heel and lead to underrunning of the horn and subsequent digital dermatitis. This is a disease that can usually be treated by drying and cleaning the affected area and correcting the environment. The cause is often unhygienic conditions such as poaching of paddocks or wet conditions and as such environmental assessment and appropriate management are critical (O'Regan and Kitchener 2005).

Fractures

Fractures are not uncommon in both captive and wild animals. These may be diagnosed as part of the osteopathic assessment but more often the osteopath is part of the rehabilitation process following fixation. Fractures can occur anywhere, but in the megafauna the limbs are typically involved. Fractures in other locations either do not require support or lead to the death of the animal. It is not uncommon to see cervical fractures in ungulates.

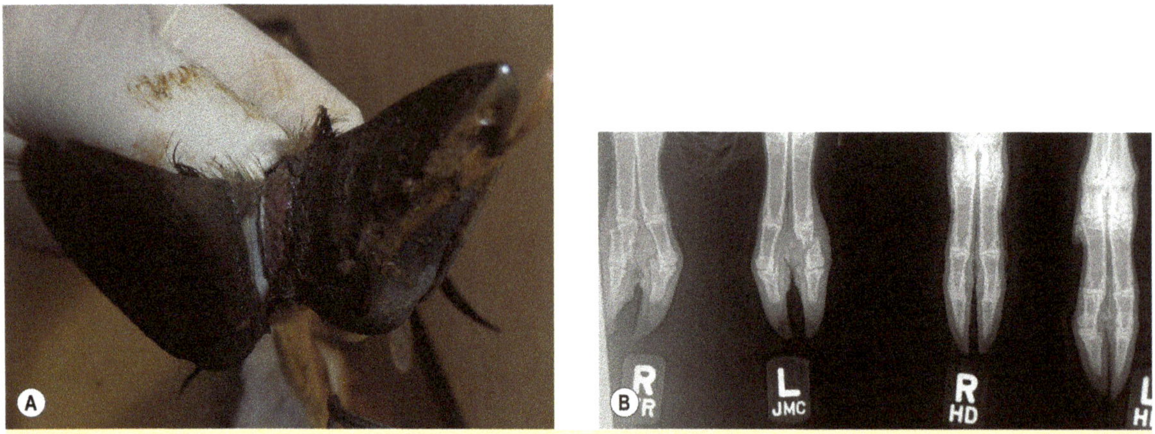

Figure 10.7
(A) A male adult blackbuck with the left forefoot showing interdigital dermatitis. (B) A dorsoventral radiographic view of the same animal with changes evident to both forefeet (left) and the left hind foot (far right). Note fractures to the lateral phalanges of the right and left forefeet

When spooked they tend to run headlong into fences, death occurring in the majority of cases.

Long bone fractures need to be assessed and supported in an appropriate fashion. Consideration of the method of fixation is not just about appropriate stabilization, but must also take into account the nature of the animal and postoperative requirements. In many cases access will be limited and implants are often left in permanently. In cases where external fixators are utilized they are often accompanied by the use of long-acting neuroleptics, which sedate the animals for long periods of time, reducing stress and facilitating handling. The osteopath must take care not to become complacent around animals receiving such agents as they are unpredictable and their use is poorly documented in captive animals. Analgesia and physical and behavioral support are critical in such cases, and osteopaths form an important part of rehabilitation in terms both of advice and hands-on treatment.

In ungulates the cause of a fracture is often not identified and can vary markedly in type. It is assumed that most occur when the animal is running and result from collision or awkward falls on uneven ground. In zebra cervical fractures are common when housing is poorly designed, and retrospective reviews may be beneficial in assessing patterns and causes as to why fractures have occurred. As part of zoo licensing requirements, zoos must undertake clinical pathological reviews and such information should be readily available.

In the great apes, fractures most commonly result from falls. Historically, fractures related to secondary hyperparathyroidism were common, but this is now limited to a small number of primates rescued from the pet trade where nutrition is often inadequate. Other causes of fractures in the great apes are fighting, especially between larger males and females, and management-related injuries such as darting or trapping limbs in hydraulic doors as they close (mostly digits). Treatment of primates is more challenging for the veterinarian due to their dextrous nature allowing them to pick out sutures and implants. Consideration needs to be given to the characteristics of the species, particularly those that are active and spend time jumping in their environment postsurgery as this will influence implant choice.

Fractures in large cats are infrequent. This author (TN) has only seen one following a darting accident, which resulted in a fractured femur. Conspecific aggression is a possible cause, but typically the animals are killed due to the nature of the species.

Infectious causes of fractures cannot be ruled out; for instance, tuberculosis is a not uncommon cause of infectious spinal fractures in cervidae (deer) (Fox 1923).

Neoplasia

Tumors of the locomotor system are not commonly reported in wild animals. They do, however, occur and should be considered in cases that are refractory to treatment or present with unusual masses or an unusual radiographic appearance (Fig. 10.8A–C). Osteosarcomas, synovial sarcomas, and fibromas have all been reported.

Myopathy

The most critical of the myopathies seen in captive animals or during wildlife handling is the group collectively known as capture myopathy. Capture myopathy describes damage to both cardiac and skeletal musculature as a result of overexertion and excessive contraction in an environment where oxygen levels are low in the muscle. It is a risk at any capture event if the induction is not well managed and is a result of speed and exertion, rather than distance run. The result varies and there are several subcategories within the cardiomyopathy complex. In peracute forms it can lead to the immediate death of the animal. The cause is a mixture of hypoxia, hyperthermia, systemic myoglobinemia, lactic acidosis, and major muscle damage (including the cardiac muscle). Animals do not always die immediately, and chronic forms can result in myoglobinemia-induced renal failure or scarring of cardiac musculature weeks or months after an event. Intermediate cases present with fever, pain, and anxiety, lameness in one or more limbs, knuckling or other neurological signs, rapid breathing, and muscular tremors. Sometimes there may be torticollis, anorexia, brown urine (myoglobinuria), paralysis, coma, and death (Blumstein et al. 2015).

In all cases the prognosis is guarded. Prevention is much more important than treatment. Treatment consists of tranquilization, preferably the use of long-acting neuroleptics, analgesia, osteopathy and muscle manipulation, fluid therapy, and nutritional support, particularly vitamin E at correct dosages.

Artiodactyls are most prone to capture myopathy, but it can potentially occur in any species.

Other myopathies have been reported, especially orthopedic-related myopathies, including avulsions and tendon injuries. Successful management is dependent on the species, timely intervention and a suitable short- to long-term plan for managing the animal. The larger the animal the more difficult it can be, especially when trying to reduce weight-bearing. One specific example is that seen in giraffe anesthesia where manipulation of the cervical spine and associated musculature during anesthesia is useful in supporting the animal during recovery. Massaging and manipulating the spine is often undertaken by the vet team but would benefit from osteopathic support to ensure effective manipulation occurs.

These are just a few examples of the more common locomotor-related pathologies that can occur. There is a large variation across the many taxonomic groups and readers are advised to review the references and current literature for current best practice when working with specific species.

General osteopathic evaluation of megafauna

Evaluation

Evaluation begins with the case history, and it will involve the head keeper and veterinary surgeon if the patient is in a collection or the hospital manager or park veterinary surgeon if the patient is in one of the conservation or national parks where the animals range more freely.

The scope of this book cannot allow for every species that you might encounter, so it has been decided to focus on elephant, rhino, giraffe, big cats, and great apes. For the various species of wolf and wild dog, please refer to Chapter 2 in general, but with the caveat that you heed all of the caution and specialist health and safety advice listed in this chapter. Ignore this at your peril.

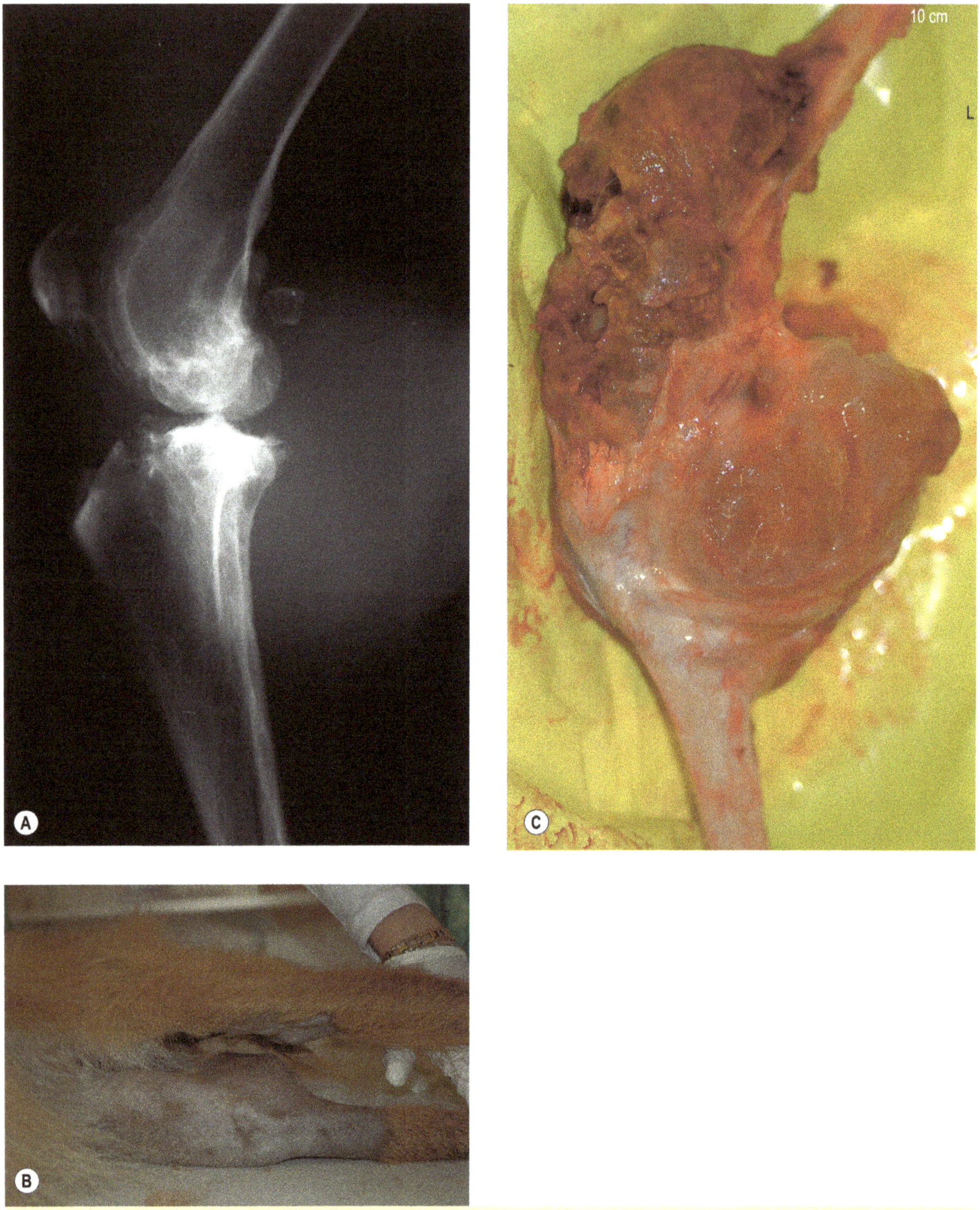

Figure 10.8
(A) A lateral radiographic view of the right stifle of a maned wolf with a synovial neoplasia. (B) The same animal shaved following radiography. (C) A postmortem dissection showing the extent of the synovial neoplastic mass.

General observation

Once the history has been assessed and the individual patient's case has been talked through with the rest of the team, the osteopath will want to view the patient in as natural a state as is possible. This is where you may have to compromise on the ideal. Observation of megafauna patients really needs to be carried out without them noticing you. Zoological research has shown that animals in collections behave differently when they are conscious that someone is watching them (BIAZA 2004).

Thermography

This is probably the best of the non-osteopathic assessment tools one can use. The main thing you need to remember with elephants is that they use their ears to help regulate body temperature by directing blood flow into and out of the ears and by fanning air down the flanks of the body.

For information on how to use thermography effectively, please refer to Chapter 1.

Elephants (Elephantidae)

Health and safety around elephants

Please refer to the section above (see page 405). Health and safety when treating elephants is particularly important and should not be ignored because of their semidomesticated nature.

Planning osteopathic treatment of elephants

All Western zoos should adhere to guidelines pertaining to specific species. These are laid down and made available by governing bodies such as the Association of Zoos & Aquariums (AZA), the British & Irish Association of Zoos & Aquariums (BIAZA), and the European Association of Zoos and Aquaria (EAZA). These guidelines define standards on all aspects of elephant care and management and should be followed by all collections that are members of these bodies.

Elephants in camps in Asia are kept in a slightly less risk-averse situation than in the Western world. For instance large bulls are handled in free contact. This will require a more dynamic "seat of the pants" form of risk assessment than we have become used to elsewhere. In this situation it is particularly important to plan treatment carefully and ensure all the team are aware of what is to be done. Even before any treatment is undertaken, the elephant team and osteopath should meet and start planning. They need to build up a relationship and know what the needs are for each group as well as for the patient.

Risk assessments should be prepared by the elephant team and communicated to and signed off by all involved with the treatment. These should at least cover:

1. A decision as to who is to have contact with the animal, i.e., handlers, osteopath, veterinary team, etc.
2. An assessment of the location. Never put yourself between anything solid and a 3,000 kg animal. Chains and ropes can trip the unwary, which can lead to an animal being spooked and hurting someone else in close proximity.
3. Most importantly, the elephant being treated must be considered in detail. What is its character? What is the risk of someone being kicked, grabbed by a trunk or hit with a tusk?
4. At least two experienced handlers capable of working with the animal must always be present for every treatment. One handler must be solely tasked with managing the animal and constantly monitoring its mood and reaction to the treatment. It must be understood by all that this person will call time out on the treatment if they feel that anyone's safety could be compromised or if the animal is at all uncomfortable with the situation.

The author (TN) has found that treatment sessions should be built up slowly so the animal can gain trust in the osteopath treating them, and the osteopath can get used to being around this particular large animal. There will be aspects of treatment that will be quite unusual for the animal and could be disconcerting for it. This is when quality elephant staff come to the fore, recognizing apprehension quickly and halting this specific part of the treatment. Come back to it at a later date. If treatments are kept positive, the elephant will start to look forward to the sessions, and will actually be pleased to see the osteopath when they arrive.

The second keeper will be tasked with the safety and monitoring of anyone not involved in the elephant team. They must be kept out of harm's way and prevented from putting themselves or others into a dangerous situation. Extreme care must be taken when working around the head of an elephant; the authors Andy Hayton and Tony Nevin have personally seen extreme reactions particularly around the jaw and throat of one animal during an initial treatment.

It cannot be stressed enough that the osteopath when treating must constantly communicate what they are doing to the handler in charge. They must always ask before moving to a different area on the animal so the handler can prepare for reactions.

A good team will work with each other during a treatment, and a huge amount of information can be obtained from the subtleties that both the osteopath and handler will be able to pick up from their respective areas, allowing a treatment to be altered very quickly to suit the needs of the animal. Elephants will give very little away when being treated, unlike horses, so a good rapport between animal, handler, and osteopath is paramount for clear communication and effective treatment.

There is a big difference between working with and around the two main species of African elephants (*Loxodonta africana*) and Asian elephants (*Elephas maximus*).

If you are working in a free contact situation, always leave any commands for the elephant to the keepers. Few elephants will respond to you, and if they do it may not be what you want from them!

African and Asian elephants have quite different behavior patterns and habits. The African elephant is generally more easily spooked and needs to be constantly monitored. The Asian elephant may appear very docile but can react suddenly. Asian elephants have been used by people over the millennia and are therefore better studied from a veterinary point of view.

It should also be noted that there are many elephants in collections that have been removed from their wild range states, some due to becoming orphaned through poaching or controlled culling. These can present with physical, developmental, and psychological problems. If orphaned at a very young age there can also be malnutrition issues affecting their musculoskeletal development.

Osteopathic observation of elephants

Observe the elephant walking. Where possible, position yourself behind, in front, and to the side, while gaining an overall impression. The use of slow motion video will often highlight gait imbalances and help you to share and evaluate your treatment responses with the rest of the care team (Fig. 10.9). Wear patterns on the soles of the feet, the general conformation, and toe growth and orientation give a good indication as to load bearing and gait.

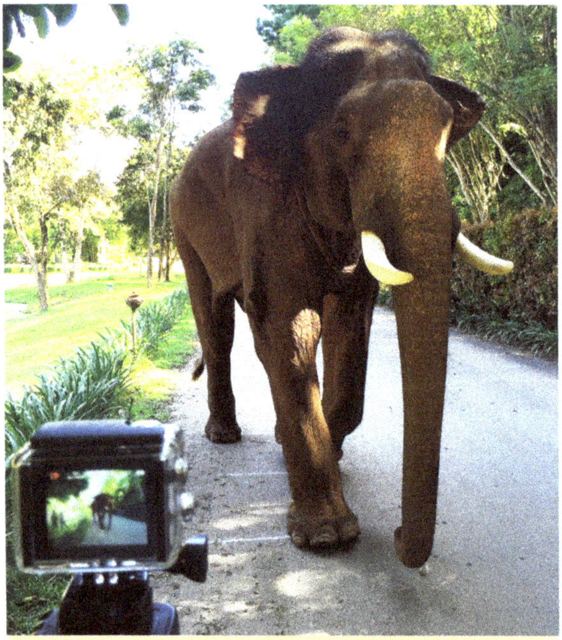

Figure 10.9
Gait analysis using slow-motion video capture to assess for lameness over a measured distance.

When observing, remember to stand further away than you would, for example, with horses. Elephants are inquisitive and have a phenomenal reach with their trunks. In order to keep them walking in a straight line you need to avoid any visual or auditory communication with them. The author advises observation first, before writing down findings afterwards, as even a clipboard can be irresistible to an elephant.

Regarding the reach of the trunk, take whatever distance you think they can touch you at and double it. Never leave any equipment lying around, as you are likely to see it being recycled!

Osteopathic palpation of elephants

As when dealing with any other species the osteopath should always have a routine. Due to the sheer size of elephants this may prove somewhat of a challenge. If the elephant can, and is willing to, ask for it to kneel down (Fig. 10.10), as well as lie on each side (Fig. 10.11) in a free contact situation. If this is not possible then palpate what you can from a standing position. Although you can stand on steps please be careful. The author ended up on his back the only time he tried this!

Use a flat hand and firm, slow pressure to assess the soft tissues. Elephants are very sensitive and can be rather ticklish. Their skin is not as thick as many people think. Many hate flies so be aware of this. Avoid getting caught by the ears and tail. Elephants can use them as very effective weapons and the author has met several keepers who have lost teeth this way.

The fingers of the trunk are highly dexterous and they can easily undo bootlaces or pick pockets. Avoid allowing an elephant to grasp your arm (or anywhere else) as this can be extremely dangerous. Above all, listen to what the keepers say and if they tell you to move don't ask questions, just move. Avoid standing directly under the head and neck of an elephant, and be aware that they can kick with remarkable speed in almost any direction.

Osteopathic treatment of elephants

All apart from one of the author's treatments have involved the patient being fully awake. Of these, most patients have been in a free contact environment and a few have been treated in a wild environment with all sorts of other animals wandering past.

Osteopathic modalities that best suit elephants vary and also depend on the animal's age and general health and well-being. If you are treating a primarily physical problem then soft tissue work, sustained positional release methods, and, to a lesser degree, articulation and mobilization techniques can be employed (Figs 10.12, 10.13, and 10.14).

For the more psychosomatic-based problems, more of the functional and involuntary mechanism (IVM)

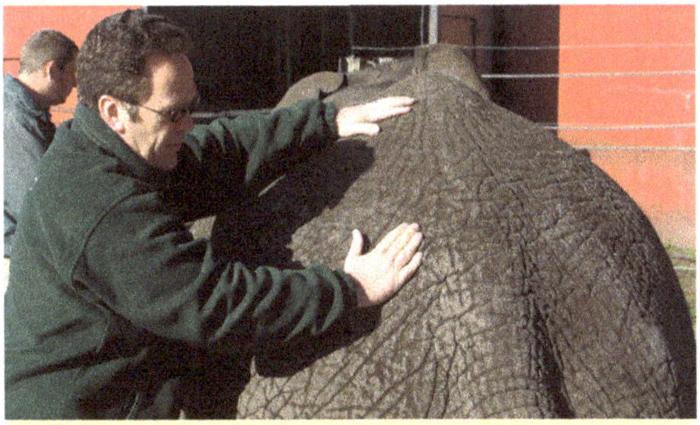

Figure 10.10
An African elephant in a kneeling position allows easier access for palpation.

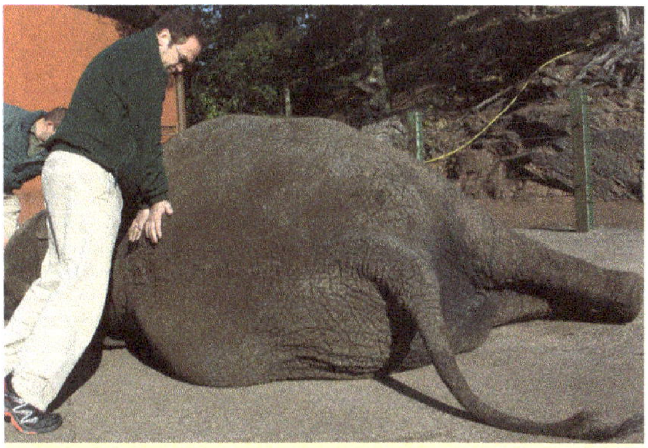

Figure 10.11
An African elephant side lying during palpation of the thoracic and lumbar paravertebral structures.

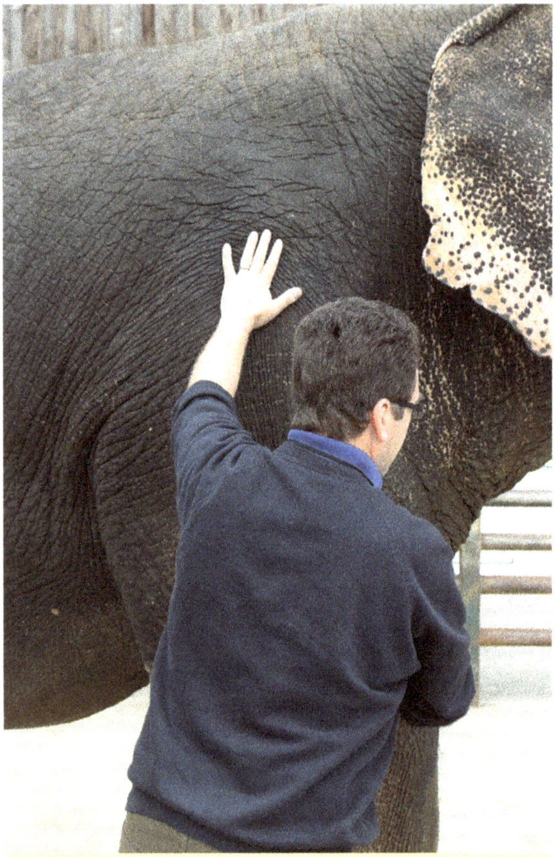

Figure 10.12
Applying firm vertical pressure against gravity to create a release in tension through the periscapular soft tissue structures.

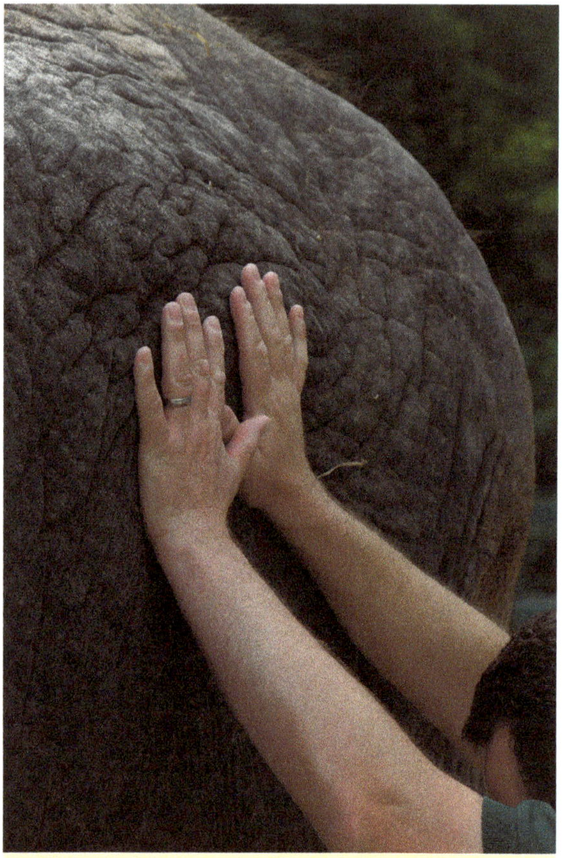

Figure 10.13
Applying a lift through the left side of the caudal rib cage to create a change in resting tension through the axial structures of the musculoskeletal system.

combined techniques, with some mild sustained positional release, and muscle inhibitory techniques work extremely well, especially in allowing relaxation around the diaphragm, frontal bones, sphenoid, and hyoid structures (Figs 10.15, 10.16, and 10.17).

With all these treatment techniques, it is important that the osteopath allows the elephant to work with him, rather than trying to force any kind of release. Although this sounds obvious, it is amazing how often this is ignored.

Ensure that you have your treatment plan set out before you begin and let the keepers know when you intend to move from one part of the elephant to another. The author would suggest starting around the shoulder and forelimb and working caudally down one side around the rear end, taking care as some elephants are not happy with having someone behind them. Then work in a cranial direction toward the head, performing any treatment work to the head and facial muscles last of all. If the elephant is lying down be aware that they can jump up much quicker than you can imagine - their reflexes are much faster than ours.

Be careful not to place your hands or fingers inside the mouth as the large molar teeth can make rather a mess of you (just as they can a two-inch thick branch)!

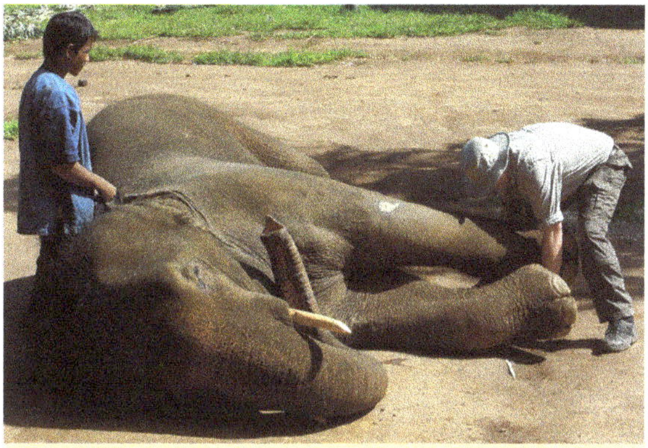

Figure 10.14
Articulation of the left forelimb of an Asian elephant with the patient side lying.

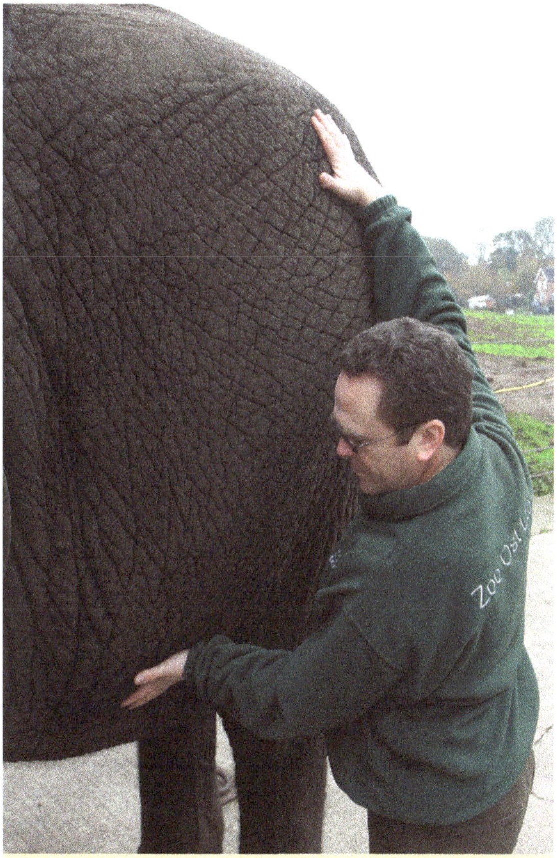

Figure 10.15
Applying inhibition to the diaphragm with the patient standing.

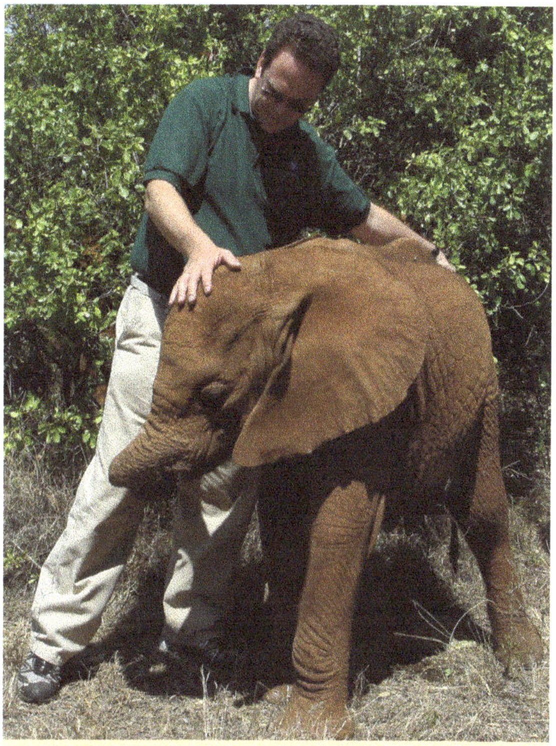

Figure 10.16
Engaging the involuntary mechanism (IVM) through the frontal bones of an orphaned African elephant calf.

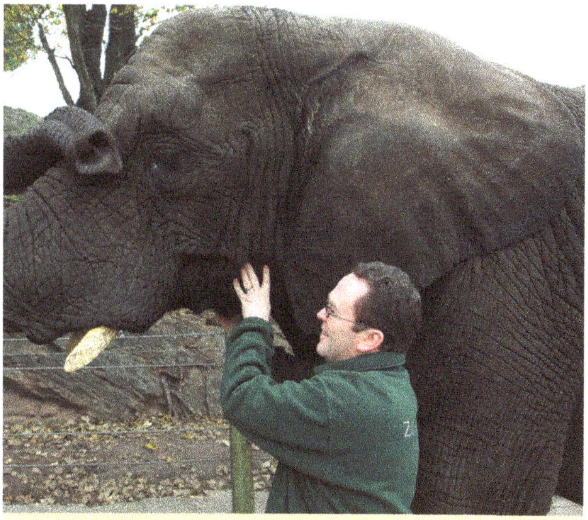

Figure 10.17
Applying a functional release through the hyoid structures of an African elephant with the patient standing.

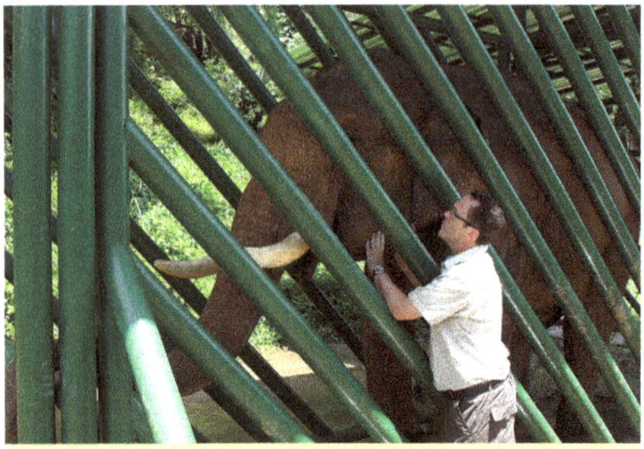

Figure 10.18
The restrictions of working in a protected contact environment, in this case with a bull Asian elephant.

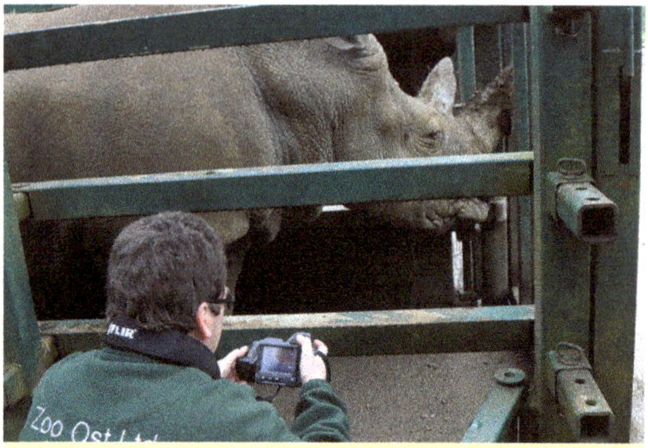

Figure 10.19
Assessing the standing posture of a bull white rhino with the aid of a medical-grade infrared thermal imaging camera..

Once an elephant gets to know you, it is very easy to lower your guard and become complacent around it. Although it makes for a more relaxed treatment environment, remember that they can, and do, have mood swings and are easily spooked by loud noises or sudden movements.

If you are treating through open bars of a protected contact environment, take care to avoid getting crushed against the metal pillars. Use your peripheral vision at all times (Fig. 10.18).

Rhinoceros (Rhinocerotidae)

Planning osteopathic treatment of rhinoceros

At the time of writing the only species you are likely to be asked to treat are the southern white rhinoceros (*Ceratotherium simum simum*), the eastern black rhinoceros (*Diceros bicornis*), and the Indian rhinoceros (*Rhinoceros unicornis*). The author (TN) did examine the last UK-held Sumatran rhinoceros (*Dicerorhinus sumatrensis*) before it was transferred to Sumatra to assist with a captive breeding program in the late 1990s.

Rhino are generally nervous and very sensitive to sound. They can be easily spooked and are unpredictable. Pay heed to their keepers and observe what they tell you.

Osteopathic observation of rhinoceros

If space allows, one of the best methods for observing these animals is from an SUV. If space precludes this then position yourself where you can gain a good impression of gait and symmetry of movement while one of the keepers encourages them with food.

Rhino should move fluidly, with relatively little movement apparent through the neck and back. Most action should occur through the limbs, although stride length is short but fast. Obviously there is movement through the spine but this is masked by the shape and muscling of these animals. Rhinos turn sharply by pivoting on their hind limbs, so that they can bring their horn(s) to bear in defence or attack. The normal carriage of the head is low in relation to the shoulders and withers (Fig. 10.19).

Osteopathic palpation of rhinoceros

Most rhinoceros cases an osteopath is likely to see will be examined and treated in a protected contact environment. This makes it much safer for the osteopath and does not seem to detract from the treatment outcome for the rhino. The author has had the privilege to work on all but two of the rhino species that are still on this planet (the northern white and Javan being the exceptions) and they have all thoroughly enjoyed being palpated. In fact, most of them will not leave you alone.

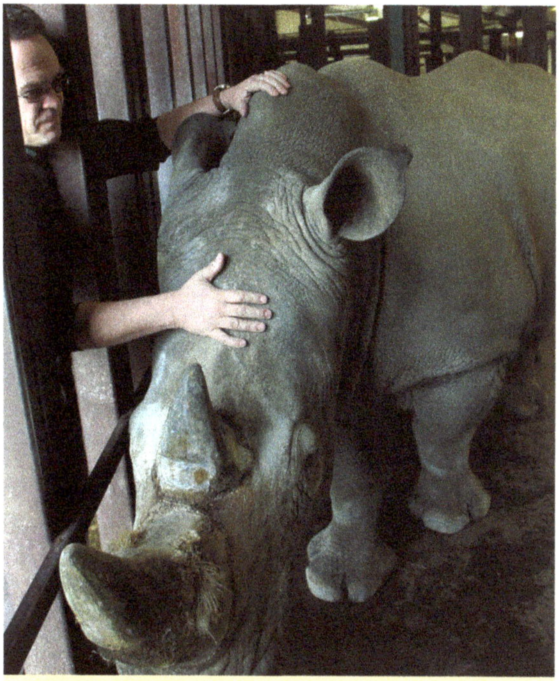

Figure 10.20
Assessing the quality of movement between the head and withers of a female white rhino in a protected contact environment.

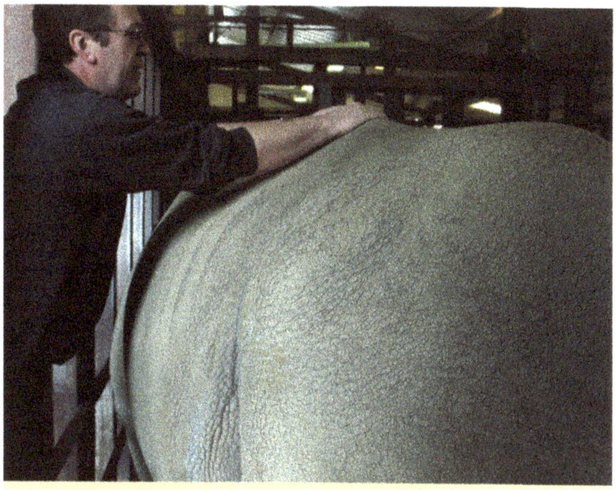

Figure 10.21
Mobility testing through the thoracic spine of a white rhino in a protected contact environment.

Where possible try to start at the shoulder and then work caudally, although many rhino will try to get you to scratch around their neck and ears. Be careful not to get caught between rhino and metal bars and pay particular attention to the horn - rhinos can turn on a dime (Figs 10.20 and 10.21).

Although rhino skin can be up to 50 mm thick it is still easy to palpate the underlying soft tissue structures.

With the Indian rhino, in particular, the large skin folds increase the surface area of the animal and, along with increased blood vessels, help to regulate the body temperature. This is of particular note when using thermal imaging.

Osteopathic treatment of rhinoceros

Rhino respond well to a mix of soft tissue work, trigger-point stimulation, sustained stretch and release techniques (Figs 10.22, 10.23, and 10.24), and also cranial osteopathy. Remember that they do not like sudden noises - even human speech can spook them - and always try to maintain contact once palpation and treatment have begun. Let the patient dictate the speed and duration of the treatment sessions. With protected contact they can walk away once they have had enough, and they will. If you are quiet and patient, however, they will tell you where they want to be treated - more than any other species the author knows.

Giraffe (Giraffa)

Until recently it was accepted that there are nine subspecies of giraffe: Angolan giraffe (*Giraffa camelopardalis angolensis*), Kordofan giraffe (*Giraffa camelopardalis antiquorum*), Nubian giraffe (*Giraffa camelopardalis camelopardalis*), South African giraffe (*Giraffa camelopardalis giraffa*), West African giraffe (*Giraffa camelopardalis peralta*), reticulated giraffe (*Giraffa camelopardalis reticulata*), Rothschild's giraffe (*Giraffa camelopardalis rothschildi*), Thornicroft's giraffe (*Giraffa camelopardalis thornicrofti*), and Masai giraffe (*Giraffa camelopardalis tippelskirchi*) (www.giraffeconservation.org). Research recently published, however, suggests that there are four separate species and one subspecies of giraffe (Fennessy et al. 2016).

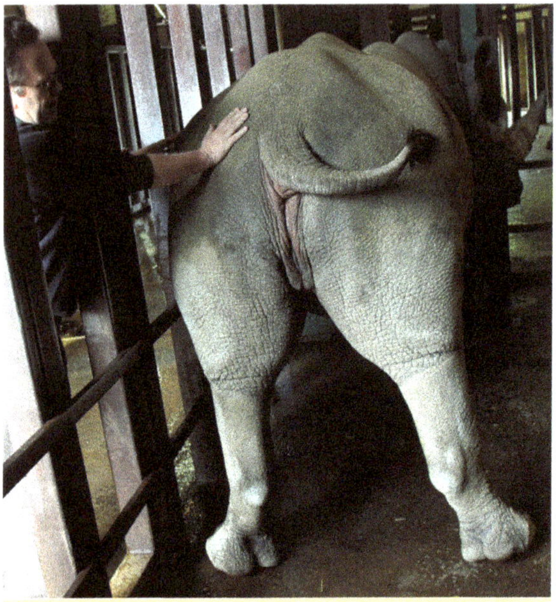

Figure 10.22
The patient is encouraged to use the practitioner as a fulcrum in order to functionally release tension throughout the body, with the contact being applied to multiple areas. In this case, the contact is around the left side of the pelvis.

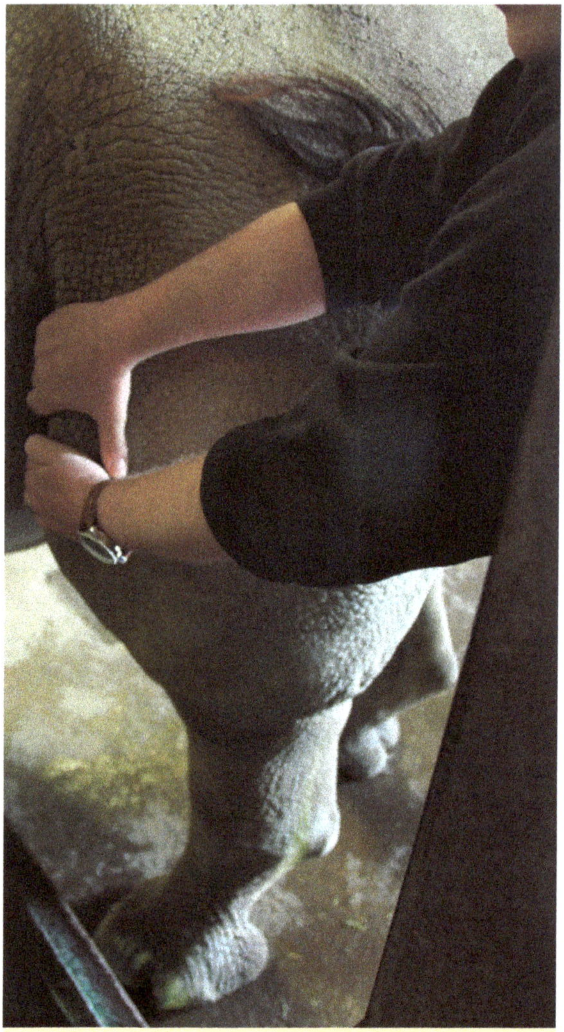

Figure 10.23
Applying cross-fiber muscle inhibition to the left hip rotators.

Some zoo and park collections have allowed a degree of cross breeding to take place, although international organizations such as the Convention on International Trade in Endangered Species of Wild Fauna and Flora (CITES) are bringing this to an end.

As an osteopath you are most likely to be asked to help with simple musculoskeletal-related issues (Fig. 10.25). In many of these cases your involvement will focus on subtle changes in husbandry rather than hands-on work.

Giraffe are generally placid but like most prey species can be rather skittish, and so observation needs to be carried out quietly. They will generally be happiest when in a group, so be sure you observe the right one!

Osteopathic observation of giraffe

Giraffe respond well to food being offered, but be prepared for the entire group to move toward the stimulus. Position yourself so that you can gain the maximum view of your intended patient and be prepared to wait while they settle. They are generally not that trusting of any changes to their routine.

Giraffe should move with a graceful undulating rhythm so look for any disruption to this pattern. Also note limb placement, but be aware that they do not appear to have the same degree of spatial awareness as horses in this regard.

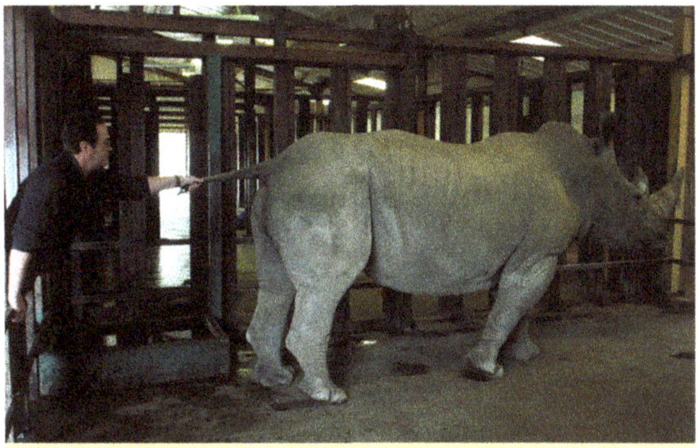

Figure 10.24
Providing sustained tail traction to allow this white rhino to alter the direction and load-bearing preference as it stretches through its entire body.

If you can view the giraffe from in front, note the eyes, ears, and ossicones, and the way the head is carried. Note whether the neck appears smooth and relatively straight and look for any signs of trauma. The head and neck are their primary weapon when fighting other giraffe.

Be aware that the angle of the scapula is nearly vertical when viewed from the side, giving the impression that the forelimbs are longer than the hind limbs (MacClintock 1973).

If you can view the giraffe from behind, look for pelvis and gluteal muscle symmetry and also limb orientation. Occasionally young bulls will repeatedly try mounting a female, and it is not uncommon to see a lame gait in these repeatedly mounted females.

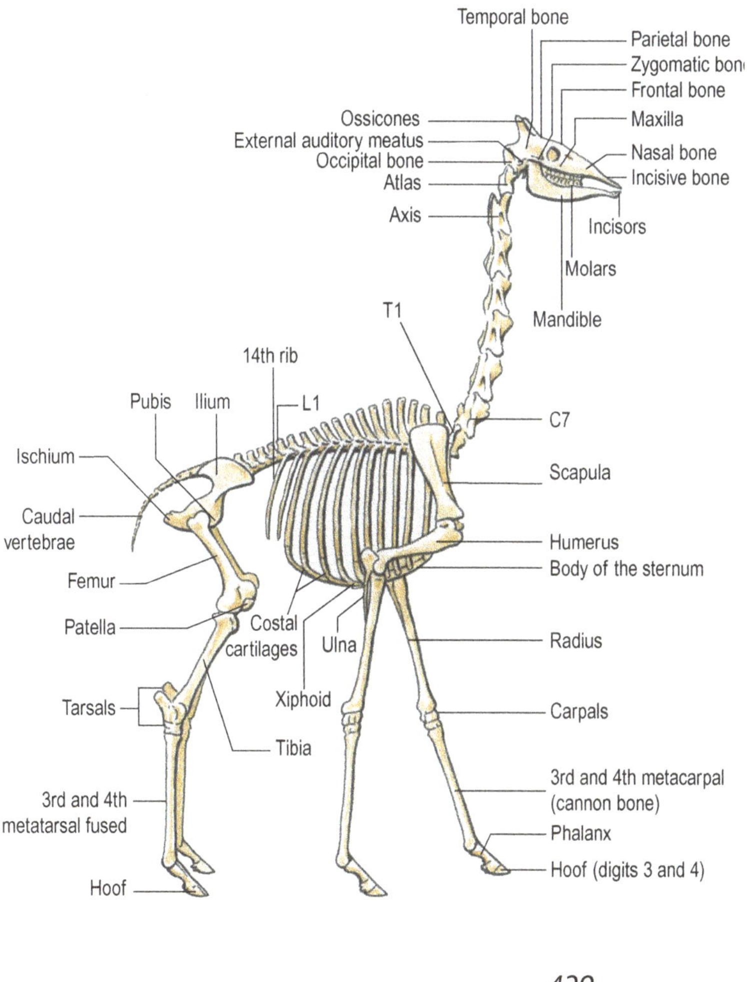

Figure 10.25
The skeleton of an adult giraffe.

Osteopathic palpation of giraffe

Except for a few cases, palpation will be rather limited. If possible, palpate the head and neck from a secure position and always watch out for the ossicones (horns), which are covered by hair but are solid underneath (Fig. 10.26). Giraffe have seven cervical vertebrae, with the bodies being the largest of any land mammal.

If you get the chance to palpate the limbs and body be aware that giraffe kick defensively with their hind legs, although the angle that they can kick forward takes the limb in an abducted arc. This makes standing in front of the forelimbs about the safest place to be if you are close up. When kicking in a backward direction there are numerous accounts from game parks in Africa of giraffe killing lion with a single kick.

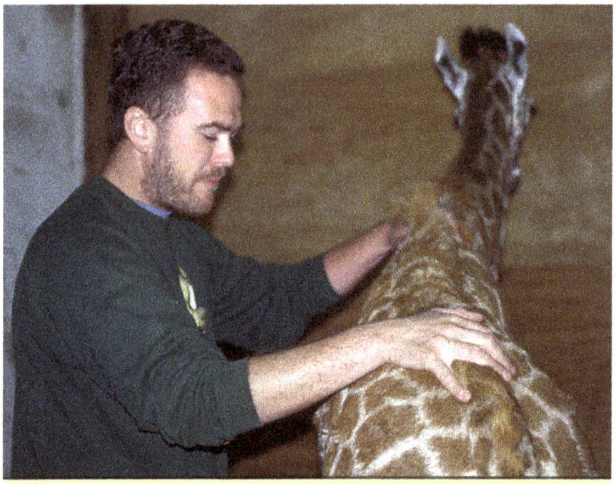

Figure 10.27
Balancing spinal ligamentous tension in a young giraffe.

Osteopathic treatment of giraffe

Due to their skittish nature the best osteopathic modalities are gentle positional release work, cranial osteopathy - as applied to human toddlers in a start-stop fashion - and some inhibitory work. Young giraffe will tolerate ligamentous balancing techniques and deeper inhibitory pressure, especially in the neck (Fig. 10.27).

These are probably the toughest species on which to perform meaningful treatment, and due to the relative problems with using general anesthesia the author (TN) has always elected to treat any giraffe conscious.

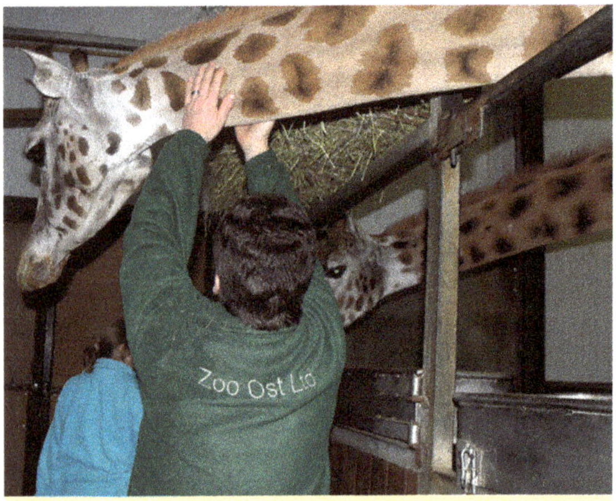

Figure 10.26
Palpating the upper cervical vertebral joints of a Rothschild's giraffe while the keeper distracts it.

Giraffe are one of the species where osteopathic observation skills are more likely to be required by veterinary departments than actual hands-on treatment. In many of the lameness cases the author has observed for veterinary surgeons, the team have collectively opted for anti-inflammatory medication combined with altered husbandry as the first line of treatment, before adding osteopathy into the mix.

Big cats (Felidae)

This section covers the African lion (*Panthera leo*), Asiatic lion (*Panthera persica*), cheetah (*Acinonyx jubatus*), Bengal tiger (*Panthera tigris tigris*), Amur or Siberian tiger (*Panthera tigris altaica*), and Sumatran tiger (*Panthera tigris sumatrae*). From an osteopathic perspective this should provide a broad enough basis for assisting with the many other members of the Felidae family.

Apart from a very few cases, these will all be treated under general anesthesia.

Osteopathic observation of big cats

Observations should be carried out in as unobtrusive a fashion as possible, and it is important to obtain and heed the advice of the section staff. Most collections will have CCTV coverage of indoor areas and sometimes some of the outdoor sections as well. Big cats are normally quite lazy, so if you see one that appears unusually active or restless you need to decide if there is a problem or if they are interested in something that is unrelated to your visit.

It is usually necessary to stimulate any cat to move. The presence of a keeper will usually cause a cat to stir, and by working together you should be able to guide the cat to walk toward an enclosure fence and walk alongside it in each direction. When it has lost interest it will usually walk away. If you need to see it run then food can be thrown into the enclosure to stimulate this.

Osteopathic palpation of big cats

The only safe course is to perform any hands-on examination with the patient anesthetized. Even if you are working with a very tame and habituated individual, the author (TN) would not advise you to handle a strange cat without chemical restraint. The author tries to combine this procedure with other health-care-related examinations such as blood testing. Be extremely vigilant as some cats are expert actors and can play at being unconscious. Do not lower your guard and do be aware of any sudden change in soft tissue tone.

In most cases you will work with the cat darted, but not intubated. The clock will be ticking and you will need to palpate in a systematic clear way to avoid wasting valuable time. The author would suggest starting with the head, and, as with small cats, check for any signs of trauma. Check the condition of the teeth (and whether they are all present), nostrils, ears, and eyes. Feel for the size and quality of the temporalis muscles before moving to the cervical and throat structures (Fig. 10.28). The author has seen one case of cervical stenosis in an African lion (*Panthera leo*) at a UK collection, where an extensive full body CT scan was used to assist with diagnosis.

Scapulae should be well muscled and move freely over their full articulation with the thorax. The forelimbs are powerfully built and can suffer trauma, as most big cats are good climbers. Check the claws and, in all species except the cheetah, make sure that you can get them to extend and retract (Fig. 10.29). Older big cats will often exhibit less muscling as well as palpable changes around the shoulder and elbow joint

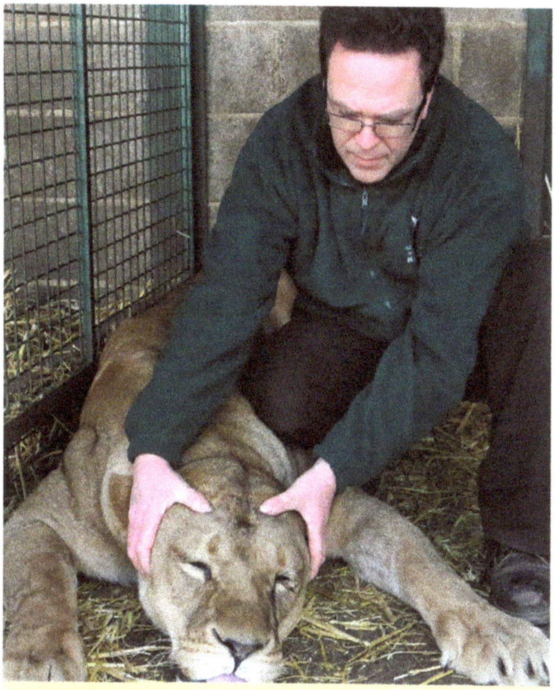

Figure 10.28
Palpating the temporalis muscles of an anesthetized lioness.

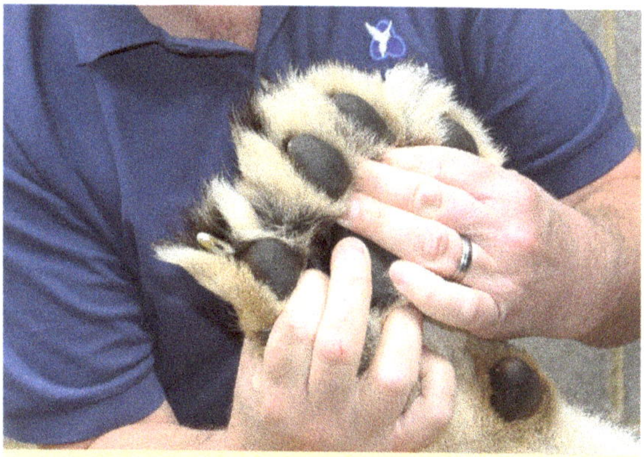

Figure 10.29
Palpation and articulation of the foot structures of an anesthetized lion.

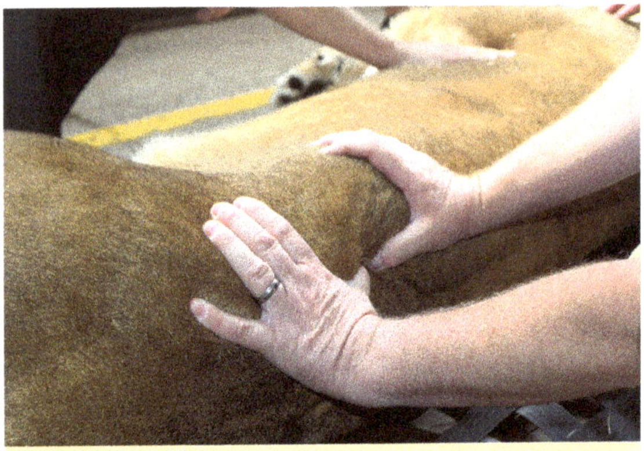

Figure 10.30
Palpation of the lumbar and thoracic spine of an anesthetized lion in side lying.

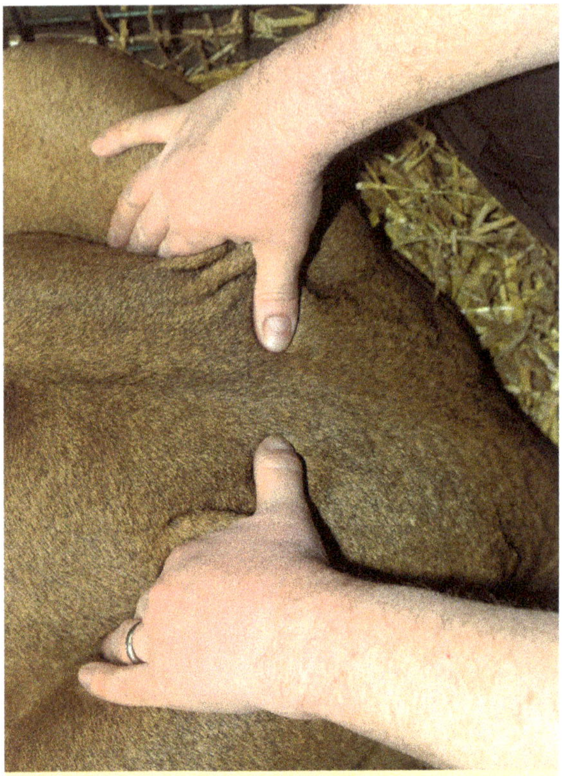

Figure 10.31
Assessing the symmetry of the tubera sacrale in an anesthetized lion.

structures. A reduced range of motion (ROM) in the carpus is also common.

Feeling in a caudal direction through the thoracic and then lumbar spine, note any changes in hair pattern around the caudal thoracic vertebrae. The author has found at least three African lions where this has coincided with disunited spinous processes or hemivertebrae or both. This was subsequently diagnosed when the individuals were radiographed (Fig. 10.30).

Like their domestic cousins, big cats tend to be heavier set over their shoulders with a fairly narrow pelvis. Their flexed hind limbs are ideally suited to their predatory role. Therefore it should be easy to palpate the important landmarks, such as the lumbosacral junction, tubera coxae, tubera sacrales, sacrum, and sacrococcygeal junctions, and the hip joints. All of these are readily palpable (Fig. 10.31).

The tail in all cats is a very important biomechanical tool, and signs of trauma can be a good guide to the general well-being of the individual.

From a biodynamic point of view, when palpating, scale up from the domestic cat with regard to landmarks, but bear in mind the subtle differences that these larger patients present. The main exception is the cheetah (*Acinonyx jubatus*). Osteopathically this resembles a cross between a cat and a greyhound. The limbs and feet are very similar to cats with the exception of the claws, which are semiextended. The back is long and dips slightly along its length, and the tail is longer in relation to the body than in the lion (*Panthera leo*) and tiger (*Panthera tigris tigris*).

Trauma to feet and claws is less of a problem for individuals held in collections, but it is important if you are treating a wild patient that will need to fend for itself.

Osteopathic treatment of big cats

Unless there is a need to remove a cat from its sleeping chamber, most treatments will be performed where it has been darted in order to maximize useable time. Remember to monitor tissue quality for signs of waking.

Due to the short time that anyone will want a cat to be anesthetized, the author would suggest blending a screening palpatory examination with osteopathic treatment. As with any chemically restrained patient there is a greater emphasis on achieving as much as the patient is willing to give during any single treatment.

The reader should refer to Chapter 3 on the cat for a general structured approach after which some of the more specific advice below may be followed. It is easy to employ general osteopathic articulatory techniques on big cats, and these techniques blend seamlessly with motion and range-of-movement testing. When treating the domestic cat, the osteopath has to continually balance handling with treatment methods. With big cats under anesthesia this is not necessary and the osteopath can employ the mix of techniques that will best suit the patient's physical condition rather than appeal to their character.

Applying slow, rhythmical neck traction can be very effective for releasing the suboccipital structures and the cervicothoracic junction and for decompression of the thoracic inlet (Figs 10.32, 10.33, and 10.34).

Inhibition around the hyoid and thyroid cartilages is very effective in aiding good temporomandibular action and occiput-atlas-axis articulation. These structures are quite narrow in relation to the width of the throat of lions (*Panthera leo*) and tigers (*Panthera tigris tigris*) (Fig. 10.35).

Long lever techniques for the limbs and their associated soft tissue attachments and bony articulations with the axial skeleton can be combined with fascial release and functional unwinding. Do not abduct limbs too far, as you will not get the same degree of guarding under anesthesia as in a conscious patient unless an area is already compromised. Also be aware of the sheer size of the claws when handling limbs. Any puncture wounds should be thoroughly cleansed, as you would with wounds from domestic cats (Fig. 10.36).

The axial spine, rib cage, and paravertebral muscles can easily be accessed with the cat lying on its side, as can the abdomen.

Specific short lever techniques can be directed at individual vertebral joints or limb joints, with limited

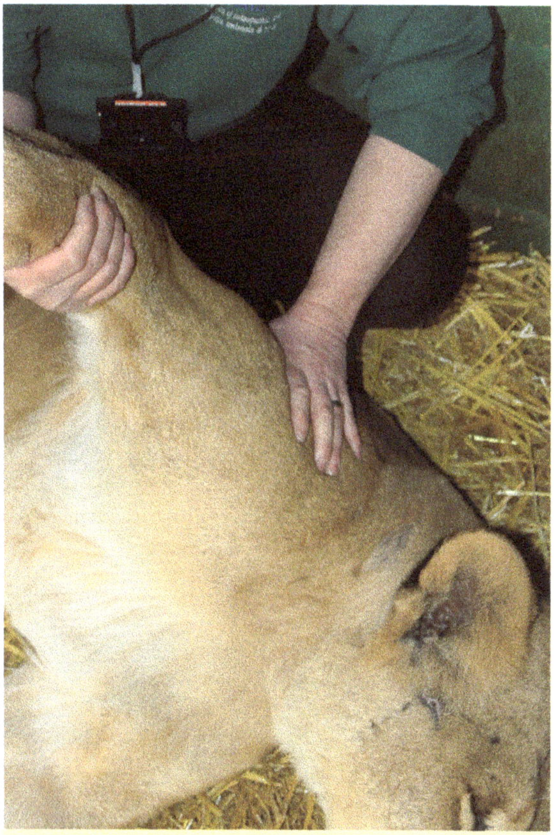

Figure 10.32
Soft tissue work to the periscapular muscles of a lion side lying with right forelimb traction.

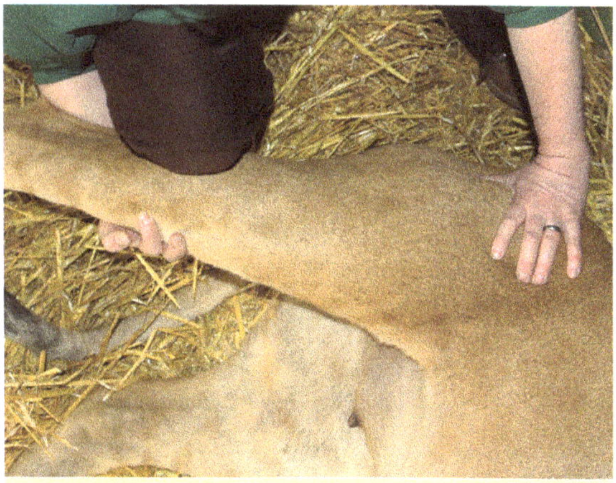

Figure 10.33
Applying a long lever approach to the right hind limb to release tension in the gluteal and hamstring muscles. The lion is side lying and anesthetized.

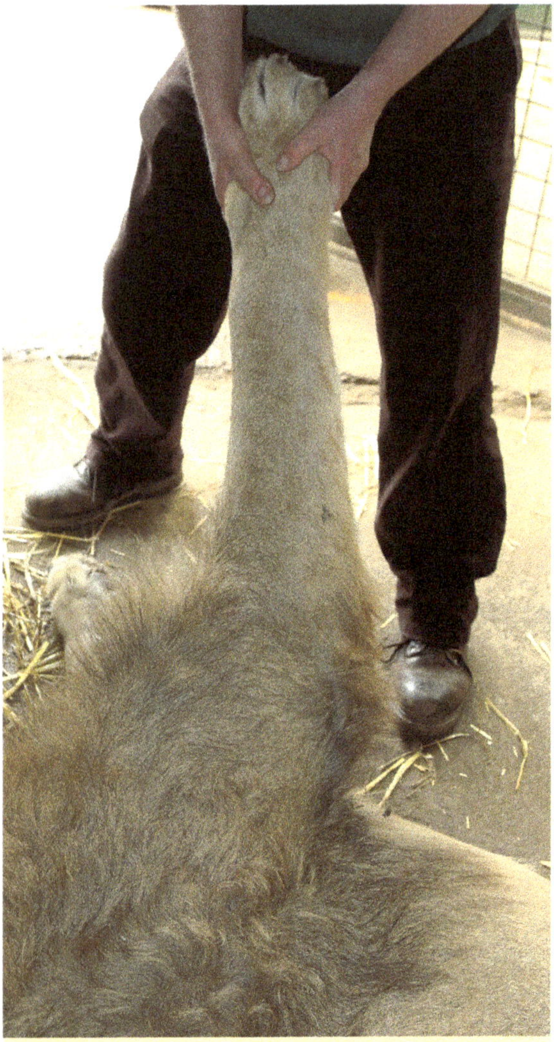

Figure 10.34
Long lever stretch and shoulder articulation with traction is applied to the right forelimb. The lion is side lying and anesthetized.

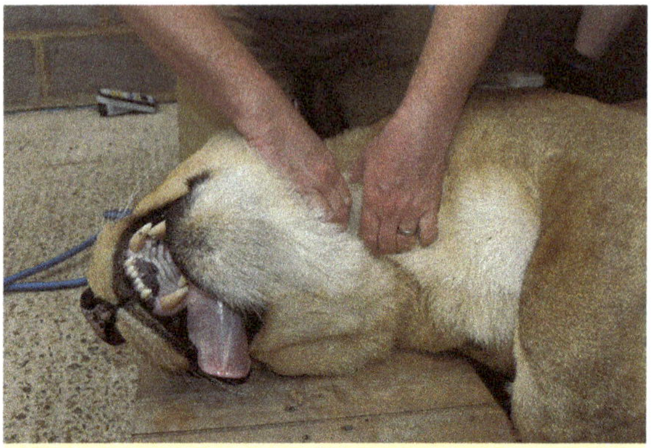

Figure 10.35
Soft tissue release method using a gentle hold around the hyoid. The lioness is side lying and anesthetized.

use of HVLAT where other techniques are deemed to be unlikely to succeed. Be aware, however, that many of the big cats that an osteopath is likely to see will be fairly old, and therefore it may be unwise to employ this technique.

The tail can provide an excellent long lever for functional release and can be used to assess the quality of movement at the end of a treatment. It forms a muscular and fascial continuum from the lumbosacral spine

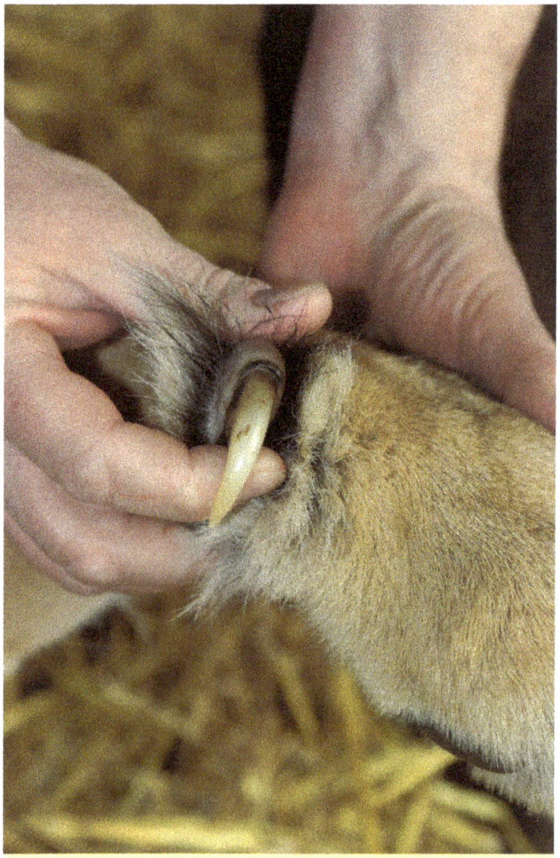

Figure 10.36
The dewclaw of a lion. Note its size when extended..

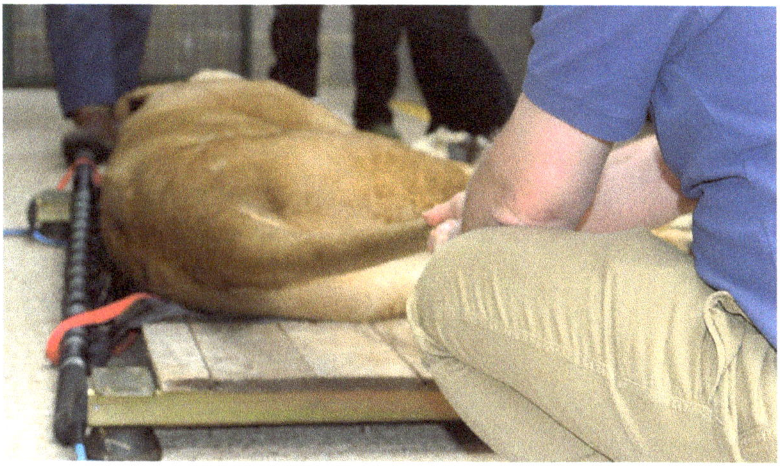

Figure 10.37
Performing a functional release using the tail. The lion is anesthetized..

where the multifidus of the lumbar spine merge to form the sacrocaudalis dorsalis medialis and lateralis muscles in the tail. If the patient is older or in poor health, avoid performing strong traction or tug techniques when working with the tail (Fig. 10.37).

Great apes (Hominidae)

The term "great apes" includes the western lowland gorilla (*Gorilla gorilla gorilla*), chimpanzee (*Pan troglodytes*), bonobo (*Pan paniscus*), Bornean orangutan (*Pongo pygmaeus*), and Sumatran orangutan (*Pongo abelii*).

It is worth remembering that most apes do not like being stared at directly. Bear this in mind when observing them as they will sometimes alter their posture toward you. You may need to spend time with them so that they become used to you. Most cases the author (TN) has treated involved watching the ape for several days before any treatment was started. Most cases you are likely to see will involve soft tissue injuries caused by playing, climbing accidents or fights. Most, if not all, will be treated under general anesthesia.

Osteopathic observation of great apes

If possible, try to observe these patients without them seeing you. Many collections have extensive CCTV systems good enough to allow a certain amount of useful observation, although in most cases you will also need to back this up with your own direct observation.

Although very similar to the human, apes possess many functional differences, such as much longer cervical vertebral dorsal spinous processes, feet that look and function more like hands, and much heavier mandibles with larger teeth and muscles of mastication (Figs 10.38 and 10.39). The forelimbs are longer than the legs, allowing them to use a quadruped form of locomotion as well as bipedal (Diogo et al. 2011). Climbing is where their biomechanical structure really shows its evolution (Gordon 1984).

When great apes walk on all fours they are plantigrade behind while preferring to weight-bear on their first interphalangeal joints in front. The muscles used for climbing are extremely powerful, and most of the cases the author has seen have involved neck and upper limb problems. Even apes that have fractured bones in their feet appear to suffer very little in the way of lameness (Figs 10.40 and 10.41).

Osteopathic palpation of great apes

When faced with one of these patients for the first time using the human model is a sound basis for assessing an ape (Diogo et al. 2011). You will of course need to factor in the different limb-length ratios and greater muscle mass, along with a more predominantly quadrupedal action.

Unless working with a very young juvenile, these cases will be examined under general anesthesia (Fig. 10.42), and so time is of the essence. Trust your

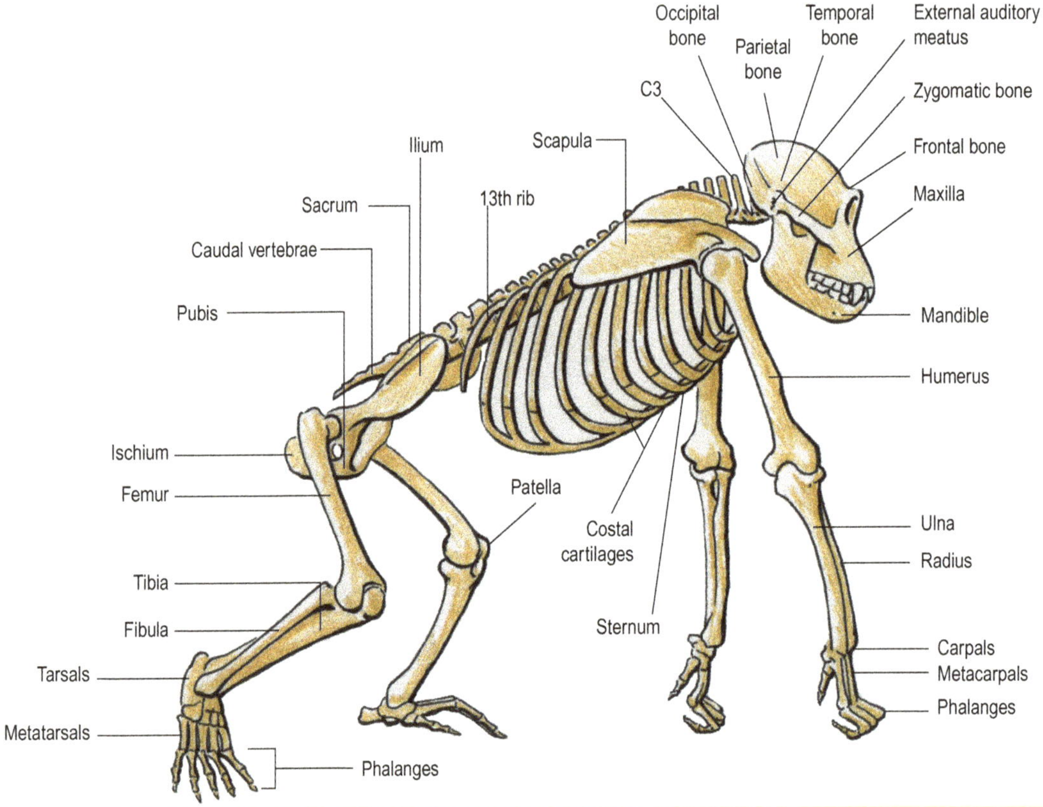

Figure 10.38
The skeleton of an adult western lowland gorilla.

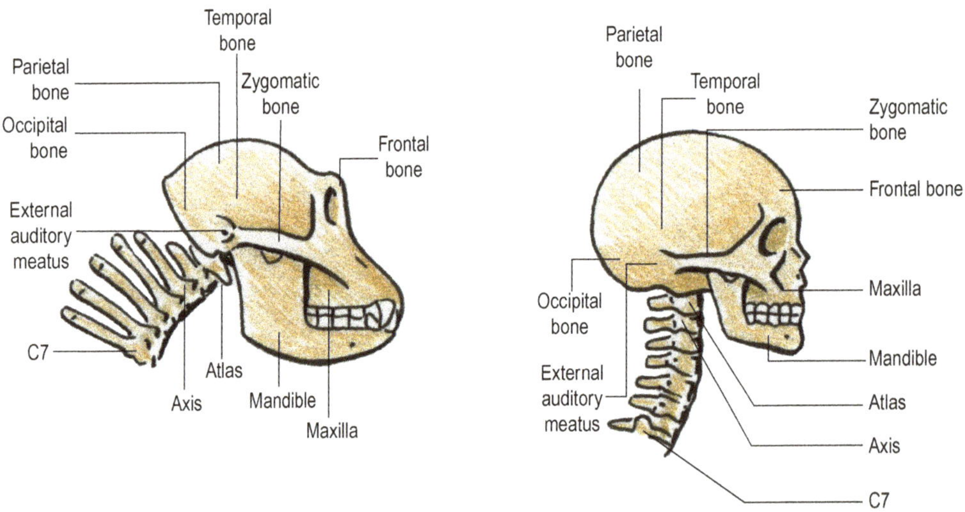

Figure 10.39
A comparison of the gorilla and human skulls..

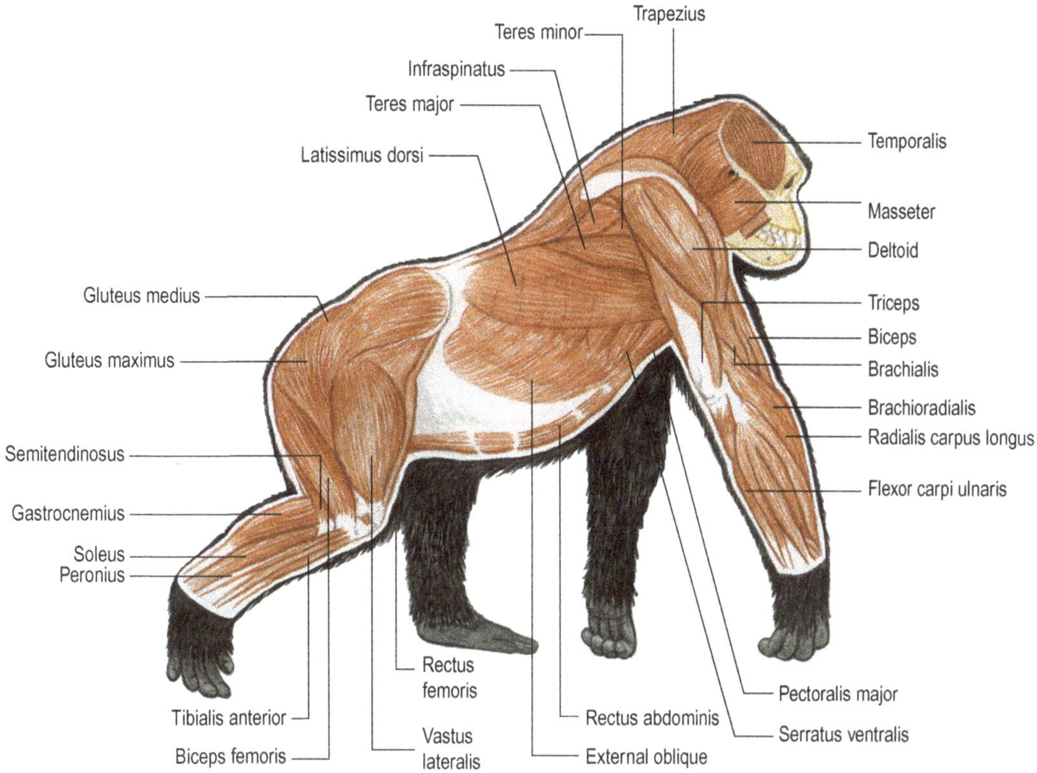

Figure 10.40
The musculature of an adult western lowland gorilla.

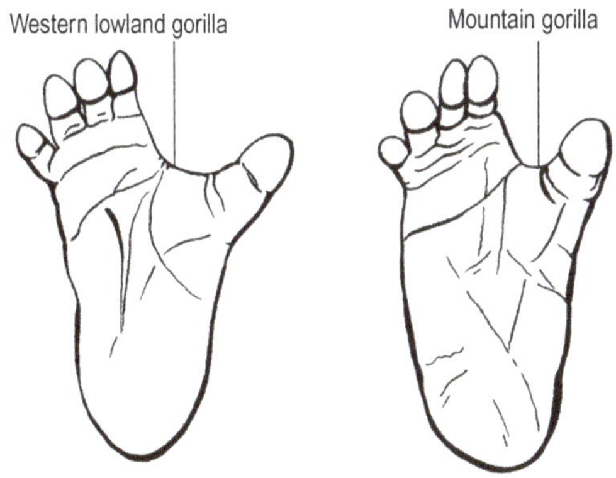

Figure 10.41
A comparison of the feet of different gorilla species.

initial findings. The soft tissues will give you all the feedback you need in order to make an accurate assessment.

If your patient is fully conscious, remember that most apes are very sensitive to touch and many are positively ticklish. Use firm contact and avoid irritation (Fig. 10.43). The normal reaction, if you do get it wrong, is for them to strike out at you, with obvious consequences. Also remember that apes possess fearsome teeth and carry many nasty bacteria in their saliva, so bites are to be avoided at all costs.

Osteopathic treatment of great apes

Most cases you examine will be the result of a traumatic incident. These respond best to articulation, mobilization, and HVLAT work. This should only be performed once normal radiographs have been obtained. Adding in myofascial and functional release work, as well as deep muscle inhibition, are the tools for treating the majority of soft tissue-related problems seen in great apes (Figs 10.44 and 10.45).

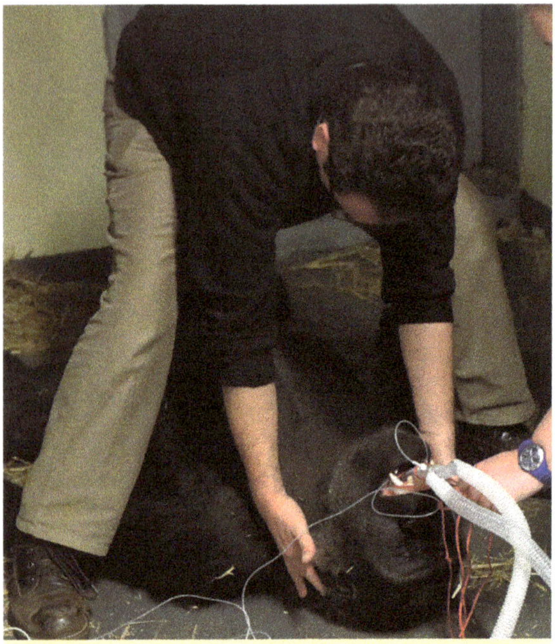

Figure 10.42
Assessing occiput–atlas–axis symmetry in a supine, anesthetized subadult western lowland gorilla.

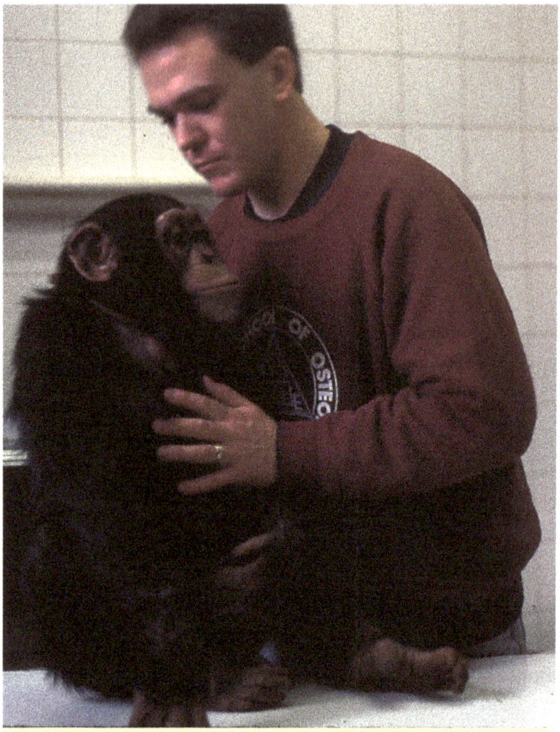

Figure 10.43
Examination of a conscious young chimpanzee. Note that in this case the patient was hand-reared and could be examined without anesthetic. Standard practice would be to anesthetize the patient.

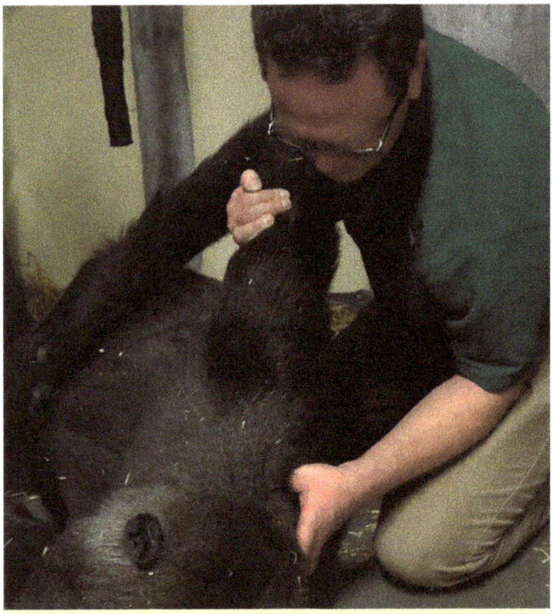

Figure 10.44
Performing right shoulder traction and lift with the patient side lying. In this case the patient is a young western lowland gorilla.

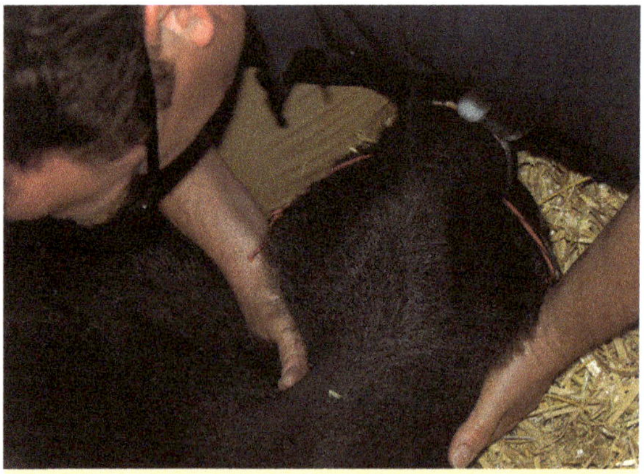

Figure 10.45
Performing a high velocity, low amplitude thrust to mobilize the upper cervical spine in an anesthetized gorilla.

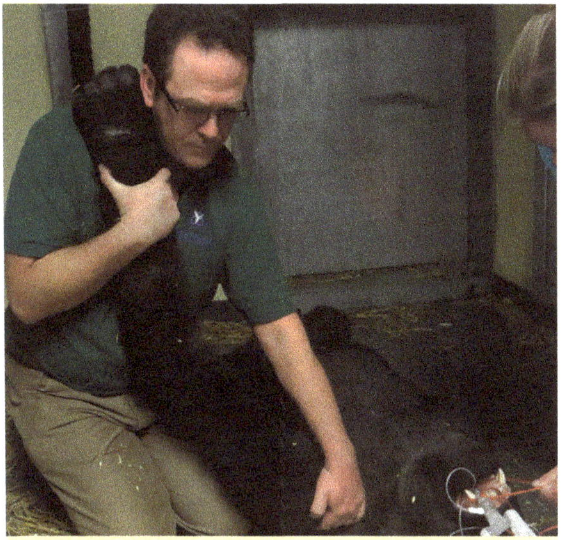

Figure 10.46
Using a long lever approach to articulate the left shoulder of an anesthetized gorilla in supine position.

When using an articulatory type of technique, as with the original general osteopathic technique (GOT) taught by classical osteopaths, work through the entire body and limbs. This is a valid system for evaluating and treating the patient simultaneously (Figs 10.46 and 10.47).

As with the human model, pay close attention to the ventral structures of the throat when treating the cervical region. Any upper limb problems will always also involve this area (Stone 1999, pp. 227-229) (Fig. 10.48.).

As with other wildlife and exotics, keep treatment times short and target the specifics at hand, although if the patient is anesthetized you will usually have sufficient time to achieve all you need to.

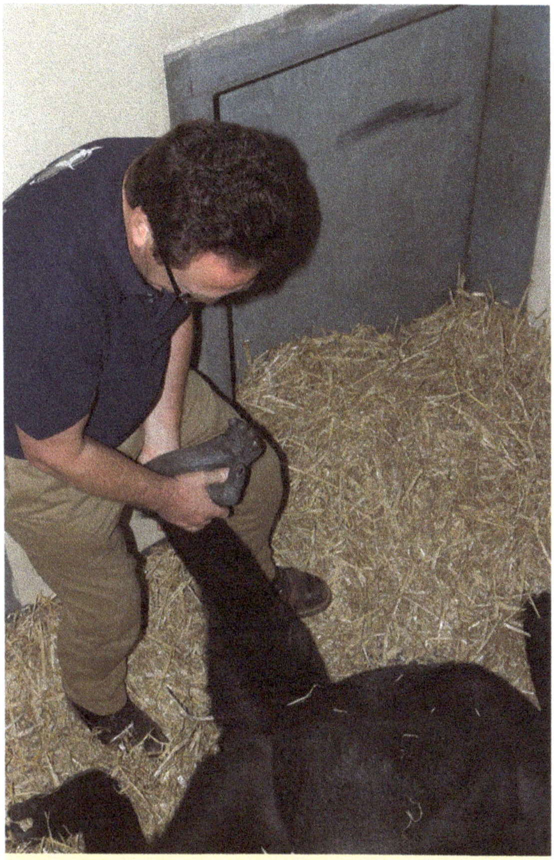

Figure 10.47
Long lever articulation using the right hind limb to assess and treat hip rotator function in an anesthetized gorilla.

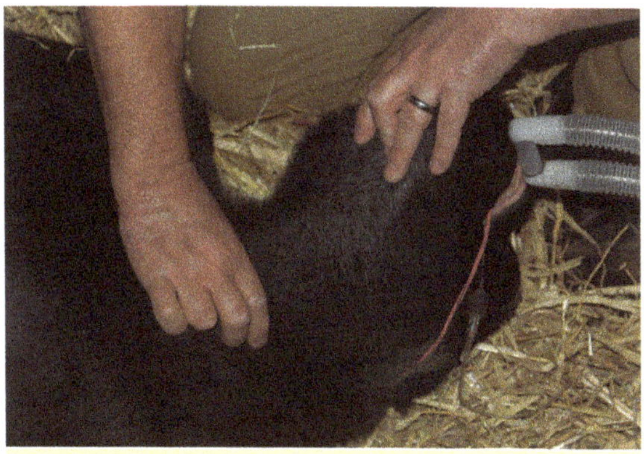

Figure 10.48
Applying a functional release approach to the hyoid and associated structures with the gorilla in supine position and anesthetized.

Case study 10.1

Asian bull elephant

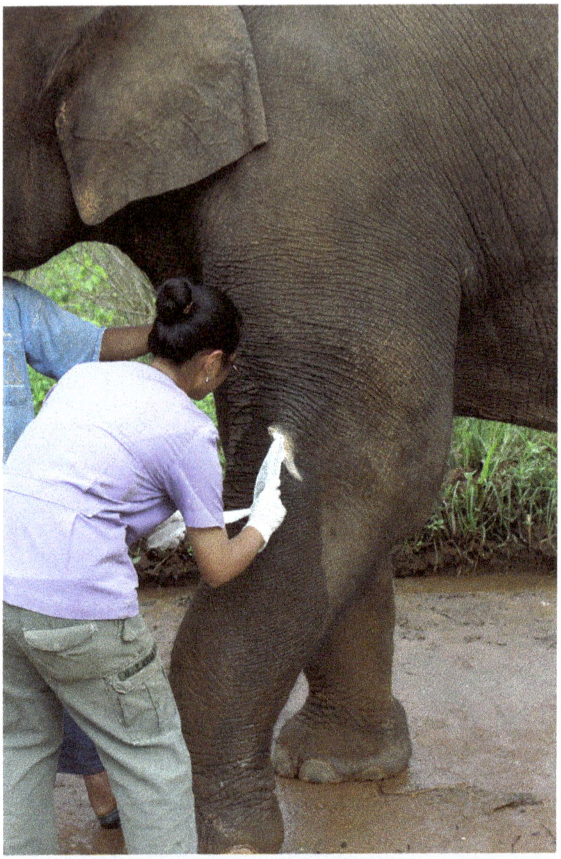

Figure 10.49
Veterinary treatment of the infected tusk wound proximal to the elbow joint of the Thai bull elephant. Note the edema in the left forelimb.

Signalment

The patient was an adolescent Thai bull elephant. He was privately owned and employed by an elephant awareness and conservation foundation that uses domesticated elephants for ethical tourist encounters.

History

The patient was involved in an elephant-on-elephant fight with a mature bull tusker. He had suffered a penetrating wound to his left forelimb proximal to the elbow joint, inflicted by a single stab of a tusk. He was lifted up and thrown backward into the surrounding undergrowth. The wound became infected and was treated locally by packing antibiotic material into the wound, which was approximately 15 cm deep. The packing was changed and the wound flushed on a daily basis by the foundation's veterinary staff. The infection and trauma also resulted in considerable edema of the forelimb, which prevented flexion at the elbow and carpus (Fig. 10.49).

Presenting signs

The patient presented with a swollen left forelimb and some muscle loss around the supraspinatus and infraspinatus muscles. He also had a slightly more roached back than is common in Thai elephants (which are generally stocky with shorter limbs than their Indian cousins). When standing he reduced the level of weight-bearing through the left forelimb.

When walking he abducted the left forelimb at the shoulder and swung the leg in an internal rotational arc with the medial toes connecting with the ground first rather than the usual heel-to-toe gait.

When asked to, he could lie down on either side, but much preferred lying on his right side with the injured limb uppermost.

Osteopathic treatment

A treatment program was devised to attempt to lower soft tissue tension to the axial musculature and then stimulate lymphatic drainage of the left forelimb. It also encouraged better freedom of movement, in normal planes, for the associated joints and structures.

Initial treatment was performed three times daily and consisted of soft tissue work through the forelimbs and periscapular structures and cervical musculature; lateral springing of the thoracic and lumbar vertebral spinous processes; functional traction through the tail;

before performing a pumping action through the solar aspect of the foot; finishing with rotational articulation of the entire left forelimb with the patient lying on his side.

Each treatment was carried out in the open air with the patient being fed sunflower seeds as an incentive to stay relaxed and still during the treatment sessions (Figs 10.50 and 10.51). Foundation members and a renowned elephant researcher observed these early treatment sessions.

After the first ten-minute session, the patient stood up and was led away in walk. He was immediately able to partially flex both the elbow and carpus with each cranial phase of the gait.

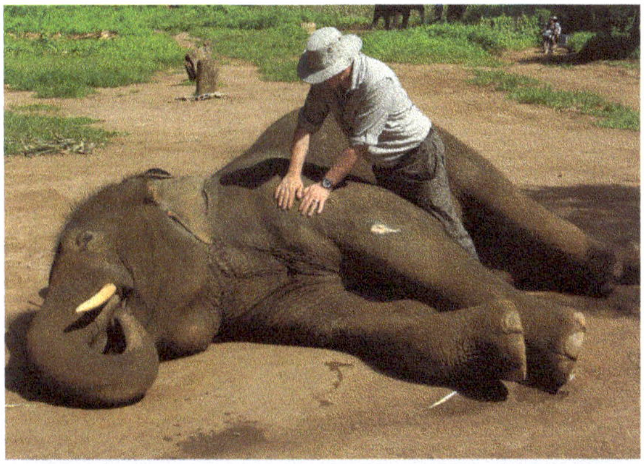

Figure 10.50
Soft tissue work around the left shoulder with the patient side lying and conscious.

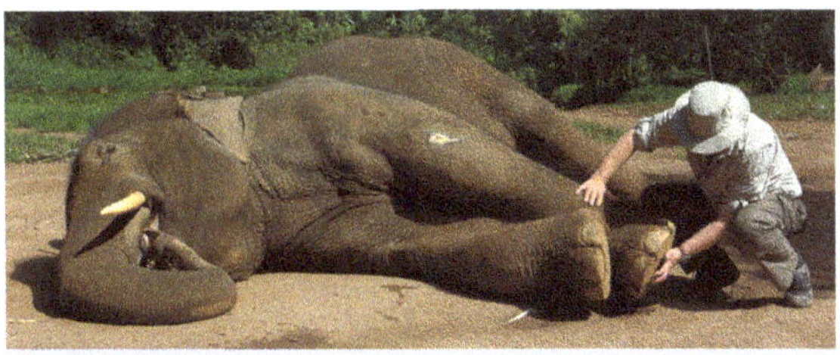

Figure 10.51
Performing a foot pump technique through the sole to stimulate lymphatic drainage to the affected limb with the patient in side lying.

Further treatment continued three times a day for seven days and was then reduced to twice daily for a further seven days. The patient's mahout (owner and handler) was shown simple techniques to continue the work while the veterinary staff continued treating the open wound as it healed. As the edema to the limb reduced and flexion improved the patient was encouraged to walk more to improve his recovery.

Outcome

The patient had received a traumatic injury to the left forelimb. He had also been physically lifted off the ground and this had resulted in an altered gait in this limb. The patient was treated on site, but only for a limited time due to the author's (TN's) work commitments. Treatment was continued by trainee veterinary students from Australia as well as by the mahout himself.

The author received updates via email for a further 12 months. The mahout left the foundation and returned after three years at which time the author was able to re-examine and treat the patient. At this time the patient had an almost normal gait and a healthy scar with little contraction evident (Fig. 10.52). The patient recognized the author and was keen to greet him. He then lay down on his side and waited to be treated, much to his mahout's amusement.

Summary

Osteopathic medicine can be extremely effective in treating trauma-based musculoskeletal problems as long as there is a commitment to treat regularly and at high session intensity.

Elephants respond well to regular short treatment sessions, ranging from five to 10 minutes long. After this they will often become restless and very little can be achieved. They are also very easy to overtreat, so care needs to be exercised to prevent this.

This patient benefited from a combined osteopathic and veterinary support package, which tackled the infection as well as the mechanical issues and inflammatory response. This was essential when one considers that treatment was undertaken in temperatures averaging 33 degrees centigrade at 95 percent humidity where infection can rapidly take over.

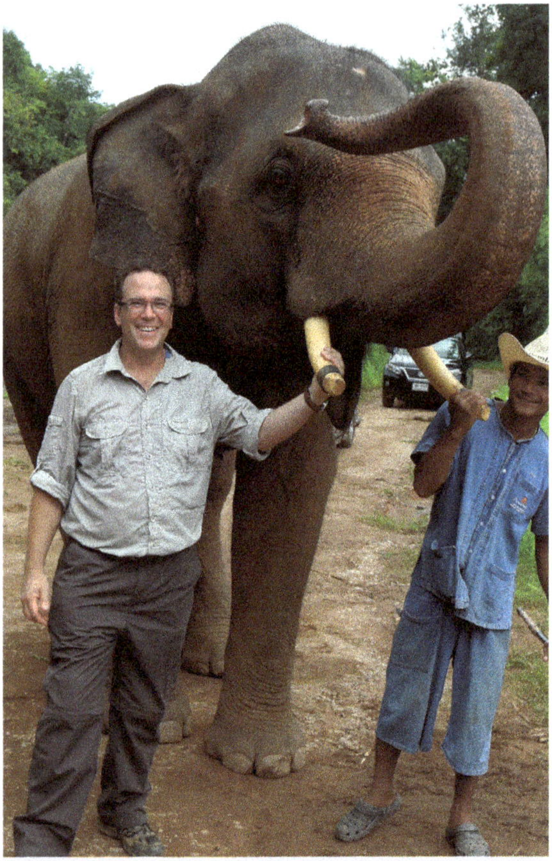

Figure 10.52
The same patient three years later, and fully grown, with the author and mahout.

The patient has continued to grow and, apart from an impressive battle scar, is left with only very minor lameness, even when viewed critically. The author was able to reassess him three years after his intensive treatment program had finished. Over a five-day period the patient was observed, palpated, and then treated in an attempt to further improve the action of the limb. Slow-motion video was used as one of the assessment tools, in addition to measuring stride distance, symmetry of movement, and ability to walk in a straight line. The video footage was shown to a group of osteopaths and a group of elephant veterinary surgeons. It was concluded that the patient improved further during this latter treatment program.

Case study 10.2

Male western lowland gorilla

Signalment

The patient was a subadult male western lowland gorilla. He was born in captivity and was 11 years old at the start of the treatment. He was living with a bachelor group of other males made up of his immediate brothers.

History

It was reported that all of the gorillas had come from another collection to allow for further breeding opportunities. On arrival at his present home Patient A was guarding his right upper limb when resting and showed a marked reluctance to use the arm for any form of locomotor function. There was documentation stating that his older brother had caused some kind of injury to him during one of their many play sessions.

He had been put on a long-term analgesic and anti-inflammatory drug regimen and the staff implemented a lameness scoring system which they were marking every morning when the gorillas moved out of their sleeping quarters. The scoring ranged from 1 to 5, with 1 indicating no lameness at all and 5 indicating inability to use the limb.

Prior to osteopathic intervention, and while on a daily dosage of diclofenac, Patient A was scoring between 3 and 4 most days and very occasionally a 5. Immediately before the first osteopathic treatment he was radiographed to ensure that there were no pathological issues. Blood samples were also taken in order to check blood cortisol levels.

Presenting signs

When observed discreetly with the rest of his group, Patient A kept his back to his older brother and maintained a certain distance. He held the right upper limb flexed and adducted across his chest with his hand resting on the ventral aspect of the left side of the chest and shoulder area. When moving on all fours he would place his elbow in contact with the ground, rather than extending the limb itself. He would alternate this with not using the limb at all when moving about the gorilla house or outdoor enclosure. His posture was hunched and his neck appeared shorter than those of his brothers (Fig. 10.53).

The author (TN) carried out an infrared thermographic scan (IRTS) on him while he was active. Despite the hair covering, there was a reduced temperature reading from the right upper limb, around the right scapula, and the ventral cervical areas.

Osteopathic treatment

For any osteopathic intervention it was necessary for Patient A to be anesthetized. Anesthesia was induced by administering ketamine via a rifle dart and was maintained by intubation and isoflurane. On the initial examination digital radiographs were taken to ensure that there was no bony pathology or obvious luxation not previously detected. Bloods were also taken to assess cortisol levels.

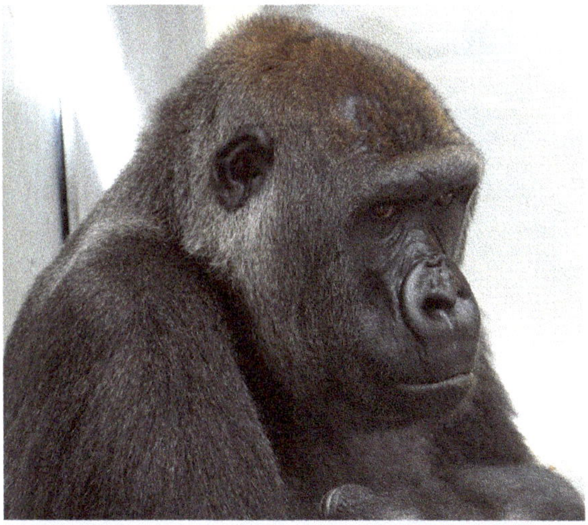

Figure 10.53
The patient sat hunched prior to the osteopathic treatment program.

Radiographic images were available almost instantly and showed no pathology (Fig. 10.54). This allowed the author to perform palpation and a joint mobility assessment. He concluded that the right shoulder area showed marked rigidity through the soft tissues. The neck musculature was so tight that it felt as though the whole structure was considerably shortened. The right upper arm measured a full 3 cm less in circumference than the left upper arm. Restrictions followed through the trapezius and latissimus dorsi with apparent fascial drag pulling into the right upper limb structure.

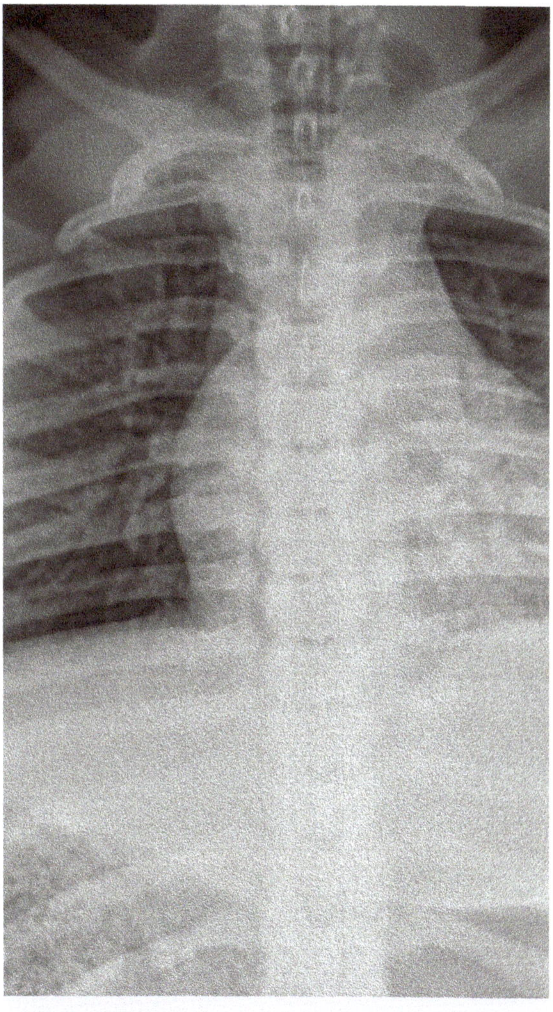

Figure 10.54
The patient's dorsoventral radiograph shows no pathology.

Osteopathic treatment began with lots of soft tissue massage and stretching followed by specific high velocity thrusts through the cranial thoracic vertebral joints and cervical vertebrae, backed up with long lever stretching and tugs through all four limbs, working through the fasciae. The thrusts used were vigorous and aimed at creating the most extreme osteopathic mobilization. The first session ended with cervical traction and functional release work around the hyoid mechanism (Figs 10.55, 10.56, 10.57, and 10.58).

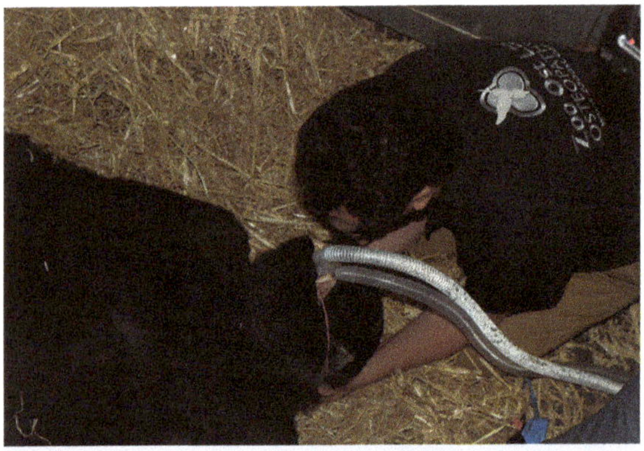

Figure 10.55
Application of suboccipital inhibition with the patient anesthetized and in the supine position.

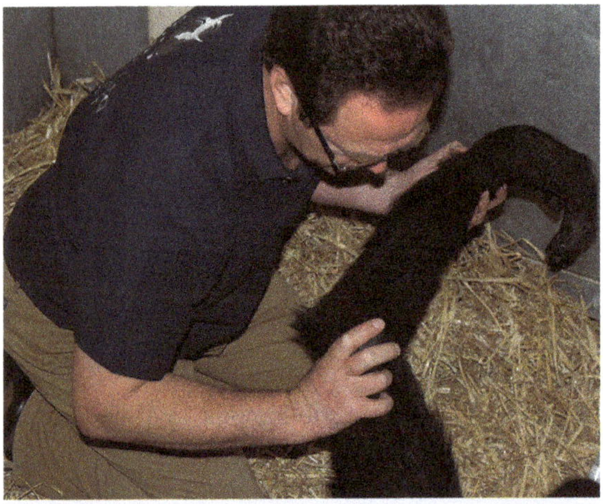

Figure 10.56
Application of right forelimb articulation with the patient anesthetized.

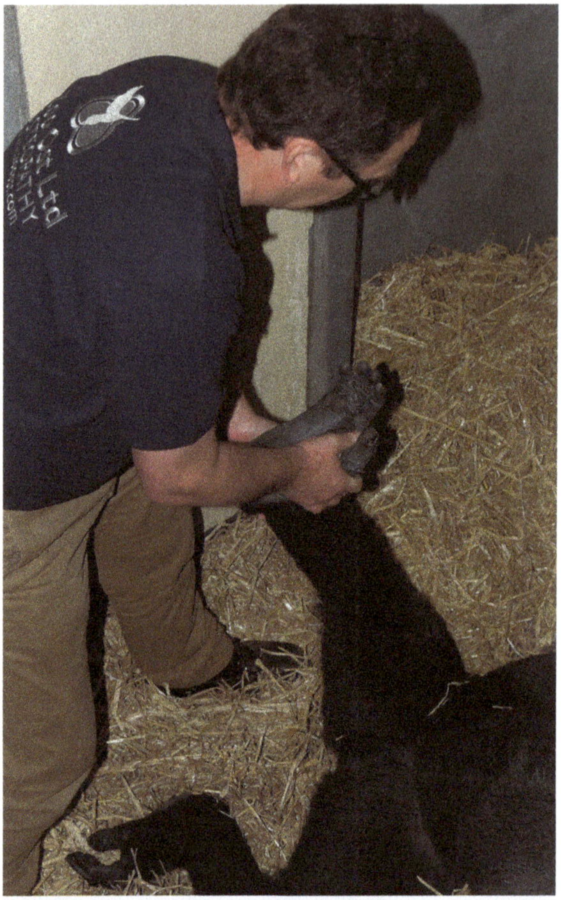

Figure 10.57
Application of right hind limb articulation with traction.

Subsequent to this treatment staff noted that when Patient A woke up and sat up they could see immediately that his neck appeared lengthened and his head carriage was much more in keeping with that of a young male gorilla.

A further six treatments have resulted in progression of the initial improvement. Patient A is now on a reducing dose of diclofenac and usually scores a 1, or occasionally a 2, on his lameness score.

Because Patient A is showing sustained improvement the frequency of osteopathic treatment has been reduced from every two months to every three months,

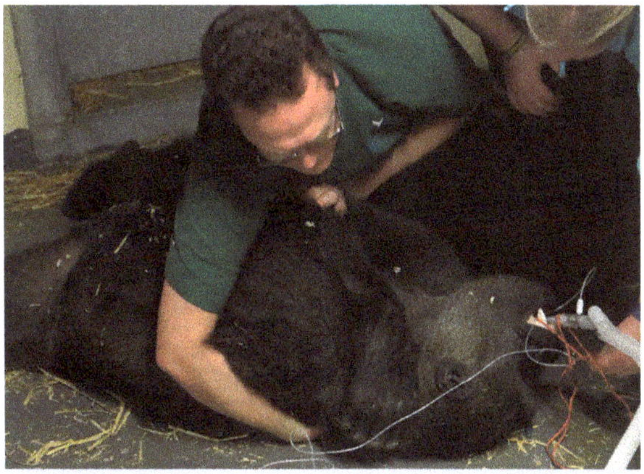

Figure 10.58
Performing HVLAT cranial thoracic spine with the patient anesthetized.

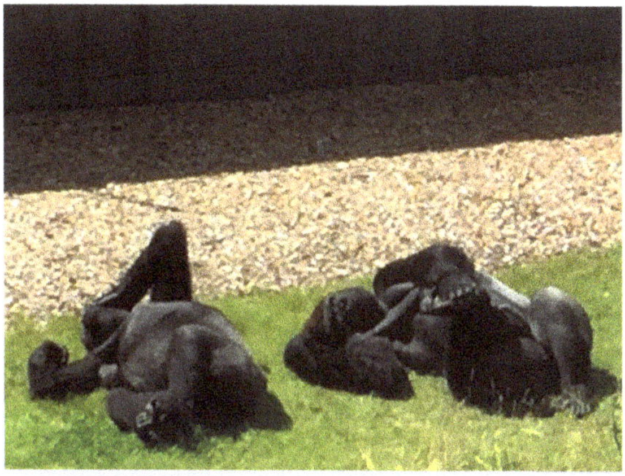

Figure 10.59
The patient sunbathing. At the end of the treatment program he had a consistent lameness score of 1 (normal).

and treatment has included monitoring and IRT scanning for the last 12 months. Patient A is now growing into an adult gorilla, and to date there are no signs of his problem returning. His personality has changed and he appears more confident and social within the group and in his interactions with the keepers and the author (Fig. 10.59).

Outcome

Patient A has responded extremely well to osteopathic treatment thus far. He is going to need further monitoring, but since any osteopathic treatment would require anesthesia treatment will be kept to a minimum. The techniques employed have been weighed against the need to achieve as much as is safely possible within a short treatment session.

Summary

This is the first documented osteopathic treatment of a gorilla, and, as with most high-value animals in a collection, there were many health and safety issues that had to be addressed before the treatment program commenced.

Working with apes can mess with the osteopath's mind as they are so similar to the human, but have considerable differences in their physical anatomy. Their weight is considerable for their size, which poses mechanical problems for the osteopath. The chronic nature of Patient A's problem meant that there was a lot of change in soft tissue quality and range of joint motion. General anesthesia was required for all treatments, which took place in the relatively cramped gorilla sleeping quarters. This was the safest place to dart him and also for him to wake up in.

By introducing osteopathy into Patient A's overall care it has been possible to reduce his dependency on diclofenac dramatically. The staff and the author have also observed that he is much more interactive within the group of bachelor gorillas.

Patient A is still under observation, and it is intended to continue trying to reduce his dependency on diclofenac to the point where he no longer requires medication. Whether this will possible, only time will tell.

Post-treatment note

As of the summer of 2018 the patient has not had any diclofenac and has no signs of his original problem. His muscular development has progressed rapidly and he appears to be very healthy and confident within the group.

References

Alexander RM, Maloiy GMO, Hunter B et al. (1979) Mechanical stresses in fast locomotion of buffalo (Syncerus caffer) and elephant (Loxodonta africana). Journal of the Zoological Society of London. November; 189 (2) 135–144.

BIAZA (British & Irish Association of Zoos & Aquariums) (2004) Proceedings of the Sixth Annual Symposium on Zoo Research, 8th and 9th July 2004 at Edinburgh Zoo, Edinburgh, UK; pp.160–211

BIAZA Elephant Welfare Group (2016) Five year report. May 2016. Healthcare, foot care and locomotion.

Blumstein D, Buckner J, Shah S et al. (2015) The evolution of capture myopathy in hooved mammals: a model for human stress cardiomyopathy? Evolution, Medicine and Public Health. July; 2015 (1) 195–203.

Brown RJ, Kupper JL, Trevethan WP, Johnston NL (1973) Fibrosarcoma in an African elephant. Journal of Wildlife Diseases. July; 9 (3) 227–228.

Caffee HH (1989) Reconstruction of the distal trunk of an African elephant. Plastic Reconstructive Surgery. 83: 1049–1051.

Chooi KF, Zahari ZZ (1988) Salmonellosis in a captive Asian elephant. Journal of Zoo Animal Medicine. March–June; 19 (12) 48–50.

Clark HW, Laughlin DC, Bailey JS, Brown TM (1980) Mycoplasma species and arthritis in elephants. Journal of Zoo Animal Medicine. 11: 3–15.

Diogo R, Pastor J, Ferrero E et al. (2011) Photographic and Descriptive Musculoskeletal Atlas of Gorilla: With Notes on the Attachments, Variations, Innervation, Synonymy and Weight of the Muscles. Boca Raton, FL: CRC Press.

Dudley R, Wood S, Hutchinson J, Weller R (2015) Radiographic protocol and normal anatomy of the hind feet in the white rhinoceros (Ceratotherium simum). Veterinary Radiology and Ultrasound. March–April; 56 (2) 124–132.

Ensley PK, Anderson M, Osborn K et al. (1994) Osteodystrophy in an orphan Asian elephant (Elephas maximus indicus). Proceedings of the American Association of Zoo Veterinarians, Pittsburgh, pp. 142–143.

Fennessy J, Bidon T, Reuss F et al. (2016) Multi-locus analyses reveal four giraffe species instead of one. Current Biology. September; 26 (18) 2543–2549.

Fowler M (2008) Restraint and Handling of Wild and Domestic Animals. London: Wiley-Blackwell.

Fowler ME (2006) Foot disorders. In: Fowler ME and Mikota SK (eds.) Biology, Medicine, and Surgery of Elephants. Ames, Iowa: Blackwell Publishing, pp. 271-290.

Fox H (1923) Disease in Captive Wild Mammals and Birds: Incidence, Description, Comparison. Philadephia: Lippincott Co.

Gordon J (1984) Structures, or Why Things Don't Fall Down. London: Penguin.

Greenough P (2007) Bovine Laminitis and Lameness. Elsevier Saunders.

Groves C, Grubb P (2011) Ungulate Taxonomy. Baltimore: Johns Hopkins University Press.

Harris M, Sherwin C, Harris S. (2008) The Welfare, Housing and Husbandry of Elephants in UK Zoos. University of Bristol. DEFRA WC05007.

Kock M, Burroughs R (2012) Chemical and Physical Restraint of Wild Animals: A Training and Field Manual for African Species. 2nd edn. South Africa: IWVS.

Kolmstetter C, Munson L, Ramsay E (2000) Degenerative spinal disease in large felids. Journal of Zoo and Wildlife Medicine. March; 31 (1) 15–19.

Liu C-H, Chang C-H, Chin S-C et al. (2004) Fibrosarcoma with lung and lymph node metastases in an Asian elephant (Elephas maximus). Journal of Veterinary Diagnostic Investigation. 16: 421–423.

MacClintock D (1973) A Natural History of Giraffes. New York: Charles Scribner's Sons.

Masters N, Turner A, Minch S, Vanlerberghe S, Sambrook L, Weller R (2013) The development of standardised systems for scoring feet and locomotion in captive elephants in the UK and Ireland. British Veterinary Zoological Society Proceedings of the Spring Meeting, 2013. The Möller Centre, Cambridge, UK, 23–24 March 2013. Diagnostics of all Zoo, Wildlife and Pet Exotic Species, pp. 13–15.

Miall LC, Greenwood F (1878) The anatomy of the Indian elephant. Journal of Anatomy and Physiology of London. 12: 385–400.

Miller RE, Fowler M (2014) Fowler's Zoo and Wild Animal Medicine, Volume 8. St. Louis, MO: Elsevier Saunders.

Montali RJ (2006) Postmortem diagnostics. In: Fowler ME and Mikota SK (eds.) Biology, Medicine, and Surgery of Elephants. Ames: Blackwell Publishing, pp. 199–209.

Nevin A (2004) The use of thermal imaging to assess osteopathic treatment of a captive Asian elephant.

BIAZA: Proceedings of the Sixth Annual Symposium on Zoo Research, 8th and 9th July 2004 at Edinburgh Zoo, Edinburgh, UK.

Nevin A (2005) Using osteopathy to treat musculoskeletal problems in two Burmese elephants. BIAZA: Proceedings of the Seventh Annual Symposium on Zoo Research, 7th and 8th July 2005 at Twycross Zoo, Warwickshire, England.

Nevin A (2012) Using IRTI to assess osteopathic treatment of two Asian elephants. The First International Congress of Osteopathy in Animal Practice, Rome.

O'Regan H, Kitchener A (2005) The effects of captivity on the morphology of captive, domesticated and feral animals. Mammal Review. December; 35 (3–4) 215–230.

Pritzker K, Kessler M (2012) Chapter 13 Arthritis, muscle, adipose tissue and bone diseases of nonhuman primates. In: Abee C, Mansfield K, Tardif S, Morris T (eds.) Nonhuman Primates in Biomedical Research, Volume 2: Diseases. 2nd edn. Elsevier Inc. Academic Press, pp. 629–697.

Rasmussen LEL (2006) Chemical, tactile, and taste sensory systems. In: Fowler ME and Mikota SK (eds.) Biology, Medicine, and Surgery of Elephants. Ames: Blackwell Publishing, pp. 409–414.

Rasmussen LEL, Munger B (1996) The sensorineural specializations of the trunk tip (finger) of the Asian elephant, Elephas maximus. Anatomical Record. September; 246 (1) 127–134.

Raven H (1950) The Anatomy of the Gorilla. New York: Columbia University Press.

Rothschild BM, Wang X, Shoshani J (1994) Spondyloarthropathy in proboscideans. Journal of Zoo and Wildlife Medicine. September; 25 (3) 360–366.

Schmidt M (1986) Elephants (Proboscidea). In: Fowler ME (ed.) Zoo and Wild Animal Medicine. 2nd edn. Philadelphia: WB Saunders, pp. 883–923.

Siegel IM (1973) Orthotic treatment of tibiotarsal deformity in an elephant. Journal of the American Veterinary Medicine Association. 163 (4) 544–545.

Shoshani J (1992) Anatomy and physiology. In: Shoshani J (ed.) Elephants: Majestic Creatures of the Wild. Emmaus: Rodale Press, pp. 66–81.

Smuts MM, Bezuidenhout AJ (1993) Osteology of the thoracic limb of the African elephant (Loxodonta africana). Onderstepoort Journal of Veterinary Research. 60 (1) 1–14.

Smuts MM, Bezuidenhout AJ (1994) Osteology of the pelvic limb of the African elephant (Loxodonta africana). Onderstepoort Journal of Veterinary Research. 61 (1) 51–66.

Stone C (1999) Science in the Art of Osteopathy: Osteopathic Principles and Practice. Nelson Thornes Ltd., pp. 227–229.

West G (2006) Musculoskeletal system. In: Fowler ME and Mikota SK (eds.) Biology, Medicine, and Surgery of Elephants. Ames: Blackwell Publishing, pp. 263–270.

INDEX

Note: Page numbers followed by f indicates figures and t indicates tables, respectively.

INDEX

D

E

F

G

H

INDEX

I

J

K

L

M

N

O

P

Q

R

S

INDEX